Advanced Health Assessment *and* Clinical Diagnosis *in* Primary Care

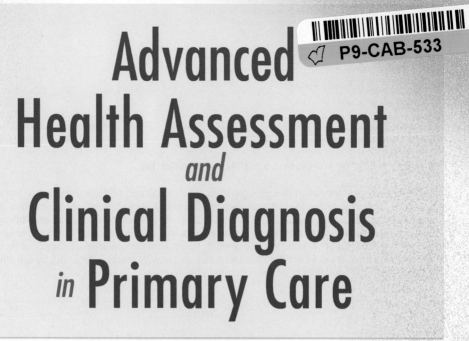

Third Edition

Joyce E. Dains, DrPH, JD, RN, FNP, BC, NAP
Manager, Professional Education for Prevention and Early Detection
The University of Texas
MD Anderson Cancer Center
Houston, Texas

Linda Ciofu Baumann, PhD, APRN, BC, FAAN
Professor
University of Wisconsin–Madison
School of Nursing
Madison, Wisconsin

Pamela Scheibel, RN, MSN, CPNP
Clinical Professor
University of Wisconsin–Madison
School of Nursing
Madison, Wisconsin

MOSBY

ELSEVIER

MOSBY
ELSEVIER

11830 Westline Industrial Drive
St. Louis, Missouri 63146

ADVANCED HEALTH ASSESSMENT AND CLINICAL
DIAGNOSIS IN PRIMARY CARE, ed 3

ISBN-13: 978-0-323-04428-8
ISBN-10: 0-323-04428-X

Notice

Knowledge and best practice in this field are constantly changing. As new research and experience broaden our knowledge, changes in practice, treatment, and drug therapy may become necessary or appropriate. Readers are advised to check the most current information provided (i) on procedures featured or (ii) by the manufacturer of each product to be administered, to verify the recommended dose or formula, the method and duration of administration, and contraindications. It is the responsibility of the practitioner, relying on their own experience and knowledge of the patient, to make diagnoses, to determine dosages and the best treatment for each individual patient, and to take all appropriate safety precautions. To the fullest extent of the law, neither the Publisher nor the Authors assume any liability for any injury and/or damage to persons or property arising out of or related to any use of the material contained in this book.

The Publisher

Previous editions copyrighted 2003, 1998

ISBN-13: 978-0-323-04428-8
ISBN-10: 0-323-04428-X

Acquisitions Editor: Sandra Clark Brown
Senior Developmental Editor: Cindi Anderson
Publishing Services Manager: Deborah L. Vogel
Senior Project Manager: Ann E. Rogers
Design Direction: Teresa McBryan
Marketing Manager: Tricia Schroeder

Working together to grow
libraries in developing countries

www.elsevier.com | www.bookaid.org | www.sabre.org

ELSEVIER   BOOK AID
International   Sabre Foundation

Printed in China
Last digit is the print number: 9 8 7 6 5 4 3 2 1

Reviewers

Carin Schofield, RN, ACNP-C
Acute Care Nurse Practitioner
Vallejo Clinic
Tullahoma, Tennessee
Adjunct Faculty
Vanderbilt University School of Nursing
Nashville, Tennessee

Marlene G. S. Sefton, PhD, APN, CNP
Assistant Professor
FNP Option Coordinator
University of Illinois at Chicago
College of Nursing
Department of Public Health, Mental Health and
    Administrative Nursing
Chicago, Illinois

Acknowledgments

No text is ever written as a solitary effort and we have many thanks to offer. We've benefited from the extraordinary support and help of friends, family, and colleagues. We'd like to acknowledge each one. Our thanks are heartfelt; we honor your place in our lives.

To our colleagues at Mosby who have continued to believe that this text is necessary and who have contributed their time, talent, and expertise—thank you. The remarkable efforts of each member of the publishing team are evident in the final product.

We'd also like to acknowledge the contributors to our first edition. Each is a superb clinician; each shared incredible expertise; and this text is richer because of them:

Katharine E. Hohol, MS, APRN, BC, APNP

Sandra K. Roof, MSN, APRN, BC, APNP

Robert W. Vogler, DSN, RN, CS, FNP

Pam Willson, PhD, RN, CS, FNP

Finally, we want to express our profound appreciation for those faculty, students, and clinicians who have found this book, for those who have shared their enthusiasm with us, and for those who have offered helpful suggestions and comments that have enhanced the content of this text. Thank you.

Joyce E. Dains
Linda C. Baumann
Pamela Scheibel

Preface

This text is designed for beginning clinicians and/or students who will be using history and physical examination skills in the clinical setting. Its purpose is to take the student to the "next step" of health assessment, that is, beyond basic history and physical examination to using a diagnostic reasoning process. The book is intended to fill the gap between basic physical examination texts and the medical texts that are aimed primarily at disease management. It is not intended as a substitute for a clinical management text nor does it address management of disorders or diseases. Rather, it is designed specifically to focus on the clinical evaluation of common problems that present in primary care settings, using the tools of history and physical examination to engage in the process of clinical diagnosis.

The third edition of this text has several changes to further assist the transition to that "next step" of health assessment. A new chapter has been added—Mood, Behavior Changes, and Psychosocial Concerns—which addresses additional and important concerns commonly seen in primary care settings. Another new chapter, The Chest Film, offers a guided approach to reading and interpreting chest x-rays. Both chapters provide an excellent educational basis for expanding and refining knowledge of advanced health assessment. We have continued to provide a list of selected references at the end of each chapter. These references support the information provided and are suggested for further in-depth learning about the problem. We have updated chapter content to reflect changes in diagnostic technology and to include emerging diseases in the differential diagnosis, where appropriate. In addition, we have increased the number of evidence-based practice guidelines. Finally, we have expanded the number of illustrations to provide graphic examples of anatomical structures and physical examination findings.

Each chapter is structured in the context of commonly occurring chief complaints rather than being based on a specific diagnosis or disease entity. Patients generally seek care for relief of symptoms and undiagnosed conditions. The initial challenge for primary care providers is to begin the process of differential diagnosis to determine the cause of a disorder, based on history and physical examination and laboratory and other diagnostic tests. However, the steps of the diagnostic reasoning process are seldom articulated in a sequence that reflects the clinician's thought process. Novice clinicians are often left to their own devices, to figure out, for example, which history questions are the most important, which should be asked first and which can be left for later, or to figure out which parts of the physical examination must be done as opposed to which will yield little information for a given complaint. This text tries to articulate the reasoning process, order the history questions in a meaningful way, and focus the physical examination for a specific chief complaint.

The diagnostic or clinical reasoning process is woven into each presenting problem. Each symptom begins with a brief introduction, providing an overview of causative mechanisms and processes. The clinical problem-solving process begins with Focused History, which walks through the thinking process involved in obtaining a pertinent, relevant, problem-specific history that will assist with differential diagnosis. The section is designed around questions that experienced clinicians ask themselves to order and organize the questions to be asked of the patient. These "self-questions" are structured according to what information the clinician needs first or most immediately about the presenting complaint, followed by self-questions that help sort through the possible differential diagnoses. The content and order of the self-questions vary, depending on the presenting problem. Sometimes the self-questions are based on what the condition is most likely to be; sometimes they are based on what is too important to miss.

For each of the self-questions there is a list of Key Questions to ask the patient or about the patient if a family member is giving the history. The Key Questions are followed by an interpretation or explanation of what the patient responses might signify. For ease of format, the Key Questions are written as though the clinician were addressing the patient. Certainly with young children and sometimes with adults, the clinician will be asking questions of another person about the patient. The intent is to convey what questions to ask, rather than to provide every possible format for each question.

Following these two sections is the Focused Physical Examination section. It instructs you in what focused physical examination to perform to assist in the diagnostic process. The section is not intended to teach basic physical examination; it assumes you know how, using the techniques of inspection, auscultation, percussion, and palpation. This section, rather, provides focus for the examination, explains how to do more advanced maneuvers, and offers an interpretation of the findings.

Following is the section titled Laboratory and Diagnostic Studies. This section provides a brief outline of what kinds of laboratory or diagnostic studies would be appropriate for the chief complaint or suspected diagnosis. Because the goal of the text is clinical diagnosis, the laboratory and diagnostic studies included are those that would be a logical starting point, although perhaps not an ending point.

The final section of each presenting complaint is the Differential Diagnosis. It contains the most common differential diagnoses for the chief complaint and summarizes, in a narrative format, the history and physical examination findings, along with the laboratory and diagnostic studies indicated. The section finishes with Differential Diagnosis table(s), mirroring the narrative summary, which can be used as a quick reference.

The focus of *Advanced Health Assessment* is primary care patients. Both adults and children are included, with divergence in questions, examination, or interpretation of findings noted where pertinent. Management of health care problems is intentionally not included. Also, no attempt is made to address all possible patient complaints but rather to seek to focus on the most common chief complaints as exemplars of the diagnostic reasoning process.

Perfecting advanced health assessment skills is a lifelong process. It is our hope that this edition continues to assist you in expanding the diagnostic reasoning process.

Joyce E. Dains
Linda C. Baumann
Pamela Scheibel

Contents

Introduction

Clinical Reasoning, Differential Diagnosis, and Evidence-Based Practice

Basic health assessment involves the application of the practitioner's knowledge and skills to identify and distinguish normal from abnormal findings. Basic assessment often moves from a general survey of a body system to specific observations or tests of function. Such an approach to assessment and clinical decision-making uses a deductive process of reasoning. For example, a specialist, when examining a patient with known hyperthyroidism, would conduct a physical examination to test for deep tendon reflexes. Brisk or hyperreflexic findings would lead the practitioner to conclude that a hyperthyroid state is a likely cause for these findings. This would greatly narrow the choices of diagnostic tests to perform and alternations in treatment to make.

Advanced assessment builds on basic health assessment yet is performed more often using an inductive or inferential process, that is, moving from a specific physical finding or patient complaint to a more general diagnosis or possible diagnoses based on history, physical findings, and laboratory and diagnostic tests. The practitioner gathers further evidence and analyzes this evidence to arrive at a hypothesis that will lead to a further narrowing of possibilities. This is known as the process of diagnostic reasoning.

DIAGNOSTIC REASONING

Diagnostic reasoning is a scientific process in which the practitioner suspects the cause of a patient's symptoms and signs based on previous knowledge, gathers relevant information, selects necessary tests, and recommends therapy. The difference between an average and an excellent practitioner is the speed and focus used to arrive at the correct conclusion and initiate the best course of treatment with minimum cost, risk, inconvenience, and delay.

By using diagnostic reasoning, the practitioner accomplishes the following:

- Determines and focuses on what needs to be asked and what needs to be examined
- Performs examinations and diagnostic tests accurately
- Clusters abnormal findings
- Analyzes and interprets the findings
- Develops a list of likely or differential diagnoses

THE DIAGNOSTIC PROCESS
The Primary Care Context

The process of assessment in the primary care setting begins with the patient stating a reason for the visit or a chief concern. Most visits to primary care providers involve concerns or symptoms presented by the patient, such as an earache, vomiting, or fatigue. The initial evidence is collected through a patient history. Demographic information, such as gender, age, occupation, and place of residence, is obtained to place the patient in a risk category that can generally rule out certain diagnoses immediately. In most primary care settings, routine vital signs are obtained, which may include height and weight, temperature, pulse, respiratory rate, blood pressure, last menstrual period, and smoking status. As the practitioner obtains the history, he or she is also making observations of the patient's appearance, interaction with family members, orientation, and physical condition and notes any unusual findings that may help focus the assessment process.

Presenting symptoms need to be explored with further questions about the (1) timing or onset, duration, and frequency; (2) anatomical location; (3) character or quality; (4) setting in which they occur; (5) severity or intensity; (6) aggravating and alleviating factors; (7) associated symptoms; and (8) patient's perception of the meaning of the symptom. The practitioner then clusters the findings into logical groups based on prior knowledge of symptom clusters associated with specific diagnoses or anatomical locations, which suggests the involvement of a specific body system.

Formulating and Testing a Hypothesis

The practitioner then formulates a hypothesis based on expertise and knowledge of probable processes, such as a pathological, physiological, or psychological process. Further interpretation of evidence refines the hypothesis to a working or probable diagnosis. Hypothesis generation, in fact, probably already began based on the patient's age, gender, race, appearance, and presenting problem. Age is the most significant variable in narrowing the probabilities of a problem. Hypothesis generation forms the context in which further data are collected. This context includes the setting in which care is delivered, such as a hospital, an outpatient setting, or another community-based setting where more than a single individual may be affected. Clinical decision-making can be filled with uncertainty and ambiguity. Because available evidence is almost never complete, hypothesis formation involves some element of subjective judgment.

The hypothesis must then be tested and assessed for the following characteristics:

1. Coherence—are the physiological linkages, predisposing factors, and complications for this disease present in the patient?
2. Adequacy—does the suspected disease encompass all of the patient's normal and abnormal findings?

3. Parsimony—is it the simplest explanation of the patient's findings? The surest way to make this determination is to ask the patient or the parents why they are seeking care and their understanding of the problem. This is a crucial step because patients must find the treatment recommendation acceptable.
4. Finally, can a competing hypothesis be eliminated? What other diseases could explain the patient's symptoms?

To confirm the hypothesis, the practitioner establishes a working definition of the problem as a basis for a treatment plan and evaluates the outcome. The goal of a clinical decision is to choose an action that is most likely to result in the health outcomes the patient desires. This step of the decision-making process involves personal preference as to whether the benefits are worth the risks involved, the cost is reasonable, and the most desired outcomes are short or long term.

Clinicians make extensive use of heuristics, or rules of thumb, to guide the inductive or inferential process of diagnostic reasoning. Heuristics are generally accurate and useful rules to make the task of information gathering more manageable and efficient—rules such as familiarity, salience, and resemblance to a patient who has a known disease. However, heuristics can, on occasion, be faulty (if the presentation is atypical or the condition is rare). The clinician must always be open to a low probability of a serious diagnosis. Heuristics can have negative effects when stereotypes or biases influence judgment. For example, assuming that a patient is heterosexual can lead to errors in clinical reasoning and differential diagnosis when evaluating the symptom of rectal pain.

EXPERT VERSUS NOVICE CLINICIANS

Students of advanced assessment have a wide variety of backgrounds, with many coming from specialized areas of clinical practice. Such students may have difficulty broadening the scope of their observations and clinical possibilities. In any case, whether specialists or not, non-experts tend to be nonselective in data gathering and in the clinical reasoning strategies they use. Experts, on the other hand, are able to focus on a problem, recognize patterns, and gather only relevant data, with a high probability of a correct diagnosis. The goal for a novice practitioner is to aim for competence and expertise.

The competent practitioner will execute the following steps:

1. *Identify the most important cues.* These cues are obtained largely through a thorough symptom analysis, functional assessment, and history to assess the patient's beliefs and understanding about the problem or representation of the illness. Research evidence shows that a person's beliefs or explanatory models of an illness or a symptom include a cause, an opinion about the timeline (acute or chronic), consequences of the condition (minor or life threatening), and some type of verbal label used to identify the cluster of symptoms or sensations (e.g., "the flu," "the blues") (Baumann and Leventhal, 1985; Kleinman et al, 1978). Clinicians need to distinguish between the presence of disease, which has a biological basis, and illness, which is the human experience of being sick that may have little correlation with the objective evidence that is available.

2. *Understand and perform advanced examination techniques.* These techniques may include special maneuvers and closer observation of fine detail during the physical examination, more in-depth interviews using valid and reliable instruments to assess the patient's risk for a specific diagnosis, and "gold standard" diagnostic tests for the identification of a specific disorder.

3. *Test differential or competing diagnoses.* A differential diagnosis results from a synthesis of subjective and objective findings, including laboratory and diagnostic tests, with knowledge of known and recognized patterns of signs and symptoms. When using the "rule-out" strategy, the clinician looks for the absence of findings that are frequently seen with a specific condition; the absence of a sensitive finding is strong evidence against the condition being present. When using the "rule-in" strategy, the clinician looks for the presence of a finding with high specificity (low false-positive and high true-negative values); the presence of this finding is strong evidence the condition is present.

4. *See a pattern in the information gathered.* A pattern or cluster of findings may emerge from the subjective and objective data. This pattern may be evident during one patient encounter or it may depend on a pattern of signs and symptoms that develops over time. Often the expert clinician can eliminate competing diagnoses only after the initial treatment prescribed is ineffective or after the symptoms either disappear sooner than expected or persist longer than expected.

DEVELOPING CLINICAL JUDGMENT

Brykcyzynski (1989) studied how advanced practice nurses developed clinical reasoning skills. In her analysis, she observed that didactic content in a lecture or a reference book often discusses the classic presentation of a patient with a specific disorder and does not acknowledge variables that are present in the actual clinical situation. Even the use of case studies has limitations because the data are presented to the reader but in actual clinical practice the practitioner has to be ready to begin the clinical reasoning process by knowing what to ask a patient (Ryan-Wenger and Lee, 1997). Thus theoretical knowledge has limitations in the exercise of expert clinical judgment. Practical knowledge requires actual experience in a situation that is contextual and transactional, and is acquired only through spending time with patients, practicing focused listening, and gaining experience in recognizing subtle cues.

NEGOTIATING GOALS AND EXPECTATIONS OF A PATIENT ENCOUNTER

It is important, especially in an ambulatory care setting, to identify the patient's goals, expectations, and resources to determine what needs to be achieved during an encounter. A patient who seeks care because of a bothersome symptom may be more interested in having the symptom relieved by a particular date than in knowing the cause or diagnostic explanation for the symptom. Other patients may want reassurance that a symptom or sign is not a serious condition and yet do not expect treatment to alleviate the sensations they are experiencing. An explicit discussion between the clinician and patient is necessary to establish what the goals and focus of an encounter will be. Goals can be mutually negotiated to assure clinicians that serious conditions can be "ruled out" and to assure patients that their needs and desires are acknowledged.

EVIDENCE-BASED PRACTICE

Evidence-based practice (EBP) is the integration of clinical judgment with the most current, relevant, and sound research evidence to guide clinical practice decisions. EBP integrates the best research evidence with clinical expertise and the patient's concerns and expectations and involves the use of simple rules of logic to apply evidence from research to an individual patient. Some of these rules include evaluating the validity and reliability of the evidence. The levels of evidence range from the "gold standard" of the randomized clinical trial to case studies, correlational studies, and expert opinion. Clinicians and patients increasingly gather evidence from web-based sources, such as the Cochrane Library, which includes databases of systematic reviews of a clinical topic,

abstracts of reviews of effectiveness, a controlled trial registry, and review methodology. These databases have gathered the "best evidence" related to clinical problems (Box 1-1). Access to web-based data requires that the practitioner develop skills in health informatics—the application of computer technology to health care delivery. Clinicians will need to develop skills in searching for and appraising information for a specific patient in a specific clinical context.

SUMMARY

In the context of primary care practice, the orientation to the patient should be holistic and general and toward the most prevalent or common conditions in a particular population group. This orientation requires that the expert practitioner develop skills in inductive reasoning to arrive at a diagnosis and treatment plan that are acceptable to the patient. Knowledge of the patient as a person over time greatly enhances the database from which the clinician works to arrive at better clinical judgments. Treatment plans in primary care settings rely on low-level technology and stress prevention, and encourage self-care behaviors as well as open and effective patient-provider communication. Practitioners need to be able to search for and evaluate the best evidence to guide practice and weigh the cost/benefit analysis of clinical decision-making and subsequent treatment plans to evaluate diagnostic efficacy. A practitioner can move from novice to expert and become more efficient in exercising clinical judgment by asking the right

Box 1-1	**Evidence-Based Practice Web Sources**	
Evidence-based practice guidelines and best practices		www.guideline.gov
Cochrane Library of systematic literature reviews about treatments and interventions		www.cochrane.org
CINAHL database on all aspects of nursing, allied health, alternative health, and community medicine		www.cinahl.com
MEDLINE database maintained by the National Library of Medicine for biomedical content for dentistry, veterinary medicine, and nursing		www.medscape.com
Online Journal of Clinical Innovations		www.cinahl.com
Agency for Healthcare Research and Quality		www.ahrq.gov
US Preventive Services Task Force		www.ahrq.gov/clinc/uspsfact.htm
British Medical Journal compendium of best available evidence		www.evidence.org

questions, seeking pertinent information from the body of scientific evidence, and using clinical reasoning to apply the best evidence to clinical practice.

CHAPTER RESOURCES

Baumann LJ, Leventhal H: I can tell if my blood pressure is up, can't I? *Health Psychol* 4:203, 1985.

Brykcyzynski KA: An interpretive study describing clinical judgment of nurse practitioners, *Schol Inq Nurs Prac Internat J* 3:75, 1989.

Eddy DM: Evidence-based medicine: a unified approach, *Health Affairs* 24:9, 2005.

Kleinman A, Eisenberg L, Good B: Culture, illness, and care, *Ann Int Med* 88:251, 1978.

Ryan-Wenger NA, Lee JE: The clinical reasoning case study: a powerful teaching tool, *Nurs Pract* 22:66, 1997.

Straus SE, Richardson WS, Glasziou P, Haynes RB: *Evidence-based medicine: how to practice and teach EBM,* St Louis, 2005, Churchill Livingstone.

Common Problems of the Head, Eyes, Ears, Nose, and Throat

Earache

Otalgia, or ear pain, is generally caused by an inflammatory process. In children, inflammation most commonly occurs in the middle ear. Adults more often have an earache from external ear conditions or from referred pain from other head and neck structures. Acute otitis media (AOM) refers to any inflammation of the middle ear and encompasses a variety of clinical conditions. Otitis media with effusion is a collection of fluid in the middle ear. This condition is also known as serous otitis media, secretory otitis, or nonsuppurative otitis. External or middle ear disorders can often be distinguished after a brief history and physical examination. If the physical findings are normal, referred pain is a likely cause. About 50% of referred pain is caused by dental problems, although other causes may include temporomandibular joint (TMJ) disorder, parotitis, pharyngitis, or cervical, mouth, or facial disorders. The most serious, although least common, cause of referred pain is nasopharyngeal cancer; this condition is more common in Asians. Figure 2-1 illustrates the structures of the ear.

DIAGNOSTIC REASONING: FOCUSED HISTORY

Is This an Acute Infection?

Key Questions
- How old are you?
- Have you had a fever?
- Have you had an upper respiratory infection?
- Have you had ear infections before?
- Is there a family history of ear infections?

Age
Age is an important clue for the cause of ear pain. The occurrence of AOM declines significantly after age 6. Increased age increases the likelihood of secondary otalgia caused by disorders of the head, face, and neck; by sinus or periodontal disease; and by malignancy.

Fever
Fever is present in 60% of all children with AOM. In infants younger than 2 months, fever with AOM is uncommon. A high fever accompanying otitis is more likely to occur as part of a systemic illness such as pneumonia or meningitis.

Upper Respiratory Tract Infection (URI)
When the mucous membranes of the nasopharynx and/or sinuses become infected, organisms are forced up the lumen of the eustachian tube. Inflammation of the mucosa or enlarged adenoids obstruct the eustachian opening so that the air in the middle ear is absorbed and replaced by mucus. This mucus creates a mechanical obstruction and can serve as a medium for bacterial growth.

Previous Infections
Infants younger than 3 months who have their first AOM run a high risk of recurrence. Seventy-one percent of children younger than 3 years have had at least one episode, and one third have had an average of three episodes. Chronic otitis media can result in anatomical changes to the tympanic membrane (TM) and middle ear ossicles, which may predispose the patient to additional ear infections.

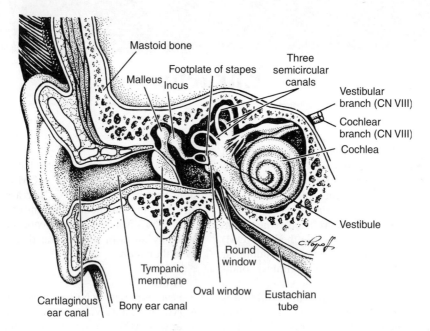

FIGURE 2-1 External auditory canal, middle ear, inner ear. (From Barkauskas VH et al: *Health and physical assessment*, ed 3, St Louis, 2002, Mosby.)

Family History

Having a sibling or parent with chronic otitis media makes it twice as likely for the illness to develop in the child. The presence of chronic otitis media may also be related to child-care practices, such as bottle propping, or environmental exposures, such as second-hand cigarette smoke.

What Environmental Conditions Might Suggest Increased Risk?

Key Questions

- Does anyone around you smoke? Do you smoke?
- If a child: Does the child attend day care?
- If a child: Does the infant take a bottle lying down?
- Have you been swimming recently?
- Have you recently been in an airplane or been scuba diving?

Smoke Exposure

Second-hand cigarette smoke exposure has been associated with a two-fold to three-fold increased risk of otitis media. Cigarette smoking leads to functional eustachian tube obstruction and decreases the protective ciliary action in the tube.

Attending Day Care

Attending a day care setting with other children is associated with an increased incidence rate of otitis media because of exposure to organisms.

Bottle Propping

In very young children, lying supine while drinking from a bottle has been associated with AOM. It is postulated that swallowing while lying down allows nasopharyngeal fluid to enter the middle ear, with subsequent infection.

Swimming

Repeated or prolonged immersion in water results in loss of protective cerumen and chronic irritation with maceration from excessive moisture in the canal. This leads to an increased occurrence of otitis externa, also called swimmer's ear.

Airplane Travelers, Divers

Barotrauma is a cause of acute serous otitis related to pressure changes from scuba diving or flying. This is often aggravated by recent upper respiratory tract infection or nasal congestion. Failure of the eustachian tube to open and equilibrate during descent results in a collection of serosanguineous fluid in the middle ear. This may be felt as ear pressure that can lead to pain, tinnitus, and temporary deafness. Swallowing, chewing, or blowing out the nose with the mouth and nose occluded can relieve symptoms.

Could This Be Related to a Systemic Disease?

Key Questions

- Do you have diabetes?
- Have you ever had dermatitis, eczema, or psoriasis?
- If a child: Does the child have a nonrepaired cleft palate?

Diabetes Mellitus

Diabetes mellitus predisposes adults to malignant otitis externa, which is a cellulitis involving the ear and surrounding tissue. Persons with diabetes are also at increased risk for otitis media and mastoiditis.

History of Seborrheic Dermatitis or Psoriasis

Chronic inflammatory dermatitis from overproduction of sebum can occur in the external canal and cause otitis externa.

Cleft Palate

Nonrepaired anomalies anatomically predispose a child to otitis media because of functional obstruction of the eustachian tubes.

What Does the Presence of Pain Tell Me?

Key Questions

- Where specifically is the pain felt? Is it in one ear or both?
- How severe is the pain? Does it interfere with sleeping, eating, or other activities?
- How long have you had this pain?
- Is the pain constant or intermittent? If intermittent, how long does it last?
- Does the pain travel (radiate) to other areas?

Location of the Pain

Pain of otitis externa is described as tenderness around the outer ear or opening to the ear canal that worsens with manipulation of the pinna. Mastoiditis is often associated with severe pain or tenderness over the mastoid bone. If the pain is bilateral, suspect otitis externa. Referred pain or pain of AOM is usually unilateral. Infants cannot assist in location of the ear pain; instead, they exhibit behavioral changes that may indicate pain, such as irritability, lethargy, poor appetite, vomiting, and diarrhea. Young children may pull or tug at their ears.

Quality of the Pain

The pain of AOM is often described as a deep pain or a blockage of the ear. Serous otitis is often painless or may be described as a bubbling, popping, or stuffy sensation in the ear. Otitis externa involves a tenderness of the outer ear or ear canal that can be accompanied by itching. A cerumen impaction creates a milder pain or vague discomfort of stuffed ears.

Quantity and Severity of the Pain

The pain of AOM is severe enough to interfere with sleep and may be suddenly relieved if the eardrum perforates. Chronic ear pain that is unresponsive to treatment may indicate a tumor.

Onset, Timing, and Duration of the Pain

TMJ pain is often described as severe pain lasting a few minutes and recurring three or four times per day, sometimes associated with headache. It is worse in the morning because nighttime teeth grinding is associated with this condition. The pain is intermittent but can be acute, related to trauma or overextension of the mouth. Chronic pain may be related to dental malocclusion or rheumatoid arthritis.

Infants may cry when sucking to indicate pain with compression and increased pressure in the ears. Nocturnal onset of otalgia from a developing infection is caused by increased vascular pressure in the reclined position, causing the TM to bulge and to stimulate pain sensation.

What Does the Presence of Discharge or Itching Tell Me?

Key Questions

- Do you have any discharge from the ear?
- Do you have any itching in the ear?

Itching or Drainage

Itching or drainage from the ear usually indicates an infection or inflammation of the external canal. Itching can also be a precursor to herpes zoster of cranial nerve (CN) V (trigeminal). Drainage may also be present after the TM ruptures from increased middle ear pressure, or it may be from exudate secondary to mastoiditis. Cholesteatoma is an epidermal inclusion cyst of the middle ear or mastoid. A perforation of the TM and associated foul-smelling discharge may occur.

What Does a History of Trauma or Injury Tell Me?

Key Questions

- Have you had any recent trauma to the ear?
- Have you had any head trauma?
- How do you clean your ears? Do you use cotton-tipped swabs?
- Do you have a history of excessive earwax?
- If a child: Does the child have a history of putting objects into ears?
- Have you had any recent insect bites around the ear?
- Have you been exposed to any loud noise?

Ear Trauma

Perforation of the eardrum can be caused by blunt or penetrating trauma. Blunt trauma might include a slap to the ear or barotrauma. Penetrating trauma to the canal or TM may be self-induced with cotton-tipped swabs or other sharp objects used to remove cerumen or to scratch the canal.

Head Trauma

Direct injury to the inner ear by fracture of the petrous temporal bone located at the base of the skull also destroys the inner ear.

Cerumen Impaction

Cerumen is a naturally wet, sticky, honey-colored wax that serves as a lubricant to protect the external ear canal. In some individuals it occurs in a dark, scaly form and accumulates in the ear canal. This accumulation may cause hearing loss, tinnitus, pressure sensation, vertigo, and infection. Self-cleaning practices can produce trauma to the canal, and cerumen-softening solutions can cause chemical irritation to the canal tissue.

Foreign Bodies

Foreign bodies, such as feathers, beads, and insects (especially cockroaches), can produce ear pain and inflammation. Children will often self-insert objects.

Insect Bites

Insect bites can lead to acute pain and tenderness of the external canal and may develop into a secondary infection.

Loud Noise

Exposure to high-pitched and loud noises for a prolonged period of time destroys the cochlear hair cells. Exposure to noisy work environments, to the operation of heavy machinery, and to loud music increases the risk of injury and eventual hearing loss.

Is Hearing Loss a Clue?

Key Questions

- Do you have any difficulty in hearing?
- Do you have any dizziness?
- Do you have any ringing in the ear?
- If a child: Do you think the child can hear normally?
- If a child: Does the child turn his or her head to listen?

Difficulty in Hearing

Complaints of hearing loss or "difficulty hearing" can indicate blockage of the ear canal by cerumen or a foreign body, inflammation of the middle or inner ear, or a neoplasm. The most frequent cause is conductive hearing loss caused by blockage of the external canal, usually by cerumen. Chronic otitis media is usually a condition of adults who have a chronic infection that may destroy the ossicles and spread to the mastoid, labyrinth, and intracranial structures, causing hearing loss. Chronic ear pain is often associated with hearing loss and ear discharge secondary to a perforated nonhealing TM.

Hearing Loss in Children

Chronic otitis media with effusion causes a conductive hearing loss in children. This loss may be caused by negative middle ear pressure, the presence of an effusion in the middle ear, or structural damage to the TM or ossicles.

Dizziness, Ringing in Ear

Hearing loss associated with dizziness, vertigo, or tinnitus may indicate a serious inner ear condition. Abnormal middle ear ventilation and middle ear effusion are the most common causes of balance disturbance in children. These symptoms are caused by reestablishment of aeration in the middle ear cavity as the effusion clears.

DIAGNOSTIC REASONING: FOCUSED PHYSICAL EXAMINATION

A correct diagnosis of ear pain requires a good view of the TM and external ear canal. Cerumen obstructions should be removed through lavage or by separating an impaction with an ear curette so that irrigation fluid can penetrate behind the impaction. The curette must be manipulated cautiously because trauma to or inflammation of the sensitive perichondrium, which lies immediately below a thin layer of epithelium in the ear canal, elicits excruciating pain and easy bleeding.

Lavage should not be performed if the medical history suggests perforation of the TM. Without visualization of the TM, however, otitis media cannot be ruled out. Lavage solution helps to soften the cerumen and can be purchased commercially in kits or a solution can be made of hydrogen peroxide and water (1:1).

Note Behaviors in Children

Otitis media is the most common childhood disorder. Young infants may exhibit nonspecific signs of irritability, poor feeding, congestion, and fever. Older infants and young toddlers are irritable, pull on the painful ear, or bang their head on the affected side. Older children will complain of an earache.

Inspect External Ears

General inspection should begin with the pinna and condition of the skin around the ear, face, and scalp. Hemorrhage over the mastoid bone (Battle's sign) may occur with a basal skull fracture. Eczematous seborrhea or psoriasis manifests as redness and scaling of the skin that can extend into the external ear canal. Pain in the opening of the ear canal and inflamed skin may suggest a bacterial infection. Fungal and yeast infections appear as white or dark patches. Furuncles or lesions secondary to trauma or irritation appear as localized areas of tenderness or swelling. A hot, swollen, and erythematous ear and surrounding skin indicate cellulitis. Redness and painful swelling over the mastoid process is a sign of infection in the mastoid air cells.

Palpate External Ears

Palpate the pinna and tragus for tenderness. In mastoiditis, the pinna is displaced forward and swelling may be present behind the ear. Palpation of the mastoid process elicits severe tenderness. Otitis externa is associated with pain on manipulation of the pinna. With referred pain, the structures will appear normal, although palpation over the TMJ may elicit tenderness, and movement of the jaw may create a clicking sound.

Palpate the preauricular and postauricular areas on the right and left simultaneously to elicit pain. Palpate anterior and posterior cervical lymph nodes and over the mastoid process. Preauricular nodes may be enlarged in AOM and otitis externa. Postauricular swelling may indicate extension of infection into the mastoid cavity.

Inspect Ear Canals

With the otoscope, observe for the patency of the canal, the condition of the skin of the ear canal, and the presence of cerumen. With cerumen impaction, no structures can be visualized. A foreign body is easily visualized. Vesicles on the external ear canal and auricle may indicate herpes zoster (Ramsay Hunt syndrome).

Visualize any discharge, noting color, consistency, and odor. Discharge is usually indicative of an active infection. However, cranial trauma with cerebrospinal fluid leakage must be kept in mind. Cheesy, green-blue, or gray discharge can be seen with otitis externa.

Inspect Tympanic Membranes

Visualize the TM, noting light reflex and anatomical structures. A normal TM is translucent and pearly gray in color. Mild diffuse redness can occur from crying or coughing. Mild vascularity is sometimes seen in the normal eardrum, especially on the handle of the malleus. Localized redness is a sign of inflammation. Scarring and effusion can cause whitening and opacification of the TM.

The contour of the normal TM is somewhat concave. Fullness or bulging indicates either increased air pressure or, more commonly, increased hydrostatic pressure within the middle ear. Fullness of the eardrum is seen first around the periphery of the TM. As pressure increases, central fullness becomes visible. Concavity or retraction of the eardrum is associated with negative middle ear pressure or postinflammatory adhesions. As the eardrum retracts, the handle of the malleus short process becomes more visible.

Myringitis is a red, inflamed eardrum without effusion. Bullous myringitis describes an extremely painful condition of small blisters on the TM caused by bacterial otitis media. Figure 2-2 illustrates the usual landmarks of a normal right TM. Chronic otitis media can lead to cholesteatoma, or a cystlike mass behind the eardrum, caused by the proliferation of squamous epithelium. The mass can grow to cause necrosis of the ossicles. Examination will reveal a collection of white granulation tissue with perforation of the TM.

Perform Pneumatic Otoscopy (Insufflation)

The normal eardrum is suspended from its margins and responds to slight pressure changes. Insufflation tests the mobility of the TM. It can be an insensitive test for otitis media if poor technique fails to create a seal. Properly performed, however, it is more reliable than visualization alone.

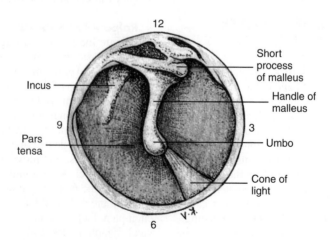

FIGURE 2-2 Usual landmarks of the right tympanic membrane with a "clock" superimposed. (From Wong DL, Perry S, Hockenberry MJ: *Maternal child nursing care*, ed 2, St Louis, 2002, Mosby.)

To perform insufflation, a large speculum is needed to create a seal. A normal finding elicits a slight motion of the TM when air is insufflated. This movement is compared with the opposite ear. A TM that has been retracted as a result of negative middle ear pressure or adhesions does not move with inflation, but rebound mobility is seen when the bulb is released. Any accumulation of liquid in the middle ear (e.g., effusion) or scarring of the TM inhibits movement when air is insufflated.

Test Hearing Acuity

Hearing acuity is tested using the whisper test and the tuning fork for the Rinne and Weber tests. The sensory function of the acoustic nerve (CN VIII) should be tested to determine whether air or bone conduction loss is present with ear pain.

The Weber test is performed with a 512-hertz (Hz) or higher frequency tuning fork. To perform the test, firmly place the vibrating tuning fork on a midline point of the skull. If there is unilateral conductive hearing loss, sound will lateralize to the ear with loss because the better ear is being distracted by ambient noise. Alternately, if the patient has unilateral sensorineural loss, the sound will lateralize to the better ear because the neural pathway is interrupted on the affected side. Equal perception of vibration can indicate normal hearing or bilateral hearing loss. The Rinne test compares air conduction with bone conduction; the ratio should be 2:1. A 20- to 30-decibel (dB) conductive loss would result in better sound transmission through bone than through air. Conductive hearing loss results when sound transmission is impaired through the external or middle ear. Sensorineural hearing loss results from a defect in the inner ear.

Examine Related Body Systems

Examine other regional body systems of the head and neck, including inspection of the conjunctivae, examination of the mucosa and patency of the nose, percussion and palpation of the frontal and maxillary sinuses for tenderness, and inspection of the posterior pharynx for lymphedema, color, and presence of exudate. Inspection of the condition of the oral mucosa—teeth and gums—will provide information about possible causes of referred pain. A focused physical examination for head and neck symptoms should include palpation of cervicofacial lymph nodes, especially the preauricular and postauricular nodes.

Perform an Intraotic Manipulation

If referred pain is suspected, conduct a more extensive neurological examination and assess for TMJ disorder. TMJ pain can be replicated by instructing the patient to open the mouth wide. Face the patient, insert a single fingertip in each ear, and pull the patient toward you as the patient is instructed to open and close the mouth. Pain will be elicited in 90% of patients with TMJ disorder.

Evaluate Cranial Nerves V, VII, and IX

Observe jaw and facial muscle movement for symmetry and strength by palpating over the masseter muscles and asking the patient to bite and clench the teeth (CN V). Assess intactness of sensation to pain and light touch using a sharp/dull stimulus over the three branches of CN V. Both CN VII (anterior two thirds) and CN IX (posterior one third) innervate taste sensation to the tongue as well as sensation to the external ear. Test taste sensation by having the patient protrude the tongue and apply sweet and salty substances separately to each half of the tongue to test CN VII and bitter and sour substances to test CN IX.

LABORATORY AND DIAGNOSTIC STUDIES

Tympanometry

Tympanometry involves inserting a probe into the external ear canal while pressure against the eardrum is continually changed to assess the mobility of the TM. The tympanogram provides an indirect measure of pressure in the middle ear. Under normal middle ear pressure, the TM absorbs the sound energy waves and produces a bell-shaped pattern that peaks when sound pressure is introduced. With positive or negative middle ear pressure, the tympanogram results in a flat pattern or an early peak pressure. Figure 2-3 illustrates examples of various tympanogram results.

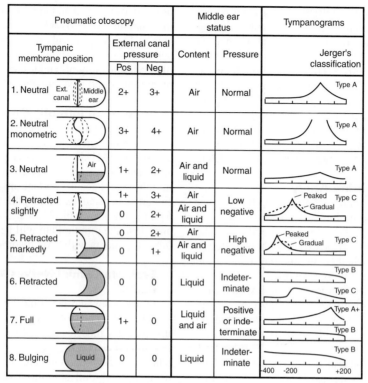

Pneumatic otoscopy				Middle ear status		Tympanograms
Tympanic membrane position		External canal pressure		Content	Pressure	Jerger's classification
		Pos	Neg			
1. Neutral	Ext. canal / Middle ear	2+	3+	Air	Normal	Type A
2. Neutral monometric		3+	4+	Air	Normal	Type A
3. Neutral	Air	1+	2+	Air and liquid	Normal	Type A
4. Retracted slightly		1+	3+	Air	Low negative	Peaked / Type C / Gradual
		0	2+	Air and liquid		
5. Retracted markedly		0	2+	Air	High negative	Peaked / Gradual / Type C
		0	1+	Air and liquid		
6. Retracted		0	0	Liquid	Indeterminate	Type B / Type C
7. Full		1+	0	Liquid and air	Positive or indeterminate	Type A+ / Type B
8. Bulging	Liquid	0	0	Liquid	Indeterminate	Type B
						-400 -200 0 +200

FIGURE 2-3   Middle ear evaluation with pneumatic otoscopy and impedance tympanograms. (From Daeschner CW Jr: *Pediatrics: an approach to independent learning*, New York, 1983, John Wiley & Sons.)

Audiometry

Audiometry assesses both the frequency and the intensity of sound that can be perceived. An air conduction audiometer transmits via earphones a pure tone that has variable frequency and intensity settings to test each ear separately. The goal of audiometry is to test the lowest decibel intensity that can be heard for each frequency tested. An individual trained in the proper technique will produce reliable, reproducible, and valid test results. A threshold of up to 20 dB is considered normal. At a higher level, hearing loss is graded as mild, moderate, moderately severe, severe, or profound.

Mastoid Process Radiography

Radiographs of the mastoid bone show clouding of the air cells when otitis media is present. Chronic mastoiditis may reveal decalcification of the bony wall between the mastoid air cells.

Computed Tomography Scanning

A computed tomography (CT) scan of the temporal bone is helpful in diagnosing cholesteatoma and congenital syndromes.

DIFFERENTIAL DIAGNOSIS

External Otitis

External otitis is more common in adults than in children and often presents as bilateral pain that worsens with manipulation of the pinna. The patient complains of a stuffed ear, and occasionally conductive hearing loss occurs. Discharge and itching that occur 1 to 2 days after swimming may be associated with otitis externa. The affected canal may be swollen shut. Palpation will often disclose enlarged preauricular or postauricular nodes.

Acute Otitis Media

AOM most often occurs in children younger than 6 years and is associated with an upper respiratory tract infection. It is an acute infection associated with ear pain and a bulging, red eardrum. The pain of otitis media is severe enough to interfere with sleep and may be suddenly relieved if the eardrum perforates. Swelling of the preauricular node is sometimes seen in children with AOM.

Serous Otitis

Serous otitis commonly occurs in children, often without pain. It is caused by a mechanical process or eustachian tube blockage that leads to inadequate ventilation of the middle ear and a collection of fluid that resembles mucus. In serous otitis, the TM may be injected and immobile, either bulging or retracted, as noted by the shape of the cone of light reflex and pneumatic otoscopy. In adults serous otitis is associated with recent upper respiratory tract infection.

Cholesteatoma

Cholesteatoma is an epidermal inclusion cyst formation in the middle ear and mastoid cavity. It is often the sequel of chronic otitis media. The formation occurs with chronic negative middle ear pressure, causing the migration of skin cells from the external ear canal through a perforation in the TM. Once established in the middle ear, the cells desquamate and form the cholesteatoma. This condition is life threatening if left untreated because it will continue to erode away medially to impinge on intracranial structures. A cholesteatoma can also occur congenitally. A cholesteatoma appears as a cyst or collection of granulation tissue on the TM, commonly located in the pars flaccida area in the superior anterior quadrant of the TM.

Mastoiditis

Mastoiditis is an infection of the soft tissue surrounding the air spaces in the mastoid bone and is connected to the middle ear space. Mastoiditis usually occurs with bacterial otitis media and is associated with fever. More advanced mastoiditis is manifested by swelling, erythema, and tenderness over the mastoid bone. Swelling can displace the position of the auricle. The swelling can extend to the facial nerve, causing paralysis, or to the labyrinth or cerebrospinal fluid, causing meningitis or brain abscess. Advanced mastoiditis requires immediate referral and surgical management.

Foreign Bodies

Foreign bodies are easily visualized on examination of the ear canal and can produce foul-smelling ear drainage secondary to infection or abscess.

Cerumen Impaction

Impaction of cerumen is likely if the patient complains of a stuffed-up ear or decreased hearing acuity. An impaction may also produce pain if cerumen is pressed against the TM. Examination will reveal cerumen that occludes the external canal.

Barotrauma

Barotrauma produces an acute serous otitis that is caused by pressure changes (e.g., in divers or airplane travelers) and is often aggravated by a recent upper respiratory tract infection or nasal congestion. Serosanguineous fluid collects in the middle ear; during descent this may be felt as ear pressure, pain, tinnitus, or temporary deafness. Swallowing, chewing, or blowing out the nose with the mouth and nose occluded can relieve symptoms.

Trauma

Blunt or penetrating trauma can perforate the TM. A hole in the TM is visible on examination, or the examiner may notice an absence of normal landmarks. A perforated eardrum does not significantly impair hearing or result in vertigo and usually heals within 4 to 6 weeks without sequelae. Assess the extent of other damage to the ear when perforation is identified.

Cervical Lymphadenitis

Anterior cervical lymphadenitis is a common cause of referred ear pain in children. This may be seen with strep throat, as well as in cases of mononucleosis with extensive cervical node swelling in adolescents or young adults.

Referred Pain From Cervical Nerves

Cervical nerves II to III innervate the skin and muscles of the neck and include the great auricular nerve, which supplies the external canals and posterior auricular area. Pain is perceived in these areas. The ear examination will be normal.

Referred Pain From Cranial Nerves

CNs associated with referred ear pain include the trigeminal nerve (CN V), which supplies the anterior portion of the auricle and tragus, the anterior and superior auditory canal, and the anterior TM, and the facial (CN VII), the vagus (CN X), and the glosso-

pharyngeal nerves (CN IX), which innervate the posterior portion of the TM and the external auditory canal. Inflammation of CN X is associated with lesions of the larynx, esophagus, trachea, and thyroid. With referred pain, the structures of the ear will appear normal.

TMJ Disorder

TMJ disorder is a common secondary cause of ear pain. Diagnosis of the disorder is likely if palpation over the TMJ elicits tenderness and movement of the joint creates a clicking sound. Results of examination of the ear are normal. Pain also increases with intraotic manipulation. TMJ pain is often worse in the morning. The pain can be acute (related to trauma or overextension of the mouth) or chronic (related to dental malocclusion or rheumatoid arthritis).

DIFFERENTIAL DIAGNOSIS OF *Common Causes of Ear Pain*

CONDITION	HISTORY	PHYSICAL FINDINGS	DIAGNOSTIC STUDIES
External otitis	More common in adults, especially those with diabetes, ear pickers, or swimmers; bilateral itching; pain	Discharge; inflamed, swollen external canal; pain with movement of pinna; TM normal or not visible	None
Acute otitis media	More common in children <6 years; those with smoke exposure, recent URI; severe or deep pain; unilateral; sensation of fullness	Red, bulging TM; fever; decreased light reflex; opaque TM; decreased TM mobility	None initially
Serous otitis	More common in children but occurs in adults with recent URI; unilateral pain; sensation of crackling or decreased hearing	Fluid line or air observed behind TM; conductive hearing loss; decreased TM mobility	Tympanogram
Cholesteatoma	Hearing loss; recent perforated TM	Pearly white lesion on or behind TM	Immediate referral
Mastoiditis	History of recent otitis media; chronic otitis pain behind ear	Swelling over mastoid process; fever, palpable tenderness, and erythema over mastoid process	Radiograph of mastoid sinuses reveals cloudiness; referral
Foreign body or cerumen impaction	Both children and adults have pain or vague sensation of discomfort; decreased hearing	Visualize foreign body or cerumen; may detect foul odor; conductive hearing loss	None

Continued

DIFFERENTIAL DIAGNOSIS OF *Common Causes of Ear Pain* —cont'd

CONDITION	HISTORY	PHYSICAL FINDINGS	DIAGNOSTIC STUDIES
Barotrauma	History of flying, diving; severe pain; hearing loss; sensation of fullness; history of recent nasal congestion	Retraction or bulging of TM; perforation of TM; fluid in canal	Tympanogram
Trauma	History of blunt trauma, penetrating trauma	Perforation of TM	Radiographs/CT scan as directed by injury
Cervical lymphadenitis	History of cervical node swelling; pain in ear common in children	Enlarged, tender, cervical lymph nodes; may see early onset of AOM in children	Throat culture if indicated; in adolescents Monospot if indicated
Cervical nerves 2, 3 (referred pain)	Pain in skin and muscles of neck and in ear canal	Dermatome evaluation for cervical nerve	None
Cranial nerves (referred pain)	History, depending on CN involved	Test function of CNs V, VII, IX, and X; ear examination normal	Radiography/CT scan, directed by CN involvement
TMJ disorder	More common in adults; 50% related to dental problems; discomfort to severe pain; unilateral; pain worse in morning	Malocclusion; bruxism; normal external and middle ear structures and function; jaw click; abnormal CN function; ear examination normal	None

CHAPTER RESOURCES

American Academy of Pediatrics and American Academy of Family Physicians: Diagnosis and management of acute otitis media, *Pediatrics* 113:145, 2004.

Ishiyama A: Why does air travel cause earache? *West J Med* 171:106, 1999.

O'Neill P: Acute otitis media, *BMJ* 319:833, 1999.

Pelton SI: Otitis media: re-evaluation of diagnosis and treatment in the era of antimicrobial resistance, pneumococcal conjugate vaccine, and evolving morbidity, *Pediatr Clin North Am* 52:711, 2005.

Pichichero ME: Acute otitis media, part I: improving diagnostic accuracy, *Am Fam Physician* 61:2051, 2000.

Sore Throat

Sore throat is most often the result of an inflammation of the mucosa of the oropharynx, secondary to an infectious cause (e.g., viral, bacterial, fungal, or spirochetal). Less commonly, sore throat may be a symptom of systemic illness, such as mononucleosis. The posterior pharynx is also vulnerable to irritants from the environment and drainage from the nose and sinuses. Thus pharyngitis begins as an inflammation of the mucous membranes with secondary involvement of the lymph node drainage system, rarely progressing to deep neck and mediastinal involvement. Throat pain can also be referred from other structures, most commonly the ears and thyroid gland.

Sore throats can be classified as those with pharyngeal ulcers and those without. The classification serves as a device to sort out those relatively few sore throats caused by specific viral or fungal infections that produce pharyngeal ulcers and those caused by agents and processes characterized by an absence of pharyngeal ulcers.

The goals of assessment and diagnosis are to identify those patients with group A β-hemolytic streptococcus (GABHS) infection (because they are at risk for rheumatic fever and glomerulonephritis), to reduce the possibility of sequelae of peritonsillar and retropharyngeal abscess, and to identify epiglottitis.

DIAGNOSTIC REASONING: FOCUSED HISTORY

Is This an Emergency?

Key Questions
- Have you been drooling?
- Have you been unable to swallow?
- Have you been unable to lie down?
- Have you been restless, unable to stay still?

- Have you been unable to carry on a conversation?

The previous complaints signal acute epiglottitis. The history is usually elicited from another individual because the ill person either is a child or is too ill to talk. Acute epiglottitis is rare, with an incidence of 10:100,000 in pediatric patients younger than 15 years and 1 to 8:100,000 adult patients. The morbidity and mortality that result from airway obstruction, however, are significant.

Symptoms of epiglottitis are sore throat, difficulty swallowing, and respiratory distress, characterized by drooling, dyspnea, and inspiratory stridor. *Haemophilus influenzae* type b is the most common pathogen. The incidence of *H. influenzae* type b epiglottitis is highest in children ages 2 to 5 years. Epiglottitis is a rapidly progressive illness with a potentially fatal outcome and must be recognized and referred immediately.

Peritonsillar abscess is also an acute infection that needs to be identified immediately for referral and treatment. The symptoms of peritonsillar abscess and cellulitis include a severe sore throat, odynophagia, trismus (spasm of the masticatory muscles and difficulty opening the mouth), and medial deviation of the soft palate and peritonsillar fold. These symptoms are caused by infection penetrating the tonsillar capsule and surrounding tissues. About 30% of patients with peritonsillar abscess require an emergency tonsillectomy.

Is the Sore Throat Related to an Infectious Cause?

Key Questions
- Is anyone else at home sick?
- Are any of your friends or co-workers sick?
- When did the pain start?
- How severe is the pain?

Exposure

Exposure to other ill individuals increases the likelihood of viral or bacterial infection. Respiratory illness caused by GABHS is spread within families, with approximately 20% of family members becoming infected. Epstein-Barr virus (EBV) is not highly contagious and requires intimate contact between susceptible individuals and symptomatic shedders of the virus. Transmission is primarily through saliva.

Onset

The sudden onset of sore throat is often caused by GABHS. The organisms invade the pharyngeal epithelium, where they multiply and cause an intense immune response. Gradual onset is more common in infectious mononucleosis. The EBV infects B lymphocytes of the pharynx with resultant dissemination throughout the lymphoreticular system, causing an immune response that is more gradual in onset

In viral pharyngitis, a sore throat begins a day or two after the onset of other illness symptoms, reaching its peak by the second or third day.

Noninfectious causes of sore throat typically have an insidious onset. The patient often is not able to pinpoint when the sore throat started but notes that it has been persistent.

Severity

Throat pain associated with streptococcal infection is usually intense. Throat pain associated with influenza and adenovirus is severe, with prominent edema of the throat. Severe throat pain with trismus and refusal to speak indicates severe peritonsillitis, which may lead to peritonsillar abscess formation (quinsy). The throat pain produced by noninfectious causes tends to be less severe and may be described as "scratchy" or "annoying."

Young children may not be able to express the sensation of a sore throat or the severity of it. Instead, they may refuse to eat or drink. Pain in the younger child, if present, more commonly indicates the presence of epiglottitis or laryngitis, abscess, diphtheria, or scarlatina.

What Does the Presence of Fever Tell Me?

Key Questions

■ Have you had a fever?
■ When did it start?
■ How high has it been?

Fever is almost always present with GABHS and is the most commonly occurring symptom in children. The fever is of sudden onset and the temperature rises above 38.5° C (101.5° F), with malaise, headache, and painful swallowing. Fever is also present in children and adults with epiglottitis.

Influenza is characterized by the abrupt onset of fever, with temperatures ranging from 37.8° C to 40° C (100° F to 104° F). Adenoviral infection in children typically presents with a temperature greater than 40° C (104° F). Patients with EBV have a low-grade fever.

Fever, followed by an interval of several days without fever and then recurrent fever, or a continuing fever for several days may indicate peritonsillar abscess.

The absence of fever suggests a noninfectious cause. Patients with candidiasis and aphthous stomatitis may also present without a fever.

What Does the Presence of Upper Respiratory Tract Symptoms Tell Me?

Key Questions

■ Do you have a cough?
■ Have you had a runny nose? What color is the drainage?
■ Do you have mucus dripping from the back of your nose down your throat?
■ Do you have any eye redness or discomfort?
■ Have your eyes been itchy or watery?
■ Have you had any hoarseness?
■ Have you been sneezing?

Cough and Rhinorrhea

Cough, rhinitis, conjunctivitis, and hoarseness rarely occur with streptococcal pharyngitis, and the presence of two or more of these signs or symptoms suggests a viral infection.

Influenza is often associated with several days of fever, cough, and rhinorrhea. Viral pharyngitis is characterized by a sore, scratchy throat, nasal congestion, rhinorrhea, and cough.

Clear nasal discharge is common in allergic pharyngitis and may produce postnasal drip that causes a sore throat.

Conjunctivitis
Conjunctivitis rarely occurs with streptococcal pharyngitis. Mild conjunctivitis is common with viral infection. Watery or itchy eyes are associated with exposure to allergens.

Sneezing
Sneezing is common with both viral infection and allergen exposure. The sneezing associated with allergic pharyngitis is more persistent and enduring, and it is often seasonal.

Hoarseness
Hoarseness is not uncommon in allergy-associated sore throat and may be present with viral infection as well. Inflammation produces laryngeal edema that results in hoarseness. Hoarseness is not typically associated with GABHS infection.

What Do the Associated Symptoms Tell Me?

Key Questions
- Do you have muscle aches?
- Have you had any nausea, vomiting, or diarrhea?

Systemic Complaints
Systemic complaints such as myalgia are common in influenza and GABHS infection. Streptococcal pharyngitis or influenza in children older than 2 years is associated with complaints of headache, abdominal pain, and vomiting.

Influenza is often associated with several days of fever and systemic symptoms such as myalgias, cough, and rhinorrhea. Pharyngitis associated with common cold viruses is also often associated with systemic symptoms such as myalgia.

Does the Presence of Risk Factors Help Me to Narrow the Cause?

Key Questions
- How old are you?
- What is your smoking history?
- What kind of work do you do?
- Do you engage in oral sex?
- Are you taking any medications?
- Do you have any chronic health problems?
- Are your immunizations up to date?

Age
Group A streptococcal infection is primarily a disease in children 5 to 15 years of age. GABHS is rare in children younger than 3 years. Influenza affects all ages, whereas parainfluenza and respiratory syncytial viruses primarily affect children.

Adenoviruses, the major viral agents isolated in exudative pharyngitis in younger children, are endemic. In military populations, adenovirus type 4 and, to a lesser extent, types 3, 7, and 21 are the most common causes of pharyngitis.

Adolescents and young adults are more likely to have a sore throat associated with mononucleosis caused by the EBV. Mononucleosis occurs in older adults but often without pharyngitis, adenopathy, or splenomegaly.

Irritant Exposures
Agents such as tobacco smoke, smog, dust, and allergens can irritate the throat. These agents cause mucosal irritation and set up the inflammatory process. People who work outdoors may have greater exposure to environmental allergens. Housekeepers may have an increased risk of exposure to dust mites or chemical irritants.

Sexual Behavior
Pharyngitis from *Chlamydia trachomatis* and *Neisseria gonorrhoeae* is more prevalent in persons with a history of orogenital sexual activity. Gonococcal pharyngitis is present in about 10% of patients with anogenital gonorrhea.

Medications and Chronic Health Problems

Immunosuppression increases susceptibility to viral agents that produce pharyngeal ulcers (e.g., herpangina, herpes simplex). Persons with diabetes and those taking broad-spectrum antibiotics are more susceptible to candidiasis. Persons with a history of gastroesophageal reflux disease (GERD) may have a sore throat secondary to reflux of gastric contents.

Immunizations

Lack of immunization to diphtheria can place a person at risk for diphtheria.

DIAGNOSTIC REASONING: FOCUSED PHYSICAL EXAMINATION

Assess Degree of Illness

Assessment of the patient begins with general observation about the severity of illness. Severe illness, with signs of upper airway obstruction such as restlessness, stridor, difficulty breathing, drooling, inability to swallow, and very high fever, signals epiglottitis and requires immediate referral. Further examination could trigger laryngospasms and lead to airway obstruction.

Inspect the Mouth

Examine the buccal mucosa, tongue, and sublingual area for the presence of ulcers. Note the location, number, size, and appearance of any lesions.

The lesions produced by the group A coxsackievirus (herpangina) first appear as small, grayish, papulovesicular lesions on the soft palate and pharynx. These progress to shallow ulcers, usually less than 5 mm in diameter.

Vincent's angina (necrotizing ulcerative gingivostomatitis) is a fusospirochetal infection of the gingiva. The gingiva appears inflamed and ulcerated, often covered with a gray slough. As the infection spreads, ulcers may appear on the oral mucosa and posterior pharynx.

Aphthous stomatitis lesions affect about 20% of the general population and are associated with immunological mechanisms.

They occur most often on the buccal mucosa, tongue, and soft palate. The lesions first appear as indurated papules and then progress to shallow ulcers. The ulcers have a yellow membrane and red halo. Herpes simplex lesions involve the anterior oral mucosa and the gums. Herpetic pharyngitis is manifested by vesicles, ulcers, or exudate of the oral and pharyngeal mucosa. Specifically, the lesions involve the tonsils, pharynx, uvula, and edges of the soft palate. Vesicular lesions may or may not be intact.

Streptococcal infection in children may cause enlarged papillae on the tongue, which gives the tongue a strawberry appearance.

Inspect the Posterior Pharynx and Observe Swallowing

Examine for edema, color, and exudate of the posterior pharynx and determine the presence, size (Table 3-1), and condition of the palatine tonsils. Good visualization is critical for accurate diagnosis. Use a good light source, and ask the patient to open wide and say "ah" but not to protrude the tongue. If you cannot view the pharynx, depress the tongue firmly with a tongue blade, far enough back to have a good view but not enough to cause the patient to gag. Use two tongue depressors to retract tissues medially and laterally when examining areas such as the retromolar region, the floor of the mouth, and the orifices of Wharton's and Stensen's ducts (Figure 3-1). The best visualization is achieved with a headlight.

Drooling may indicate peritonsillar abscess or epiglottitis partially occluding the pharynx and esophagus. Only occasionally can the red, swollen epiglottis be visualized above the base of the tongue. If you suspect epiglottitis, do not examine the pharynx because manipulation may precipitate

Table 3-1	Grading Tonsillar Size
GRADE	**TONSIL LOCATION**
1	Behind pillars
2	Between pillars and uvula
3	Touching uvula
4	Extending beyond midline of oropharynx

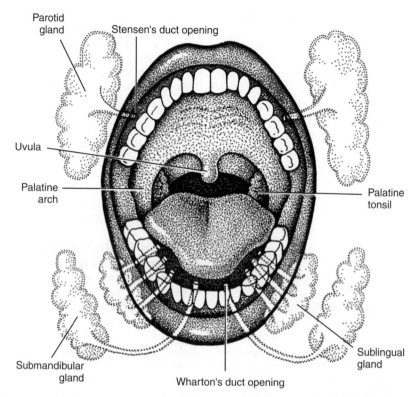

Parotid gland
Stensen's duct opening
Uvula
Palatine arch
Palatine tonsil
Submandibular gland
Wharton's duct opening
Sublingual gland

FIGURE 3-1 Anatomical structures of the mouth. (From Barkauskas VH et al: *Health and physical assessment*, ed 3, St Louis, 2002, Mosby.)

laryngospasms and airway obstruction. Refer the patient immediately for specialist evaluation and further diagnosis, which may involve soft tissue radiography of the head and neck and laryngoscopy.

Edema of the affected tonsil, with movement of the tonsil toward midline, indicates peritonsillar abscess. Diphtheria may appear as a thick, gray tonsillar exudate or pseudomembrane, spreading to the tonsillar pillars, uvula, soft palate, posterior pharyngeal wall, and larynx. The exudate is not easily removable and bleeds easily.

Pharyngeal or tonsillar exudate can be present with either a bacterial or a viral infection. A yellowish exudate of GABHS pharyngitis is often present. Generally the exudate of viral agents tends to be whiter than that from GABHS.

A bright red uvula and the presence of petechiae on the posterior pharynx and palate indicate group A streptococcal pharyngitis. "Doughnut lesions," or red, raised hemorrhagic lesions with a yellow center, are highly diagnostic of streptococcal pharyngitis.

Postnasal drainage can irritate the posterior pharynx and should be observed for color. Purulent drainage that is yellow or greenish is associated with infectious sinusitis. White curdlike patches that bleed on scraping are characteristic of oral candidiasis.

When examination reveals normal findings, suspect a systemic referred cause for the sore throat, particularly acute otitis media, sinusitis, or thyroiditis.

Palpate the Cervicofacial Lymph Nodes

In streptococcal pharyngitis, the anterior cervical lymph nodes are often enlarged and tender. In viral infections, the posterior cervical nodes are more often enlarged. Lymphadenopathy is a cardinal sign of infectious mononucleosis, with more than 90% of patients having enlarged posterior cervical nodes.

Inspect the Nasal Mucosa

Red, swollen turbinates indicate an infectious process, whereas pale, boggy turbinates indicate an allergic process. The presence of mucoid discharge occurs in allergic rhinitis. Purulent discharge suggests infectious sinusitis.

Inspect the Conjunctivae

Injected conjunctivae associated with a sore throat may indicate pharyngoconjunctival fever. It is caused by an adenovirus and is often associated with nonpurulent discharge, fever, and pharyngitis. It frequently occurs in epidemics. Mild conjunctivitis in the presence of itching eyes and with a clear watery discharge is associated with an allergic process.

Inspect the Tympanic Membrane

Evidence of otitis media with effusion may indicate nontypical *H. influenzae* acute otitis media (conjunctivitis-otitis syndrome). Earache can be caused by referred pain, especially from the tonsils.

Palpate the Thyroid

Acute thyroiditis is associated with a sore throat in the presence of a normal throat examination but with an enlarged and tender thyroid gland.

Inspect the Skin

Evidence of a fine maculopapular erythema that has a generalized distribution with accentuation in the skinfolds, circumoral pallor, and sparing of the palms and soles indicates scarlet fever. The rash characteristically is followed by a fine desquamation, starting at the hands.

Auscultate the Lungs

Mycoplasma pneumoniae is frequently associated with sore throat in adolescents and young adults. If pneumonia is present, palpation, percussion, and auscultation of the lungs reveal an area of consolidation and adventitious breath sounds (see Chapter 11 for further discussion of the lung examination).

Palpate the Abdomen

Splenomegaly is found in about half the cases of mononucleosis, although hepatomegaly is rare. GERD may be associated with palpable upper epigastric tenderness.

LABORATORY AND DIAGNOSTIC STUDIES

The laboratory evaluation of sore throat is generally limited to the identification of GABHS. Other infectious causes, such as gonorrhea or diphtheria, are rare, and testing is conducted only if the history indicates exposure. It is important to diagnose streptococcal pharyngitis so it can be treated promptly with antibiotics, avoiding serious sequelae such as peritonsillar abscesses or rheumatic fever.

Rapid Screening Tests

A throat swab is a rapid screen for streptococcal antigens and should be done if GABHS is suspected. If it is positive, the patient is treated without follow-up cultures. If the swab is negative, a throat culture is obtained. The test has a sensitivity of 75% to 85% and a specificity of 95% to 98%.

The Monospot is a rapid slide test that detects heterophil antibody agglutination; it is not specific for EBV. It is most sensitive 1 to 2 weeks after symptoms appear and remains positive for up to 1 year. If chronic fatigue syndrome is being considered as a differential diagnosis, specific EBV antibody tests should be considered.

Culture

A throat culture to detect GABHS is the "gold standard" of diagnosis, with a 10% or lower false-negative rate. When obtaining a culture, first remove crusts from lesions, taking care to touch only the throat or tonsils with the sterile swab. Avoid touching the tongue. Roll the throat swab over one tonsil, proceed across the posterior pharynx, and then swab the other tonsil. A culture for gonorrhea can confirm a diagnosis of gonococcal pharyngitis.

ASO Titer

GABHS produces enzymes that include streptolysin. An ASO titer is a serological test that detects the presence of a previous streptococcal infection. This titer does not increase until 1 to 6 months postinfection, so it is of no diagnostic value. It is used to aid in the diagnosis of streptococci-associated infections, such as rheumatic fever, glomerulonephritis, and pericarditis. A caution, however, is that in as many as 50% of positive streptococcal cultures, an elevated ASO titer postinfection will not be found.

Complete Blood Cell Count With Differential

Test results that show 50% lymphocytes and at least 10% atypical lymphocytes confirm the diagnosis of mononucleosis.

Computed Tomography Scan

Suspicion of an obstruction or swelling of the throat should be referred for further radiographic evaluation with a computed tomography scan.

Nasal Smear

Nasal cytology can be performed on nasal secretions obtained by having the patient blow the nose into a paper or by using a cotton-tipped swab to obtain secretions from the nose. The presence of eosinophils on a nasal smear stained with Wright's stain viewed under a high-power microscope suggests an allergic, inflammatory process.

DIFFERENTIAL DIAGNOSIS

Pharyngitis Without Ulcers

Epiglottitis

Epiglottitis is caused by infection with *H. influenzae* type b that produces inflammation and edema of the epiglottis and the surrounding areas, obstructing the flow of air. The edematous epiglottis may be pulled into the larynx during inspiration and can completely occlude the airway. Symptoms are respiratory distress, sore throat, difficulty with secretions, drooling, pain on swallowing, and a toxic appearance. The infection occurs in both children and adults.

Peritonsillar/Retropharyngeal Abscess

A peritonsillar abscess, also called quinsy, is a collection of pus between the tonsil and the capsule of the tonsillar pillar. This condition occurs in children but is more common in adults, especially in persons with a history of recurrent tonsillitis. The patient's presenting symptoms usually include a history of respiratory symptoms, difficulty swallowing, otalgia, malaise, fever, and cervical lymphadenopathy. On examination there may be trismus; asymmetrical swelling of the uvula, tonsils, or posterior pharynx; or a visible abscess. Children's presenting symptoms typically include fever, toxic appearance, refusal to swallow, drooling, and stridor. Children with retropharyngeal abscess are usually under the age of 4 and need immediate referral.

Viral Pharyngitis

Most sore throats are caused by viral infections. Patients usually display systemic symptoms of malaise, fever, headache, cough, and fatigue. The pharynx is usually erythematous, or it may be pale, boggy, and swollen. There usually is no tonsillar or pharyngeal exudate or tonsillar enlargement present, although infection with an adenovirus may produce pharyngeal exudate. The presence of concomitant upper respiratory tract symptoms such as cough and congestion makes the diagnosis of viral pharyngitis more likely than that of streptococcal pharyngitis. Common cold viruses cause sore throats most frequently during the colder months of the year.

Streptococcal Pharyngitis

The major differential diagnoses for sore throat will be viral or bacterial infection. Fewer than 10% of adults and 30% of children who seek care for sore throat symptoms have streptococcal tonsillopharyngitis. However, reliance on clinical impression to arrive at a specific diagnosis is problematic. The symptoms most likely to occur with streptococcal pharyngitis include a fever with a temperature of 38.5° C (101.5° F) or higher, tonsillar exudate, anterior cervical adenopathy, and a history of recent exposure. The incidence of streptococcal pharyngitis increases from 10% in the summer and fall to 40% during the winter and early spring. GABHS cannot be reliably diagnosed on the basis of signs and symptoms, and even when cultures are obtained, a causative agent may not be identified in 50% of patients. Table 3-2 shows the groups at risk for GABHS.

Mononucleosis

Mononucleosis causes about 5% of sore throats. It is most often a disease of young adults, and the causative agent is EBV in more than 90% of cases. History reveals a gradual onset, low-grade fever, mild sore throat, posterior cervical lymphadenopathy, and pronounced malaise and fatigue. Diagnosis can be confirmed with a positive Monospot test and a complete blood cell count that shows greater than 50% lymphocytosis. Splenomegaly occurs in about 50% of cases, and palatine petechiae are a less common symptom. GABHS occurs concomitantly in 10% to 20% of cases.

Gonococcal Pharyngitis

This is a fairly rare form of pharyngitis that can occur in patients who are at risk (i.e., those with a history of orogenital sexual activity). The patient may have no symptoms. Examination shows an exudative pharyngitis with bilateral cervical lymphadenopathy. Diagnosis is confirmed through Gram staining or culture.

Inflammation

Inflammatory sore throat occurs in the presence of sinusitis or exposure to local irritants. The patient often complains of a postnasal drip and allergic symptoms (itchy, watery eyes; runny nose). On examination, the patient may have sinus tenderness. The pharynx may be swollen or pale, and posterior drainage may be apparent. The patient has no fever or lymphadenopathy. Patients with allergies report symptoms that regularly follow seasonal patterns.

Table 3-2	Groups at Risk for Group A β-Hemolytic Streptococcus (GABHS) Pharyngitis	
RISK FACTORS	**DIAGNOSTIC TESTS**
High Risk Tonsillar exudate Temperature >38.5° C (101.5° F) Cervical lymphadenopathy Existing valvular rheumatic heart disease	None; treat on basis of risk factors
Presumed Strep Scarlet fever Strep epidemic Antibiotics already started	None; treat
Medium Risk Exudate, nodes, or fever present Prior rheumatic fever "Low risk" by PE but <25 years old and no URI Person with diabetes Recent "strep" exposure	Rapid strep screen; if positive, treat; if negative, do culture; treat if culture positive; do not treat if culture negative
Low Risk No exudate, nodes, or fever	Rapid strep screen; if positive, treat; if negative, do not culture; do not treat if culture negative

PE, Physical examination; *URI,* upper respiratory tract infection.

Pharyngitis With Ulcers

Herpangina

Herpangina is an infection caused by the coxsackievirus. The patient complains of a painful sore throat, fever, and malaise. Headache, anorexia, and neck, abdomen, and extremity pain may occur. Within 2 days of onset, small, grayish, papulovesicular lesions appear on the soft palate and pharynx. These progress to shallow ulcers, usually less than 5 mm in diameter. Outbreaks occur during the summer months. Coxsackievirus peaks in August, September, and October, although some cases occur during the winter months. It is more common in children and in immunosuppressed patients. Diagnosis is based on symptoms and characteristic oral lesions. An antibody titer can confirm diagnosis.

Vincent's Angina

Vincent's angina is caused by a fusospirochetal infection that results in necrotizing ulcerative gingivostomatitis. The patient's symptoms include painful ulcers, foul breath, and bleeding gums. Without secondary infection, there usually is no fever. On examination, gray, necrotic ulcers without vesicles are apparent on the gingivae and interdental papillae. Gram staining shows spirochetes and confirms the diagnosis.

Aphthous Stomatitis

Aphthous stomatitis, or "canker sores," appears as discrete ulcers without preceding vesicles. The ulcers are located on the inner lip, tongue, and buccal mucosa. Lesions last about 1 to 2 weeks. The cause of the lesions is unknown, but immunological mechanisms play a major role.

Herpes Simplex

Herpes simplex virus (HSV) type 1 (can also include HSV type 2) is an infection manifested by fever, headache, sore throat, and lymphadenitis. Characteristic clusters of yellow vesicles appear on the palate, pharynx, and gingiva. Lesions last 2 to 3 weeks. Recurrent lesions are characterized by prodromal symptoms of burning, tingling, or itching. Active lesions are usually painful. Recent studies indicate that infections afflict about 20% to 45% of the U.S. population.

Candidiasis

Candidiasis is a yeast infection that produces white plaques over the tongue and oral mucosa with erythema; the plaques bleed when scraped. *Candida* infection occurs commonly in otherwise normal infants in the first weeks of life; in immunocompromised persons, including those with diabetes; and in persons taking antibiotics or using inhaled steroids.

DIFFERENTIAL DIAGNOSIS OF *Common Causes of Sore Throat*

CONDITION	HISTORY	PHYSICAL FINDINGS	DIAGNOSTIC STUDIES
Pharyngitis with Ulcers			
Aphthous stomatitis	Oral trauma, ill-fitting dentures; painful ulcers vary in size; absence of other symptoms	Shallow ulcers, no vesicles; indurated papules that progress to 1-cm ulcers; ulcer has yellow membrane and red halo; no fever or nodes	None
Herpes simplex infection	History of trauma to mucosa; pain, fever, headache	Perioral lesions; lymphadenitis; vesicles on palate, pharynx, gingiva	Viral culture
Candidiasis	Immunosuppressed; persons taking antibiotics or with diabetes; sore mouth/throat	Curdlike white plaques that bleed when scraped off	KOH smear shows hyphae; culture

Continued

DIFFERENTIAL DIAGNOSIS OF *Common Causes of Sore Throat —cont'd*

CONDITION	HISTORY	PHYSICAL FINDINGS	DIAGNOSTIC STUDIES
Pharyngitis Without Ulcers			
Epiglottitis	Sore throat, difficulty with secretions, odynophagia (seen in pediatric patients <2 years), unable to lie flat, unable to talk	Respiratory distress, drooling, toxic appearance; DO NOT EXAMINE PHARYNX	Refer immediately
Peritonsillar/ retropharyngeal abscess	History of recurrent tonsillitis; sore throat, difficulty swallowing, respiratory tract symptoms, fever, malaisea	Orthopnea, dyspnea, symmetrical swelling, abscess, trismus	Refer immediately: CT scan; head and neck radiographs; laryngoscopy
Viral pharyngitis	Scratchy, sore throat, malaise, myalgias, headache, chills, cough, rhinitis	Erythema, edema of throat, tender posterior cervical nodes	None
Group A β-hemolytic streptococcal pharyngitis	Most common in persons 5-15 years; known exposure; fall/winter season; sudden onset of fever, severe sore throat, and malaise; absence of cough and upper respiratory tract symptoms	Temperature >38.5° C (101.5° F); exudate; anterior cervical lymphadenopathy	Positive rapid strep antibody screen; strep culture
Mononucleosis (Epstein-Barr virus)	Young adults; slow onset of malaise, low-grade fever, mild sore throat	Presence/absence of pharyngeal exudate, palatine petechiae, posterior cervical lymphadenopathy, splenomegaly	Positive Monospot; CBC with differential; >50% leukocytes
Gonococcal pharyngitis	History of orogenital sexual activity; may be asymptomatic	Pharyngeal exudate; bilateral cervical lymphadenopathy	Gram stain; gonorrhea culture
Inflammation	Exposure to irritants; postnasal drip; allergic symptoms	Sinus tenderness, pale or swollen pharynx, postnasal drainage visible, no fever or lymphadenopathy	Eosinophils in nasal secretions with allergies
Pharyngitis With Ulcers			
Herpangina (coxsackievirus)	More common in children; immunosuppressed; painful throat; fever, malaise	Lymphadenopathy; small grayish papulovesicular lesions on soft palate and pharynx, progressing to shallow ulcers, usually <5 mm in diameter	Serology
Fusospirochetal infection (Vincent's angina)	Poor oral hygiene; painful ulcers, foul breath, bleeding gums	Gray necrotic ulcers without vesicles on gingival margins and interdental papillae	Gram stain reveals spirochetes

CT, Computed tomography; *CBC,* complete blood cell count.

CHAPTER RESOURCES

Darrow DH, Siemens C: Indications for tonsillectomy and adenoidectomy, *Laryngoscope* 112:8, 2002.

Ebell MH et al: The rational clinical examination: does this patient have strep throat? *JAMA* 284:2912, 2000.

Gerber M: Diagnosis and treatment of pharyngitis in children, *Pediatr Clin North Am* 52(3):729, 2005.

Richardson MA: Sore throat, tonsillitis, and adenoiditis, *Med Clin North Am* 83:75, 1999.

Tierney LM, McPhee SJ, Papadakis MA: *Current medical diagnosis & treatment*, ed 44, New York, 2005, McGraw-Hill.

Nasal Symptoms and Sinus Congestion

Concern about symptoms of the "common cold" accounts for a significant proportion of primary care visits by both children and adults, especially in the winter months. Symptoms include nasal congestion, rhinorrhea, postnasal drip, sneezing, itchy nose, watery and itchy eyes, and frontal headache. Severe symptoms are associated with ageusia (loss of taste) and anosmia (loss of smell).

The nose humidifies, warms, and filters inspired air. The nasal turbinates promote turbulent airflow that causes particulate matter to fall on the mucosa, where it is swept away by ciliated pseudostratified columnar cells to the nasopharynx. Rhinitis, or inflammation of the mucous membranes, is a frequent nasal symptom that is caused by bacterial or viral infection, a response to allergens, or a response to medication or extremes in environmental temperature.

Nasal polyps, septal deviation, or congenital anomaly can cause nasal obstruction. In children, nasal obstruction is very frequently unilateral and may be secondary to a foreign body inserted into the nose.

Respiratory epithelium lines the paranasal sinuses and creates drainage into the nasal cavity via the superior meatus and middle meatus. The maxillary sinus is the most frequently involved paranasal sinus because its ciliated cells carry maxillary sinus drainage against gravity. When drainage systems become impaired as a result of mucosal edema, mechanical obstruction, or impaired ciliary activity, viruses and bacteria proliferate.

The paranasal sinuses include the frontal, ethmoid, maxillary, and sphenoid (Figure 4-1).

Most sinus infections are caused by bacteria common to the nasopharynx that proliferate when local or systemic defenses are impaired. The most common causative organisms producing bacterial sinusitis in both adults and children are *Streptococcus pneumoniae* and *Haemophilus influenzae*. Sinusitis may also be associated with allergies and asthmatic exacerbations or with contiguous infection of the mouth or face.

DIAGNOSTIC REASONING: FOCUSED HISTORY

What Are the Primary Symptoms That Will Help Me Narrow the Possibilities?

Key Questions
- How long have these symptoms been present?
- Do you have a history of nasal or sinus problems?
- Do the symptoms occur at any particular time of the year or season?
- Is there a family history of allergies or asthma?
- Do you have other symptoms?

Acute Symptoms
Acute symptoms of rhinitis or sinus congestion, usually lasting 48 to 72 hours, are caused by edematous mucosa obstructing the sinus ostia. If a person has no previous history of similar symptoms but has systemic symptoms such as fever, myalgias, and chills, acute infectious rhinitis caused by rhinoviruses or parainfluenza virus is likely.

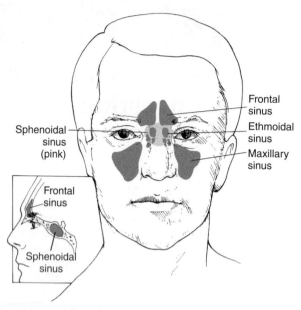

FIGURE 4-1 Anterior and lateral views of the paranasal sinuses. (From Barkauskas VH et al: *Health and physical assessment*, ed 3, St Louis, 2002, Mosby.)

Chronic Symptoms

Chronic rhinitis lasting weeks to years is rarely infectious; rather it is often associated with anatomical abnormalities that impair the sinus drainage system, although the mucociliary clearance mechanisms are normal.

Allergic Symptoms

Suspect allergic rhinitis if a person describes seasonal occurrence of nasal symptoms, associated with sneezing, wheezing, and itchy or burning eyes. A distinguishing feature of the allergic individual is the propensity to develop sustained IgE response after antigenic stimulation. IgE is an antibody capable of interacting with target cells that release mediators on contact with specific antigens. This reaction is the manifestation of an allergy.

Persons with perennial allergies have an allergen present in the environment on a year-round basis from sources such as animal dander, house dust, mold, feathers, and cockroaches. Seasonal allergies usually occur in early spring (tree pollens), early summer (grass pollens), and early fall (weed pollens). A family history of asthma or allergies is frequently associated with allergic rhinitis. Other symptoms may include a sensation of head stuffiness, ear discomfort, fatigue, and a scratchy or mild sore throat.

If I Suspect Sinus Problems, What Do I Need to Know?

Key Questions

- Do you have a history of sinus problems?
- Do you have pain? Please point to the areas of pain.
- Do your symptoms change with position changes?
- How long have you had these symptoms?

Acute Symptoms

Acute sinusitis is an abrupt onset of infection of one or more of the paranasal sinuses, and it occurs when the sinus ostia become obstructed, usually after an upper respiratory tract infection. Sinusitis is frequently associated with a sore throat, often irritated by postnasal discharge, facial or tooth pain, or headache over the affected sinus, as well as morning periorbital swelling, fever, and malaise. Other less common causes include anatomical abnormality, adenoid hypertrophy, and contiguous infection, such as a dental abscess or periorbital cellulitis.

Location of Pain

An adult patient with sinusitis most often complains of a prolonged cold with symptoms of nasal congestion and facial pain. Children rarely complain of headache or facial pain. The location of pain may indicate which sinus is involved. Pain of maxillary sinusitis occurs over the sinuses and is sometimes perceived as a maxillary toothache. Frontal sinusitis produces a frontal headache that is worse on morning wakening. Ethmoid sinusitis causes pain that refers to the vertex, forehead, or occipital or temporal region, whereas the pain of sphenoid sinusitis is perceived on the top of the head.

Position Change

Maxillary sinusitis produces pain that worsens with bending or leaning forward. The postnasal discharge associated with sinusitis produces a cough that worsens while lying down.

Chronic Symptoms

In children chronic sinusitis is defined as the presence of symptoms for longer than 30 days. The cause can be prolonged obstruction of the osteomeatal complex, which leads to dysfunction of ciliary motility and movement of mucus within the sinuses. Local factors that cause mechanical obstruction include adenoid hypertrophy, conchae bullosa, nasal polyps, foreign bodies, and nasal deviations.

Do Associated Symptoms Provide Any Clues?

Key Questions

■ Do you have other acute symptoms such as cough, fever, or muscle aches?
■ Do you have other chronic symptoms, such as eye pain, bad breath, or fatigue?

Other Acute Symptoms

Acute bacterial infection of the nasal and sinus mucosa is characterized by the presence of purulent nasal discharge. Acute rhinitis caused by a bacterial or viral infection produces systemic symptoms such as fever, myalgia, and chills. Allergic rhinitis is associated with sneezing, nasal congestion, clear and profuse rhinorrhea, and pruritus of the nose, palate, pharynx, and middle ear. Eye complaints include conjunctival irritation, itching, erythema, and tearing. Ear complaints involve a feeling of fullness in the ears with popping. Sinus complaints are pressure and/or pain of the cheeks, forehead, or behind the eyes.

Acute sinusitis in children involves the presence of symptoms for less than 30 days, a persistent cough, fever with a temperature greater than 39° C (102.2° F) for more than 3 days, and malodorous breath. The maxillary and ethmoid sinuses are most commonly affected, with the frontal sinus occasionally and the sphenoid sinus rarely affected.

Chronic Symptoms

Chronic sinusitis involves long episodes of inflammation or repeated infections that lead to anatomical destruction. The recurrent symptoms interfere with daily activities and are not relieved with nonpharmacological measures or over-the-counter medications. Patients often complain about a cold that does not go away, eye pain, halitosis, chronic cough, fatigue, anorexia, malaise, and low-grade fever.

Is It Viral or Bacterial?

Key Questions

■ What color is your nasal drainage?
■ How long have you had these symptoms?

Acute rhinitis caused by a bacterial or viral infection produces yellow or green purulent nasal discharge. Watery or clear discharge occurs with allergic reactions. Symptoms of viral upper respiratory tract infections in children persist 5 to 10 days and then gradually subside. Many children may have up to eight colds per year.

Are Symptoms Unilateral or Bilateral?

Key Question

■ Is the symptom on one side or both sides? Infectious rhinitis and allergic rhinitis are usually bilateral. Unilateral symptoms are more indicative of an anatomical cause, such as nasal polyps, septal deviation, or a foreign body (typically occurs in children).

Are There Risk Factors That Will Narrow the Diagnosis?

Key Questions

■ Do you smoke?
■ Are you exposed to others who smoke?
■ Do you have any other health problems?
■ Have you had a recent history of head or facial trauma?
■ Have you been diving or swimming?
■ Have you been exposed to infections in day care, school, or work settings?
■ Are you pregnant?

Smoking History

Smokers have an increased risk of sinusitis. Smoking can lead to the production of more tenacious mucus and to temporary paralysis of the nasal cilia. Exposure to passive smoke causes an increased risk of upper and lower respiratory tract infections.

Trauma History

Nasal trauma or fracture may lead to nasal congestion. A rare but serious post-trauma cerebrospinal fluid rhinorrhea can be present. Up to 80% of head injuries involve the paranasal sinuses.

Diving and Swimming

Sinusitis from diving or swimming is secondary to barotrauma, infection from contaminated water, or an allergic response to chlorine.

Exposure

Exposure to viral infections increases when children are exposed to other children. The spread of a virus occurs via direct secretion of droplets or via contaminated wet objects.

Pregnancy

The hormonal changes of pregnancy can cause nasal congestion.

Is the Patient Using Any Drugs That Would Cause Nasal Congestion?

Key Questions

■ Are you using nasal sprays or drops?
■ Do you use cocaine or other drugs?
■ What other medications are you taking?

Nasal Spray

The use of topical sympathomimetic sprays or drops for more than 1 week can lead to rebound nasal congestion or vasodilation after short periods of vasoconstriction. The use of decongestants and antihistamines with low ambient humidity leads to excessive dryness and impaired ciliary function.

Drug Use

Chronic or acute cocaine use can also cause rebound nasal congestion. Nasal congestion associated with conjunctivitis and irritation of the eyes may be seen in persons who abuse drugs via inhalation.

Medications

Oral contraceptives, phenothiazines, angiotensin-converting enzyme (ACE) inhibitors, and β-blockers may cause nasal congestion.

Is There Systemic Disease Present?

Key Questions

■ Have you noticed any other general body symptoms?
■ Do you have any chronic health problems?

Systemic Disorders

Systemic causes of decreased mucociliary clearance include cystic fibrosis, ciliary dyskinesia syndrome, and immunoglobulin deficiency. Persons with congenital or acquired immune deficiencies, such as diabetes mellitus, leukemia, acquired immunodeficiency syndrome, and cystic fibrosis, have an increased risk of developing acute and chronic sinusitis. Hypothyroidism, acromegaly, Horner syndrome, neoplasm, and granulomatosis disorder can also cause nasal symptoms.

DIAGNOSTIC REASONING: FOCUSED PHYSICAL EXAMINATION

Perform a General Inspection

Note the patient's general appearance. Observe for signs of impaired mental status. A severe unremitting or new-onset headache, vomiting, or alteration in consciousness requires consideration for immediate referral.

Take Vital Signs

Persons with acute viral rhinitis or acute sinusitis may be afebrile or have a low-grade fever. Persons with allergic rhinitis are afebrile. The presence of mouth breathing suggests chronic nasal obstruction caused by hypertrophied pharyngeal lymphoid tissues.

Inspect the Face

Children with chronic allergic conditions have an allergic "salute"; this is a crease on the nose from continued wiping up of nasal drainage. Allergic "shiners" are dark circles under the eyes suggestive of venous congestion and stasis. Observe for facial symmetry and signs of periorbital edema. Periorbital cellulitis is the most common serious complication of severe bacterial sinusitis.

Perform a Regional Examination of the Head and Neck

Examine the eyes (including visual acuity), ears, and cervicofacial lymph nodes. Complications of severe fulminate sinusitis are rare and are caused by the direct spread of infection, secondary to destruction of the wall between the sinuses and the orbit. Symptoms can include a sudden increase in pain, acute edema of the eyelids, periorbital edema and erythema, decreased visual acuity, diplopia, and displacement of the eye laterally. The patient may experience pain on testing

of extraocular muscles. These symptoms mandate immediate referral.

Observe for symptoms of coryza (acute rhinitis) as well as ear and eye drainage. Erythematous tympanic membranes are seen in acute viral rhinitis.

Examine the Mouth and Teeth

Examine the teeth for the presence of abscesses, especially the first and secondary maxillary molars and the alveolar margin of the teeth. Tenderness elicited by tapping on the maxillary teeth with a tongue blade may indicate dental root infection or maxillary sinusitis. Mouth breathing is associated with hypertrophied gingival mucosa and halitosis. Halitosis can also be a sign of dental abscess or sinusitis.

Children with acute viral rhinitis have mild erythema of the tonsils and posterior pharynx. If there is vasomotor rhinitis, mucus is present in the posterior pharynx.

Test for Smell

Severe nasal congestion or ethmoid sinusitis causes anosmia.

Inspect Condition of Nasal Mucosa and Turbinates

Use a nasal speculum and head mirror to optimally visualize the condition of the nasal mucosa and turbinates. A topical vasoconstrictive agent may be needed to shrink the swollen mucosa to visualize the middle meatus.

In infants and young children, the nares tend to open forward, and tilting the tip of the nose up with the thumb and directing the light into the nares will allow inspection of the nasal cavities.

Pale, boggy turbinates are seen with allergic rhinitis. Inflamed mucous membranes are seen with acute coryza or hay fever. Allergic rhinitis may also produce a violet-colored mucous membrane. Ulceration of the nasal mucosa may be found in persons who abuse drugs by inhalation.

Inspect for Masses

Observe for the presence of nasal polyps, which look like skinned grapes and are usually bilateral and hang from the middle turbinate into the lumen of the nose. Septal deviation or anatomical anomalies may predispose to infection. Nasal septum deviation can also lead to nasal obstruction. Squamous cell carcinoma usually occurs unilaterally. Masses that increase in size and pulsate on Valsalva maneuver may indicate an encephalocele or a meningocele.

Note the Presence and Color of Any Discharge

Pus in the ostium of the middle turbinate suggests a bacterial sinusitis. Cerebrospinal fluid (CSF) drainage will increase in a forward position. Identify CSF by testing nasal drainage for glucose and protein levels comparable to those of CSF. Foul-smelling nasal discharge is a characteristic feature of sinusitis of dental origin. Foul-smelling unilateral purulent discharge may indicate a foreign body in the nasal cavity.

Transilluminate the Sinuses

Light will pass through air-filled sinuses. Transillumination is used to assess the presence of fluid in the frontal and maxillary sinuses and cannot be used to examine the ethmoid or sphenoid sinuses. Normal transillumination of the frontal sinus rules out frontal sinusitis in 90% of cases. Complete opacity of sinuses suggests infection. However, the results of transillumination are often nonspecific, such as reduced illumination, and do not lead to a diagnosis.

Transillumination of maxillary sinuses can be done in two ways. Place a transilluminator over the infraorbital rim, blocking light from the examiner's vision with the free hand, and judge the amount of light transmission (opaque, dull, normal) through the hard palate. This should be performed in a completely darkened room. Dentures must be removed. A second method is to place the transilluminator in the patient's mouth, sealing the lips, and observe the amount of light transmitted through the maxillary sinuses. Frontal sinuses can be transilluminated by placing the instrument below the supraorbital rim.

Palpate and Percuss Frontal and Maxillary Sinuses for Tenderness

Percuss and palpate the cheeks for tenderness and swelling, indicating maxillary sinusitis of dental origin. To assess the frontal sinuses, exert pressure over the eyebrow or slightly upward pressure under the brow to assess for tenderness. Direct percussion may elicit tenderness over the affected sinus.

Test for Facial Fullness and Pressure

Bending forward from the waist (with head dropping downward) or performing a Valsalva maneuver will worsen the symptoms if a partial or complete sinus obstruction is present.

Examine the Lungs

Auscultate the lungs for signs of wheezing, rales, and loudness of breath sounds. Peak flow volume or PO_2 saturation as measured using a pulse oximeter will detect the presence of reactive upper airway disease.

Perform Neurological Testing if Indicated

To detect any complications from sinusitis, assess neurological and cranial nerve function if the patient appears severely ill. Severe complications of sinusitis are cavernous sinus thrombosis and brain abscesses.

LABORATORY AND DIAGNOSTIC STUDIES

Nasal Smear

A nasal smear performed to look for eosinophils confirms the diagnosis of allergic rhinitis. Nasal scraping of the surface epithelium along with a sample of secretions is more reliable in detecting the presence of eosinophils than is the sampling of secretions alone. Either method can be used to detect the presence of neutrophils. Specimens are graded using a semiquantitative scale of 0 to 4+, based on the concentration of cells. Table 4-1 illustrates the diagnostic classifications found with varying nasal smears.

Table 4-1	Diagnostic Classifications of Nasal Smear Specimens
NASAL SMEAR	**DIAGNOSTIC CLASSIFICATION**
Increased eosinophils	Allergic or nonallergic eosinophilia; aspirin intolerance
Increased basophils	Same as above; nonallergic basophilia
Increased neutrophils	
With intracellular bacteria	Nasopharyngitis; sinusitis
With ciliary tophthoria	Viral upper respiratory tract infection (URI)
With fungi	Fungal URI
With no bacteria	Irritant reaction
Bacteria (2-4+)—intracellular	Nasopharyngitis or sinusitis
No eosinophils or basophils, 2+ or fewer neutrophils, few bacteria	Normal finding

From Mygind N, Naderio R: *Allergic and non-allergic rhinitis,* Copenhagen, Denmark, 1993, Munksgaard International Publishers.

Sinus Radiographs

Radiographs are not routinely indicated but may be obtained in patients who have severe symptoms, fail to respond to treatment, or have chronic and recurrent sinusitis. Severe symptoms may indicate complications of sinusitis, such as orbital cellulitis, brain abscess, osteomyelitis, or cavernous sinus thrombosis. A sinus radiographic series consists of four views: an anteroposterior (Caldwell) view of the ethmoid sinus, a view (Chamberlain) of the frontal sinus, a lateral view of the sphenoid and frontal sinuses, and an occipitomental (Waters) view of the maxillary sinuses.

Computed Tomography Scan

A computed tomography (CT) scan shows air, bone, and soft tissue and optimally facilitates definition of regional anatomy and the extent of disease. A CT scan is done when sinusitis becomes chronic and does not respond to symptomatic or antibiotic treatment. A CT scan may also show causes for chronic sinusitis by visualizing many disorders not detected by plain films, such as facial fractures, nasal polyps, cysts, chronic mucosal thickening, temporomandibular joint (TMJ) disorders, foreign bodies, and tumors.

Magnetic Resonance Imaging

Magnetic resonance imaging (MRI) is an excellent technique for imaging soft tissue pathology of the face and neck, especially neoplastic conditions. CT does not delineate soft tissue pathology as well as MRI.

Sinus Aspiration

Sinus aspiration is the only way to confirm the diagnosis of bacterial sinusitis and is performed by an otolaryngologist. A trocar is introduced into the maxillary sinus through the upper gingival recess.

Allergy Skin Testing

Results of skin testing can confirm immunological disease and identify specific antigens responsible for allergic rhinitis, which may come from exposure to irritants in the patient's environment. The presence of serum IgE antibody suggests an allergic response.

DIFFERENTIAL DIAGNOSIS

Infectious Rhinitis

Infectious rhinitis is an acute condition frequently associated with a history of recent upper respiratory tract infection. A definitive sign of this condition is the presence of yellow or green purulent discharge and red nasal mucosa.

Allergic Rhinitis

Allergic rhinitis is distinguished by a recurrent rhinorrhea with clear watery mucus, sneezing, and pruritus. Nasal turbinates are pale and swollen. Family history of allergies is often positive. About 25% of the population has some type of allergy. IgE-mediated reactions to aeroallergens are based on a combination of history, physical examination, and skin tests. Nasal smears can be tested for the presence of eosinophils to confirm an allergenic response.

Seasonal allergies are associated with short bursts of intense exposure to an allergen that creates symptoms consistent with a histamine-mediated response, such as pruritus, swelling, sneezing, and rhinorrhea. A common seasonal allergy is pollenosis or hay fever. A history or pattern of symptoms and exposure is critical in diagnosis.

Perennial allergies are caused by continuous exposure to allergens associated with chronic congestion. Common indoor allergens are animal dander, dust mites, and cockroaches. Outdoor allergens include grasses, trees, pollens, and weeds.

Nonallergic Rhinitis

Nonallergic rhinitis can be associated or not associated with eosinophilia on nasal smear. Nonallergic rhinitis with eosinophilia syndrome (NARES) is a diagnosis based on nasal cytology and involves symptoms similar to allergic rhinitis without an identifiable allergen cause. A history will reveal aspirin or nonsteroidal anti-inflammatory drug intolerance and rhinorrhea. Noneosinophilia is associated with any other nonallergic cause of rhinitis.

Rhinitis Medicamentosa

Drug-induced rebound congestion can follow the long-term use of topical nasal decongestants. Rhinitis medicamentosa is also used to describe nasal symptoms secondary to other medications, such as nasal congestion associated with hormone changes of pregnancy. Other drugs that have vasodilatory effects include antihypertensives that interfere with adrenergic neuronal function and hormones in oral contraceptives. Nasal vasoconstriction response is completely abolished after the administration of reserpine.

Acute Sinusitis

Acute sinusitis is characterized by purulent nasal discharge, postnasal drip, and localized facial pain over the sinus involved. It often follows a viral upper respiratory tract infection. However, symptoms such as halitosis, reduced sense of smell, or morning cough have been reported in children in the absence of facial pain. Physical examination will elicit localized tenderness to palpation or percussion over the affected sinus. Pressure and pain will increase in a forward-bending position. Purulent discharge may be visible in the posterior pharynx or may be seen emerging from the ostia of the middle turbinate. Transillumination will indicate unilateral or bilateral obstruction. Ciliary function is impaired with infection and may not be completely restored for 2 to 6 weeks. The diagnosis of sinusitis in children requires two of three major criteria (cough, purulent nasal discharge, or purulent pharyngeal drainage) or one major and two minor criteria (sore throat, wheezing, foul breath, facial pain, periorbital edema, headache, earache, fever, and toothache).

Chronic Sinusitis

An incompletely treated acute sinusitis can lead to a chronic condition. The patient presents with persistent symptoms of low-grade infection and intermittent acute exacerbations typical of acute sinusitis. Symptoms are recurrent and not controlled with over-the-counter or nonpharmacological remedies. Multiple pathogens may be causative organisms, with the most common being *Moraxella catarrhalis, H. influenzae,* and *S. pneumoniae.* Sinus radiographs or CT scan will reveal mucosal thickening of 5 mm or greater. Allergy testing may reveal a perennial allergy that creates chronic inflammation.

Nasal or Sinus Obstruction

A history of aspirin intolerance or asthma with polyps is associated with obstruction. Acute obstruction suggests edema secondary to infection, allergic response, exposure to irritants, or foreign body (in children). Chronic obstruction may be secondary to congenital deformity, nasal polyps, or septal deviation. In infants, congenital choanal atresia can cause obstruction.

Nasal Polyposis

This syndrome has multiple causative factors, including a history of asthma and aspirin intolerance. The polyps are translucent grape-like growths that are mobile, rarely bleed, and prolapse into the nasal cavity. The resulting obstruction can be associated with chronic sinusitis. Any suspicious polyps should undergo a biopsy.

Osteomyelitis of the Frontal Bone

Osteomyelitis can occur as a complication of sinusitis. Osteomyelitis occurs in children and young adults and may follow head trauma or scuba diving. *Staphylococcus pyogenes* or anaerobic streptococci are causative organisms. Patients appear severely ill and may have edema of the upper eyelid and puffy swelling over the frontal bone. Diagnosis is by radiography and blood culture.

DIFFERENTIAL DIAGNOSIS OF *Common Causes of Nasal Symptoms and Sinus Congestion*

CONDITION	HISTORY	PHYSICAL FINDINGS	DIAGNOSTIC STUDIES
Infectious rhinitis	Perennial but more common in winter months; recent URI	Red, swollen mucosa; purulent discharge	Nasal smear for neutrophils, intracellular bacteria
Allergic rhinitis	Family history of allergies; sneezing; recurrent pattern; more common in children and young adults	Pale, boggy mucosa; rhinorrhea with clear, watery mucus	Nasal smear for eosinophils; allergy testing
Nonallergic rhinitis	No allergenic cause identified	Similar to allergic rhinitis	Absence of eosinophilia on nasal cytology
Rhinitis medicamentosa	History of medication use: oral contraceptives, nasal sprays, antihypertensives; nasal congestion	Swollen mucosa; clear mucus or dry mucosa	None
Acute sinusitis	Smoker; recent URI; winter months; frontal headaches made worse with forward bending; sensation of fullness or pressure	Purulent discharge; maxillary toothache on percussion, postnasal drainage; decreased transillumination	None
Chronic sinusitis	History of previous sinus infections; dull ache or no pain; persistent symptoms	Same as above; decreased or no transillumination; obstruction such as deviated septum, polyps	Sinus radiographs; CT scan; sinus aspiration and culture
Obstruction	History of asthma, aspirin intolerance; foreign body in children; tumor in adults; infants with choanal atresia: difficulty feeding; cyanosis if bilateral	Increased pain with forward motion or Valsalva; pain with percussion and palpation of sinuses; no transillumination; septal deviation	Sinus radiographs; CT scan
Nasal polyposis	History of asthma, aspirin intolerance	Presence of polyps	May require biopsy
Osteomyelitis of frontal bone	History of head trauma, diving	Appears severely ill; periorbital and frontal edema	Sinus and skull radiographs; blood culture

URI, Upper respiratory tract infection; *CT,* computed tomography.

CHAPTER RESOURCES

Gendo K, Larson EB: Evidence-based diagnostic strategies for evaluating suspected allergic rhinitis, *Ann Intern Med* 140:4, 2004.

Leung A, Kellner J: Acute sinusitis in children: diagnosis and management, *J Pediatr Health Care* 18:72, 2004.

Nash D: Sinusitis, *Pediatr Rev* 22:111, 2001.

Novelline RA: *Squire's fundamentals of radiology,* ed 6, Cambridge, Mass, 2004, Harvard University Press.

Seller RH: *Differential diagnosis of common complaints,* ed 4, Philadelphia, 2000, Saunders.

Skoner DP: Allergic rhinitis: definition, epidemiology, pathophysiology, detection and diagnosis, *J Allergy Clin Immunol* 108(1 suppl):S2, 2001.

Zacharisen M: Pediatric sinusitis, *Immunol Allergy Clin North Am* 25:313, 2005.

Hoarseness

Hoarseness is a disturbance of the normal voice pitch by processes that affect the structure or function of the vocal cords. It is a term used to describe an unnaturally rough, harsh, or deep voice. Voice is the sound produced when the vocal folds are approximated and expired airflow between the cords causes them to vibrate. The sound produced by the larynx is amplified by the pharynx, oral cavity, sinuses, and nasal cavity and is modified by movements of the tongue, uvula, and soft palate. Hoarseness may be an early sign of local disease or a manifestation of a systemic illness. Hoarseness is a cardinal symptom for laryngeal disease.

The larynx is a musculocartilaginous structure lined with a mucous membrane connected to the superior part of the trachea and to the pharynx inferior to the tongue and hyoid bone. It is the sphincter that guards the entrance into the trachea and functions secondarily as the organ of voice. Nine cartilages connected by ligaments and eight muscles form the larynx. The lower portion of the thyroarytenoid muscle forms the true vocal fold, or folds, which are highly elastic and account for the extraordinary versatility of the voice and the wide range of pitch, volume, and quality. The glottis is the triangular opening between the true vocal cords. The supraglottic area includes the ventricular folds (false vocal cords), aryepiglottic folds, and the epiglottis (Figure 5-1). The epiglottis is the lidlike cartilaginous structure that overhangs the entrance to the larynx and serves to prevent food from entering the larynx and trachea while swallowing.

Many benign conditions cause hoarseness, such as functional disorders from voice overuse. Functional causes are unrelated to organic disease and may have a psychosocial component, such as restraint in expressing anger, or crying, or a history of psychological trauma.

However, persistent hoarseness for more than 3 weeks in an adult and 1 week in a child may indicate secondary changes to the vocal cords. These changes may be caused by structural changes resulting from palsies, polyps, or cysts; laryngeal neoplasm; or congenital disorders of the larynx. Hoarseness may also be a symptom of systemic disease, such as hypothyroidism, or a symptom of inflammation caused by a variety of processes. Many forms of laryngitis that appear alike on physical examination may have very different causes; critical clues to the specific etiology for laryngitis depend on a careful history.

DIAGNOSTIC REASONING: FOCUSED HISTORY

Is the Hoarseness Acute or Chronic?

Key Questions
- How long has the symptom been present?
- Has this happened before? Is it recurrent?
- Is it getting worse?

Duration
Symptoms of less than 3 weeks' duration are considered to be acute; the most likely cause is a viral upper respiratory tract infection. Inflammations secondary to acute viral infection or voice overuse are the most common causes of acute laryngitis. Chronic symptoms suggest structural change in the larynx or hoarseness secondary to disorders such as gastroesophageal reflux disease (GERD) or systemic disease. If the duration

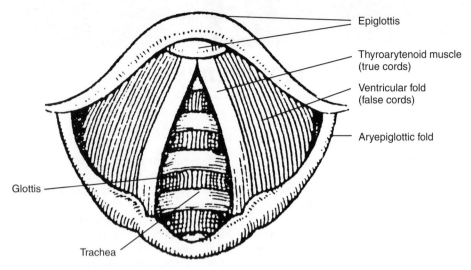

Epiglottis

Thyroarytenoid muscle
(true cords)

Ventricular fold
(false cords)

Aryepiglottic fold

Glottis

Trachea

FIGURE 5-1 Laryngoscopic view of the interior of the larynx. (Modified from Greene MCL, Mathieson L: *The voice and its disorders*, ed 5, London, 1989, Whurr Publishers.)

of hoarseness is longer than 3 weeks, referral to an ear, nose, and throat specialist is indicated to evaluate for neoplasm, most often squamous cell carcinoma, because chronic laryngitis is rarely of an infectious etiology.

Recurrence
Recurrent episodes of hoarseness may indicate allergies or sinusitis with postnasal drip.

Progression
Progressive hoarseness usually indicates a lesion such as a laryngeal or hypopharyngeal cyst.

What Does the Onset of Hoarseness Tell Me?

Key Questions
- How did the hoarseness develop?
- Is there any history of trauma to the throat?
- Have you had any recent surgery around the throat or neck?

Onset
An acute onset of hoarseness is usually the result of infection or trauma. The trauma can be from direct injury (foreign body,

accidents) or overuse from screaming. The overuse can be gradual, resulting in progressive hoarseness and vocal cord changes. This hoarseness is worse in the afternoon or evening.

Hoarseness from birth may indicate a congenital problem, such as laryngeal web, cyst, palsy, or angioma. Newborns with aphonia or a hoarse cry that does not resolve may have a congenital anomaly, papilloma, or vocal cord paralysis.

Trauma
External trauma to the throat is a rare cause of hoarseness but can result in hematoma formation in the laryngeal soft tissues. There can also be mucosal lacerations, arytenoid cartilage dislocation, or fracture of the laryngeal cartilage. Internal trauma can occur with intubation associated with surgery, as occurs when an endotracheal tube catches on laryngeal structures and is pushed against resistance.

Surgical History
Tonsillectomy, thyroidectomy, or rhinoplasty can alter the quality of the voice secondary to structural change and scarring. Cardiac surgery has also been cited as a

cause of injury when the vagus nerve (cranial nerve [CN] X) is damaged in its course around the aorta.

Does the Presence of Risk Factors Help Narrow the Diagnosis?

Key Questions

- Have you had a recent cold or upper respiratory tract infection?
- Do you have allergies or asthma?
- Do you smoke? How long have you been a smoker?
- How much alcohol do you drink?
- Describe your voice habits, such as singing, talking, and shouting.
- Are you frequently exposed to dust, fumes, or loud noise?
- Are your immunizations up to date?

Upper Respiratory Tract Infection

Acute laryngitis, epiglottitis, and acute laryngotracheobronchitis (croup) are sequelae from a viral upper respiratory tract infection (URI) that can result in vocal cord inflammation. Postnasal discharge that is thick and purulent may pool around the larynx and cause chronic secondary edema. Nasal congestion that leads to mouth breathing produces laryngeal dryness, with resultant hoarseness on arising in the morning.

Children who have epiglottitis are not hoarse, but, as the epiglottis swells, the voice becomes muffled and drooling is observed.

Allergies and Asthma

Poorly controlled or undiagnosed asthma can result in a chronic cough with subsequent hoarseness. Allergies can cause chronic or recurrent irritation and swelling of both the upper and lower airways. Children who have a history of allergies can develop vocal cord edema and inflammation and hoarseness.

Smoking

Cigarette smoking is the most significant risk factor for laryngeal cancer. Smoking is also a risk factor for acute or chronic laryngitis because smoke irritates all mucous membranes and impairs ciliary function, causing pooling of secretions around the larynx.

Alcohol Consumption

Chronic consumption of hard liquor is a direct irritant to the throat and is associated with laryngeal cancer.

Voice Habits

Voice misuse occurs when the true vocal cords are forced to vibrate under undue stress and tension. Voice abuse is exuberant overuse and can lead to inflammation of the larynx and edema, hemorrhage, or vocal cord polyps. A gradual progression of hoarseness may go unnoticed by the patient. Often a precipitating incident (such as shouting, excessive speaking, or singing) produces acute laryngitis. Specific questions may need to be asked to make the patient aware of conditions that lead to voice abuse, such as the following:

- Have others noticed a change in the quality of your voice?
- Do you talk frequently to persons who are hard of hearing?
- Do you yell at children?
- Do you work in an environment that is noisy or contains dust or fumes?
- Have you attended a recent sporting event?

Exposures

Patients who are chronically exposed to work environments that contain dust, fumes, or a high noise level that leads to chronic voice abuse are at increased risk for laryngeal cancer.

Immunizations

Laryngeal diphtheria should be considered in patients who have failed to update their diphtheria immunization. Updating the tetanus-diphtheria (Td) immunization is recommended every 10 years after the primary immunization series is completed. Laryngeal diphtheria usually develops as a downward progression of the tonsillar-pharyngeal membrane.

What Other Clues Will Help Narrow the Diagnostic Possibilities?

Key Questions

- Does the hoarseness change during the day?
- Is it painful?

■ What other symptoms are present?

■ Do you have a neurological disorder?

Timing

Hoarseness that is altered by a position change suggests a mobile lesion such as a pedunculated polyp. Patients with myasthenia gravis have a normal voice in the morning with progressive hoarseness throughout the day.

Pain

Pain may be associated with an inflammatory process, such as a viral URI or GERD. Pain occurs late in laryngeal cancer. Neurological and hormonal causes do not usually produce pain.

Associated Symptoms

The presence of cough, shortness of breath, weight loss, dysphagia, ear pain, or throat pain should raise concerns about neoplasm, systemic disease, or neurological causes. Hormonal disorders, such as hypothyroidism, will also produce signs and symptoms that vary in severity, according to the duration and degree of hormone deficiency. Early symptoms of hypothyroidism include cold intolerance, heavy menses, weight gain, dry skin, fatigue, and constipation. Later signs and symptoms include hoarseness, very dry skin, hair loss of lateral eyebrows, and neurological symptoms such as delayed deep tendon reflex recovery, depression, and mental confusion.

Neurological Disease

Patients with Parkinson's disease, myasthenia gravis, or amyotrophic lateral sclerosis have progressive dysarthria and dysphagia.

As neurological disease progresses, patients will develop a chronic cough and throat clearing caused by microaspiration of pooled secretions.

Gastroesophageal Reflux Disease

Reflux of gastric contents causes inflammation of the posterior larynx, especially the arytenoid mucosa. The patient may also report a habit of frequent throat clearing and a sensation of a lump in the throat. Chronic cough or throat clearing further damages already irritated vocal folds. In children, GERD presents with dysphagia, vomiting, and failure to thrive.

DIAGNOSTIC REASONING: FOCUSED PHYSICAL EXAMINATION

Listen to the Quality of Voice

Acoustic evaluation criteria for voice include range (monotonic to extremely variable), loudness (soft to loud), pitch (low-pitched voice requires more effort to produce adequate volume; also sudden changes in pitch), register (temporary loss of voice because of abductor spasm), and quality (roughness, breathiness, and hoarseness). Table 5-1 lists common criteria used in evaluating the voice.

Examine the Respiratory System

If the patient is able to cough and laugh but cannot speak, this indicates a functional problem, because coughing and laughing require total adduction of the vocal cords. Auscultate the lungs for quality of breath sounds, asthmatic wheezing, and signs of consolidation.

Table 5-1	**Diagnostics Used in Evaluating Voice**	
ACOUSTIC QUALITY	**MEASUREMENT**	**DISORDER**
Range	Monotonal to extremely variable	Monotonal: Parkinson's disease, depression
Loudness	Soft to loud	Environmental, psychological, systemic disease
Pitch	Low to high; glottal, raspy to falsetto	Variable: puberty
		Low: male gender, overuse
Register	Presence of voice	Vocal fatigue, overuse
Quality	Breathy to resonant	Vocal cord mass, paresis, bowing, atrophy

Perform a General Inspection

Note hair distribution, especially signs of hair loss over lateral eyebrows and hair loss on scalp, to assess thyroid function. Look for the placement of the trachea and thyroid gland. Bulges or asymmetry of the neck suggest a tumor. A head and neck hemangioma or lymphangioma increases the possibility of a similar laryngeal lesion as the source of hoarseness.

Examine the Head and Neck

Examine the oral, pharyngeal, and nasal mucosa for signs of excessive dryness, inflammation, or infection. Excessive mucosal dryness, including the conjunctiva, may be secondary to medication use, such as decongestants and antidepressants, or may be a symptom of an autoimmune disorder such as Sjögren's syndrome.

Otoscopy may indicate otitis media with effusion, contributing to hearing loss, a factor to be considered in voice abuse. Inspect the nasal mucosa for color, edema, and purulent discharge, and examine the nasal septa for deviation that may cause obstruction. Hypertrophic tonsils and severe dental abnormalities (malocclusion, cleft palate) can contribute to hoarseness.

Any indication of airway obstruction associated with hoarseness is a potentially life-threatening situation. Do not perform a physical examination of the pharynx if you suspect acute epiglottitis. Examination may trigger laryngospasms and airway obstruction. Refer immediately for emergency treatment and airway support.

Examine the larynx indirectly using a laryngeal mirror. Patient cooperation is critical. Ask the patient to open the mouth wide and extend the neck while protruding the tongue. The mirror is advanced to contact and lift the uvula while the patient breathes through the mouth. Focus the light on the mirror after the mirror is angled to visualize the larynx. Ask the patient to say "e" or "a" to observe movement. Sometimes the epiglottis obscures visualization. Direct examination of the larynx with a laryngoscope requires the skill and experience of a specialist.

Observe the larynx for the presence of secretions and evidence of ulcers, polyps, masses, edema, or redness. Observe for vocal cord motion, especially adduction and abduction of vocal cords, and the presence of spasm or tremor.

Assess Cranial Nerve Function

Most of the CNs play a part in speech and voice production, and any disease process that affects neurological function, especially vocal cord paralysis, may affect the voice. Specifically examine CNs V, VII, VIII, IX, X, XI, and XII.

Assess Hearing (Cranial Nerve VIII)

Voice or whisper testing for hearing acuity is the first level of hearing screening. An audible whisper is approximately 20 decibels (dB), and normal speech is about 50 dB. Patients with neurosensory hearing loss may use abnormally loud speech.

Palpate Lymph Nodes

Palpate the cervicofacial lymph nodes. Tender nodes indicate inflammation; nontender nodes may indicate neoplasm. Enlarged nodes in the deep cervical chain in the absence of other symptoms may indicate laryngeal cancer.

Palpate Thyroid

Palpate the thyroid for size, tenderness, and crepitus by moving the thyroid cartilage across the cervical spine.

LABORATORY AND DIAGNOSTIC STUDIES

Flexible Fiberoptic Laryngoscopy

Laryngoscopy allows direct examination of the hypopharynx and larynx. A local anesthetic is applied to the oral or nasal mucosa, and the instrument is passed through the nose or oral cavity for excellent visualization of laryngeal structures. Laryngoscopy is also performed using a general anesthetic.

Radiography

Lateral view radiographs of soft tissues of the neck are used to evaluate structures for abnormalities.

Barium Esophagography

This contrast radiographic technique can be used to differentiate between mechanical lesions and motility disorders, providing important information about the latter in particular. For patients with esophageal dysphagia and a suspected motility disorder, barium esophagoscopy should be performed first.

DIFFERENTIAL DIAGNOSIS

Acute Laryngitis

Acute laryngitis is a self-limiting condition caused by a viral infection, environmental irritants, postnasal drainage secondary to poorly controlled allergic rhinitis, or voice overuse. The loudness and quality of voice are affected, and the patient may complain of a sore throat. Hoarseness often progresses throughout the course of the day. Indirect examination of the larynx reveals redness and edema of the vocal cords. Physical pathology may be absent in mild cases.

Acute Epiglottitis

Adults will complain of severe and rapidly progressing symptoms of sore throat, dyspnea, and hoarseness. In children, there is no cough or hoarseness, and drooling with a forward leaning posture is observed. This condition is most commonly associated with *Haemophilus influenzae* infection. Voice quality is froglike. The patient will also have a high temperature and be anxious, fearful, and restless with respiratory distress.

Trauma

Any swelling in response to trauma, directly to the larynx or indirectly to the throat, will cause hoarseness. Swelling might be secondary to head and neck surgery, such as dental surgery, tonsillectomy, or thyroidectomy. Postintubation trauma may be acute if secondary to inflammation or chronic if neurological or structural damage is irreversible. Mucosal abrasion or ulcer may be caused by direct trauma to the larynx and is associated with painful phonation and a breathy voice.

Acute Laryngeal Edema

Laryngeal edema may be one symptom in a generalized allergic response that involves the lips, tongue, and other hypopharyngeal structures. Drug reactions and food allergies, especially to seafood and nuts, often precipitate this response. This condition is a medical emergency because of the high risk of airway obstruction.

Laryngotracheobronchitis (Croup)

Subglottic edema is caused by a viral infection, most often parainfluenza 1 virus that can obstruct the airway. This condition is most common in children ages 3 months to 3 years of age and is more prevalent in the fall and winter. It is associated with a barking cough, dyspnea, wheezing, low-grade fever, and hoarseness. Inspiratory stridor occurs abruptly because of narrowing of the passage, causing negative pressures generated on inspiration. Physical examination can determine the degree of respiratory distress, such as color, stridor, nasal flaring, and level of consciousness.

Chronic Laryngitis

This condition is associated with a combination of chronic exposure to working conditions with high levels of dust, fumes, or noise; hard liquor consumption; cigarette smoking; and a history of frequent and persistent cough. Physical examination reveals edema or nodules of the vocal cords.

Polyps

Vocal cord polyps develop as a result of chronic inflammation from voice abuse, allergies, or GERD. The voice quality is breathy. With dependent polyps, the patient may report that symptoms of hoarseness change with position.

Neoplasm

Laryngeal cancer usually occurs in patients who have a long history of cigarette smoking and alcohol consumption. Hoarseness is characterized by a raspy or harsh voice. Physical examination may reveal leukoplakia, or a white scaly appearance of the vocal cords. Patients do not usually complain of pain until carcinoma is advanced. Pain secondary to ulceration is late and is often perceived as ear pain, especially when swallowing.

Gastroesophageal Reflux Disease

Patients with GERD will complain of retrosternal burning (heartburn) that radiates upward. The regurgitation of gastric acid is exacerbated by consuming large meals, lying in a supine position, or bending over. Patients may describe a sour taste, experience salivary hypersecretion, have painful swallowing, or have a chronic cough or habit of throat clearing. Physical examination will be normal or epigastric tenderness may be elicited by abdominal examination. Inflammation or ulceration may be visible on the vocal cords.

Hypothyroidism

One symptom of hypothyroidism is a low, gravelly voice. The degree of hoarseness depends on the severity of thyroid deficiency. Usually the diagnosis of hypothyroidism is suspected when other symptoms are present, such as cold intolerance; rough, scaly skin texture; weight gain; and signs such as bradycardia and prolonged deep tendon reflex recovery. Risk factors for hypothyroidism include increased age, postpartum in women, and a family history of thyroid disease. The thyroid gland may be nonpalpable or enlarged. Examination of the larynx may reveal edema or polyps. An elevated serum thyroid-stimulating hormone (TSH) level will confirm the diagnosis.

Vocal Cord Paralysis

Paralysis is usually unilateral and produces a weak, breathy voice. A unilateral abductor paralysis on the left side is caused by pressure on the vagus or recurrent laryngeal nerve by a mass of malignant glands in the superior mediastinum or carcinoma of the thyroid or esophagus.

Psychogenic Hoarseness

Patients with psychogenic hoarseness will have a low, breathy voice caused by voluntarily abducting the vocal cords during phonation. Physical examination will be normal. Psychogenic hoarseness may follow a traumatic event.

Laryngeal Papillomas

These are the most common laryngeal lesions that occur during childhood. Most patients are between the ages of 2 and 7 and present with hoarseness. Occasionally papillomas, caused by the human papillomavirus, are seen in newborns.

DIFFERENTIAL DIAGNOSIS OF *Common Causes of Hoarseness*

CONDITION	HISTORY	PHYSICAL FINDINGS	DIAGNOSTIC STUDIES
Acute laryngitis	Voice overuse, exposure to environmental irritants, recent URI	Voice quality: aphonia, cervical lymphadenopathy; pharyngitis; edema and redness of vocal cords	None, if duration of hoarseness is <3 wk
Acute epiglottitis	Adults: rapid onset of sore throat, dyspnea, hoarseness; child: drooling, forward-leaning posture	Voice quality froglike; fever, signs of respiratory distress; drooling	Possible airway support; lateral and AP radiographic views of neck
Trauma	Hoarseness after intubation; direct throat trauma or foreign body	Subluxation of cricoarytenoid joint	Lateral and AP radiographic views of neck; laryngoscopy
Acute laryngeal edema	History of food or drug allergy	Edema of lips, tongue, and hypopharynx; observe for respiratory distress; voice quality breathy	Possible airway support

Continued

DIFFERENTIAL DIAGNOSIS OF *Common Causes of Hoarseness—cont'd*

CONDITION	HISTORY	PHYSICAL FINDINGS	DIAGNOSTIC STUDIES
Laryngotracheobronchitis (croup)	Children 3 mo to 3 yr; recent URI	Barking cough, low-grade fever, wheezing, hoarseness; edema of vocal cords; observe for signs of respiratory distress	None initially, airway support may be necessary
Chronic laryngitis	Chronic history of smoking and alcohol use; exposure to environmental irritants; chronic cough; duration of hoarseness >3 wk	Edema of vocal cords; nodules may be present	Lateral and AP radiographic views of neck; laryngoscopy
Polyps	History of allergy; voice abuse, GERD, smoker; duration of symptoms >3 wk; progressive hoarseness, worse at end of day, but near normal in morning; hoarseness may change with position	Polyps visible on vocal cords	ENT referral for biopsy
Neoplasm	Smoking, airborne exposure, chronic alcohol use, history of chronic cough, hoarseness for >3 wk	Tracheal deviation; pain with advanced tumor; hoarseness may be only sign	ENT referral for biopsy
GERD	History of upper GI burning and cough especially at night; chronic use of alcohol, NSAIDs, or aspirin; history of ulcer disease, smoker, age <45 yr; frequent throat clearing	May have epigastric tenderness on palpation; vocal cord inflammation or ulcers	Referral for endoscopy if symptoms not relieved with medication or dietary alterations
Hypothyroidism	Presence of systemic symptoms such as cold intolerance, weight gain, fatigue; age >65 yr; postpartal women; family history of thyroid disease	Normal or enlarged thyroid gland, coarse hair, very dry skin, prolonged DTR recovery	TSH, free T_4 index
Vocal cord paralysis	Chronic cough; inspiratory or expiratory stridor with exertion	Breathy, weak, soft voice; abnormal movement (usually unilateral) of vocal cords; examination may suggest specific CN involvement	Refer for ENT evaluation
Psychogenic hoarseness	History of psychiatric illness or psychological trauma	Breathy, low voice; larynx will appear normal	As indicated to rule out other causes (i.e., lateral and AP radiographic views of neck); laryngoscopy
Laryngeal papillomas	Children 2-12 yr and may occur in infants; history of maternal human papillomavirus; may be recurrent, progressive	Faint cry, severe stridor, voice change, or complete aphonia	Refer for ENT evaluation

URI, Upper respiratory tract infection; *AP,* anteroposterior; *GERD,* gastroesophageal reflux disease; *GI,* gastrointestinal; *ENT,* ear, nose, and throat; *NSAIDs,* nonsteroidal anti-inflammatory drugs; *DTR,* deep tendon reflex; *TSH,* thyroid-stimulating hormone; T_4, thyroxine; *CN,* cranial nerve.

CHAPTER RESOURCES

Banfield G, Tandon P, Solomons N: Hoarse voice: an early symptom of many conditions, *Practitioner* 244:267, 2000.

Dejmclere PH: Voice problems in children: pathogenesis and diagnosis, *Int J Pediatr Otorhinolaryngol* 49(suppl):S311, 1999.

Garrett CG et al: Hoarseness, *Med Clin North Am* 83:115, 1999.

Hartnick CJ: Congenital laryngeal anomalies: laryngeal atresia, stenosis, webs, and clefts, *Otolaryngol Clin North Am* 33:1293, 2000.

Malhotra A: Viral croup, *Pediatr Rev* 22:5, 2001.

McMurray JS: Medical and surgical treatment of pediatric dysphonia, *Otolaryngol Clin North Am* 33:1111, 2000.

Wiatrak BJ: Congenital anomalies of the larynx and trachea, *Otolaryngol Clin North Am* 33:91, 2000.

Red Eye

The term red eye is used to denote a myriad of ocular entities. The anatomical location in and around the eye and the probable cause of the eye disorder provide an important framework to use in assessment. General anatomical locations are the ocular adnexa, conjunctiva, cornea and anterior segment, and posterior eye (Figure 6-1).

The eye has two major defense mechanisms. The first is tears, which contain immunoglobulin A and lysozymes that provide an important washing action. The second defense mechanism is a conjunctival immune system of lymphocytes, plasma cells, and neutrophils. Inoculation of the eye with virulent organisms or trauma disrupts these normal defense mechanisms, leading to a red eye.

Although most cases of red eye are caused by viral or bacterial conjunctivitis, other possibilities exist, including trauma, glaucoma, systemic disease, and congenital anomalies. Determining the etiology is an important step in assessment of the condition.

DIAGNOSTIC REASONING: FOCUSED HISTORY

Is This a Chemical Emergency?

Key Question
- Did you get a chemical into your eye?

Chemical Injury
Chemical burns of the conjunctiva and cornea represent one of the true ocular emergencies. Alkali burns usually result in greater damage to the eye than acid burns because alkali compounds penetrate ocular tissues more rapidly.

All chemical burns require immediate and profuse irrigation and immediate referral to an ophthalmologist. Irrigate the eye with water while obtaining a history of the incident and possible chemical contact.

Could This Be Caused by an Orbital Infection?

Key Questions
- Do you notice any swelling or tightness around the eye(s) or of the eyelid(s)?
- Does it hurt to move your eye?
- Do you have a fever?
- Have you had a recent sinus infection?

Swelling, Redness, and Fever
Orbital or periorbital cellulitis can present with conjunctivitis and signal a medical emergency. They can occur as a complication of sinusitis. Complaints of swelling, redness, and fever should alert you to these conditions. Both conditions require immediate referral; orbital cellulitis is life threatening.

Pain on Attempted Motion of the Eye
Orbital cellulitis causes pain on movement because of the collection of pus between the periosteum and the wall of the orbit. The inflammation continues to all tissues in the orbit, and proptosis and impairment of ocular motility are seen.

Recent Sinus Infection
Sinusitis is the most common predisposing condition in patients with orbital cellulitis. The ethmoid sinuses are most commonly involved, with the maxillary sinus the next most common site of infection.

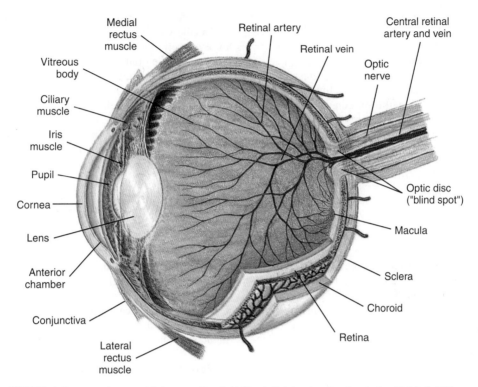

FIGURE 6-1 Anatomical structures of the human eye. (From Seidel HM et al: *Mosby's guide to physical examination*, ed 6, St Louis, 2006, Mosby.)

Can I Rule in or Rule out Trauma?

Key Question

■ How was your eye injured (e.g., foreign body, chemical, blow, stab, cut)?

Blunt trauma to the ocular adnexa can cause lid swelling and/or discoloration. Rupture of the globe, fractures of the orbital bones, and internal bleeding may also be possible. Sharp trauma to the area can cause lacerations of the lid and underlying lacerations of the globe. Internal bleeding may be subconjunctival (between the conjunctiva and sclera) or intraocular (hyphema). The cornea may have a foreign body and/or abrasions.

History of forceful trauma causing laceration or perforation of the globe is a surgical emergency and should be immediately referred without manipulation of the eye or eyelid.

Is This an Acute or Chronic Condition?

Key Questions

■ How long has the eye been red?
■ Did the redness start abruptly, or was it gradual?
■ Have you had this redness before? When?

Onset

An abrupt onset of redness typifies trauma, chemical burn, foreign body, ultraviolet (UV) exposure, or contact lens problems. Onset over a few hours may indicate infection from adjacent structures (periorbital, orbital, or sinuses). Onset over a few days is characteristic of conjunctivitis. Acute redness can be caused by infection of the conjunctiva and/or eyelids. Common causative organisms include *Staphylococcus aureus*, *Streptococcus pneumoniae*, group A *Streptococcus, Haemophilus influenzae,* and *Neisseria gonorrhoeae.*

Recurrence

Recurrent redness is often the result of allergic conjunctivitis from a hypersensitivity reaction to a specific antigen. Iritis from systemic causes can also produce recurrent redness because of collagen destruction.

Can I Narrow the Problem by Location?

Key Question

■ Does one eye (or do both eyes) bother you?

Unilateral redness is more likely to indicate trauma or infection. Bilateral redness is more likely to indicate an allergy or an underlying systemic process. Blepharitis, inflammation of the eyelids, causes itching and crusting of the lash line and is usually bilateral. A hordeolum (sty) produces redness at the base of eyelashes and is usually unilateral. A chalazion is a chronic granulomatous inflammation of the meibomian gland. It is found in the mid eyelid, often on the conjunctival side, and is usually unilateral. Some conditions can present with either unilateral or bilateral symptoms. Conjunctivitis often starts in one eye and then spreads to the other eye. Subconjunctival hemorrhage is often unilateral but may involve both eyes. Herpetic infection may be unilateral or bilateral.

A unilaterally painful, inflamed eye with photophobia and often a foreign body sensation without a history of significant trauma may indicate acute glaucoma.

What Does the Presence or Absence of Pain Tell Me?

Key Questions

■ Do you have pain in your eye? How severe is the pain?
■ Does it hurt when you move your eye?
■ Does it feel like there is something in your eye?

Location of Pain

Decide whether the pain is coming from the eye itself or is referred from surrounding structures. The ophthalmic nerve innervates the lid, conjunctiva, cornea, and uveal tract. The retina, vitreous, and optic nerve are less well innervated and seldom are a source of pain. Referred pain can originate from contiguous structures or from inflamed structures innervated by the meningeal branches of the ophthalmic nerve.

Severity of Pain

Bacterial conjunctivitis causes minimal pain; most patients complain of discomfort from the discharge and matting. There may be an itching/burning pain with allergy, moderate pain with iritis, and severe pain with corneal abrasion/ulcer. Constant, boring, throbbing pain, often severe enough to interfere with sleep, can result from ocular inflammation associated with iritis, acute glaucoma, and scleritis.

Foreign Body Sensation

A foreign body in an eye is a likely cause of pain. Viral causes of conjunctivitis produce a gritty sensation in the eye. A scratchy sensation often accompanies conditions that lead to dry eye, such as Sjögren's syndrome. Patients who over-wear contact lenses frequently complain of pain in the eye, caused by corneal hypoxia, several hours after removing the contacts.

Do I Need to Worry About Vision Changes?

Key Questions

■ Have you noticed any loss of vision?
■ Have you had any blurred vision, double vision, halos, or floaters?

Visual Decrease or Loss

Distinguish visual loss from blurry vision caused by the discharge associated with conjunctivitis. No decrease in vision is seen in bacterial and allergic conjunctivitis, beyond that reasonably related to blurring from the

Box 6-1	Differential Diagnosis Based on Symptoms of Pain and Visual Loss		
RED EYE (NO PAIN OR VISUAL LOSS)	**RED EYE (PAINFUL)**		
		VISION NORMAL	**VISION IMPAIRED**
Conjunctivitis		Episcleritis	Iritis
Subconjunctival hemorrhage		Keratitis	Glaucoma
Episcleritis		Cluster headache	Orbital cellulitis
		Corneal abrasion	Scleritis
		Corneal ulcer	Corneal abrasion
			Keratitis
			Corneal ulcer

heavy discharge. Vision is mildly decreased in iritis but markedly decreased in acute glaucoma and with corneal abrasions/ulcers. Box 6-1 lists differential diagnoses based on symptoms of pain and visual loss (also see Chapter 7).

Sudden diminution in or loss of visual acuity is an ocular emergency and may indicate corneal or uveal tract disorders, acute glaucoma, or orbital cellulitis.

Blurring

True blurring is caused by an ocular problem. When the cornea, lens, aqueous humor, or vitreous is hazy, vision blurs and often there is dazzle in bright light. Some patients describe both refractive errors and double vision as "blurred vision." Heavy discharge associated with conjunctivitis can also produce perceived blurring of vision.

Double Vision

True double vision becomes single vision when one eye is covered. Sudden onset usually indicates a neurological problem. Chronic diplopia may be caused by muscular problems. Monocular diplopia usually indicates either corneal or lens changes.

Halos

Halos result from prismatic effects. They can be visual signs of corneal edema caused by an abrupt rise in corneal or intraocular pressure (acute glaucoma). Less serious causes are water drops in the cornea or lens (seen in corneal edema or cataract).

Floaters

Floaters and/or flashing lights occur with vitreoretinal traction. The traction may progress to a retinal tear or detachment. With a tear, patients may complain of spaghetti-like strands floating in their vision. With a detachment, patients will give a history of blurred or blackened vision over several hours that progresses to complete or partial monocular blindness.

What Does the Presence or Characteristics of the Discharge Tell Me?

Key Questions

- Do you have any discharge from your eye?
- Is the discharge from one eye or both eyes?
- What are the color, consistency, and characteristics of this discharge?

A watery, nonpurulent discharge usually indicates allergic conjunctivitis. A mucoid (stringy or ropy) discharge is also common with allergic conjunctivitis. In allergic conjunctivitis the discharge is usually bilateral. Discharge that is purulent or mucopurulent may indicate bacterial conjunctivitis and often affects both eyes. Copious purulent discharge may be caused by *N. gonorrhoeae* infection. Viral conjunctivitis discharge is watery and may affect only one eye. Corneal abrasions and ulcers also produce watery/purulent discharge and are usually unilateral.

In the neonate who is 24 hours old, mucoid or purulent discharge indicates chemical conjunctivitis from prophylactic instillation of silver nitrate and other medications. Severe, bilateral purulent conjunctivitis 3 to 7 days after birth may indicate gonococcal infection of the eye. Discharge that is seen 5 to 30 days postpartum may indicate chlamydial conjunctivitis.

What Does the Presence of Photophobia Tell Me?

Key Question

■ Does light bother you/hurt your eye(s)?

Photophobia usually indicates ocular inflammation or irritation. Intraocular inflammation (iritis or generalized uveitis) causes pain on pupillary changes and thus leads to the avoidance of bright light. This symptom may be mild and often is not reported unless the patient is questioned specifically about this symptom. There is no photophobia with bacterial conjunctivitis. In infants and young children, photophobia signals a serious condition, such as juvenile arthritis, intraocular tumors, congenital glaucoma, herpetic keratitis, or trauma.

What Other Things Do I Need to Consider?

Key Questions

■ Has there been any swelling?
■ Do you have excessive tearing?
■ Do your eyes itch?
■ Does the itching occur at different times of the year?
■ Has there been a cough and fever?

Swelling

The orbital septum is a continuation of the periosteum of the bones of the orbit. It extends to the margins of both the upper and lower eyelids. Any conditions occurring in these areas can cause swelling. Secondarily, the skin of the eyelids is a very thin subcutaneous tissue that is musculofibrous and contains no fat. Thus the eyelid can allow a considerable amount of fluid to accumulate in a short period of time. Swelling and erythema under, and associated with, the medial canthus of the affected eye may indicate dacryocystitis. Swelling of the lids may be associated with inflammation, local infection, or trauma. Periorbital swelling may indicate cellulitis.

Tears

The lacrimal gland, which is situated in the upper lateral orbit, produces tears that are then carried across the eye to the puncta on the nasal side of the upper and lower lids. Obstruction of the passage of tears via the nasolacrimal duct to the nose causes regurgitation of fluid down the cheek (tearing). Epiphora (excessive production of tears) is common with viral conjunctivitis, corneal abrasions, infantile glaucoma, and nasal lacrimal duct stenosis.

Itching and Tearing

The hallmark of an allergic conjunctivitis is itching and tearing disproportionate to findings. Vernal conjunctivitis is seasonal, recurrent, and bilateral. Itching is intense in the spring and fall months.

Cough and Fever

Bacterial conjunctivitis is not associated with a fever. Otitis-conjunctivitis syndrome begins with a low-grade to moderate fever, mucopurulent rhinorrhea, and a cough. Three or 4 days after the onset of fever, the individual wakes up with the eyelashes crusted together. Ear complaints begin the same day as eye symptoms. Viral conjunctivitis, seen as slight crusting along the lid margins, may be seen with upper respiratory tract infections.

DIAGNOSTIC REASONING: FOCUSED PHYSICAL EXAMINATION

Test Visual Acuity

In adults and children older than $3^1/_2$ years, use a Snellen, Tumbling E, or Lippman chart. In children, the referral standard is 20/40 or worse in both eyes or a two-line difference between eyes. Retesting before referral of children is suggested because the child may perform better (within normal limits) on the second examination.

For children younger than $3^1/_2$ years, use an ophthalmoscope. Darken the room. Stay at arm's length from the child and look at the eyes at a distance of 1 m or greater. When the child looks at the light, look at both red reflexes simultaneously and compare them. They should be red and equal in coloration. This indicates that the vision and binocular alignment are good and that no major pathology of the cornea, lens, vitreous, or retina is present. If the reflexes are not equal, a referral is required to an ophthalmologist.

Test Visual Fields

Testing of visual fields assesses the function of the peripheral vision and the central retina, optic pathways, and cortex. The peripheral field is damaged in glaucoma and by tumors or vascular lesions involving the visual fibers from the chiasm to the occipital cortex.

Inspect the Lids and Lid Margins and Periorbital and Orbital Tissues

Note redness or swelling of the lids. Look for lid lesions. Inspect the lid margins. Evert the lids and note appearance.

Unilateral inflammation of the lids and periorbital tissues without proptosis or limitation of eye movement characterizes periorbital cellulitis. If proptosis and/or limitation of eye movement is present, orbital cellulitis is the cause.

Erythematous swelling without systemic signs may be caused by contact dermatitis. All exposed skin should have the same coloring. Magenta discoloration of the eyelid is caused by *H. influenzae.*

A lid that is injected, swollen, and irritated may be so because of an underlying disease process in the conjunctiva, cornea, sclera, or intraocular area.

Examine for the presence of focal or diffuse inflammation. Blockage of the glands along the lash line may produce localized or diffuse redness or flaking of the skin as a result of staphylococcal or seborrheic causes.

Lids that appear to have follicular changes (small aggregates of lymphocytes) in the palpebral conjunctiva are commonly seen with viral conjunctivitis. Lids that have large, flattened, cobblestone-like papillary lesions of the palpebral conjunctivae are characteristic of vernal conjunctivitis.

Inflammation of the lid margins in all four lids and with associated loss of eyelashes is common in children; this condition is known as blepharitis. The lashes are waxy, scaling, red, and irritated, and the eyes have slightly swollen lid margins.

Eye pain with no external inflammation suggests referred causes, such as sinusitis, carotid artery aneurysm, temporal arteritis, migraine or cluster headache, or trigeminal neuralgia. Optic neuritis can also cause eye pain without inflammation.

Observe for Entropion and Ectropion

Entropion occurs when the eyelid margin turns inward. The eyelashes contact the corneal and conjunctival surfaces, and the patient complains of discomfort. Scarring can occur.

Ectropion occurs when the eyelid margin turns outward. A pool of stagnant tears results and does not allow proper mechanical protection of the cornea and conjunctiva. The exposed tarsal conjunctiva is also susceptible to repeated trauma.

Evert the Eyelid if Indicated by History

Eversion of the eyelid is necessary to detect a possible foreign body. This is done by first having the patient look down. Hold the upper eyelashes straightforward. Push down on the upper tarsal border with a cotton-tipped applicator. The lid everts. Hold the eyelid in this position by moving fingers to the brow. To undo, hold the lashes and pull gently forward while asking the patient to look up.

Inspect the Conjunctiva

Note bilateral or unilateral redness and the location of redness on the conjunctiva. Distinguish between peripheral or circumcorneal injection (ciliary flush). Ciliary flush is the deep conjunctival or episcleral blood vessel injection around the limbus (junction between the cornea and conjunctiva), dilating in response to corneal disease or injury. It is frequently associated with keratopathy, uveitis, and episcleritis/scleritis. Abrasions and ulcers of the cornea cause increased redness of the globe around the corneal limbus, appearing as a reddish ring surrounding the cornea. Note any discharge. Look for visible lesions or foreign bodies on the conjunctiva.

Conjunctival inflammation as a result of infection causes a red eye with peripheral injection that is maximal toward the fornix (the fold between globe and lid). Peripheral injection involves the bulbar conjunctiva without edema or exudate, and the cornea is spared.

Look for swelling of the conjunctiva (chemosis). Fluid can accumulate beneath the loosely attached bulbar conjunctiva, causing it to balloon away from the globe. Chemosis occurs most frequently and dramatically with hyperacute bacterial conjunctivitis.

Subconjunctival hemorrhage causes a bright red splash of blood that is visible on the conjunctiva and sclera. Without a history of trauma or bleeding diathesis and no presence of retinal hemorrhage, the cause may be intravascular pressure from coughing, sneezing, or straining.

Systemic autoimmune processes such as juvenile rheumatoid arthritis, serum sickness, and Stevens-Johnson syndrome may cause conjunctivitis. Perilimbal conjunctival injection is seen in juvenile rheumatoid arthritis.

A localized degenerative process of the substantia propriae of the conjunctiva, known as pinguecula, may invade the superficial cornea. These are yellow, elevated nodules of fibropathic material that are usually adjacent to the cornea on the nasal side.

Look at the palpebral conjunctiva and the fornices for foreign bodies and pterygia, which are neovascularized structures that can encroach on the cornea and form a pannus that interferes with vision.

Inspect the Sclera

Note the color. The sclera gives the eye its white appearance. Inflammation (scleritis) causes a dusky red color.

Examine the Cornea

Test the corneal light (red) reflex. Note if the cornea is hazy or has opacities. Look for visible foreign bodies.

The normal cornea is transparent, with blood vessels only at the limbus (the junction between cornea and conjunctiva). Illumination of the cornea tangentially may show abnormalities, such as abrasions or foreign bodies. These imperfections of the corneal surface will produce an abnormal light reflex or a break in the image as the light reflects off the cornea. The blood vessels around the limbus dilate in response to corneal disease or injury.

Topical application of fluorescein to the cornea that reveals dendrite ulcers should lead you to suspect herpes simplex virus.

Examine the Iris, Pupil, and Lens

Note pupil size and equality. Note transparency of lens. Test pupillary reaction (direct and consensual). Note any photophobia.

The anterior chamber should contain only clear aqueous humor. Trauma may cause blood to accumulate in the chamber; this is known as a hyphema. The shock wave produced by the sudden compression and decompression of the cornea is transmitted through the eye and may result in a tear in the ciliary body. Disruption of the anterior arterial circle of this structure produces bleeding that accumulates. The hyphema appears as a bright red or dark red fluid level between the cornea and iris or as a diffuse murkiness of the aqueous humor. Pus may also accumulate in this space in association with corneal infection. This is known as hypopyon. All hyphemas are abnormal and must be referred to an ophthalmologist.

The pupil is the central aperture of the iris. It floats in the aqueous humor and divides the anterior segment into anterior and posterior chambers, which communicate throughout the pupillary aperture. It slides freely on the anterior surface of the lens when dilating and contracting. Conditions that affect this anatomy cause pupil abnormalities. Inflammation of the iris (iritis) causes reduction in the reactive capacity of the iris and inequality of pupils. Acute increased intraocular pressure causes the space in the anterior chamber to become very shallow, resulting in a dilated, fixed, oval pupil.

The lens is normally transparent and not visible on inspection; however, any visible clouding of the lens as seen through the pupil is indicative of cataract formation.

Perform Ophthalmoscopy

When looking for the red reflex, note any corneal opacity as well as the depth of the opacity. Corneal opacities move in the opposite direction of the ophthalmoscope, lens opacities stay still, and vitreous opacities move in the same direction as the ophthalmoscope. Corneal clouding (edema) is seen with glaucoma.

Look for a large and deepened cup if you suspect glaucoma. Early in the course of the disease, the ophthalmoscopic examination may be normal. Do not use mydriatic agents if you suspect glaucoma.

Test Extraocular Movements

Test eye movement in all six fields of gaze. Note pain or restriction. Inflammation or underlying periostitis and impaired venous drainage as a result of reactive inflammation cause restrictive eye movement and proptosis (exophthalmos). Decreased range of motion can also occur with orbital cellulitis.

Palpate the Lid/Lacrimal Puncta

Observe for edema and note pain or tenderness on palpation. The lacrimal puncta should be turned backward slightly to catch the pool of tears in the inner canthus. Tears should not spill over the cheeks. Note if gentle palpation of each lacrimal sac produces any material that regurgitates into the eye. Unilateral swelling over the lacrimal sac on the lid margin at the side of the nose because of infection or obstruction of the lacrimal drainage system is common. Infection of the meibomian glands of the eyelids (hordeolum or internal sty) and the glands of Zeis or Moll (hordeolum or external sty) produces pain on palpation. Internal sties are generally large and very tender and may point to the conjunctiva or epidermis portion of the lid. External sties are small and superficial and point only to the epidermis side.

Granulomatous inflammation of a meibomian gland nodule that is firm and not tender and has no inflammatory signs is a chalazion.

Examine the Tympanic Membranes

Examination of the tympanic membrane is necessary because of the frequent association with atypical *H. influenzae* acute otitis media (conjunctivitis-otitis syndrome).

Palpate Preauricular Nodes

The preauricular nodes are usually palpable with a viral infection of the eyes. Palpable adenopathy is uncommon in acute bacterial conjunctivitis but may occur in hyperacute infection caused by *N. gonorrhoeae* or *Neisseria meningitidis*.

LABORATORY AND DIAGNOSTIC STUDIES

Fluorescein Staining

Dendrite etchings on the anterior portion of the cornea are seen in herpes infection. Nodules near the limbus with surrounding hyperemia are seen in keratoconjunctivitis. Hypertrophy of the dorsal conjunctiva with elevated grayish areas near the limbus is consistent with vernal conjunctivitis. Under a blue light, a corneal abrasion and foreign body will stain bright green with fluorescein.

Culture

Cultures are not usually required in patients with mild conjunctivitis of suspected viral, bacterial, or allergic origin. However, bacterial cultures should be obtained in patients with severe, chronic, or recurrent conjunctivitis. Moisten a sterile alginate (not cotton) swab with sterile saline and wipe the lid margin or conjunctival cul-de-sac. The culture medium is then inoculated directly with the swab tip. Place on solid medium, writing R for right eye, L for left eye, and Z for another culture site. The tip of the applicator may then be broken off and dropped into the tube of liquid culture medium.

Cultures should be taken before instilling topical anesthetics because preservatives will reduce the recovery of some bacteria.

Gram Stain

Gram-positive cocci in pairs may indicate *Streptococcus pyogenes*. Gram-negative diplococci indicate *N. gonorrhoeae*. Large gram-negative diplobacilli indicate *Moraxella catarrhalis; H. influenzae* stains as gram-negative coccobacilli.

Complete Blood Cell Count

A complete blood cell count with differential can be done to establish the presence of a systemic infection. An increase in white blood cells and bands is seen with systemic infection.

Blood Cultures

Blood cultures are obtained for any suspected orbital cellulitis or when there is reason to suspect a clinically significant bacteremia. *H. influenzae, Streptococcus pneumoniae, Staphylococcus aureus, Streptococcus pyogenes,* or anaerobes are possible infecting organisms.

Computed Tomography Scanning

A computed tomography scan is used to determine the presence and extent of an abscess and/or to localize the site of infection in the periorbital region as well as in the sinuses.

Intraocular Pressure

Intraocular pressure is measured with a Schiøtz tonometer. The technique is as follows: after instillation of a local anesthetic agent, the patient is placed in a supine position and asked to look directly upward. The lids are held separated, and the instrument is placed gently in a vertical position directly over the cornea, with the plunger placed on the cornea. A reading on the scale is then taken. A pressure elevated greater than 21 mm Hg is seen in acute closed-angle glaucoma.

DIFFERENTIAL DIAGNOSIS

Lacrimal Sac

Dacryocystitis

Infection of the lacrimal sac occurs secondary to obstruction. In infants, it is a complication of congenital dacryostenosis. In adults, duct obstruction results from nasal trauma, deviated septum, hypertrophic rhinitis, and mucosal polyps. The patient experiences pain, swelling, and redness around the lacrimal sac with tearing. Conjunctivitis, blepharitis, and leukocytosis are associated with an acute condition; with a chronic condition, the only symptom may be slight swelling of the sac. Pus may regurgitate through the punctum.

Eyelids

Blepharitis

Blepharitis is the most common inflammation of the eyelids. It usually involves the lid margins and frequently is associated with conjunctivitis. It is bilateral and not painful, and it has no associated photophobia. The lids are inflamed, and scaling of the lid margins is seen. Loss of eyelashes occurs late. Visual acuity is unimpaired.

Hordeolum

Hordeolum is caused by infection of the glands of Zeis or Moll along the lash line. It develops acutely and manifests as a palpable indurated area along the lid margin, with a purulent center and surrounding erythema. It spontaneously drains within 1 to 2 weeks. Patients experience swelling of the eyelid and localized lid pain.

Chalazion

A chalazion is a granulomatous reaction in the meibomian gland on the tarsal plate of the lid. This is usually a chronic condition. The lesion is usually painless and indurated. When symptoms are present, they include pruritus and redness of the involved eye and eyelid.

Entropion and Ectropion

Malposition of the eyelid causes local irritation and may be a cause of red eye. In entropion the lid is turned inward; in ectropion the lid is turned outward.

Conjunctiva

Bacterial Conjunctivitis

S. aureus, S. pneumoniae, group A *Streptococcus, H. influenzae,* and *N. gonorrhoeae* most commonly cause bacterial conjunctivitis. The onset is gradual, begins unilaterally, and often becomes bilateral. The patient usually complains of a scratchy sensation instead of pain. There is generally no photophobia. Examination reveals peripheral injection, purulent discharge, and matted eyelids. Visual acuity is not affected, although the presence of discharge may produce "blurring" of vision.

Viral Conjunctivitis

Occurring most commonly in young adults, viral conjunctivitis is caused by such viruses as adenovirus, picornavirus, rhinovirus, and herpesvirus. The onset is gradual and unilateral early in the course and then may become bilateral. The patient complains of a scratchy, rather than painful, sensation. On examination, peripheral injection with watery discharge is apparent. Visual acuity is intact. Lids may have follicular changes (small aggregates of lymphocytes) in the palpebral conjunctiva.

Allergic Conjunctivitis

Allergic conjunctivitis is a chronic, seasonal condition caused by hypersensitivity reaction to a specific allergen. It is bilateral, itchy, and painless. The conjunctival injection is peripheral. There is ropy, mucoid discharge. The palpebral conjunctiva has a cobblestone appearance. Visual acuity is unaffected.

N. gonorrhoeae Conjunctivitis

The *N. gonorrhoeae* organism can produce a bacterial conjunctivitis in newborns. It is bilateral, with very purulent discharge 48 to 72 hours after birth. Although rare in adults, it can occur through direct transmission via finger contact or via contact of the eyes in a nonchlorinated swimming pool. The infection has an abrupt onset and is characterized by copious purulent discharge that reaccumulates after being wiped away. In addition to redness and irritation, the patient has marked conjunctival injection, chemosis, lid swelling, and tender preauricular adenopathy. The condition warrants immediate ophthalmic referral.

Chemical Conjunctivitis

Chemical conjunctivitis occurs with instillation of chemical prophylaxis in the neonate. A bilateral reaction occurs within the first 24 hours.

Subconjunctival Hemorrhage

Subconjunctival hemorrhage is usually the result of a small blood vessel rupture in the conjunctival tissue and frequently develops after episodes of coughing or straining. It is painless although often frightening to the patient. Visual acuity is not impaired.

Anterior Chamber
Hyphema

Hyphema is caused by blood in the anterior chamber of the eye, usually produced by trauma to the eye. The patient has a marked decrease in vision, with red blood cells present diffusely throughout the anterior chamber. A settled layer of blood present inferiorly or a complete filling of the anterior chamber is possible, obscuring the visual examination of the posterior chamber. The pupil is irregular and poorly reactive.

Sclera
Episcleritis

Often a benign inflammatory condition of the covering of the sclera, episcleritis is bilateral, with mild stinging. Peripheral injection is present. There is no discharge, but some lacrimation and photophobia may be present. Visual acuity is unimpaired.

Scleritis

Inflammation of the sclera can result in severe destructive disease. It is usually a unilateral inflammatory condition associated with rheumatoid arthritis, systemic immunological disease, or other autoimmune disorders. There is pain and ciliary injection. Lacrimation is present, and visual acuity is variable.

Cornea
Keratitis

Bacterial, fungal, and viral organisms can cause infection of the cornea. Moderate to severe eye pain is present, there is some discharge, and visual acuity is decreased. Pupils are equal and normal, but the cornea appears cloudy. Peripheral injection is present and diffuse. A ciliary flush is also present.

Corneal Abrasion

Corneal abrasion may be superficial, lying on top of the anterior surface of the cornea, or it may be subtarsal and become implanted on the palpebral conjunctiva, causing the cornea to become irritated when the patient blinks. The patient usually has a history of a foreign body on the anterior surface of the eye. The abrasion causes moderate to severe pain with discharge present. Visual acuity may be normal or decreased; photophobia is present; and pupil size and reaction are normal. Fluorescein stain is taken into the ulcer and can be seen under a Wood's lamp.

Herpetic Infection

Caused by the herpes simplex virus, this infection occurs unilaterally or bilaterally. The patient's presenting symptoms are pain, photophobia, and diffuse or ciliary injection. Discharge is variable, and visual acuity is markedly decreased. Dendrites are seen on fluorescein staining.

Herpes zoster can cause inflammation and scarring of the cornea, with conjunctivitis and iritis. In some cases the retina and optic nerve are involved. Severe or chronic outbreaks of herpes zoster may cause glaucoma, cataract formation, double vision, and scarring of the cornea. Patients with suspected ocular herpes infection (simplex or zoster) should be referred to an ophthalmologist.

Orbit
Periorbital Cellulitis

The patient's presenting symptoms include unilateral swelling of lid, redness, fever, and hotness. The conjunctiva is clear, the eye moves freely, and vision is not impaired.

Orbital Cellulitis

The patient's symptoms include unilateral lid swelling, fever, and pain. Examination reveals proptosis, chemosis, and conjunctivitis. There is limitation of eye motion on testing of extraocular movements. The patient appears ill. This condition is life threatening and requires immediate intervention.

Uveal Tract
Iritis

Characterized by inflammation of the iris and ciliary body, iritis may be idiopathic and develop in response to coexistent conjunctivitis, keratitis, or eye trauma, or it may occur with chronic inflammatory or infectious processes. Eye pain is moderate and aching, visual acuity is decreased, and photophobia is present. There is minimal eye discharge, the affected pupil is smaller, and the cornea appears normal. There is central redness of the eye, with ciliary flush present.

Glaucoma
Acute Closed-Angle Glaucoma

The patient's presenting symptoms include unilateral, deep eye pain and photophobia. There may be a complaint of halos around visualized objects. There is ciliary injection with tears and decreased visual acuity. The pupil is mid dilated and has decreased reactivity to light. The cornea is cloudy. There is diffuse redness of the eye with an intraocular pressure of greater than 21 mm Hg. This condition requires emergency referral.

◤ DIFFERENTIAL DIAGNOSIS OF *Common Causes of Red Eye Complaints*

CONDITION	HISTORY	PHYSICAL FINDINGS	DIAGNOSTIC STUDIES
Eyelids			
Lacrimal Sac			
Dacryocystitis	Unilateral, acute onset; pain	Swelling and redness around lacrimal sac; tearing; may have pus through punctum	CBC, leukocytosis
Blepharitis	Bilateral, gradual onset; no pain	Lids inflamed; scaling on margins; visual acuity okay; loss of lashes (late)	None

Continued

DIFFERENTIAL DIAGNOSIS OF *Common Causes of Red Eye Complaints* —*cont'd*

CONDITION	HISTORY	PHYSICAL FINDINGS	DIAGNOSTIC STUDIES
Hordeolum/sty	Unilateral; pain	Swelling of eyelid; indurated lesion with central pus and surrounding erythema	None initially; if repeated, screen for diabetes
Chalazion	Unilateral, chronic; painless	Indurated lesion on tarsal plate of lid; may have pruritus and redness of involved eye and eyelid	None
Entropion/ectropion	Unilateral or bilateral	Lid turned inward or outward; local irritation and tearing; peripheral injection	None
Conjunctiva			
Bacterial conjunctivitis	Gradual onset, unilateral early, bilateral late; scratchy (no pain); photophobia	Peripheral injection; purulent discharge; matted eyelids; visual acuity okay	None initially; if not better with treatment, obtain culture and sensitivities; Gram stain
Viral conjunctivitis	Gradual onset, unilateral early, bilateral late; scratchy (no pain)	Peripheral injection; watery discharge; visual acuity okay; follicular changes (small aggregates of lymphocytes) in palpebral conjunctiva	Same as for bacterial conjunctivitis
Allergic conjunctivitis	Chronic; seasonal; bilateral; itchy (no pain)	Peripheral injection; ropy, mucoid discharge; cobblestone mucosa; visual acuity okay	Fluorescein staining; hypertrophy of dorsal conjunctiva with elevated gray areas near limbus with vernal conjunctivitis
N. gonorrhoeae conjunctivitis	Bilateral; newborn	Purulent discharge 48-72 hours after birth	Culture on Thayer-Martin plate; Gram stain
Chemical conjunctivitis	Bilateral	Neonate: within first 24 hours	None
Subconjunctival hemorrhage	Unilateral; painless; coughing or straining	Splash of blood in conjunctiva or sclera; visual acuity okay	None
Anterior Chamber			
Hyphema	Unilateral; trauma to eye	Red blood cells in anterior chamber; visual acuity decreased; pupil irregular and poorly reactive	Refer to ophthalmologist
Sclera			
Episcleritis	Bilateral; mild stinging	Peripheral injection; no discharge; visual acuity okay	None
Scleritis	Unilateral; deep, boring pain	Ciliary injection, teary; visual acuity variable; photophobia	Associated with systemic immunological disease
Keratitis	Bilateral; moderate to severe pain	Discharge; pupils normal; cornea cloudy; visual acuity decreased	Test for bacterial, fungal, viral infection
Corneal abrasion/ foreign body	Unilateral; pain/photophobia	Diffuse injection; tears; visual acuity variable	Fluorescein stain positive
Herpetic keratitis	Unilateral or bilateral; pain; photophobia	Ciliary flush; discharge; visual acuity markedly decreased	Fluorescein stain shows dendrites

Continued

DIFFERENTIAL DIAGNOSIS OF *Common Causes of Red Eye Complaints —cont'd*

CONDITION	HISTORY	PHYSICAL FINDINGS	DIAGNOSTIC STUDIES
Orbit			
Periorbital cellulitis	Unilateral	Swelling of lid; fever, redness; conjunctiva clear; eye moves freely; vision not impaired	CBC—leukocytosis, blood cultures
Orbital cellulitis	Unilateral; pain	Proptosis; lid swelling; chemosis; conjunctivitis; limitation of eye motion	CBC, blood cultures; CT scan; life threatening
Uveal Tract			
Iritis	Unilateral; moderate aching pain; photophobia	Tearing; affected pupil smaller; cornea normal; ciliary flush	Refer
Glaucoma			
Acute closed-angle glaucoma	Unilateral; deep pain; photophobia; halos	Ciliary injection; tears; visual acuity decreased	Tonometry; emergency referral

CBC, Complete blood cell count; *CT,* computed tomography.

CHAPTER RESOURCES

Alessandrini EA: The case of the red eye, *Pediatr Ann* 29:112, 2000.

Bal SK, Hollingworth GR: Red eye, *BMJ* 331:7514, 2005.

Greenberg M, Pollard Z: The red eye in childhood, *Pediatr Clin North Am* 50:105, 2003.

Jain A, Rubin PA: Orbital cellulitis in children, *Int Ophthalmol Clin* 41:71, 2001.

Leibowitz HM: The red eye, *N Engl J Med* 343:345, 2000.

Rietveld RP, ter Riet G, Bindels PJ, Sloos JH, van Weert HC: Predicting bacterial cause in infectious conjunctivitis: cohort study on informativeness of combinations of signs and symptoms, *BMJ* 329:7459, 2004.

Simon JW: Commonly missed diagnoses in the childhood eye examination, *Am Fam Physician* 64:623, 2002.

Wald E: Periorbital and orbital infections, *Pediatr Rev* 25:312, 2004.

Vision Loss

For vision to occur, light is transmitted through the eye to photoreceptors in the retina that collect light and send neural impulses to the brain. These impulses are then processed to give information on what is being seen. Vision loss occurs with any interruption in this visual pathway such as opacification of the cornea, lens, or vitreous body (see Figure 6-1 for the anatomical structures of the eye). Vision loss also occurs when light energy cannot be converted into neural impulses, such as in glaucoma, retinal detachment, ischemic optic nerve atrophy, and pituitary or occipital tumors. In all cases, subnormal vision requires evaluation by an ophthalmologist. However, knowledge of the causes of vision loss can provide important clues to the diagnosis of these conditions.

DIAGNOSTIC REASONING: FOCUSED HISTORY

Is This a True Vision Loss?

Key Questions

- Has there been a loss of vision, or is the vision blurred?
- Does the patient look at you?
- If a child: Does the child's eye wander?

Blurring of Vision

Distinguish between loss of vision and loss of visual acuity. Vision loss is the absence of vision, completely or partially, in one or both eyes. Blurriness refers to a change in the acuity of vision. The most common cause of visual acuity change is refractive error.

Ability to Focus

Patients who are without sight have no ocular alignment and commonly manifest a gross searching and wandering nystagmus. Nystagmus in the first year of life suggests bilateral vision loss until proved otherwise. In infancy, vision loss is a common cause of nystagmus.

Visual Fixation

Even though the visual system is incompletely developed at birth, most infants can see and will demonstrate visual interest when stimulated by a human face. At birth the infant will have visual fixation present, and by 2 months of age fixation will be well developed. Any parental concern about a child's visual functioning is an important history finding.

Is This an Emergency That Requires Immediate Intervention?

Key Questions

- Was the loss of vision sudden?
- Is the loss in one or both eyes?
- Is the loss complete or partial?
- Is there any pain with the loss of vision?
- Are there other symptoms associated with the loss, such as a flash of light?
- Was the loss momentary or persistent?

Onset

Sudden loss of vision suggests a vascular etiology. Sudden vision loss is considered to be a result of occlusion of the central retinal artery until proved otherwise. In occlusion of the central retinal artery, the patient notes that vision is lost suddenly, and light cannot be distinguished from dark. Loss of vision in one eye indicates that the problem is anterior to the chiasm; hemianopic field defects in both eyes suggest a postchiasmal lesion (Figure 7-1).

Occlusion of the artery is an emergency and requires immediate treatment.

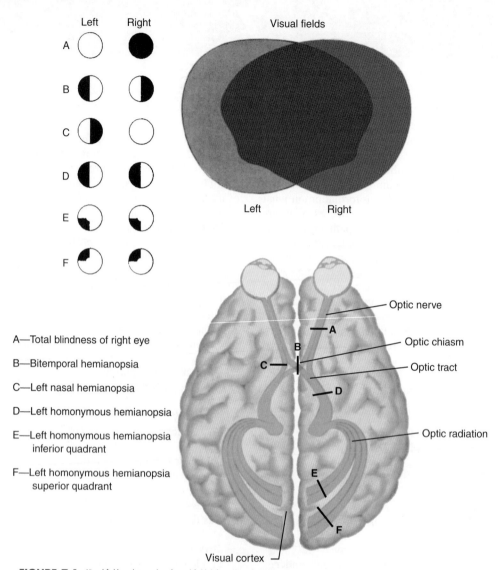

FIGURE 7-1 Visual fields and examples of visual field defects along the optic nerve, optic chiasm, optic tracts, and optic radiations in the cortex. (From Rudy EB: *Advanced neurological and neurosurgical nursing,* St Louis, 1984, Mosby.)

Pain

Sudden loss of vision with eye pain and photophobia indicates pathology of the cornea, iris, and ciliary body. Sudden loss of vision with a red painful eye may indicate acute-angle glaucoma (see Chapter 6). Inflammation, demyelinization, or degeneration of the optic nerve causes pain on movement of the eye and is thought to be the result of general inflammation of the posterior portion of the orbit or inflammation of the optic nerve (cranial nerve II). Retrobulbar neuritis is the most common disease in this category.

A common cause of sudden loss of vision without pain is vitreous hemorrhage. The patient describes floaters that begin to drift in front of the eye, followed by a red glow. The vision gradually fades until only light and dark are distinguished. Painless vision loss is also associated with macular degeneration, retinal detachment, diabetic retinopathy, and anterior ischemic optic neuropathy.

Other Symptoms

In children acute optic neuritis rarely occurs as an isolated condition and is usually a manifestation of a neurological or systemic disease such as meningitis, viral infection, or demyelinizing diseases. It may also be associated with lead poisoning and long-term use of certain drugs, most notably chloramphenicol or vincristine.

Flash of Light With Loss of Vision

Patients who have retinal detachment describe a flash of light shortly before loss of vision. Some patients describe a veil over the eye either just before or immediately after the flash. The reason for the flashes is that detachment of the retina causes mechanical stimulation of the rods and cones as it tears away from the pigment epithelium and floats free.

Patients whose retinae pull away but do not detach experience the same flash of light as those with retinal detachment. They may also experience momentary total or partial loss of vision in the affected eye.

Transient Loss of Vision

Some patients with migraine headache experience a scotoma, or an area of impaired vision within the visual field, before the onset of the headache. The scotoma may be either positive (the patient sees a light spot or scintillating flashes [e.g., scintillating scotoma]) or negative (the patient experiences a blind spot). Scotoma may be prodromal to a migraine headache. Profound anxiety can produce a transient loss of vision or a perceived loss of vision.

Can I Rule Out Trauma?

Key Questions

- Is there a history of head trauma?
- Is there a history of eye trauma?
- Has there been a chemical or thermal injury?

Head Trauma

Loss of vision is most likely to occur after trauma to the occiput. The vision loss is sudden and complete, but vision usually returns in a matter of hours. Severe head trauma with skull fracture but without direct damage to the eyeball can result in loss of vision that occurs immediately or shortly thereafter. Occasionally a patient can have good vision in the affected eye after the accident and subsequently loses vision as a result of severe retrobulbar hemorrhage. In children, trauma is the most common cause of retinal detachment. Shaken baby syndrome may result in retina and vitreous hemorrhage.

Eye Trauma

Blunt trauma occurs when an object larger than a tennis ball or hockey stick, for example, or smaller than a golf ball or champagne cork, for example, impacts the bony orbit of the eye. High-velocity injuries to the eye are not always immediately obvious. Small perforations or penetrations of the cornea may appear similar to corneal abrasions. Sharp trauma includes impact from a sharp object that may perforate the cornea, leaking fluid from the eye.

Cataract formation is a result of major trauma to the eye in children. Opacification of the lens may result from a blunt or penetrating injury.

Chemical or Thermal Trauma

Alkaline burns from household cleaners and lawn and garden products can cause irreversible vision loss. Exposure to extreme heat or flames may damage the cornea and eyelids.

Minutes make a difference with chemical trauma to the eye—treat first and examine later. Wash the eye with water or normal saline solution immediately.

Is the Vision Loss Because of a Chronic Problem?

Key Questions

- How long has vision loss been present?
- Has vision decreased over time?

Progression of Vision Loss

Slowly progressive degenerative disease of any part of the eye may cause progressive vision loss. Progressive loss of visual acuity and color vision can be seen with optic gliomas, the most frequently occurring tumor of the optic nerve in childhood. A history of neurofibromatosis can be found in 25% of patients. Children who have surgery for cataracts are especially at risk for glaucoma. Glaucoma may cause chronic loss of vision. Age-related macular degeneration is associated with decreased reading vision (see Chapter 6).

Is This Related to a Genetic, Familial, or Intrauterine Risk?

Key Questions

- Is there a family history of vision or eye problems?
- Is there a history of maternal, intrapartum, or neonatal conditions?

Family History

A family history of retinoblastoma, congenital cataracts, or metabolic or genetic disease is a risk factor for visual and ocular abnormalities. Retinoblastoma occurs in 12% of children with a family history. Hereditary congenital cataracts occur in 10% to 25% of children with a family history. Autosomal dominant inheritance is the most common cause.

Maternal, Intrapartum, and Neonatal Risks

Infants at risk for vision problems are those who are premature; have been on oxygen therapy; are low birth weight; or have mothers who have had rubella, infections related to HIV/AIDS and toxoplasmosis, rubella, cytomegalovirus, and herpes simplex—known as the TORCH complex of infections. These conditions during pregnancy may produce blindness at birth or vision loss later in life. Down syndrome is associated with cataracts. Children with galactosemia develop cataracts in infancy. Children with galactokinase deficiency develop cataracts in the first decade of life.

Is the Loss Because of a Systemic Disease?

Key Question

- Do you have any chronic disease?

Chronic Disease

Neurodegenerative disease and juvenile rheumatoid arthritis can cause visual changes. Prolonged treatment with systemic steroids almost invariably results in the formation of posterior subcapsular cataracts. Marfan syndrome may cause dislocated lens.

Could This Be an Anatomical Problem?

Key Questions

- Do the eyes cross?
- If a child: Does the child squint, especially in the sun?
- Do the eyes appear symmetrical?
- Are the eyes bulging or sunken?

Eye Alignment

Amblyopia is impaired vision in an eye that appears to be structurally normal. It is defined in one of the following three ways:

1. Strabismic amblyopia occurs when one eye is out of alignment and the fovea of that eye receives an image that is different from that received in the opposite eye. The brain suppresses the image in the deviating eye to avoid diplopia and visual confusion.
2. Refractive amblyopia occurs when the refraction of each eye is so different that the child uses the eye that focuses the best, resulting in poor development of the other eye.
3. Deprivation amblyopia is anything that prevents an image from being received clearly by the retina. Conditions such as severe ptosis, congenital cataracts, or vitreous opacity may cause this.

Squinting

Squinting blocks out the outer rays from the object, resulting in a smaller amount of distortion, and increases the chance of being able to more clearly perceive the image on the retina. This often occurs with strabismus. Excessive squinting in bright light may indicate glaucoma.

Exophthalmos

Bilateral exophthalmos is protrusion of the eyeballs that occurs with hyperthyroidism. Lid lag is observed on downward gaze as a lag in the falling of the lid with the globe as it moves downward. Unilateral exophthalmos may indicate a tumor located behind the eye.

Enophthalmos

Enophthalmos is the backward displacement of the eyeball in the eye socket, leading to a sunken appearance. It is caused by starvation, dehydration, or trauma.

Ptosis

With ptosis, the eyelid margin is at or below the pupil. The eyelid appears to be drooping and interferes with vision. Ptosis may indicate a lesion of the oculomotor nerve (cranial nerve III), a neuromuscular weakness, or a congenital condition.

Is There a Pattern to the Vision Loss?

Key Question

■ When does the vision loss occur?

Pattern of Vision Loss

Retinitis pigmentosa is characterized by progressive disorganization of the pigment of the retina, usually accompanied by a decrease in the number of retinal vessels and some degree of optic atrophy. Night blindness is often the first symptom of vision loss. A progressive loss of vision may occur over decades.

Individuals who are extremely myopic often experience a reduction in vision at nighttime and may refer to that condition as "night blindness." Vitamin A deficiency or the result of retinotoxic drugs, such as quinine, can cause night blindness.

Can I Associate the Vision Loss With Developmental Delay in the Child?

Key Questions

■ If a child: Is there a history of developmental delay?
■ If a child: Is there a change in school performance?

Developmental Delay

Decreased vision can result in developmental delays. Motor development requires good visual cues and depth perception. Poor school performance may be the first indication of vision loss related to refractory errors and progressive myopia in some children. Craniopharyngiomas may compress the optic nerve system, causing a decrease in visual acuity and a decrease in school performance (Box 7-1).

Box 7-1	Normal Development of Vision and Eye Movements

Age	Normal Vision and Eye Movements
Birth (term)	Fixation
	Poor following
	Intermittent strabismus frequently present
	Visual acuity 20/400 to 20/600
1 mo	Horizontal following to midline
	Normal alignment
	Visual acuity 20/300
2 mo	Vertical following begins
	Normal alignment
	Visual acuity 20/200
3 mo	Good horizontal and vertical following
	Normal alignment
	Visual acuity 20/100
	Accommodation begins
	Binocularity detectable
6 mo	Visual acuity 20/20 to 20/30
	Binocularity well developed
8 to 10 yr	End of sensitive period for amblyopia

From Monte M: The eye in childhood, *Am Fam Physician* 60:907, 1999.

DIAGNOSTIC REASONING: FOCUSED PHYSICAL EXAMINATION

Clue: Children become increasingly threatened the closer the examiner comes to their face. The least-threatening assessment should be done first.

Assess for Visual Acuity

Visual acuity for distance vision in adults and children older than 4 years is tested using the Snellen or Tumbling E chart. Test each eye separately, with and without corrective lenses. A Rosenbaum pocket card held 15 inches from the eyes is used to test near or reading vision.

To test for central vision in infants, observe the infant's eyes as they follow large objects, such as the face or hand of the examiner, in various gazes. In children ages 1 to 3 years, use the cover/uncover test and observe the corneal light reflex.

Any child who has a difference of one line between the two eyes must be referred. Vision of 20/50 for 5 year olds and 20/40 for children 6 years and older requires referral. Retest using the Snellen chart before referring because children tend to do better on a second examination (Table 7-1).

Table 7-1	Pediatric Eye Evaluation Screening Recommendations for Primary Care Providers, Nurses, Physician's Assistants, and Trained Lay Personnel	
RECOMMENDED AGE FOR SCREENING*	**SCREENING METHOD**	**CRITERIA FOR REFERRAL TO AN OPHTHALMOLOGIST**
Newborn to 3 mo	Red reflex[†]	Abnormal or asymmetrical
	Inspection	Structural abnormality
6 mo to 1 yr	Fix and follow with each eye	Failure to fix and follow in cooperative infant
	Alternate occlusion	Failure to object equally to covering each eye
	Corneal light reflex	Asymmetrical
	Red reflex[†]	Abnormal or asymmetrical
	Inspection	Structural abnormality
3 yr (approximately)	Visual acuity[‡]	20/50 or worse or two lines of difference between eyes
	Corneal light reflex/cover-uncover	Asymmetrical ocular refixation movements
	Red reflex[†]	Abnormal or asymmetrical
	Inspection	Structural abnormality
5 yr (approximately)	Visual acuity[‡]	20/40 or worse or two lines of difference between eyes
	Corneal light reflex/cover-uncover	Asymmetrical/ocular refixation movements
	Stereoacuity[§]	Failure to appreciate stereopsis
	Red reflex[†]	Abnormal or asymmetrical
	Inspection	Structural abnormality
Older than 5 yr	Visual acuity[‡]	20/30 or worse or two lines of difference between eyes
	Corneal light reflex/cover-uncover	Asymmetrical/ocular refixation movements
	Stereoacuity[§]	Failure to appreciate stereopsis
	Red reflex[†]	Abnormal or asymmetrical
	Inspection	Structural abnormality

Reprinted with permission from the American Academy of Ophthalmology: *Pediatric Eye Evaluations Preferred Practice Pattern*, © 1997, American Academy of Ophthalmology, Inc.

*Note: These recommendations are based on expert opinion.

[†]Physician or nurse responsibility.

[‡]Figures, letters, "tumbling E," or optotypes.

[§]Optional: Random Dot E Game (RDE), Titmus Stereograms (Titmus Optical, Inc., Petersburg, Va), Randot Stereograms (Stereo Optical Company, Inc., Chicago).

Assess Lids, Pupils, and Orbits

Note the position of the eyelids. Eyelids that droop (ptosis) may cause vision loss. Assess for the symmetry of each eye, and observe for a transparent cornea.

The appearance of a white pupil (leukokoria) may indicate a cataract, retinoblastoma, persistent hyperplastic primary vitreous (PHPV) retinal detachment, vitreous hemorrhage, or intraocular inflammation, such as by *Toxocara canis,* which is a roundworm that is contracted from dogs and invades the liver, abdomen, and eyes.

Pupil size is smaller in infants and older adults. Five percent of people will have noticeable differences in pupil size (physiological anisocoria). However, many types of central nervous system diseases also cause differences in pupil size.

Enlargement of the pupil may be caused by ocular injury, acute glaucoma, systemic parasympatholytic drugs, and dilating drops. Constriction of the pupil is seen in iris inflammation and patients with glaucoma who are treated with pilocarpine. Irregularity of the pupil contour is invariably abnormal, occurring in iritis, syphilis of the central nervous system, trauma, and congenital defects.

Inspect for Nystagmus

On far lateral gaze, some eyes will develop a rhythmic twitching motion (nystagmus) in the direction of gaze followed by a drift back. This is a normal finding. However, nystagmus is a neurological sign that may indicate disease or structural changes in the vestibular-cerebellar-oculomotor system. Pathological nystagmus is seen when the movement is in the same direction, regardless of the direction of gaze. Nystagmus in the first year of life suggests bilateral vision loss until proved otherwise.

Assess Visual Fields

Testing of the visual fields assesses the function of the peripheral vision and central retina, the optic pathways, and the cortex. The peripheral field is damaged in glaucoma and by tumors or vascular lesions involving the visual fibers from the chiasm to the occipital cortex. A central vision loss is decreased visual function surrounded by normal function. Hemianopsia is a visual defect in the right and left halves of the visual field; this is due to a lesion involving the chiasm. In homonymous hemianopsia, the same half of the visual field of each eye is affected by a lesion posterior to the chiasm (see Figure 7-1).

Test Corneal Light Reflex

The corneal light reflex test is used to detect strabismus. Alignment of the eyes is most easily demonstrated by observing the reflection of a light on the cornea. The light should fall in each eye at the same point. An asymmetrical light reflex will be present in a deviating eye or in an eye with an asymmetrical contour.

Perform a Cover/Uncover Test

Have the patient look with both eyes at a specific point. With one eye covered, watch the uncovered eye. If this eye moves to fix on the point, it was not aligned before the other eye was covered and a heteropia, or deviation of an eye, is present. If the uncovered eye does not move, alignment is present and this is referred to as orthophoria. Repeat the test for the other eye.

Perform an Alternating Cover/Uncover Test

Alternate the cover rapidly on each eye and note any movement of the eyes. Perform this test to discover a latent tendency for misalignment of the two eyes, a condition referred to as heterophoria.

Use the Amsler Grid

An Amsler grid is used to test for distortion of central vision. The patient is asked to wear reading glasses, and the chart is held 15 inches from the eyes. Ask the patient to stare at the dot and tell you if the lines around the dot are curved or bent. Distortion, called metamorphopsia, is found in age-related macular degeneration or central vision loss (Figure 7-2).

Test for Extraocular Movements

Extraocular movements test six pairs of ocular muscles and three cranial nerves (III, IV,

RIGHT

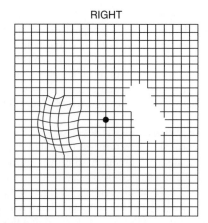

FIGURE 7-2 Example of metamorphopsia and a scotoma projected on an Amsler grid. (From Hampton GR, Nelson PT: *Age-related macular degeneration principles and practice*, New York, 1992, Raven Press.)

and VI). Strabismus is any condition in which the normal binocular alignment of the eyes to a single point in any and all fields of gaze is disturbed; there is an imbalance in neuro-muscular sensory and motor control of the extraocular muscles. Half of patients with strabismus also have amblyopia.

Paralytic strabismus is a deviation in the direction opposite the muscle involved. Double vision is usually a symptom but may not be present if the condition occurred at an early age and the child suppressed the vision in one eye or developed a compensatory head malposition.

Nonparalytic strabismus is present when the angle of deviation is the same in all cardinal fields of gaze.

Obtain a Direct and Consensual Pupillary Response

In monocular blindness, the affected eye will have no direct pupil response but will react consensually to stimulation of the opposite eye. Stimulation of the blind eye, however, will not cause consensual reaction of the opposite normal eye.

Perform an Ophthalmoscopic Examination

Examination of the optic disc can rule out optic atrophy, papilledema, and glaucoma.

Death of the fibers of the optic nerve results in disappearance of the vessels of the disc, leading to pallor or whiteness of the disc.

Observe for a red light reflex, especially in the early days and months of life. If the red reflexes are not equal, refer to an ophthalmologist. To obtain a red reflex in a newborn or young infant, swaddle and then hold the child. Position the ophthalmoscope diopter at 0, direct it to the eye, and gently swing or slightly parachute the infant. The vestibular system usually triggers the infant's eyes to open because of the maneuver.

In older children and adults, darken the room and instruct the patient to stare at an object or a glow sticker in the distance. When the child looks at the ophthalmoscope light, look at both red reflexes simultaneously and compare them. A uniform red glow equal in color is normal. Absence of a red reflex indicates that some abnormality is blocking the transmission of light through the eye.

The earliest sign of papilledema is a hyperemic disc cause by increased venous pressure. The dilated vessels leak their contents. The fluid leak causes elevation of the disc, which may spread beyond the disc margins, making the edges of the disc appear swollen or indistinct. In glaucoma, one sees a glaucomatous cup. The disc edge appears to be displaced slightly backward, causing a cup shape.

Hemorrhages scattered in the vitreous cavity tend to disperse and absorb light. A red reflex is not seen; only darkness will be seen. This is a common finding in advanced diabetic retinopathy.

LABORATORY AND DIAGNOSTIC STUDIES

Ophthalmoscopy With Pupillary Dilation

Direct ophthalmoscopy allows a view into the retina and optic nerve. More of the peripheral posterior segment is seen when the eye is dilated with a mydriatic drug.

Clue: If the iris seems abnormally close to the cornea, dilation is contraindicated because of the risk of inducing acute-angle closure glaucoma.

Tonometry

A tonometer is a device that measures intra-ocular pressure. Intraocular pressure greater than 21 mm Hg is considered a high-risk factor for glaucoma.

Fluorescein Dye

Fluorescein dye is used to detect the presence of abrasions or a foreign body on the corneal surface. If the corneal epithelium has been disturbed, fluorescein will pool within these areas and stain the hydrophilic stoma. A stain showing a dendritic pattern indicates herpes infection.

DIFFERENTIAL DIAGNOSIS

Early detection and treatment of vision and eye diseases yield immense benefits.

Strabismus and Amblyopia

The most common causes of vision loss in children are amblyopia and strabismus. Amblyopia, or lazy eye, is reduced visual acuity in one eye that is not correctable with lenses. It is caused by incomplete visual system development when a refractive error is not corrected in childhood. Strabismus is a condition in which the two eyes do not point in the same direction when the patient is looking at a distant object. These conditions cause vision loss in 2 out of every 100 children. The risk of the development of amblyopia is greatest during the first 2 to 3 years of life, but the potential for recurrence exists until visual development is complete at 9 years of age.

Refractive Errors

Refractive errors are a common visual disorder of childhood, occurring in 20% of children by 16 years of age. Permanent visual impairment may result if optical correction is not provided at an appropriate age.

Myopia (nearsightedness) is when the cornea and lens of the eye focus the image in front of the retina. Hyperopia (farsightedness) is a refractive error in which the focus of an image is behind the retina. Hyperopia can be corrected to some degree by adjustment of the natural lens (accommodation)

normally done for near-focusing. The use of accommodation can cause visual fatigue, discomfort, and headache.

Astigmatism

Astigmatism is an irregularity in the refractive system of the eye that prevents light from being focused onto the retina. It can be secondary to the shape of the cornea or lens and is usually correctable with lenses.

Cataracts

A cataract is any opacity of the crystalline lens of the eye. There are many causes of cataracts, and they can be defined by onset, cause, or anatomy.

Congenital cataracts are inherited in an autosomal dominant form and are associated with intrauterine infections by the TORCH complex of organisms. Cataracts of infancy and childhood occur in 1 per 1000 live births, and congenital glaucoma occurs in 1 per 10,000 live births.

Adult cataracts are a major cause of visual impairment in the elderly because with time, the human lens begins to develop opacities. Cataracts can be caused by galactosemia, metabolic disorders (e.g., diabetic cataracts), and trauma (e.g., from heat or blunt trauma); steroid-induced cataract formation is also possible. The first sign of opacities is the inability to focus on near objects (presbyopia) and altered color vision.

Optic Neuritis

Optic neuritis occurs more often in younger adults, 20 to 50 years old, and in women; it is typically monocular. It is often idiopathic and may be associated with multiple sclerosis, post viral infection, and granulomatous inflammatory conditions. Vision loss occurs over a few hours to days and is extremely variable. Visual field loss includes central scotoma in 90% of patients. In the majority of patients, pain is present that precedes the vision loss and is worse with eye movement.

Optic Nerve Hypoplasia

This visual disorder affects the optic nerve, the bundle of fibers that transmits signals from the retina to the brain. It is a nonprogressive disorder in which the optic nerve is 25% smaller than the normal size. Some children have a loss of peripheral vision while others lose central vision.

Injury

More than 100,000 eye injuries occur annually in the general population, of which 90% are preventable with the use of protective eyewear. Exposure to long periods of high heat or blunt trauma to the eye globe can result in cataracts.

Retinoblastoma

This is the most common intraocular tumor of childhood; it occurs bilaterally in 30% of cases. A common symptom is strabismus. Retinoblastoma is inherited in an autosomal dominant manner. Early lesions are flat, transparent, or white masses in the retina. The tumor can spread to the brain through the optic nerve or into the bone marrow.

Retinopathy of Prematurity

This condition is seen in premature infants and refers to the changes of ischemia, blood vessel growth, and fibrosis that occur because of inadequate oxygen delivery to the peripheral retina. The vessels of the retina normally complete vascularization by 40 weeks of gestation. Infants who are born before this time may have incomplete vascularization with subsequent poor vessel development and visual impairments. Infants smaller than 1500 grams (g) are at greatest risk.

Central Retinal Artery Occlusion

Patients with this condition have a sudden onset of severe vision loss in one eye. There is no associated pain. The loss is caused by plaque lodging at the level of the lamina cribrosa. On physical examination a few hours after occlusion, the retina becomes edematous and white or opaque. There is a reddish orange reflex from the intact choroidal vascular and foveola that creates a "cherry red spot" that contrasts with the surrounding white retina. With time the retinal artery opens and the retina edema clears.

Glaucoma

Glaucoma is loss of vision because of increased pressure in the eye; it is characterized by defects in the visual field and optic nerve damage and most often associated with an increased intraocular pressure. It is the second leading cause of blindness in the United States. The condition is painless, and symptoms appear in late stages. Ophthalmic examination reveals pathological cupping of the optic disc that may be asymmetrical. Patients with intraocular pressures above 21 mm Hg should be referred to an ophthalmologist (Box 7-2).

Retinal Detachment

This condition occurs when the neurosensory retina is separated from the retinal pigment epithelium. About half of patients will have brief flashes of light (photopsia) or floaters (entopsia). It is caused by a collection of fluid beneath the neurosensory retina, traction from fibrovascular elements associated with diabetic retinopathy, or trauma. Nearly 95% of detachments are treatable.

Macular Degeneration

Age-related macular degeneration is the leading cause of blindness in the United States. It may be asymptomatic or associated with gradual loss of central vision. Risk factors include advanced age, family history, cigarette smoking, hyperopia, and hypertension. There are two forms of pathological macular degeneration. The exudative form results in rapid vision loss caused by the development of a subretinal pigment epithelial neovascular membrane. The nonexudative form is associated with gradual loss of central vision.

Diabetic Retinopathy

Diabetic retinopathy is a retinovascular disease that occurs in two forms. Nonprolif-

Box 7-2	**Adult Vision Screening**

Vision acuity should be assessed intermittently after age 40 with no optimal interval recommended. Routine screening for glaucoma by primary care providers is not recommended.

erative retinopathy is characterized by micro-aneurysms, macular edema, lipid exudates, and intraretinal hemorrhages. In proliferative retinopathy, blood vessels regenerate on the retina. The patient may be asymptomatic or have decreased vision or floaters.

Uveitis

Uveitis is a general term used to describe inflammatory activity of the iris, ciliary body, and choroid. Symptoms vary according to cause and severity, but most patients experience some decrease in vision, light sensitivity, and tearing. Pain may be variable. Acute uveitis lasts less than 3 months, but the condition may have a chronic recurrent pattern.

Optic Nerve Glioma

Optic nerve gliomas are present in two forms. In the adult, they are malignant glioblastomas; in the child, they are benign pilocytic astrocytomas. They appear in children younger than age 10 and are highly associated with neurofibromatosis, a condition associated with café au lait lesions of the skin. In children, gliomas may appear as rapid onset of vision loss with headache. Of the malignant optic nerve gliomas, nearly 75% present with unilateral, rapidly progressive vision loss with pain.

Craniopharyngioma

Craniopharyngiomas are tumors that arise from squamous epithelial cells of the brain. They are most common in the first two decades of life but also may occur in adults 50 to 70 years old. Children's presenting symptoms include headache and visual disturbance caused by increased intracranial pressure. Nystagmus and bitemporal hemianopias are pathognomonic for this tumor. In the older patient, visual deficit is common in the presence of normal optic discs.

Chemical or Thermal Trauma

A chemical burn is an ophthalmic emergency. Alkaline solutions denature eye proteins and lyse cell membranes, allowing the chemical to penetrate the eye. Acid burns may also cause severe damage, but the acid solution precipitates proteins, decreasing the amount of penetration damage.

Congenital Infection

Congenital TORCH infections may cause vision problems in infants. Postnatal screening is performed to diagnose a TORCH infection.

DIFFERENTIAL DIAGNOSIS OF *Common Causes of Loss of Vision*

CONDITION	HISTORY	PHYSICAL FINDINGS	DIAGNOSTIC STUDIES
Strabismus	Family reports child's eyes cross, family history	Extraocular movements abnormal, cover/uncover test positive	Refer
Amblyopia	May have history of premature birth, Down syndrome, cerebral palsy, hydrocephalus	Vision decreased in one eye	Refer
Refractive errors	Sitting close to television, squinting	Loss of visual acuity	Screen with Snellen, Tumbling E, or figures; refer
Cataracts	Blurred vision, glare, distortion and change in color perception, increased age, history of infection, trauma, or chronic disease	Whitish appearance of pupil, bilateral or unilateral	Refer

Continued

DIFFERENTIAL DIAGNOSIS OF *Common Causes of Loss of Vision—cont'd*

CONDITION	HISTORY	PHYSICAL FINDINGS	DIAGNOSTIC STUDIES
Optic neuritis	History of multiple sclerosis, viral infection, pain with eye movement, rapid vision loss	Decreased visual acuity, reduced color perception, afferent pupil defect and central scotoma	Refer
Optic nerve hypoplasia	History of vision loss, may have central vision but no peripheral vision	Optic nerve is one half to one third normal size, pale to gray in color, surrounded by yellow halo	Refer
Injury, penetrating injury	History suggesting head or eye trauma (blunt or sharp)	Directed by history	Refer because of high incidence of penetrating injury
Retinoblastoma	Family history, child 2 years old or younger	Partial or absent red reflex, strabismus	Refer
Nystagmus	History of eyes moving repetitively, searching	Rhythmic, repetitive oscillation of eyes	Refer
Retinopathy of prematurity	Premature birth <36 weeks, 1500 g, oxygen administered, may be a twin	Abnormalities of retinal vessels	Refer
Central retinal artery occlusion	Sudden onset of painless vision loss, may come and go	Macular edema, cherry red spot; may see vessel narrowing	Refer
Glaucoma	Most often painless, gradual vision loss, blurring, and halos; more common in older adults; history of systemic disease	Decreased visual acuity; may have increased intraocular pressure on palpation of eye globe	Refer for tonometry
Retinal detachment	Sensation of flashing light accompanied by shower of floaters; history of trauma to head or face	Retina markedly elevated; appears gray with dark blood vessels; may lie in folds	Refer
Macular degeneration	Older than 60 years, decreased central vision, blue eyes, image larger in one eye	Hyaline (drusen) deposits on retina near macula, gray-green areas of pigment under retina, decreased visual acuity	Amsler grid
Diabetic retinopathy	History of diabetes, floaters, gradual vision loss	Venous dilation, retinal hemorrhages	Refer
Uveitis	History of infection or chronic inflammation, mild to moderate pain, photophobia, tearing	Findings vary according to cause and severity	Refer
Optic nerve glioma	Dimness of vision with loss of fields; may be unilateral rapid vision loss with pain	Visual field defects, optic atrophy	Refer
Craniopharyngioma	Unilateral vision loss, headache, child or adult	Funduscopic examination may be normal	Refer
Chemical burn	History of acid or alkaline exposure	Treat first, then examine	Immediate eye irrigation and referral
Thermal burns	History of exposure to high heat, occupational risk	Corneal opacities	Refer
Congenital infections	TORCH, maternal exposure to measles	Retinitis, optic nerve hypoplasia	Screen for TORCH, refer

CHAPTER RESOURCES

Anonymous: Glaucoma: early detection can minimize vision loss, *Mayo Clin Health Lett* 23:7, 2005.

Coles WH: *Ophthalmology: a diagnostic text*, Baltimore, Md, 1989, Williams & Wilkins.

Harvey PT: Common eye diseases of elderly people: identifying and treating causes of vision loss, *Gerontology* 49:1, 2003.

Norton I: Practical ophthalmology—a survival guide for doctors and optometrists, *Emerg Med Australas* 17:5, 2005.

Thompson L, Kauffman L: The visually impaired child, *Pediatr Clin North Am* 50:225, 2003.

Tierney LM, McPhee SJ, Papadakis MA: *Current medical diagnosis & treatment*, ed 44, New York, 2005, McGraw-Hill.

Common Problems of the Skin

CHAPTER 8

Rashes and Skin Lesions

Dermatological problems result from a number of mechanisms, including inflammatory, infectious, immunological, and environmental (traumatic and exposure induced). At times, the mechanism may be readily identified, such as the infectious bacterial etiology in impetigo. However, some dermatological lesions may be classified in more than one way. Most insect bites, for example, involve both environmental (the bite) and inflammatory (the response) mechanisms. Awareness of the potential mechanism of any skin rash or lesion is most helpful in identifying the risk a person may have for other illnesses. For example, persons with eczema are also frequently at risk for or have other atopic conditions, notably asthma and/or allergies. Thousands of skin disorders have been described, but only a small number account for the vast majority of patient visits.

Evaluation of rashes and skin lesions depends on a carefully focused history and physical examination. For this, the provider needs to be familiar with the characteristics of various skin lesions; anatomy, physiology, and pathophysiology of the skin; clinical appearance of the basic lesion; arrangement and distribution of the lesion; and clinicopathological correlations. Common symptoms associated with specific lesions, such as itching or fever, are also important to know. It is necessary to quickly identify life-threatening diseases and those that are highly contagious. Ultimately, competence in dermatological assessment involves recognition through repetition.

DIAGNOSTIC REASONING: INITIAL FOCUSED PHYSICAL EXAMINATION

Initial Inspection

Dermatological assessment is similar to the assessment of most other body systems in that it depends on patient history and physical assessment. However, sometimes a brief initial physical assessment preceding the history can assist in the development of the initial differential diagnosis, followed by a focused history and further physical examination.

Morphological Criteria

Examination involves the classification of the lesion based on a number of morphological features. Evaluation should be systematic. Generally, each of the following morphological features should be analyzed (examples are listed in Tables 8-1 and 8-2 and Figures 8-1 and 8-2):

- Identify the location of the lesion(s).
- Identify the distribution of the lesions as localized, regional, or generalized.
- Identify whether the lesion is primary (appearing initially) or secondary (resulting from change in a primary lesion).
- Identify the shape of the lesion and any arrangement if numerous lesions are present.
- Describe the margins (borders).
- Describe the pigmentation, including variations.
- Palpate to assess texture and consistency.
- Measure the size of an individual lesion or estimate size if lesions are numerous or widespread.

Table 8-1 Morphological Criteria of Rashes and Skin Lesions

NATURE OF LESION	DESCRIPTION	EXAMPLES
Primary Lesions (develop initially in response to change in internal or external environment of skin)		
Macule	Discrete flat change in color of skin; usually <1.5-cm diameter	Freckle, lentigo, purpura
Patch	Discrete flat lesion (large macule); usually >1.5-cm diameter	Pityriasis rosea, melasma, lentigo
Papule	Discrete palpable elevation of skin; <1-cm diameter; origin may be epidermal, dermal, or both	Nevi, seborrheic keratosis, dermatofibroma
Nodule	Discrete palpable elevation of skin; may evolve from papule; may involve any level of skin from epidermis to subcutis	Nevi, basal cell carcinoma, keratoacanthoma
Plaque	Slightly raised lesion, typically with flat surface; >1-cm diameter; scaling frequently present	Psoriasis, mycosis fungoides
Wheal	Transient pink/red swelling of skin; often displaying central clearing; various shapes and sizes; usually pruritic and lasts <24 hr	Urticaria
Tumor	Large papule or nodule; usually >1-cm diameter	Basal cell carcinoma, squamous cell carcinoma, malignant melanoma
Pustule	Raised lesion <0.5-cm diameter containing yellow cloudy fluid (usually infected)	Folliculitis, acne (closed comedones)
Vesicle	Raised lesion <0.5-cm diameter containing clear fluid	Herpes simplex, herpes zoster, contact (irritant) dermatitis
Bulla	Vesicle >0.5-cm diameter	Bullous pemphigoid, contact (irritant) dermatitis, blisters of second-degree sunburn
Cyst	Semi-solid lesion; varies in size from several mm to several cm; may become infected	Sebaceous cyst
Secondary Lesions (appear as result of changes in primary lesions)		
Crust	Dried exudate that may have been serous, purulent, or hemorrhagic	Impetigo, herpes zoster (late phase)
Scale	Thin plates of desquamated stratum corneum that flake off rather easily	Xerosis, ichthyosis, psoriasis
Excoriation	Shallow hemorrhagic excavation; linear or punctate; results from scratching	Contact (irritant) dermatitis
Lichenification	Thickening of skin with exaggeration of skin creases; hallmark of chronic eczematous dermatitis	Chronic eczema
Erosion	Partial break in epidermis	Herpes simplex or zoster, pemphigus vulgaris
Fissure	Linear crack in epidermis	Xerosis, angular cheilitis, severe eczema
Distribution of Lesions		
Localized	Lesion appears in one small area	Impetigo, herpes simplex (e.g., labialis), tinea corporis ("ringworm")
Regional	Lesions involve specific region of body	Acne vulgaris (pilosebaceous gland distribution), psoriasis (extensor surfaces and skinfolds)
Generalized	Lesions appear widely distributed or in numerous areas simultaneously	Urticaria, disseminated drug eruptions

Continued

Table 8-1	Morphological Criteria of Rashes and Skin Lesions—cont'd	
NATURE OF LESION	**DESCRIPTION**	**EXAMPLES**
Shape/Arrangement		
Round/discoid	Coin or ring shaped (no central clearing)	Nummular eczema
Oval	Ovoid shape	Pityriasis rosea
Annular	Round, active margins with central clearing	Tinea corporis, sarcoidosis
Zosteriform (dermatomal)	Following nerve or segment of body	Herpes zoster
Polycyclic	Interlocking or coalesced circles (formed by enlargement of annular lesions)	Psoriasis, urticaria
Linear	In a line	Contact dermatitis
Iris/target lesion	Pink macules with purple central papules	Erythema multiforme
Stellate	Star shaped	Meningococcal septicemia
Serpiginous	Snakelike or wavy line track	Cutanea larva migrans
Reticulate	Netlike or lacy	Polyarteritis nodosa, lichen planus lesions of erythema infectiosum
Morbilliform	Confluent and salmon colored	Rubeola
Border/Margin		
Discrete	Well demarcated or defined; able to draw a line around it with confidence	Psoriasis
Indistinct	Poorly defined; having borders that merge into normal skin or outlying ill-defined papules	Nummular eczema
Active	Margin of lesion shows greater activity than center	Tinea species eruptions
Irregular	Nonsmooth or notched margin	Malignant melanoma
Border raised above center	Center of lesion depressed compared to edge	Basal cell carcinoma
Advancing	Expanding at margins	Cellulitis
Associated Changes Within Lesions		
Central clearing	Erythematous border surrounds lighter skin	Tinea eruptions
Desquamation	Peeling or sloughing of skin	Rash of toxic shock syndrome
Keratotic	Hypertrophic stratum corneum	Calluses, warts
Punctation	Central umbilication or dimpling	Basal cell carcinoma
Telangiectasias	Dilated blood vessels within lesion blanch completely; may be markers of systemic disease	Basal cell carcinoma, actinic keratosis
Pigmentation		
Flesh		Neurofibroma, some nevi
Pink		Eczema, pityriasis rosea
Erythematous		Tinea eruptions, psoriasis
Salmon		Psoriasis
Tan-brown		Most nevi, pityriasis versicolor
Black		Malignant melanoma
Pearly		Basal cell carcinoma
Purple		Purpura, Kaposi's sarcoma
Violaceous		Erysipelas
Yellow		Lipoma
White		Lichen planus

Table 8-2 | Descriptive Dermatological Terms

LESION*		CHARACTERISTICS	EXAMPLES
Annular		Ring shaped	Ringworm
Arcuate		Partial rings	Syphilis
Bizarre		Irregular or geographic pattern not related to any underlying anatomic structure	Factitial dermatitis
Circinate		Circular	
Confluent		Lesions run together	Childhood exanthems
Discoid		Disc-shaped without central clearing	Lupus erythematosus
Discrete eczematoid		Lesions remain separate Inflammation with tendency to vesiculate and crust	Eczema
Generalized grouped		Widespread Lesions clustered together	Herpes simplex
Iris		Circle within circle; bull's-eye lesion	Erythema multiforme (iris)
Keratotic		Horny thickening	Psoriasis
Linear		In lines	Poison ivy dermatitis
Multiform papulosquamous reticulated		More than one type of shape or lesion Papules or plaques associated with scaling Lacelike network	Erythema multiforme psoriasis Oral lichen planus
Serpiginous		Snakelike, creeping	Cutaneous larva migrans
Telangiectatic		Relatively permanent dilation of superficial blood vessels	Osler-Weber-Rendu disease
Universal zosteriform†		Entire body involved Linear arrangement along nerve distribution	Alopecia universalis Herpes zoster

*Examples of different configurations of skin lesions and their descriptions are contained within Table 8-1. (From Swartz MH: Textbook of physical diagnosis: history and examination, ed 3, Philadelphia, 1998, WB Saunders.)
†Also known as dermatomal.

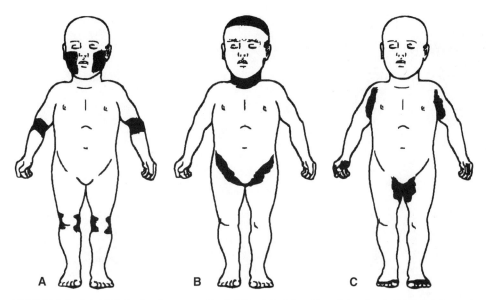

FIGURE 8-1 Typical distribution of papulosquamous eruptions in children. **A**, Atopic dermatitis: usually located on cheeks, creases of elbows, and knees. **B**, Seborrheic dermatitis: usually located on scalp, behind ears, in thigh creases, and in eyebrows. **C**, Scabies: usually located on axillae, webs of fingers and toes, and intragluteal area. (From Berkowitz CD: *Pediatrics: a primary care approach*, ed 2, Philadelphia, 2000, WB Saunders.)

Examination in a systematic manner, and in part before obtaining the majority of the history, provides greater relevance to the data. Gloves are not necessary unless there are open, draining, or exudative lesions.

DIAGNOSTIC REASONING: FOCUSED HISTORY

Is the Rash Associated With an Immediate Life-Threatening Condition?

Key Questions

- Do you have a fever?
- Are you short of breath, or do you have difficulty swallowing?
- Is the rash tender with fever and mucosal involvement?

Fever

Fever is common in viral exanthems (rashes), and the accompanying condition is usually not life threatening. However, fever, irritability, hypotension, and a macular or petechial rash may indicate meningococcemia. Treatment needs to be immediate to be lifesaving.

Allergic Reaction

Urticarial allergic reactions may be associated with angioedema (swelling) of the extremities, face, lips, tongue, and/or airway; cough; wheezing; shortness of breath; or heart palpitations. The sooner symptoms occur after the exposure to the allergen, the more severe is the reaction. Treatment needs to be instituted immediately.

Rash With Fever and Mucosal Involvement

Toxic epidermal necrolysis (Stevens-Johnson syndrome) is a tender, morbilliform, erythematous rash accompanied by fever, conjunctivitis, oral ulcers, and diarrhea. Immediate hospitalization is required to treat exfoliation of large areas of skin. The condition is usually drug induced.

Is the Rash Acute or Chronic (Recurrent)?

Key Questions

- How long have you had this rash?
- Have you ever had a rash like this before?

Macule

Papule

Plaque

Wheal

Nodule

Vesicle

Bulla

Pustule

Cyst

Scale

Excoriation

Fissure

Ulcer

Crust

Atrophy

0   1   2   3   4
cm

FIGURE 8-2 Types of skin lesions. (From Seidel HM, Ball JW, Dains JE, Benedict GW: *Mosby's guide to physical examination*, ed 4, St Louis, 1999, Mosby.)

Onset

The diagnosis of skin lesions is initially aided by categorizing the lesion as acute versus chronic or recurrent. Acute eruptions, such as urticaria or various fungal rashes (tinea), are classified as such because they have a tendency to be self-limiting or to not recur after effective treatment. Chronic rashes, such as psoriasis or eczema, may persist or be recurrent with exacerbations and remissions. Box 8-1 shows common rashes categorized by duration. Ascertain the duration of the eruption at presentation; however, the initial occurrence of a chronic rash may present acutely. Conversely, an acute eruption not optimally treated may present as a chronic problem.

Where Is the Rash in Its Evolution?

Key Questions

- What did this look like initially?
- Has the rash changed? If so, how?
- Has it spread? Where?

Initial Presentation

Most skin lesions evolve over time, although this varies from minutes with urticaria to weeks or even months with psoriasis or mycosis fungoides.

Change in Lesion

Determining whether there has been a change from the initial appearance of a lesion provides diagnostic clues. The eruption of pityriasis rosea classically begins with a "herald patch," a single, scaly, erythematous patch usually on the trunk, followed within days by a regional outbreak of numerous smaller erythematous patches, thus providing a key diagnostic clue. The rash may look like that of ringworm, but it appears too quickly to be ringworm. Another example of evolutionary change is the eruption of herpes simplex virus (HSV), which begins with small vesicles that later umbilicate, possibly ooze, and eventually crust before healing. A rash may appear in different ways, depending on the point at which evaluation is sought.

Spread

The way in which a rash spreads is helpful in diagnosing the specific rash. There are three general ways in which a rash can spread: centripetal, or moving to the center; centri-

---

Box 8-1 | Duration of Rash

Acute	Chronic
Allergic or contact dermatitis	Acne vulgaris
Candida dermatitis (diaper rash, intertrigo)	Bullous pemphigus
Erythema infectiosum (fifth disease)	Eczema
Erythema multiforme	Erythema nodosum
Fixed drug eruptions	Kaposi's sarcoma
Folliculitis	Mycosis fungoides
Herpes simplex virus (HSV)*	Polyarteritis nodosa
Herpes zoster/varicella zoster (HZ)	Psoriasis
Impetigo	Rosacea
Infestations (scabies, pediculosis)	Seborrheic dermatitis
Insect bites	Systemic lupus erythematosus
Kawasaki disease	
Pityriasis rosea	
Septicemia (meningococcal)	
Scarlet fever	
Tinea (corporis, pedis, versicolor)	
Urticaria*	
Viral exanthems (measles)	

*Occasionally recurrent.

fugal, or moving away from the center; and caudal, or moving down.

What Does the Presence of Pruritus Tell Me?

Key Question

■ Does it itch?

Itching

All dermatoses can be classified into three groups: a small group that always itches, those that never itch, and an intermediate group in which itching is variable (Box 8-2). Pruritus is often reported to be worse at night; during the day, pruritus is less troublesome because the patient is distracted by daily routines. It is only at bedtime that the slightest sensation of pruritus becomes overwhelming; this is because the patient is focusing on trying to sleep. Once the patient scratches the area, histamine is released from the inflammatory cells (especially mast cells), and this causes more pruritus and an itch/scratch cycle is established.

Swimmer's itch occurs in areas unprotected by a swimsuit. Sea bather's itch occurs in areas under the swimsuit. Nocturnal pruritus most typically occurs in scabies infestations. Itching in the absence of rash may be an important clue to internal disease.

What Does Associated Pain Tell Me?

Key Questions

■ Is it painful or sore?
■ Does it burn?

Pain

Pain is a rare symptom. The classic painful rash is associated with herpes zoster (HZ), including postherpetic neuralgia, although severe psoriasis or eczema, when associated with fissures and bleeding, may be described as painful by some patients. Soreness is a more common symptom and may be associated with numerous rashes. Tender erythema may be associated with toxic epidermal necrolysis.

Burning

Burning is infrequently reported. It is most notable preceding the rash in herpesvirus infections (e.g., HSV or HZ).

What Do Associated Symptoms Tell Me?

Key Questions

■ Do you have a fever? Sore throat? Headache?
■ How are you feeling in general?

Fever, Sore Throat, and Headache

Fever may be a common presenting complaint in infectious diseases accompanied by rash, such as HZ, erythema infectiosum, scarlet fever, or Kawasaki disease. Similarly, malaise, sore throat, nausea, or vomiting may occur with mononucleosis.

General Health

In a patient with a maculopapular eruption, the two most common causes are drug reaction and viral illness. Inquire about viral symptoms, such as fever, malaise, and upper respiratory tract or gastrointestinal symptoms.

Box 8-2	Itching: Comparison		
Always Itch	**May Itch**		**Never Itch**
Atopic dermatitis	Psoriasis		Warts
Urticaria	Impetigo		Neurofibromatosis
Insect bites	Tinea		Vitiligo
Scabies	Pityriasis rosea		Nevi
Pediculosis			
Lichen planus			
Chickenpox			

Are There Possible Contacts or Sources of Contagion?

Key Questions

- Does anyone with whom you live or have close contact have something similar? If so, how long have they had it?
- Have you traveled recently? Where?
- What do you do for a living? What are your hobbies or leisure activities?
- Do you have any pets? Have you been around animals?

Living Situation

Explore the patient's living situation. The geographic details of his or her daily activities may help provide diagnostic clues, particularly for rashes caused by infectious or infestation mechanisms. Children, in particular, may contract scabies, pediculosis (lice), or impetigo by direct contact in school or daycare.

Travel

A patient may develop a rash weeks or months after a travel exposure. Diseases endemic to other parts of the world may present with rash, such as erythema nodosum, which is common in Southeast Asia, or leprosy, which is common in Africa, Southeast Asia, and South America. Both eruptions may also occur secondary to tuberculosis. Camping trips to wooded areas may result in a bite by a deer tick, causing Lyme disease. The resultant skin eruption in Lyme disease is known as erythema chronicum migrans (ECM), which begins 4 to 20 days after the bite of the tick; only a third of patients remember being bitten.

Other Exposures

Outdoor occupations or leisure activities may expose persons to a variety of rashes and lesions, including insect bites and allergic or contact dermatitis from poison ivy or chemical substances. People exposed to animal skins contaminated with *Bacillus anthracis* can develop cutaneous anthrax, characterized by lesions that evolve from a papule, through a vesicular stage, to a depressed eschar. Sun exposure can also worsen chronic eruptions, such as rosacea or the malar butterfly rash in systemic lupus erythematosus (SLE). Ringworm is common in farmers and ranchers who work with cattle.

Pets

Fleabites produce an urticarial lesion with a central punctum. The reaction is an immunological one, making it different in each individual. Bites are usually on the legs. New lesions may appear daily, and itching is variable but sometimes intense. Fleas on a cat or dog are usually the culprits. An atypical form of scabies may be transmitted from dogs to humans and usually presents only as a single lesion.

Is There Anything That Exacerbates or Triggers the Reaction?

Key Questions

- Does anything seem to make this worse?
- Do you have any known allergies?

Triggers

Patients often easily identify aggravating factors. Any rash involving vasodilation will become more vivid and likely more pruritic with heat exposure, whether via sunlight, sweating, or a hot shower. Localized eruptions, especially on the hands or forearms, prompt many patients to consider chemicals or other products as causes. Persons with eczema whose hands are frequently exposed to water are vulnerable to the development of irritant eczema on the exposed skin. Foods occasionally exacerbate skin lesions. Rosacea is a vasomotor instability disorder characterized by exacerbation with dietary consumption of vasodilators, such as coffee, tea, alcohol, or spicy foods. Stress, whether physiological (e.g., menstruation, pregnancy) or psychological, is widely believed to trigger or worsen many chronic rashes, especially eczema and psoriasis. Stress also may facilitate recurrent eruptions of HSV.

Could This Rash Be Caused by a Medication?

Key Questions

- Are you taking any medications (prescription or over-the-counter medications)?
- Do you have any medication allergies?

Medication

There are four types of dermatological effects of drugs: side effects (e.g., photodermatitis), allergic reactions (e.g., urticaria, fixed drug eruptions, or morbilliform eruptions), commensal skin eruptions (e.g., pityriasis versicolor in a patient on systemic corticosteroids), and worsening of existing skin eruptions (e.g., tinea eruptions mistakenly treated as eczema with topical corticosteroids). Medications used after the onset of a rash may be irritants or sensitizers and worsen the condition.

Is There a Significant Dermatological Family History?

Key Question

■ Does anyone else in your family have chronic skin problems?

Family History

A family history of dermatological problems may add insight to the diagnosis. Atopic disease (atopic dermatitis, asthma, hay fever) tends to cluster in families. Psoriasis, seborrheic dermatitis, and rosacea are also frequently noted to have a familial inheritance pattern. Multiple café au lait spots with a positive family history for neurofibromatosis can help identify children with this dominantly inherited disease.

DIAGNOSTIC REASONING: FOCUSED PHYSICAL EXAMINATION

Look at All the Skin and Mucous Membranes

A "peephole" diagnosis should be avoided; the whole organ should be examined. If the patient is not fully undressed, relevant lesions could be missed. However, it is useful to select one typical well-defined lesion to describe in detail, followed by an orderly and sequential system of examination so that no areas of the body are missed. The feet should always be examined in the presence of hand dermatitis so as not to miss a hypersensitivity reaction to a tinea infection or a concomitant hand tinea. Erythema in dark-skinned persons may be difficult to appreciate; it often is seen as postinflammatory hyperpigmentation.

Inspect for Distribution

Determine if the lesion is widespread or localized, unilateral or bilateral, symmetrical or asymmetrical. Symmetrical lesions commonly have internal causes (e.g., eczema, psoriasis, acne); asymmetrical lesions have external causes (e.g., bacterial or fungal infections, allergic contact eczema). Is the lesion predominantly on the flexor (atopic eczema) or extensor (psoriasis) surfaces? Determine if the distribution is confined either to protected areas or to light-exposed areas, such as in collagen-vascular diseases, photosensitive reactions to drugs, and airborne contact dermatitis. Is the lesion predominantly centrifugal (affecting the extremities, as seen in erythema multiforme, Rocky Mountain spotted fever, and insect bites) or centripetal (sparing the extremities and concentrated on the trunk)? Intertriginous distribution (neck, axilla, groin) is found in candidiasis, some inflammatory fungal infections, and some forms of psoriasis.

Inspect the Mouth

Drug eruptions from sulfonamides, penicillin, streptomycin, quinine, and atropine often have associated mucosal erosions and crusts. Mucosal involvement is common in hand and foot lesions (e.g., hand-foot-and-mouth disease), herpes, and syphilis.

Inspect the Hair

In children, a triad of hair loss, scaling, and lymphadenopathy is diagnostic of tinea capitis. A high index of suspicion is warranted in inner-city urban areas, where the condition is common.

Palpate the Skin

Palpate skin lesions to assess for tenderness, texture and consistency, firmness, fluctuance, and depth. Smooth skin has no felt irregularity. Uneven skin has fine scaling or some warty lesions. Rough skin feels like sandpaper and is characteristic of keratin/horn or crusts. Assessing the superficial skin for texture is done by palpation with the fingertips. Deeper palpation is done using the thumb and index fingers. Soft skin feels like the lips, normal skin like the cheeks, firm skin like the tip of the nose, and hard skin like the forehead. The depth of the lesion determines if it is on the surface or located within the dermis or the subcutaneous tissue. An indurated base is a thickening in the depths of the lesion rather than on the surface.

Palpate the Regional Lymph Glands

Many viral exanthems present with rash and lymphadenopathy. Palpation of the regional lymph glands may be of assistance in the diagnosis if neoplasm is suspected.

Perform an Abdominal Examination

The detection of hepatic or splenic enlargement may assist in the diagnosis of a systemic cause of skin disorders.

LABORATORY AND DIAGNOSTIC STUDIES

Diascopy

Diascopy is used to assess for blanching on pressure and is accomplished by pressing a glass or clear plastic slide on the lesion. Diascopy is most helpful in evaluating purpuric lesions: blood that is outside vessels (as in petechiae) will not blanch, whereas that entrapped within dilated vessels (as in telangiectasias) will demonstrate this phenomenon.

Wood's Light

Long-wave ultraviolet (UV) light is used in the diagnosis of lesions caused by fungal infections. Many, but not all, fungal rashes fluoresce. *Trichophyton,* dermatophytes that are frequently identified in tinea eruptions, do fluoresce; *Microsporum,* which may also be responsible for tinea eruptions, does not.

Skin Scraping and Potassium Hydroxide Preparation

Microscopically examine a sample of cells retrieved from a lesion, assessing for the presence of fungal or dermatophytic spores and hyphae. The lesion should be gently scraped using a scalpel (collect cells from an active area such as the border of the lesion); the cells are treated with a drop of 20% potassium hydroxide (KOH) and then warmed or allowed to stand a few minutes to soften the keratin. The addition of 40% dimethyl sulfoxide (DMSO) to the KOH solution accelerates diagnosis. Chlorazol Black E stain highlights fungal hyphae as dark blue-black against a light gray background.

Tzanck Smear

In a Tzanck smear, an indirect test for herpesvirus infections (HSV, HZ), cells are retrieved by swabbing the base of a lesion (usually a vesicle), smearing it onto a glass slide, and then staining it with Giemsa or Wright's solution. Examined microscopically, the presence of multinucleated giant cells confirms the diagnosis.

Bacterial Culture

In taking a bacterial culture, exudate from a lesion is collected on a sterile swab and then cultured for growth. Gram stain may also be done. Once a bacterial isolate is known, antibiotic sensitivity testing is performed.

Viral Culture

For a viral culture, cells from the base of a lesion (usually a vesicle) are collected on a Dacron swab and cultured for identification of viral infections, particularly HSV or HZ.

Punch Biopsy

In a punch biopsy, a tissue sample is assessed histopathologically for identification. Select a punch size about 2 to 3 mm larger than the lesion or sample an active area if the lesion is large. Gently swirl while exerting slight downward pressure on the punch. When well into the dermis, remove the punch and excise the sample at its base. The defect may be closed with electrocautery or suture(s) or left open to heal by second intention. Place the sample in a preservative such as formaldehyde solution.

Excisional Biopsy

In excisional biopsy, a tissue sample is assessed histopathologically for identification. Excise the entire lesion, usually making an elliptical incision around the lesion beyond its margins. Excise the base and close the defect with sutures or cauterize bleeding vessels. Place the sample in preservative.

DIFFERENTIAL DIAGNOSIS

The following conditions represent many of the most common skin eruptions observed in primary care. Consult a dermatology text for a complete review.

Follicular Eruptions
Acne Vulgaris

Acne presents as a chronic eruption of the pilosebaceous unit, with noninflammatory (open and closed comedones) and/or inflammatory (papules, pustules, cysts) lesions, and is most commonly a problem of adolescents. Its distribution follows that of the sebaceous glands—face, neck, chest, back, and upper arms. Neonatal acne first occurs between 2 and 4 weeks of age, lasting until 4 to 6 months of age. Persistence beyond 12 months may indicate endocrine dysfunction. African Americans and other dark-skinned persons need aggressive treatment to prevent postinflammatory hyperpigmentation.

Rosacea

Rosacea is a vasomotor instability disorder characterized by sebaceous gland hypertrophy, papules, pustules, persistent erythema, and telangiectasias. It shows a predilection for the face.

Infectious Eruptions
Impetigo

Impetigo presents as a superficial pustular, bullous, or nonbullous eruption, followed by crusting (often honey colored). The causative organism is usually *Staphylococcus* or *Streptococcus*. Contagion occurs via direct inoculation. It is typically a localized eruption that may occur anywhere on the body, with a predilection for the face and trunk.

Folliculitis

Folliculitis is a superficial pustular infection of the hair follicles. Causative organisms are usually *Staphylococcus* and occasionally *Streptococcus* or gram-negative organisms, including *Pseudomonas, Klebsiella,* and *Proteus*. It is typically a localized eruption that may occur anywhere on the body, with a predilection for hairy areas and flexural regions.

Furuncle

A furuncle, often referred to as a "boil," is a more extensive infection secondary to a folliculitis (see Folliculitis).

Carbuncle

A carbuncle is an abscess of conjoined or adjacent furuncles (see Furuncle).

Macular and Papular Eruptions
Erythema Infectiosum (Fifth Disease)

Fifth disease, also known as "slapped cheek disease," presents as a systemic illness of sudden onset characterized by a coalescing, red, maculopapular eruption on the face. A reticular eruption occurs on the extremities 2 to 3 days later. The causative organism is parvovirus B19. This is a self-limiting condition.

Children with underlying hemolytic anemia may experience an aplastic crisis.

Measles (Rubeola)

Measles are caused by a viral exanthem, and the systemic illness that results is characterized by a fine, erythematous, morbilliform eruption on the face that spreads rapidly to the trunk and becomes confluent and reticulate. Cough, purulent coryza, photophobia, and fever precede the rash. This is a self-limiting condition.

Rubella

Rubella results from a viral exanthem similar to measles and starts as fine macules and papules on the face and progresses caudally. Lymphadenopathy of postauricular nodes is characteristic of this disease.

Pityriasis Rosea

Pityriasis rosea presents with a rapidly evolving papulosquamous eruption of possible viral etiology. An initial "herald patch" is characteristic, followed within days by numerous faintly erythematous patches on the trunk and upper extremities ("T-shirt and shorts" distribution). The patches demonstrate fine scaling, and mild to severe pruritus may be present. It is more common in the spring and fall and among adolescents. In African American children, the eruption may consist only of occasional oval lesions along the cleavage lines. The remaining lesions are discrete, scattered follicular or nonfollicular papules over the trunk and proximal extremities. The face may also be involved.

Scarlet Fever

Scarlet fever is a systemic illness associated with group A β-hemolytic *Streptococcus* (GABHS) (strep throat). It is characterized by a macular erythema of the face (flushing), except around the mouth (circumoral pallor), followed by a disseminated fine papular erythema (scarlatiniform), which may then desquamate. The rash is intensified in the flexor folds (Pastia's lines). Associated symptoms are sore throat, malaise, fever, circumoral pallor, and a white or strawberry tongue.

Roseola

Roseola is a viral infection caused by human herpesvirus 6 (HHV-6). It is characterized by 2 to 3 days of sustained fever in an irritable infant who otherwise appears well. Mild edema of the eyelids and posterior cervical lymphadenopathy are occasionally seen. After the patient's temperature decreases, a pink, morbilliform, cutaneous eruption appears transiently and fades within 24 hours. This is a self-limiting condition.

Vesicular and Bullous Eruptions
Hand-Foot-and-Mouth Disease

Coxsackievirus A16 is the causative organism of this viral exanthem and systemic illness. Painful mouth ulcers followed by painful white vesicles with a surrounding erythema on the fingers, palms, toes, and soles characterize the condition. Patients usually have a low-grade fever, sore throat, and malaise for 1 to 2 days. Some develop submandibular or cervical lymphadenopathy. This is a self-limiting condition.

Insect Bites

Mosquito and horsefly bites can cause a common blistering reaction that is surrounded by faint erythema, central pallor if swollen, and usually a visible central punctum. The bites may be arranged in groups if they are multiple. The lesions are pruritic and/or sore; the condition is self-limiting.

Herpes Simplex Virus

HSV lesions have vesicles (solitary or grouped) that are surrounded by an erythematous base, with discrete, well-demarcated areas that later crust. The condition is associated with soreness and/or pain and may be preceded by tingling. There is a predilection for lips and genitalia. Recurrences in the same location are common and usually milder.

Herpes Zoster (Shingles)

HZ lesions present as clustered vesicles that are surrounded by an erythematous base, with discrete, well-demarcated lesions that later crust. Intense burning and pain often precede the eruption. There is a predilection for dermatomal distribution.

Varicella Zoster (Chickenpox)

Varicella lesions are discrete vesicles with a disseminated distribution; lesions develop in crops or in succession. Vesicles later crust, and occasionally secondary impetigo develops. The illness is associated with malaise and fever. This is a self-limiting condition.

Fungal Infections
Candidiasis

A yeastlike fungus that produces rashes at a variety of sites causes candidiasis; these rashes are called vulvovaginitis, thrush, intertrigo (groin, axilla, gluteal), and diaper dermatitis. The lesion is an erythematous maculopapular eruption that is well demarcated, occasionally with satellite lesions (pinpoint papules) at the periphery with maceration in moist areas. It is associated with mild to intense pruritus; the causative organism usually is *Candida albicans*.

Tinea

Tinea is a fungal eruption that causes rashes at a variety of sites: body (corporis), foot (pedis), beard (barbae), groin (cruris), and scalp (capitis). Lesions have erythematous scaling areas with a discrete border and central clearing that is often associated with pruritus or soreness. The causative organisms are *Trichophyton, Microsporum,* and *Epidermophyton.*

Pityriasis (Tinea) Versicolor

Pityriasis versicolor is a yeast infection characterized by a macular eruption of many colors, hypopigmentation to hyperpigmentation, and fine scaling. Macules begin insidiously, may take weeks to months to fully develop, and may coalesce. The condition is usually asymptomatic but occasionally pruritic. There is a predilection for a sebaceous gland distribution (neck, trunk). The causative organism is *Pityrosporum orbiculare* (*Malassezia furfur*). Repigmentation may take years or may never occur. Recurrences are common.

Immunological and Inflammatory Eruptions

Eczema

Eczema is a chronic relapsing inflammatory condition that can take several forms (atopic, nummular, or dyshidrotic). Eczema is characterized by erythematous macules, papules, and vesicles that occasionally weep and/or crust. When severe, eczema may be associated with fissuring and bleeding. It is associated with mild to intense pruritus. In dark-skinned persons, scaling and dryness associated with eczema give an "ashy" appearance to the skin.

Contact/Allergic Dermatitis

Contact dermatitis is an inflammatory reaction to many substances (e.g., poison ivy, nettles). Papulovesicular or bullous eruption surrounded by erythema, with weeping of exudate (noncontagious), is characteristic of the condition. It may be associated with moderate to intense pruritus.

Psoriasis

Psoriasis is a chronic, relapsing autoimmune disorder characterized by well-demarcated erythematous plaques, patches, and papules, which typically present with silvery scales. There is a predilection for the elbows, knees, hands, nails (pitting), scalp, and gluteal cleft. The condition may be pruritic

or sore. The lesions may demonstrate Auspitz sign: pinpoint bleeding when the surface is scraped.

Seborrheic Dermatitis

Seborrheic dermatitis is a chronic, relapsing disorder characterized by erythematous scaling patches, which are poorly demarcated and may be pruritic. There is a predilection for the scalp, face, central chest, and genitals. The condition is aggravated by cold weather, dry skin, and stress.

Allergic Reactions
Erythema Multiforme

Erythema multiforme is an immune complex disorder involving the skin and occasionally the mucous membranes. Iris (target) lesions appear on the extremities and desquamation often follows. Common causes include medications (especially sulfonamides, penicillins, barbiturates, salicylates), histoplasmosis, mycoplasma, HSV, mononucleosis, hepatitis B, and malignancies. It is often self-limited. A severe form, Stevens-Johnson syndrome, is characterized by widespread involvement with vesicobullous lesions. It involves the mucous membranes, conjunctiva, and urethra and possibly the lungs, gastrointestinal tract, and kidneys.

Urticaria

Urticaria is characterized by a well-demarcated, usually disseminated, eruption that is evanescent over minutes to about 24 hours. The condition usually has an asymmetrical distribution.

Neoplastic Eruptions
Malignant Melanoma

Melanoma is an aggressive cancer with a tendency for rapid spread and early metastasis. Characterized by asymmetry (half of a mole or lesion does not look like the other half), melanoma has an irregular, scalloped, or not clearly defined border with a color that varies or is not uniform (whether the color is tan, brown, black, white, red, or blue). The diameter is usually larger than 6 mm. However, any change in the size of a mole should be viewed with suspicion. The three most significant risk factors for the development of melanoma include history of melanoma in a first-degree relative, a large number of moles (more than 50 to 100), and atypical moles as designated by biopsy. Other factors that increase the risk of melanoma include adulthood, blond or red hair, blue or light-colored eyes, changed or persistently changing mole, Caucasian race, fair complexion, freckles, personal history of melanoma, immunosuppression, inability to tan, severe sunburns in childhood, and presence of a congenital mole.

Basal Cell Carcinoma

Basal cell carcinoma usually appears as a small, fleshy bump or nodule on the head, neck, or hands. Occasionally, these nodules may appear on the trunk of the body, usually as flat growths. These basal cell tumors do not spread quickly. It may take many months or years for one to reach a diameter of $1/2$ inch. Untreated, the carcinoma will begin to bleed, crust over, and then repeat the cycle. Although this type of cancer rarely spreads to other parts of the body, it can extend below the skin to the bone and cause considerable local damage. The cure rate for basal cell carcinoma (sometimes referred to as nonmelanoma carcinoma) is 95% when properly treated.

Squamous Cell Carcinoma

Squamous cell carcinoma presents as an indurated papule, plaque, or nodule with a thick scale that is often eroded, crusted, or ulcerated. It can be found on sun-exposed skin surfaces, in areas of radiodermatitis, or on old burn scars. Although slow growing, squamous cell carcinomas arising on the lip, mouth, or ears may be associated with regional lymphadenopathy and metastasis. If promptly and properly treated, it has a cure rate of 95%.

DIFFERENTIAL DIAGNOSIS OF *Common Causes of Rashes and Skin Skin Lesions*

CONDITION	CHARACTERISTICS	DISTRIBUTION/ PROGRESSION	ASSOCIATIONS	DIAGNOSTIC STUDIES
Follicular Eruptions				
Acne vulgaris	Comedones and/or papules, pustules, cysts	Face, neck, back, chest, upper arms	Onset of puberty, topical steroids, anabolic steroids, systemic corticosteroids, lithium, phenytoin	Usually none
Rosacea	Flushing, persistent redness, sebaceous hyperplasia, erythematous papules, telangiectasias, ocular involvement in up to 40%	Symmetrical, usually face only; may involve eyes	Topical steroids, systemic corticosteroids	Usually none
Infectious Eruptions				
Impetigo	Vesicular infection; honey-colored crusts and erosions	Face; any area of body with a minor wound, especially excoriated lesions	Scratching as a result of insect bites, atopic dermatitis, scabies	Bacterial culture
Folliculitis	Superficial perifollicular papules and pustules	Any hair-bearing body surface, but especially scalp, beard, legs, axillae	Shaving, hot tubs, contact with mineral oils, occlusive dressings	Bacterial culture

Continued

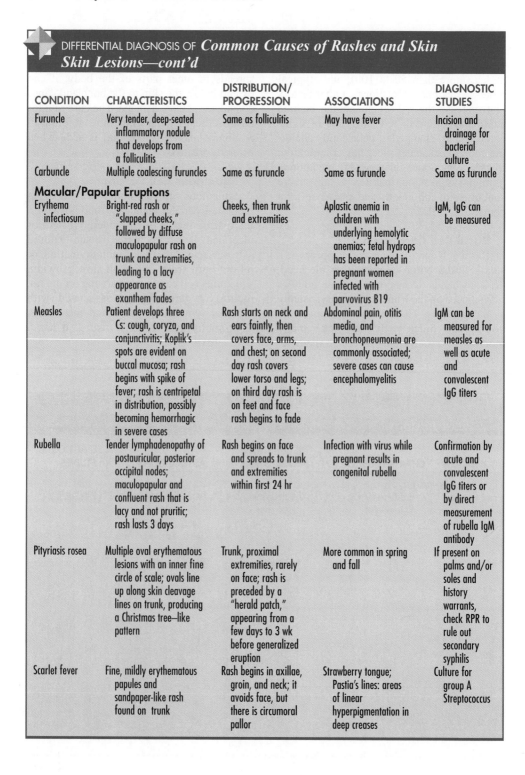

DIFFERENTIAL DIAGNOSIS OF *Common Causes of Rashes and Skin Skin Lesions—cont'd*

CONDITION	CHARACTERISTICS	DISTRIBUTION/ PROGRESSION	ASSOCIATIONS	DIAGNOSTIC STUDIES
Furuncle	Very tender, deep-seated inflammatory nodule that develops from a folliculitis	Same as folliculitis	May have fever	Incision and drainage for bacterial culture
Carbuncle	Multiple coalescing furuncles	Same as furuncle	Same as furuncle	Same as furuncle
Macular/Papular Eruptions				
Erythema infectiosum	Bright-red rash or "slapped cheeks," followed by diffuse maculopapular rash on trunk and extremities, leading to a lacy appearance as exanthem fades	Cheeks, then trunk and extremities	Aplastic anemia in children with underlying hemolytic anemias; fetal hydrops has been reported in pregnant women infected with parvovirus B19	IgM, IgG can be measured
Measles	Patient develops three Cs: cough, coryza, and conjunctivitis; Koplik's spots are evident on buccal mucosa; rash begins with spike of fever; rash is centripetal in distribution, possibly becoming hemorrhagic in severe cases	Rash starts on neck and ears faintly, then covers face, arms, and chest; on second day rash covers lower torso and legs; on third day rash is on feet and face rash begins to fade	Abdominal pain, otitis media, and bronchopneumonia are commonly associated; severe cases can cause encephalomyelitis	IgM can be measured for measles as well as acute and convalescent IgG titers
Rubella	Tender lymphadenopathy of postauricular, posterior occipital nodes; maculopapular and confluent rash that is lacy and not pruritic; rash lasts 3 days	Rash begins on face and spreads to trunk and extremities within first 24 hr	Infection with virus while pregnant results in congenital rubella	Confirmation by acute and convalescent IgG titers or by direct measurement of rubella IgM antibody
Pityriasis rosea	Multiple oval erythematous lesions with an inner fine circle of scale; ovals line up along skin cleavage lines on trunk, producing a Christmas tree–like pattern	Trunk, proximal extremities, rarely on face; rash is preceded by a "herald patch," appearing from a few days to 3 wk before generalized eruption	More common in spring and fall	If present on palms and/or soles and history warrants, check RPR to rule out secondary syphilis
Scarlet fever	Fine, mildly erythematous papules and sandpaper-like rash found on trunk	Rash begins in axillae, groin, and neck; it avoids face, but there is circumoral pallor	Strawberry tongue; Pastia's lines: areas of linear hyperpigmentation in deep creases	Culture for group A Streptococcus

DIFFERENTIAL DIAGNOSIS OF *Common Causes of Rashes and Skin Skin Lesions—cont'd*

CONDITION	CHARACTERISTICS	DISTRIBUTION/ PROGRESSION	ASSOCIATIONS	DIAGNOSTIC STUDIES
Roseola	High fever for 3-4 days in infants and young children; as fever returns to normal, a diffuse maculopapular rash erupts	Rash begins on trunk and quickly spreads to arms, face, neck, and legs	Posterior cervical lymphadenopathy	None
Vesicular and Bullous Eruptions				
Hand-foot-and-mouth disease	Systemic illness caused by coxsackievirus A16; painful white vesicles with surrounding red halo	Painful mouth ulcers followed in 24 hr by painful vesicles on fingers, palms, toes, and soles	Low-grade fever, sore throat, and malaise; cervical and submandibular lymphadenopathy possible	Tzanck smear
Insect bites	Flea bites most common; intensely pruritic eruption, usually in groups of three	Lower legs, but may appear anywhere on body if pets allowed on furniture or beds	Exposure to dogs or cats or to carpeted areas previously in contact with infected animals	Confirmatory biopsy occasionally needed
Herpes simplex virus	Primary infection with grouped vesicles on an erythematous base at site of inoculation; regional lymphadenopathy; may be preceded by prodrome of tingling, itching, burning, or tenderness	Can occur anywhere on body, but most common areas are genitals and thighs, mouth, lips, and chin; may be disseminated in patients who are immunocompromised	Other STDs, HIV; triggered by sun, stress, fatigue, fever, trauma	Tzanck smear, viral culture; screen for other STDs, HIV if history warrants
Herpes zoster	Unilateral pain, itching, or burning preceded by 3-5 days of eruption of vesicles or bullae; followed by crusting and erosions	May occur anywhere on body but is unilateral, following a dermatomal pattern; requires prompt referral to ophthalmologist if eye involved (Note: see lesion on tip or side of nose for indication)	Immunosuppression, older age, local trauma in children	Viral culture (not Tzanck smear)
Varicella zoster	Generalized pruritic vesicular lesions that are in different stages of healing; erythematous vesicles, ruptured vesicles, and crusted vesicles with scabs	Lesions usually begin on trunk and spread to face and proximal extremities	Herpes zoster occurs with reactivation of virus	ELISA titers can confirm acute infection

DIFFERENTIAL DIAGNOSIS OF *Common Causes of Rashes and Skin Skin Lesions—cont'd*

CONDITION	CHARACTERISTICS	DISTRIBUTION/ PROGRESSION	ASSOCIATIONS	DIAGNOSTIC STUDIES
Fungal Infections				
Candidiasis	Beefy-red, well-demarcated plaques, often with scaling edge and satellite lesions; intertriginous areas may also show erosions and maceration	Diaper area in infants, body folds, mucosal surfaces, nails, and nail folds	Immunocompromised, diabetes, steroid inhalants, pregnancy, oral contraceptives, antibiotics, systemic and topical steroids	KOH, culture
Tinea	Variable, depending on body part affected; hair: scaling, hair loss, pustules; skin: red, scaly patch that may develop central clearing; feet: vesicles or bullae	Skin, hair, feet, nails	Immunocompromised, systemic corticosteroids, farmers and others with animal contact, hot humid weather with tight clothing or occlusive footwear	KOH, culture
Pityriasis (tinea) versicolor	Variably colored white to pink to brown scaling, round or oval macules of varying sizes; often coalescing to form large areas of discoloration	Upper trunk, axillae, neck, upper arms, abdomen, thighs, genitals	Heat, humidity, tropical climates, exercise, systemic corticosteroids, seborrheic dermatitis	KOH shows hyphae and spores in "spaghetti and meatballs" pattern
Immunological/Inflammatory Eruptions				
Eczema/atopic dermatitis	Erythema, papules, vesicles, scaling, excoriations, crusts, pruritus always present	Symmetrical; infant: face, flexures; children: flexural creases; adults: may be discrete round patches or be regionalized to specific area	Personal or family history of asthma, seasonal allergies, and eczema; secondary colonization with *S. aureus* or HSV	Serum IgE; culture for bacteria or HSV if indicated
Contact/allergic dermatitis	Vesicles and erosions with edema and inflammation, giving way to crusts and lichenification; pruritus	Localized, often asymmetrical; may be generalized with airborne allergens/poison ivy; linear pattern with plant dermatitis	Occupational, recreational pursuits	Patch testing
Psoriasis	Well-demarcated, ham-colored plaques and papules with silvery scale; chronic, recurrent pruritus is common	Favors elbows and knees, scalp; intertriginous areas may involve nails	Streptococcal infection, arthritis, HIV infection, medications, alcohol, family history	ASO titer or strep culture if indicated; HIV if indicated; biopsy
Seborrheic dermatitis	Chronic scaling, flaking, erythematous dermatitis; variable pruritus	Areas where sebaceous glands are most active: face, scalp, eyebrows, eyelashes, body folds, ear folds, presternal area, mid and upper back, genitalia	Atopic history, HIV infection	HIV if indicated

DIFFERENTIAL DIAGNOSIS OF *Common Causes of Rashes and Skin Skin Lesions—cont'd*

CONDITION	CHARACTERISTICS	DISTRIBUTION/ PROGRESSION	ASSOCIATIONS	DIAGNOSTIC STUDIES
Allergic Reactions				
Erythema multiforme	Hypersensitivity reaction seen as annular target or iris lesions	Begins on upper extremities and trunk	Herpesvirus, *Mycoplasma pneumoniae* infections, drugs (especially sulfonamides)	Skin biopsy may assist in diagnosis if caused by Stevens-Johnson syndrome; chest film for *Mycoplasma*
Urticaria	Transient wheals that may be acute or chronic (lasting >6 wk); individual lesions tend to come and go within hours; pruritic	Localized, regional, or generalized	Angioedema may also be present, may be life threatening; chronic infection, SLE, lymphoma	Biopsy; general medical workup to rule out underlying systemic disease in chronic urticaria
Neoplastic Eruptions				
Malignant melanoma	Asymmetrical border, irregular, has color variation within lesion and is >6 mm	Anywhere on body, including scalp	Usually asymptomatic, unless bleeding, ulceration, discharge present	Skin biopsy, excisional biopsy
Basal cell carcinoma	Papular or nodular lesions, with raised pearly borders and numerous superficial telangiectases	Sun-damaged areas; also seen in covered areas when there is genetic predisposition to basal cell carcinoma	Usually asymptomatic	Skin biopsy
Squamous cell carcinoma	Indurated papule, plaque, or nodule; may be eroded, crusted, or ulcerated	Sun-damaged areas, areas of radiodermatitis, old burn scars; can occur anywhere on body	Usually asymptomatic; can be associated with HPV, immunosuppression, topical nitrogen mustard, oral PUVA, chronic ulcers, industrial carcinogens, arsenic	Skin biopsy, excisional biopsy

STD, Sexually transmitted disease; *HIV*, human immunodeficiency virus; *ELISA*, enzyme-linked immunosorbent assay; *HSV*, herpes simplex virus; *HPV*, human papillomavirus; *SLE*, systemic lupus erythematosus; *PUVA*, psoralen plus ultraviolet A (light therapy); *RPR*, rapid plasma reagin.

CHAPTER RESOURCES

Gable EK: Pediatric exanthems, *Prim Care* 27:353, 2000.

Goroll AH, Mulley AG: *Primary care medicine*, ed 5, Philadelphia, 2006, Lippincott Williams & Wilkins.

Jackson R et al: The diagnosis of skin disease, *Dermatol Nursing* 11:275, 1999.

Jaffe R: Atopic dermatitis, *Prim Care* 27:503, 2000.

McKinnon HD: Evaluating the febrile patient with a rash, *Am Fam Physician* 62:804, 2000.

Morgan-Glenn P: Scabies, *Pediatr Rev* 22:322, 2000.

Reifsnider E: Common adult infectious skin conditions, *Nurse Practitioner* 22:17, 23, 26, 1997.

Sanfilippo AM, Barrio V, Kulp-Shorten C, Callen JP: Common pediatric and adolescent skin conditions, *J Pediatr Adolesc Gynecol* 16:5, 2003.

Common Problems of the Cardiovascular System

Chest Pain

The first task in the evaluation of a patient with chest pain is to determine if the pain is a life-threatening condition, such as ischemic heart disease, aortic dissection, or pulmonary embolism (PE). Myocardial ischemia and myocardial infarction (MI) are life-threatening causes of chest pain and must be assessed rapidly so emergent treatment can be initiated. Aortic dissection is a rare but equally catastrophic cardiovascular cause of chest pain that also must be diagnosed quickly. If acute ischemic heart disease is an unlikely cause, other causes of acute chest pain should be considered, such as pulmonary, gastrointestinal (GI), or psychological conditions, musculoskeletal causes, or other conditions such as pericarditis. A significant proportion of patients whose presenting symptoms include acute chest pain have esophageal spasm or gastroesophageal reflux disease (GERD); however, harmless conditions may mimic more serious disease. Pericarditis and valvular diseases such as aortic stenosis and mitral valve prolapse are less emergent causes of cardiac pain.

Clue: A quick diagnosis of acute myocardial infarction greatly increases the patient's chances of survival.

Pain in any organ or system can be the result of inflammation, obstruction/restriction, or distention/dilation. All pain arising from the GI, musculoskeletal, respiratory, cardiac, and pulmonary systems transmits to the same spinal cord segments, T1 through T5, making identification of the specific origin of discomfort difficult. Many causes of noncardiac chest pain relate to chest anatomy, specifically skin, muscles, ribs and cartilage, pleura, lungs, esophagus, mediastinum, and thoracic vertebrae.

In children, chest pain is rarely associated with serious organic disease. The most common causes of chest pain in children are costochondritis, trauma and muscle strain to the chest wall, and respiratory conditions associated with cough. Chest pain from cardiac disease is relatively rare in children. However, patients and families often associate chest pain with heart disease and can be anxious about the condition because of reports of sudden death in young athletes.

DIAGNOSTIC REASONING: FOCUSED HISTORY

The identification of potentially acute life-threatening situations must be determined immediately. Once you have determined that there is no immediate risk of severe oxygen deprivation to vital organs (e.g., MI, aortic dissection, and PE), proceed with a focused history (Table 9-1).

PE is a life-threatening cause of acute chest pain, accompanied by the sudden onset of dyspnea.

First, Is This a Life-Threatening Condition?

Key Questions

- Can you describe the pain? What does it feel like, e.g., dull, sore, stabbing, burning, squeezing?
- When did it start?
- What were you doing when it started?
- How long have you had the pain?
- What other symptoms have you noticed?

Characteristics of Pain

Typical anginal pain is described as substernal heaviness, pressure, or a squeezing sensation that is provoked by exertion and

Table 9-1	Differentiating Ischemic From Nonischemic Chest Pain	
FACTORS	**ISCHEMIC ORIGIN**	**NONISCHEMIC ORIGIN**
Character of pain	Constricting, squeezing, burning, heavy feeling	Dull or sharp pain
Location of pain	Substernal, midthoracic; radiates to arms, shoulders, neck, teeth, forearms, fingers; interscapular	Left submammary and hemothorax areas
Precipitating factors	With exercise, excitement, stress, after meals	Pain after exercise; provoked by specific body movements or deep breaths

Modified from Selzer A: *Principles and practices of clinical cardiology,* ed 2, Philadelphia, 1983, Saunders.

relieved with rest or nitroglycerin. The substernal pain or discomfort may radiate to the left shoulder and down the left arm and may extend to the neck and lower jaw. An abrupt tearing pain, located in the anterior or posterior chest, characterizes aortic dissection. It may migrate to the arms, abdomen, back, or legs.

PE, pneumothorax, and pneumonia may all present with chest pain. The patient with PE is able to point to the area of pain over the affected lung and usually describes a gripping, stabbing pain that is moderate to severe in intensity. The pain may radiate to the neck or shoulders.

Patients experiencing a pneumothorax most frequently report mild to severe chest pain of sudden onset located in the lateral thorax and radiating to the ipsilateral shoulder. The quality of pain is described as sharp or tearing. Chest pain of pneumonia is located over the area of infiltration and does not radiate. It frequently has a burning or stabbing quality and is associated with cough (see Chapter 12).

Remember that chest pain is subjective and that prior experience, personal attitudes, and cultural values form the patient's perception of pain. The severity of the chest pain may not be an indication of the severity of the condition.

Assessment of the severity of the pain is often made easier by the use of rating scales that use 1 to 10 or happy to sad faces (see Figure 13-1).

Onset of Pain

Onset. Determine if the onset of pain is sudden or gradual and what the patient's

activity was at the time of onset. The typical onset of angina occurs during exercise, exertion, or emotional stress. It is relieved by rest or nitroglycerin. Chest pain of MI may occur at any time and is not relieved by rest or nitroglycerin. Sudden onset of chest pain and dyspnea is common with PE. In a pneumothorax, the patient may report that severe coughing, exertion, or straining suddenly precipitated the chest pain. Chest pain caused by pneumonia occurs gradually over several hours or days. Chest pain in adolescents that occurs after activity but not at any other time may indicate organic cardiac disease.

Most MIs occur in the morning hours, with a peak on Mondays. Patients might also report acute chest pain hours after heavy exertion, such as snow shoveling, other physical activity, or sexual intercourse.

In children, ask about recent choking episodes or swallowing a foreign body when the pain increases with attempts to swallow. Pain that usually occurs when lying down after eating is associated with GERD. Trauma to the chest wall from a fall or strenuous activity may cause rib fractures or chest contusions.

Duration. The most life-threatening conditions produce an acute onset of chest pain. The more chronic the pain, the less likely it is that a specific cause will be found. Intermittent chest pain that occurs frequently probably indicates a more serious problem, such as angina, than one episode of brief, mild pain.

Associated Symptoms

The person experiencing an acute MI frequently reports nausea, vomiting, diaphoresis, shortness of breath, and syncope. PE is often associated with shortness of breath, apprehension, hemoptysis, and chest pain that increases with deep breathing. Fever, cough, and thick sputum production usually accompany chest pain caused by pneumonia.

Does the Patient Have Risk Factors for Coronary Artery Disease?

Key Questions

- How old are you?
- Do you smoke?
- Do you have high blood pressure, diabetes, or heart disease?
- Do you have a history of myocardial infarction?
- Has anyone in your family had a heart attack or stroke before the age of 60?

Risk Factors

According to the report of the U.S. Preventive Services Task Force, clinically significant coronary artery disease (CAD) is uncommon in men under 40 and premenopausal women, but risk increases with advancing age. The presence of risk factors such as smoking, hypertension, diabetes, high cholesterol level, obesity, and family history of heart disease increases the risk of CAD. The National Cholesterol Education Program (2001) identifies the following major risk factors for CAD: cigarette smoking, hypertension, low high-density lipoprotein (HDL) cholesterol level (<40 mg/dl), a family history of premature coronary heart disease, and age (men 45 years and older; women 55 years and older). In addition, a lipoprotein panel after fasting should be obtained that includes low-density lipoprotein (LDL) (<100 mg/dl is optimal) and total cholesterol values (<200 mg/dl is desirable).

If This Is Not a Life-Threatening Condition, What Does a Description of the Pain Tell Me?

Key Questions

- Is the pain acute or chronic?
- What were you doing when the pain first occurred?

- Point to where the pain is located. Does it spread to any other part of your body?
- What seems to trigger the pain?
- Does the pain awaken you from sleep?

Acute or Chronic

Once life-threatening causes of acute chest pain are ruled out, sudden-onset pain may be associated with trauma or musculoskeletal injury or inflammation. Chronic, gradual-onset chest pain is rarely an emergent situation. Chest pain may be the sequelae to an upper respiratory tract infection. Pain from GERD often occurs at night or after a large meal.

Location and Character of Pain

Pain arising from the thoracic skin and other superficial tissues, such as that associated with furuncles, contusions, and abrasions, is sharply localized.

Irritation of the intercostal nerves can result in a neuritis that produces sudden onset of a stabbing, burning pain, and tenderness that is easily located at the intercostal spaces and along inflamed nerves with three maximal pain points: adjacent to the vertebrae, in the axillary lines, and along the parasternal lines. Pain may be severe when the patient breathes deeply, coughs, or moves suddenly.

Dorsal root irritation associated with herpes zoster may present with intense burning or knifelike pain along the spine to the lateral thoracic wall and the anterior midline. This pain may restrict movement of the trunk and respirations. Generally this pain is continuous and increases in severity.

Nerve root pain is caused by mechanical irritation or edema of the nerve root. This pain can be felt at the point of irritation but is frequently referred to points along the peripheral course of the nerve. If the dorsal root is involved, the dorsal radicles in the proximity of the spinal cord are implicated. Thoracic spinal segment root pain is often referred to the lateral and anterior chest wall and is seen with spinal diseases and thoracic deformities.

Costal cartilage that loosens from the fibrous attachment and curls upward off the end of the cartilage on the inner aspect of the rib causes localized pain and tenderness over the eighth, ninth, and tenth ribs on either side. The pain is dull and aching but may be acute, paroxysmal, or stabbing.

Musculoskeletal pain is produced by irritation of tissues and transmitted through the sensory nerves. The stimulus travels through the nerve to the dorsal ganglion up the spinal afferent pathway to the central nervous system.

Bone pain results from irritation of sensory nerve endings in the periosteum and is intense and well localized. Chronic diseases affecting the bone marrow may cause a poorly localized pain of varying severity. Ribs are common sites for metastatic malignant deposits, probably because of their rich vascularity. When metastasis expands to the rib and involves the periosteum, pain results. Referred pain from a nerve dermatome is described as intense, aching, and boring back pain.

When tumors involve the mediastinum, chronic aching or dull substernal chest pain is produced by pressure of the tumor against the spine or ribs.

Lung pain is caused by the involvement of adjacent structures. The trachea and large bronchus are innervated by the vagus nerve (cranial nerve X). The finer bronchi and lung parenchyma are free of pain innervation, and therefore extensive disease may occur in the periphery of the lungs without pain until the process extends to the parietal pleura. Pleural pain results from the loss of normal lubricating function and irritation of the serous membranes of the pleura. Pleuritic pain indicates that the thoracic pathology involves the pleural surfaces. It is a sharply localized, cutting sensation that is accentuated with respiratory movement and is present all the time. Diaphragmatic pleural pain may be referred to the base of the neck or abdomen. Children often report chest pain from tachyarrhythmias because they are unable to differentiate between true pain and the unusual sensation of the arrhythmia. Cardiac causes of chest pain in children are usually associated with congenital anomalies or acquired diseases of the coronary artery such as Kawasaki disease.

Sleep

Distinguish between awakening with pain and awakening from pain. Awakening because of pain signals a more serious problem of organic origin such as cardiac ischemia. Psychogenic chest pain in adolescents commonly accompanies sleep disturbances.

What Do Associated Symptoms Tell Me?

Key Questions
- Do you have a cough or a change in your usual cough?
- Do you bring up sputum? If so, how much and what color?
- Do you have a fever?
- Are you lightheaded or dizzy?
- Do you feel like your heart is racing?

Cough and Sputum Production

Chest pain associated with cough and colored sputum production is usually caused by an acute infection such as pneumonia. Pain results from a pleural effusion or the collection of fluid in the pleural space. Sputum associated with pneumonia can be dark green, rust color, or red. Frequent lower respiratory tract infections can be caused by congenital heart disease with large left-to-right shunts and an increase in pulmonary blood flow. Children and older adults with persistent cough may experience chest pain related to the musculoskeletal strain associated with coughing. Asthmatic persons can develop chest pain from straining of the chest wall muscles caused by tachypnea, coughing, or retraction.

Fever

Fever may indicate pneumonia, myocarditis, or PE. Elderly and immunosuppressed persons may not have fever, even with bacterial infections.

Lightheadedness, Dizziness, or Fainting

Arrhythmias caused by hypoxia, trauma, or electrical shock may cause insufficient coronary blood flow and chest pain. Premature atrial tachycardia (PAT) may cause lightheadedness. Diastole is shortened in PAT, and thus cardiac output is decreased.

Most cases of syncope in adults are caused by cardiac problems such as structural heart disease, arrhythmias, and coronary insufficiency. Most cases of syncope in children are benign and are the result of breath holding, orthostatic syncope, hyperventilation, or vasosyncopal episodes.

Palpitations

Caffeine, stress, and hormonal changes may cause the sensation of a rapid or forceful heartbeat. Mitral valve prolapse may present with a history of palpitations. β-Adrenergic agents or theophylline can cause arrhythmias, including supraventricular tachycardia, which may be perceived as palpitations.

Is the Pattern of Pain Related to Activity and Position Change?

Key Questions

- Describe your recent physical activities.
- Have you had any injury to the chest?
- Does chest movement or position make the pain better or worse?

Recent Activities

Recent strenuous exercise (especially weight lifting) or horseplay can strain the pectoral, trapezius, latissimus dorsi, serratus anterior, and shoulder muscles. Rib fractures and musculoskeletal strains and contusions can cause significant chest pain, especially with movement. Musculoskeletal disorders are the most common cause of chest pain in children and younger adults.

Decreased exercise tolerance may result from significant heart disease such as shunts, arrhythmias, or CAD. In children, congenital coronary anomalies may arise abnormally (as from the pulmonary artery), take an abnormal course, or have fistula connections to other structures, resulting in exertional chest pain. These conditions are rare and difficult to diagnose.

Any episode of moderate to severe chest pain during or after exercise should be investigated as cardiac in origin.

History of Chest Trauma

A careful history of preceding activities should be obtained to detect any recent muscle strain. Posttraumatic pericardial effusion may develop 1 to 3 months after chest trauma. Blunt injury can cause hemothorax, pneumothorax, soft tissue injury, and rib fracture. A ruptured spleen can cause irritation of the phrenic nerve, producing shoulder pain.

Pain With Movement

Pain of cardiac origin, except for pericarditis, is not affected by respiration. Pain on inspiration suggests pleural etiology. A sharp, pleuritic pain relieved by sitting upright and leaning forward suggests pericarditis. Pain that is aggravated by chest wall movement, especially along the sternal border, is most frequently costochondritis; adults and children may experience this inflammatory condition of the costal cartilage. Lying flat, consuming alcohol, taking aspirin, eating spicy meals, and wearing tight clothing often precipitate the pain of esophagitis. Frequently, patients report that this pain occurs after lying down following eating a meal.

Is There a Gastrointestinal Origin for the Patient's Chest Pain?

Key Questions

- Does the pain get better or worse from eating?
- Do you have blood in your stools?
- Have you vomited any blood?

Food Association

Differentiating between esophageal and cardiac origin of chest pain can present a challenge because the character and location of the pain may be very similar. Nitroglycerin may relieve both the pain of angina and the pain of esophagitis. In these instances, an electrocardiogram may be indicated.

Esophagitis is the most frequent GI cause of chest pain. Patients describe this pain as "heartburn," or a dull, burning sensation in the epigastric and retrosternal area. The esophagus is more pain sensitive in its proximal portion. Therefore chest pain that is temporally related to eating meals or particular foods should suggest esophagitis.

Associated symptoms of a sour taste in the mouth and mild nausea may or may not be associated with esophagitis. An esophageal tear or spasm causes more acute, severe chest pain, described as a "tearing" or "crushing" sensation. Frequently the patient experiencing pain of GI origin will report mild to moderate chest pain occurring intermittently over days to months.

Peptic ulcer and cholecystitis may cause chest pain intermittently. Hematemesis (blood in the emesis) or hematochezia (blood in the stool) frequently accompanies peptic ulceration. Cholecystitis is frequently reported as right anterior chest pain that radiates to the shoulder or upper back.

Acute pancreatitis should be considered if the chest pain is excruciating and constant, and reported in the left upper quadrant of the abdomen radiating to the chest, shoulder, and arm. Pancreatitis is often accompanied by hypotension. Physical examination and diagnostic tests are necessary to differentiate it from chest pain of cardiovascular origin.

Could This Pain Be From a Systemic Cause?

Key Questions
- Do you have any skin problems?
- Do you have any chronic health problems?

Skin Symptoms
If the patient reports persistent unilateral chest pain of pruritic, burning, or stabbing quality, consider herpes zoster. This pain will follow the distribution of a cervical or thoracic nerve root. A vesicular rash in the area of pain is characteristic; this rash occurs several days after the occurrence of chest pain.

Systemic Conditions
Chest muscle pain may be caused by localized inflammation of the muscles in collagen diseases such as polymyositis, fibromyalgia, or systemic lupus erythematosus. Arthritic inflammatory changes of the cervical and thoracic spine and shoulders may produce upper chest pain. This pain is aggravated by range of motion of the affected joints.

Sickle cell disease (SCD) may cause chest pain. In sickle cell anemia, the erythrocytes become rigid and "sickle," leading to capillary occlusion and sickle cell crisis. The heart increases the stroke volume to compensate for the anemia. The heart gradually dilates and heart failure ensues. Chest pain in a patient with SCD can also originate from acute coronary syndrome (ACS). In this condition, chest pain, fever, dyspnea, and cough are caused by infarction of lung tissue or an infectious agent.

Marfan syndrome is a hereditary connective tissue disease. Cardiovascular involvement occurs in more than 50% of persons by age 21. Mitral valve involvement is common, with auscultatory findings of mitral regurgitation and mitral valve prolapse. Marfan syndrome is associated with an increased risk for aortic dissection.

What Does the Family History Tell Me?

Key Questions
- Has anyone in your family had heart disease, chest pain, or sudden death from cardiac arrest?
- Has anyone in your family been born with heart problems?

Family History
History of congenital heart disease in close relatives increases the chances of its occurrence in a child. When one child has the condition, the risk of siblings having the condition increases by one third. Essential hypertension and CAD show a strong family pattern. Hypertrophic cardiomyopathy has a positive family history with autosomal dominant transmission in one third of patients.

What Is the Emotional State of the Patient?

Key Questions
- In the past 6 months, have you had a spell or an attack in which you suddenly felt frightened, anxious, or very uneasy?

■ In the past 6 months, have you had a spell or an attack in which for no apparent reason your heart suddenly began to race, you felt faint, or you could not catch your breath?

Panic Disorder

Two questions can be a highly sensitive screen for panic disorder. A "yes" answer to either of the preceding questions is a positive screen for panic disorder. Patients with anxiety or depression often describe feelings of chest heaviness or tightness that can last for days, unrelated to exertion or rest. Patients may also report difficulty taking a deep breath.

DIAGNOSTIC REASONING: FOCUSED PHYSICAL EXAMINATION

A focused physical examination of the patient experiencing chest pain will provide objective data for the assessment. A thorough examination of the cardiovascular, pulmonary, upper GI, and upper body musculoskeletal systems is essential.

Clue: The electrocardiogram (ECG) greatly improves the accuracy of the diagnosis of acute chest pain and should be obtained early in the assessment if cardiac causes are suspected.

Observe General Appearance

Initial observation of the patient will provide clues to the severity of the problem. Observe the patient for grimacing, diaphoresis, pallor, cyanosis, tachypnea, use of accessory muscles for breathing, splinting of chest wall, and unequal chest wall excursion. Persons experiencing an MI may be diaphoretic, pale, and anxious. Patients manifesting PE appear diaphoretic and anxious; respirations are rapid; splinting of the chest is common; and peripheral cyanosis may be present. Persons with fractured ribs or significant chest wall contusions splint their chest walls and take shallow breaths to avoid aggravating pain with respiratory expansion.

Observe the height and weight of a child. Abnormal findings for age may indicate chronic disease.

Measure Vital Signs and Respiratory Patterns

Vital signs for persons experiencing angina may be within normal ranges. Frequently, however, with acute MI, blood pressure is elevated and cardiac arrhythmias are present. If cardiogenic shock ensues, hypotension will occur.

The patient with aortic dissection may be hypotensive with unequal peripheral pulses. Pericarditis may be accompanied by fever, rapid and shallow respirations, and hypertension. Myocarditis may present with fever, respiratory distress, and paradoxical pulse.

In heart failure, decreased stroke volume reduces the systolic blood pressure, and compensatory vasoconstriction maintains a constant diastolic pressure. This may result in a decreased pulse pressure.

Pneumothorax is manifested by tachypnea and unequal chest wall excursion. The patient with pneumonia may also be tachypneic, with signs of infection that include fever and a productive cough.

In children, chest pain with tachycardia and hypotension is generally caused by hypovolemia secondary to a hemothorax, hemopneumothorax, or vascular injury. Pain may also be caused by rhythm disturbance.

The rate, rhythm, and depth of respirations in patients experiencing costochondritis, GI disease, or herpes zoster are not usually altered.

Hyperventilation can cause chest pain as a result of hypercapnic alkalosis or coronary artery vasoconstriction. Most hyperventilation is associated with a stressful event or emotional upset; however, aspirin overdose, severe pain, and diabetic ketoacidosis may be organic causes.

Inspect the Skin

Cool, pale, moist skin may accompany an acute MI, PE, or aortic dissection. Observe the skin overlying the area of chest pain for signs of a vesicular rash of herpes zoster. Petechial rash on the face and shoulders may be a sign of protracted coughing as a result of pneumonia, asthma, or upper respiratory tract infection. Bruises may indicate trauma or abuse.

Sweat on the forehead of an infant may indicate congenital heart disease (CHD). A decrease in cardiac output causes a compensatory sympathetic overactivity, resulting in a cold sweat on the forehead. Examine the color of the mucous membranes, conjunctivae, soft palate, lips, and tongue for central cyanosis.

Palpate Trachea and Chest

Tracheal shift can occur with pneumothorax and, in children, with atelectasis involving a significant portion of one lung. To assess the trachea for lateral displacement, position your index finger first on the right side of the suprasternal notch and then the left. If the trachea has shifted to the side, you will feel the wall on one side but only soft tissue on the other. In a pneumothorax, the trachea is deviated to the opposite side during exhalation and toward the side of the pneumothorax during inspiration. The trachea is displaced toward a lung that is atelectatic, with the displacement exaggerated during inspiration.

Palpate the entire chest wall for tenderness, depressions, or bulges. Fractured ribs and contusions will result in tenderness to palpation and possible deformity. Palpate each costochondral and chondrosternal junction. Costochondritis will be manifested by pain with palpation over the cartilage between the sternum and the ribs. Palpation and range of joint motion may elicit arthritis pain in the shoulder or cervical spine. Musculoske-

letal chest pain is usually reproduced with palpation or by moving the arms and chest through a variety of positions. Subcutaneous emphysema may be palpable at the neck or upper chest wall. Rib pain on palpation in children without a reported history of trauma may indicate child abuse.

To check the chest wall for symmetry, first test for diaphragmatic excursion of both the anterior and the posterior thorax between the eighth and tenth ribs. As the patient takes a deep breath, each hand should move the same distance from the spine. Pneumothorax, pneumonia, and fractured ribs may alter this finding.

Percuss the Chest

Percussion in the area of pneumothorax will result in a hyperresonant sound of an air-filled cavity. Areas of infiltration, as in pneumonia, will produce a dull or flat sound.

Auscultate Breath Sounds

Instruct the patient to breathe through the mouth slowly and deeply. Auscultate systematically from the lung apexes to the lower lobes anteriorly, posteriorly, and laterally (Table 9-2).

Auscultation of bronchial or bronchovesicular breath sounds over the peripheral lungs may indicate consolidation. If breath sounds are diminished over all lung fields, suspect chronic obstructive pulmonary disease (COPD). Obese patients may have

Table 9-2	**Normal Breath Sounds**		
BREATH SOUND	**LOCATION**	**QUALITY**	**INSPIRATION/EXPIRATION RATIO**
Bronchial	Heard on chest over sternum and on back between scapulae	Loud, high pitched	Expiration longer than inspiration
Bronchovesicular	Heard over bronchi at first and second intercostal spaces anteriorly and between scapulae posteriorly	Loud, medium pitched	Equal inspiratory and expiratory phases
Vesicular	Heard over most of peripheral lung fields	Soft, low pitched	Inspiration longer than expiration

breath sounds that are difficult to auscultate. Breath sounds will be inaudible in areas of pneumothorax.

Auscultate for Adventitious Sounds

Adventitious lung sounds are superimposed on normal sounds and can be auscultated over any area of the lung field during inspiration or expiration. Documentation of abnormal lung sounds should include the type of sound heard, location, and changes during both inspiration and expiration phases of respiration.

Crackles or rales are discontinuous popping sounds heard most often during inspiration. Any disease process that increases peripheral airway resistance, obstructs the peripheral airway, or causes a loss of elastic recoil will produce crackles. They indicate the presence of fluid, mucus, or pus in the smaller airways. Fine crackles are soft and high pitched. Medium crackles are louder and lower pitched. Crackles may be heard over the site of a PE.

Wheezing is frequently described as a whistling sound and can be heard during inspiration, expiration, or both. The sound is high pitched and musical. Wheezing indicates that there is fluid in the large airways, such as in severe heart failure; more often it is associated with bronchospasm, as seen in asthma. Wheezing occurs on exhalation because that is when small airways collapse. During inhalation, the negative pressure in the chest tends to hold open the airways. However, during exhalation, positive pressure in the alveoli is conducted from the outside of the small airways and tends to collapse them. The sound is usually polyphonic; this means that multiple slightly different high-pitched sounds are heard at the same time. Most of the causes of wheezing affect many small airways at the same time; each one collapses at a slightly different time, creating a slightly different tone. The presence of a single-tone wheeze suggests a single area of blockage, such as with a foreign body. A prolonged expiratory phase of respiration is produced by intrathoracic airway obstruction associated with lower respiratory tract involvement.

Rhonchi are continuous, deep-pitched, coarse breath sounds usually heard during expiration. They are generated by turbulent air passing through secretions in large airways. Rhonchi may be present when the patient has pneumonia.

Pleural friction rub is a grating or squeaking sound heard in the lateral lung fields during inspiration and expiration. It indicates that inflamed parietal and visceral pleural linings are rubbing together.

If abnormal lung sounds are detected, additional auscultation for bronchophony, egophony, and whispered pectoriloquy are indicated (see Chapter 11).

Auscultate Heart Sounds

Auscultate for normal heart sounds in all positions, identifying S_1, S_2, rate, and rhythm. Identification of myocardial ischemia cannot be reliably performed by physical examination alone. An ECG or stress ECG must be obtained to assess electrical conduction and the condition of myocardial function. Abnormal sounds, such as a new, transient, paradoxical S_2 during pain, are a useful sign of coronary ischemia. A transient, paradoxical S_2 could indicate a transient left ventricular dysfunction, chronic heart failure, or left bundle-branch block. A transient S_3 (ventricular gallop) or mitral regurgitation murmur at the apex can occur occasionally with myocardial ischemia or congestive heart failure. An S_4 (atrial gallop) typically indicates a stressed heart, which may be the result of hypertension, MI, or CAD causing heart failure. A summation gallop is the result of an S_3, S_4, and rapid rate; this may also occur with heart failure. Abnormal rhythms, including tachycardia, bradycardia, and irregular rhythms, are often heard during MI. ECGs are necessary to identify the specific rhythm.

Also note any murmurs and their location, grade, and radiation. Incompetent heart valves produce murmurs and may be the cause of heart failure. In children, a loud murmur, best audible at the upper right sternal border or upper left sternal border with a thrill, may indicate a congenital heart defect.

Aortic diastolic murmur may be present with a dissecting aorta.

Midsystolic click/late systolic murmur (honk) is heard with mitral valve prolapse. The patient must be examined in both the supine and upright positions to elicit the characteristic sounds.

Observe the Spine for Evidence of Scoliosis

Persons with scoliosis are at increased risk for pulmonary problems because of structural variations that may cause compression of intrathoracic contents.

Examine the Abdomen

Auscultate for bowel sounds. Palpate the abdomen for tenderness and masses. Epigastric pain with palpation may occur with esophagitis or peptic ulcer disease. Cholelithiasis or cholecystitis may be manifested by pain on palpation in the right upper quadrant. Pancreatitis may produce left upper quadrant tenderness.

Examine the Extremities

Clubbing of the fingers may be an indication of chronic hypoxia resulting from congenital heart disease in children or COPD in adults. Peripheral cyanosis indicates hypoxia if accompanied by central cyanosis. Consider exposure to a cold environment or anxiety if peripheral cyanosis is observed. Lower extremity edema is a sign of heart failure or venous stasis. Note the progression of the edema or whether there is pitting edema up the leg.

Absent peripheral pulse(s) may be a sign of atherosclerotic vessel disease or dissecting aortic aneurysm. Compare the quality of the pulses bilaterally.

LABORATORY AND DIAGNOSTIC STUDIES

Diagnostic tests are usually indicated when cardiovascular, pulmonary, or GI pathology is the suspected cause of chest pain. Musculoskeletal and neurological causes of pain usually do not require diagnostic tests.

Electrocardiogram

An ECG can add objective data to the diagnostic process in evaluating chest pain. ECGs are most valuable when there is a previous ECG with which to compare the findings or when serial ECGs are obtained. ST segment elevation or depression indicates the presence of injured myocardium. T wave inversion will demonstrate the presence of ischemia. The appearance of both strongly supports ischemia but is not diagnostic of CAD. Arterial spasm, pericarditis, and electrolyte imbalance can also cause these variations from normal. Q waves are indicative of myocardial muscle loss but are not diagnostic of CAD.

Evidence of ischemia is not always obvious on an ECG even when the patient is reporting anginal pain.

Treadmill Exercise Testing

Persons experiencing intermittent chest pain who have a normal ECG and are not taking digoxin should have an exercise stress ECG for diagnostic and prognostic purposes. Treadmill exercise testing uses a standardized protocol of increasing workload with continuous ECG recording. Stress tests provide information on myocardial function determined by blood flow. An important objective of stress testing is to identify patients who have a high risk of severe (left main or three-vessel) CAD. The sensitivity of the test ranges from 65% to 70%.

Exercise Myocardial Perfusion Imaging

This imaging has greater accuracy than the standard treadmill test when the resting ECG is abnormal. Because of its higher sensitivity, the test is able to localize and characterize the extent of myocardial ischemia and to provide direct measurement of other variables, such as left ventricular function. This test is more costly than a treadmill test.

Cardiac Enzymes

Levels of creatinine kinase-MB (CK-MB) isoenzyme rise above normal within 4 hours after an MI and will peak at around 24 hours. The patient who has had an MI will have a CK-MB result that is five or more times the normal value. Cardiac troponins T and I are sensitive and specific markers of myocardial injury and are more predictive of future coronary events. Levels of cardiac troponins

T and I are affected less than those of CK-MB in the first 12 hours following an acute MI but the troponin levels remain elevated for 7 to 10 days after the cardiac event.

Echocardiography

An echocardiogram is a noninvasive test for examining the heart that provides information about the position, size, and movements of the valves and chambers as well as the velocity of blood flow by means of reflected ultrasound. This test is used to determine biological and prosthetic valve dysfunction and pericardial effusion, to evaluate velocity and direction of blood flow, to furnish direction for further diagnostic study, and to monitor patients with cardiac disease over an extended period.

Ventilation/Perfusion Lung Scan

With PE, the blood supply distal to the embolus is restricted. Imaging will show poor or no visualization of the affected area. The ventilation scan demonstrates movement or lack of movement of air in the lungs. The perfusion scan demonstrates blood supply to the affected area of the lungs. The ventilation/perfusion scan is reported as one of three categories: normal, high probability, and nondiagnostic. A normal scan is characterized by even distribution of the radiotracer throughout both lungs and rules out significant pulmonary emboli; no additional diagnostic tests are required. A high-probability scan is represented by multiple segmental or larger defects with normal ventilation in at least one area of abnormal perfusion. This is also known as a ventilation/perfusion mismatch. When a scan does not fit into either the normal or the high-probability category, the study is considered to be nondiagnostic, and further investigation is required.

Pulmonary Angiography

A pulmonary angiogram (arteriogram) is necessary if an embolectomy is considered. Radiographic contrast medium is injected into the pulmonary arteries, and the vasculature is visualized. This test can detect emboli as small as 3 mm in diameter. The test sensitivity is 98%, and the specificity is 96%. This test is the gold standard for diagnosing PE, but it is expensive and carries a small risk of cardiac arrhythmias, anaphylaxis, and death.

Arterial Blood Gases

Arterial blood gases (ABGs) are obtained to detect respiratory alkalosis resulting from hyperventilation, decreased carbon dioxide pressure (Pco_2), and sometimes decreased oxygen pressure (Po_2) (hypoxemia). Hypoxemia often correlates with the extent of the lung area occluded in a PE.

Radiography

Pneumothorax and pneumonia can be identified by chest radiography. Pneumothorax reveals evidence of pleural air, whereas pneumonia is seen on radiographs as a parenchymal infiltrate. Chest radiography with suspected PE is usually nonspecific; it may be normal or an elevated hemidiaphragm or pulmonary infiltrate may be present. Rib radiographs will confirm rib fracture.

Cervical and thoracic spine and shoulder radiographs may show degenerative joint changes.

Computed Tomography (CT) Scanning

Computed tomography (CT) scans produce cross-sectional images of anatomical structures without superimposing tissues on each other. They show the different characteristics of tissue structures within solid organs. Aortic dissections and tumors of the lung and pancreas can be detected with CT scans.

Magnetic Resonance Imaging

Magnetic resonance imaging (MRI) is a noninvasive technique that produces cross-sectional images of the body through exposure to magnetic energy sources. It does not involve radiation and is used to differentiate healthy and diseased body tissues. It is useful in detecting tumors, infection sites, and diseased vessels.

Activated Partial Thromboplastin Time and Prothrombin Time

Activated partial thromboplastin time (aPTT) is a clotting test that screens for coagulation disorders and is used to monitor the effectiveness of heparin therapy. Prothrombin time (PT) measures a potential defect in stage II of the clotting mechanism through analysis of the clotting ability of five plasma coagulation factors. PTs are commonly ordered to measure the effects of oral anticoagulant therapies. Ineffective anticoagulation therapy places the patient at risk for PE. These tests may also be ordered to search for the cause of PE.

Serum Amylase and Lipase

Amylase is an enzyme that helps convert starch to sugar; it is produced in the pancreas, liver, salivary glands, and fallopian tubes. If there is inflammation of the pancreas or salivary glands, increased levels of amylase enter the bloodstream. Lipase is the enzyme responsible for the breakdown of fats to fatty acids and glycerol. The pancreas is the main source of lipase. Pancreatic damage results in elevated serum lipase levels. Therefore, determining the levels of serum amylase and lipase is useful in the diagnosis of pancreatitis. Amylase levels return to normal before lipase levels.

Abdominal Ultrasound

Abdominal ultrasound is a noninvasive procedure to visualize solid organs. It is useful in detecting masses, fluid collections, and infection. Pancreatitis and gallbladder disease may be detected with ultrasound.

Bronchoscopy

Bronchoscopy permits visualization of the trachea, bronchi, and select bronchioles. It is useful to diagnose tumors, hemorrhage, and trauma; to obtain brushings for cytological examinations; and to remove foreign bodies from the lower respiratory tract.

Complete Blood Cell Count

A complete blood cell count is obtained to detect an elevated white blood cell count that occurs with infection. Hemoglobin and hema-

tocrit levels are useful if anemia is suspected as an underlying cause of chest pain.

Esophageal pH

When GERD is suspected, 24-hour esophageal pH monitoring is performed to document pathological acid reflux.

Endoscopy

Upper endoscopy with biopsy is necessary to document the type and extent of tissue damage in GERD. A normal endoscopy, however, does not rule out mild gastric reflux disease.

Erythrocyte Sedimentation Rate

The erythrocyte sedimentation rate value will be elevated with inflammation, such as in arthritis and pericarditis. The test is not specific for a particular disease.

DIFFERENTIAL DIAGNOSIS

Common Causes of Emergent Chest Pain

Acute Myocardial Infarction

Assessment of the patient experiencing acute chest pain must first focus on the potential diagnosis of MI to facilitate prompt initiation of treatment to limit infarct size. The patient with an acute MI generally describes a sudden onset of pain at rest. It is a persistent, often severe, deep, central chest pain and may radiate, as does angina, to the throat or neck, across both sides of the chest to the shoulder, and/or down the medial aspect of either or both arms. Rest or nitroglycerin does not relieve the pain. The chest pain is often associated with a number of other nonspecific noncardiac complaints, such as shortness of breath, nausea, vomiting, and diaphoresis.

The quality of the pain or discomfort may be similar but is generally more intense than any previously experienced anginal symptoms. Patients may also express a sense of impending doom. Quick review for positive risk factors (older than 45 years for men and older than 55 years for women, cigarette smoker, hyperlipidemia, hypertension, diabetes, obesity, history of CAD, family history of CAD) is useful. There may be some objective evidence of an MI, including skin pallor, cool diaphoretic skin, and possible transient paradoxical S_2. The patient may be hypertensive or hypotensive.

The patient experiencing severe chest pain or suspected of having an MI should be placed on a cardiac monitor as soon as possible. Observe for premature ventricular contractions and classic electrocardiographic changes that indicate MI, including ST segment elevations, T wave inversions, and Q waves. Performing a 12-lead ECG and determining levels of cardiac isozymes will help confirm or rule out an MI.

Aortic Dissection

The patient often is in a great deal of distress, describing the unrelenting chest pain as ripping and tearing and radiating to the interscapular region, jaw, neck, or lower back. Physical examination reveals severe hypertension and unequal or absent peripheral pulses. Chest radiography demonstrates a wide mediastinum with extension of the aortic wall beyond the calcific border. A CT scan or MRI may be ordered, but aortography remains the gold standard. Patients with suspect aortic dissection should be referred for emergent care.

Acute Coronary Insufficiency

Acute coronary insufficiency refers to those situations in which chest pain is caused by lack of oxygen to the myocardium but there is no evidence of infarct. The patient reports severe, oppressive, constricting, retrosternal discomfort lasting longer than 30 minutes. The patient may report prior history of MI or angina. The ECG may show intermittent ischemic changes or be normal. Cardiac isozymes are normal.

Pulmonary Embolus

Patients presenting with PE usually report sudden onset of severe sharp, crushing, nonradiating chest pain if there is an embolus impacted in a major artery. Infarction of the pulmonary parenchyma closer to the pleural surface will cause pleuritic chest pain. This pain is most often accompanied by the sudden onset of dyspnea and hemoptysis. Patients frequently express feelings of impending doom.

A review of risk factors will likely reveal one or more of the following: older age, prior venous thromboembolism, prolonged immobility or paralysis, cancer, heart failure, other chronic disease, pelvic or lower extremity surgery, recent pregnancy or delivery, obesity, oral contraceptive use, or varicose veins. Physical findings include restlessness, tachycardia, tachypnea, fever, diminished breath sounds, crackles and/or wheezes, and possible pleural friction rub. There may be signs of thrombophlebitis of the extremities. Initial diagnostic tests should include chest radiograph and ECG; these may both be normal but if clinical signs still point to PE, referral for consultation and further tests, including ABGs, venous Doppler studies, ventilation/perfusion scans, and pulmonary angiography, are indicated.

Pneumothorax

Pneumothorax can be a life-threatening event, especially if the patient has underlying COPD or asthma. The patient reports sharp or tearing chest pain that may radiate to the ipsilateral shoulder. Sudden onset of shortness of breath is also associated with spontaneous pneumothorax. Objective findings include decreased or absent breath sounds on the affected side, tachycardia, tachypnea, and possible deviated trachea. A chest radiograph is needed to evaluate the possible complete or partial collapse of the lung.

Arrhythmias

Patients report palpitations and/or forceful heartbeats. These arrhythmias can be the result of myocardial ischemia, cocaine abuse, or conditions such as prolapsed mitral valve or anxiety. Syncope associated with palpitations indicates a more serious cardiac arrhythmia.

Congenital Coronary Anomalies

The coronary arteries may arise abnormally, take an abnormal course, or have fistulous connections to other structures, resulting in exertional chest pain that may lead to sudden death in the young athlete. The child or adolescent may have a history of moderate to severe chest pain during or after exercise. Family history of sudden death at an early age, heart disease, or seizures, a prior history of lightheadedness or loss of consciousness during exercise, and tall and lanky body type, with double-jointedness, are risk factors. Referral to a pediatric cardiologist is warranted.

Common Causes of Nonemergent Chest Pain

Stable Angina

Stable angina refers to chest pain typically described as substernal chest pressure or heaviness, radiating to the left shoulder and arm, neck, or jaw. The pain onset is usually gradual, brought on and exacerbated by exercise and stress; it is associated with nausea, diaphoresis, and shortness of breath and is alleviated with rest and/or nitroglycerin. Pain typically lasts 2 to 10 minutes. Physical examination is usually normal. An S_4 gallop may be transiently present during an episode of pain. Tests for angina include performing an ECG during an episode of pain, which may show ST segment depression and T wave inversions, or the findings may be normal.

Myocarditis

Myocarditis is an inflammation of the myocardium and is commonly caused by viruses. The heart is unable to contract properly because the inflammatory process interferes with the contractile function of the myocardial cells and eventually leads to cell death. It is frequently accompanied by pericarditis. The chest pain is caused by ischemia or arrhythmia. Patients have fever and dyspnea and may have evidence of heart failure. Heart murmurs and friction rubs may be heard. Chest radiographs show cardiomegaly.

Pericarditis

The pain associated with pericarditis is described as sharp, located in the center of the chest, short-lived, episodic, and radiating to the back in the trapezial area. The pain is worse when the patient is supine and sitting, whereas leaning forward often reduces the intensity of the pain. Shallow breathing may be an associated symptom in an effort to avoid pain. Dyspnea may be present with compression of the bronchial tree by a large pericardial effusion. Risk factors for pericarditis include recent viral or bacterial infection, recent MI, uremia, myxedema, and history of autoimmune disease. Objective signs include fever before the onset of pain, tachycardia, and pericardial friction rub. The rub is pathognomonic for pericarditis but is found in only 60% to 70% of patients with pericarditis. Diagnostic tests show elevated white blood cells and erythrocyte sedimentation rate and diffuse ST segment elevation in the early stages. Chest radiography may be normal or show effusion with an increase in cardiac shadow.

Aortic Stenosis

Aortic stenosis may cause exertional chest pain. Associated symptoms include fatigue, palpitation, dyspnea on exertion (DOE), dizziness, and syncope. Physical examination will reveal a loud, harsh crescendo-decrescendo murmur best heard at the second right intercostal space with the patient leaning forward. The murmur may radiate to the neck and is often associated with a thrill. An echocardiogram will provide diagnostic evidence of aortic stenosis.

Mitral Regurgitation

Symptoms of mitral regurgitation are similar to those of aortic stenosis; they include exertional substernal chest pain, fatigue, palpitation, dizziness, DOE, and syncope. The murmur associated with mitral regurgitation is holosystolic and blowing and often is heard best at the apex in the left lateral position. The murmur decreases with inspiration and may radiate to the left axilla and occasionally to the back. Again, echocardiography will provide evidence of mitral regurgitation.

Pneumonia

Signs and symptoms of pneumonia include pleuritic chest pain; a productive, moist cough with dark sputum; shortness of breath; and fever and chills. Risk factors include ineffective cough reflex, inability to swallow, the elderly, or the very young. Auscultation of the lungs reveals diminished breath sounds over affected areas, and crackles and wheezes may be heard. Rales and rhonchi are frequently heard on auscultation of the lungs. Dullness with percussion is heard over areas of consolidation. Vocal fremitus is positive. In addition, physical findings may include tachycardia, tachypnea, bronchophony, and egophony. Chest radiography, sputum culture, and ABGs will further support the diagnosis of pneumonia. Follow-up chest radiographs are indicated after pneumonia because lung tumors can be hidden by pneumonia. The very young and very old are most often hospitalized for observation and treatment of pneumonia. Healthy adults are usually managed on an outpatient basis.

Mitral Valve Prolapse

Patients with chest pain from mitral valve prolapse report a range of symptoms, including arrhythmias, palpitations, and anxiety. Physical examination may be normal, or a midsystolic click can be heard over the apex while the patient is sitting or squatting. An echocardiogram will provide evidence of mitral valve prolapse.

Pleuritis

Pleuritic chest pain occurs suddenly and is worsened by deep breathing, coughing, and sneezing. Pleuritic chest pain may be a manifestation of pneumonia or may represent pleural inflammation, especially following a viral upper respiratory tract infection. Physical examination of the chest may be normal, or a pleural friction rub may be heard over the area of inflammation. The patient's respiration rate is normal, but respirations are often shallow or guarded. Unless pneumonia is suspected, no diagnostic tests are indicated. If signs and symptoms of pneumonia are absent, the cause of pleuritic chest pain is more likely of viral etiology.

Esophagitis

Esophagitis or esophageal spasm symptoms often mimic angina. In fact, sublingual nitroglycerin may also relieve the symptoms, but usually relief takes longer than the 3 to 5 minutes for angina to be relieved. Patients frequently report that the pain is worse after eating spicy foods or large meals or if they lie down after eating. They may report a sour taste in their mouth. Physical examination is normal except for possible epigastric tenderness with palpation. The most reliable way to detect reflux as the cause of chest pain is to correlate episodes of chest pain with results of 24-hour esophageal pH monitoring.

Chest Trauma

Rib fractures usually follow trauma. Pain is made worse by deep breathing. The patient's respirations are shallow, and pain is exacerbated by palpation in the area of the fracture. Chest or rib radiographs will confirm suspected rib fractures.

Costochondritis and Tietze's Syndrome

Costochondritis and Tietze's syndrome are both identified by severe pain with palpation along the anterior cartilage where the ribs meet the sternum. Deep breathing and movement of the chest wall intensify the pain. In Tietze's syndrome, swelling also occurs along this border.

Herpes Zoster

Herpes zoster is manifested by unilateral chest pain that follows a dermatome. The pain is usually described as burning, stabbing, or pruritic. Early in the course of the disease, no objective manifestations are present. As the course of herpes zoster progresses, a vesicular rash appears in the area of pain (see Chapter 8).

Peptic Ulcer Disease

Subjective manifestations of peptic ulcer disease include episodes of pain 1 to 3 hours after eating. The pain may awaken the patient at night and is frequently relieved by antacids or eating. The patient may report hematemesis and/or melena. A complete blood cell count may show iron-deficiency anemia. Personal or family history of ulcer disease may be a risk factor, as well as cigarette smoking and alcohol abuse. Upper GI radiography and endoscopy are diagnostic tests that can confirm peptic ulcer disease.

Cholecystitis

Cholecystitis is reported as colicky, intermittent epigastric or right upper quadrant pain that often follows a high-fat meal. Nausea and vomiting may accompany the pain, which often radiates to the right infrascapular area. Physical examination may show a positive Murphy's sign, as indicated by tenderness in the region of the gallbladder. The gallbladder may be distended and palpable. Gallbladder ultrasonography is the most important diagnostic test in the evaluation of this problem.

Acute Pancreatitis

Acute pancreatitis occurs as the sudden onset of severe, steady upper epigastric or left upper quadrant abdominal pain, which frequently radiates to the left anterior chest, shoulders, or back. The pain is worse in the supine position. The patient appears restless, and pain can be associated with nausea and severe vomiting, hypotension, and unexplained shock. Left upper quadrant abdominal pain with palpation is present. The laboratory test most frequently used to confirm this diagnosis is determination of serum amylase and lipase levels. A rise in amylase level is seen 2 to 12 hours after the onset of symptoms. The lipase level returns to normal slower than the amylase level and thus is more useful in diagnosing pancreatitis later in its course. Pancreas ultrasonography and CT are necessary to show positive evidence of pancreatitis.

Lung and Mediastinal Tumors

Lung and mediastinal tumors may be manifested by chest pain. Associated symptoms include shortness of breath, cough, and hemoptysis. Pneumonia is often the initial diagnosis, and persistence of symptoms after treatment may lead to further investigation for tumors. Risk factors include a smoking history and family history of cancer. Physical examination may be normal or reveal diminished breath sounds in the area of the tumor. Dull sounds on percussion of the chest may be an objective manifestation of a chest mass. Chest radiography and CT of the chest are diagnostic tools to identify these lesions. Bronchoscopy is performed to obtain a biopsy.

Cocaine Use

Cocaine increases the metabolic requirement of the heart for oxygen and decreases the supply of oxygen, producing myocardial ischemia and chest pain. Cocaine causes adrenergic stimulation, thus increasing heart rate, blood pressure, and left ventricular contractility. Concomitantly, myocardial oxygen supply declines because of cocaine-induced vasoconstriction of the coronary arteries. ECGs, serial cardiac enzymes, and urine drug screens are useful diagnostic tools.

Psychogenic Origin

Adults and adolescents with a history of a recent stressful situation may present with chest pain. Physical examination is negative.

Pleurodynia

Group B coxsackieviruses may cause pleurodynia. Presentation is usually a sudden, severe onset of stabbing, paroxysmal pleuritic pain over the lower rib cage and substernal area. Deep breathing aggravates the pain. Fever, headache, malaise, and unproductive cough are usually present. The chest examination is negative except for pleuritic friction rub in 25% of cases. The condition lasts from 1 to 14 days.

Precordial Catch Syndrome

Recurrent brief episodes of sudden, sharp, but not distressing pain occurring at rest or during mild exercise may indicate precordial catch syndrome. It is localized near the apex of the heart and along the left sternal border or beneath the left breast. It is seen in adolescents and is benign in nature.

DIFFERENTIAL DIAGNOSIS OF *Common Causes of Emergent Chest Pain*

CONDITION	HISTORY	PHYSICAL FINDINGS	DIAGNOSTIC STUDIES
Acute myocardial infarction	Severe, oppressive, constricting retrosternal discomfort, radiating to left or right arm, neck, and/or jaw, lasting >30 min; diaphoresis, dyspnea, nausea; history of CAD, cigarette smoker, positive family history of CAD, history of elevated lipids	Hypertension or hypotension, cardiac arrhythmia, paradoxical S_2	Serial ECGs, serial cardiac enzymes, nuclear scan
Aortic dissection	Sudden, tearing pain in anterior or posterior chest; migrates to arms, abdomen, and legs	Pulse deficits, hypertension; possible neurological changes in legs; aortic diastolic murmur	Echocardiogram, angiography, CT scan/MRI, emergency referral
Acute coronary artery insufficiency	Severe, constricting retrosternal chest pain lasting >30 min; anxiety, diaphoresis, dyspnea; prior history of angina or MI	Restlessness, cool and clammy skin, tachycardia	ECG, isoenzymes
Pulmonary embolus	Acute onset; sense of doom; pleuritic pain, restlessness; mild to severe pain; hemoptysis; history of DVT, recent trauma to lower extremity, surgery; oral contraceptives	Fever, dyspnea, cough, tachycardia, tachypnea, diminished breath sounds; crackles, wheezing	PT/aPTT, ABGs, chest radiograph, ventilation/perfusion scans
Pneumothorax	Sharp or tearing pain, may radiate to ipsilateral shoulder; dyspnea; children with asthma, CF, or Marfan syndrome at risk	Tachycardia; diminished breath sounds; crackles, wheezing	Chest radiograph, ABGs
Arrhythmias	Palpitations, dizziness, forceful heartbeats; history of CHD, fever, and medications (sympathomimetics and β-adrenergic agents); history of cocaine abuse	SVT = tachycardia of 150-250 beats/min, sinus or ventricular tachycardia, irregular pulse	ECG during episode, Holter 24-hour ECG
Congenital coronary anomalies	In children and adolescents, history of moderate to severe chest pain during or following exercise; family history of early sudden death	May have murmurs, clicks, decreased lower extremity pulses, irregular pulse, BP	ECG, referral to pediatric cardiologist

ECG, Electrocardiogram; *CAD*, coronary artery disease; *CT*, computed tomography; *MRI*, magnetic resonance imaging; *MI*, myocardial infarction; *DVT*, deep venous thrombosis; *PT*, prothrombin time; *aPTT*, activated partial thromboplastin time; *ABG*, arterial blood gas; *CF*, cystic fibrosis; *CHD*, coronary heart disease; *SVT*, supraventricular tachycardia; *BP*, blood pressure.

DIFFERENTIAL DIAGNOSIS OF *Common Causes of Nonemergent Chest Pain*

CONDITION	HISTORY	PHYSICAL FINDINGS	DIAGNOSTIC STUDIES
Stable angina	Substernal chest pressure following exercise or stress and relieved by rest or nitroglycerin; nausea, SOB, diaphoresis, sternal chest pressure	Normal examination; possible transient S_4	ECG during episode of chest pain
Myocarditis	Chest pain; history of fever, dyspnea	Heart murmur, friction rub, fever	ECG, chest radiograph
Pericarditis	Sharp, stabbing pain referred to left shoulder or trapezius ridge, usually worse during coughing or deep breathing; may be relieved by sitting forward; history of viral or bacterial infection, autoimmune disease	Fever before onset of pain, tachycardia, pericardial friction rub	WBC, ESR, ECG, chest radiograph
Aortic stenosis	Chest pain on exertion, substernal and anginal in quality; fatigue, palpitations, DOE, dizziness, syncope	Radial pulse diminished; narrow pulse pressure; loud, harsh, crescendo-decrescendo murmur heard best at second right ICS with patient leaning forward; thrill	Echocardiogram, ECG, chest radiograph
Mitral regurgitation	Exertional chest pain, fatigue, palpitations, dizziness, DOE, syncope	Holosystolic, blowing, often loud murmur heard best at apex in left lateral position and decreases with inspiration; murmur may radiate to axilla and possibly back	Chest radiograph, ECG, echocardiogram
Pneumonia	Productive cough of yellow or green or rust sputum, dyspnea, pleuritic pain	Fever; tachycardia, tachypnea; inspiratory crackles; vocal fremitus; percussion dull or flat over area of consolidation; bronchophony; egophony	Chest radiograph, sputum cultures, ABGs
Mitral valve prolapse	Chest pain, varies in location and intensity; palpitations; anxiety; nonexertional pain of short duration; history of Marfan syndrome	Arrhythmias, possible midsystolic click heard over apex; heard best while patient is in sitting or squatting position; thoracoskeletal deformity common in children	ECG, echocardiogram
Pleuritis	Mild, localized chest pain, worse with deep breathing; recent URI	Shallow respirations, local tenderness, pleural friction rub	None initially
Esophagitis	Substernal pain worse after eating and lying down; sour taste in mouth	Epigastric pain with palpitation	Esophageal pH
Chest trauma (rib fracture)	History of injury or trauma; pain with deep breaths; splinting of chest wall	Shallow respirations; chest wall pain on palpitation	Chest radiograph

Continued

DIFFERENTIAL DIAGNOSIS OF *Common Causes of Nonemergent Chest Pain —cont'd*

CONDITION	HISTORY	PHYSICAL FINDINGS	DIAGNOSTIC STUDIES
Costochondritis	Pain along sternal border, increases with deep breaths; history of exercise, URI, or physical activity	Pain with palpitation over costochondral joints; normal breath sounds	None
Herpes zoster	Unilateral chest pain; painful rash	Normal breath sounds; vesicular rash along dermatome	None
Peptic ulcer disease	Epigastric pain 1 to 2 hours after eating, may be relieved by antacids; hematemesis and melena; risk factors include smoking and alcohol overuse	Tenderness to palpitation in epigastric area; signs of hypovolemia	Upper GI radiograph, upper endoscopy, CBC
Cholecystitis	Right upper quadrant abdominal pain radiating to right chest, often after eating high-fat meal; nausea and vomiting	Positive Murphy's sign; palpable gallbladder	Gallbladder ultrasound
Acute pancreatitis	Severe left upper quadrant abdominal pain radiating into left chest; pain worse in supine position; nausea, vomiting, fever	Left upper abdominal pain with palpation; hypotension	Serum analysis, pancreas ultrasound or CT scan
Lung tumors	Chest pain, SOB, cough, hemoptysis, history of cigarette smoking; history of pneumonia	Normal exam or diminished breath sounds over tumor and dull percussion sound over tumor	Chest radiograph, CT scan of chest, bronchoscopy
Cocaine use	Chest pain, SOB, diaphoresis, nausea; may relate to substance use	Tachycardia, hypertension	ECG, serial cardiac enzymes, drug screen
Psychogenic origin	Precordial chest pain, history of stressful situations	Normal exam	ECG, chest radiograph
Pleurodynia	Severe, acute onset, stabbing, paroxysmal, pleuritic pain over lower rib cage and substernal edge; headache, malaise, nonproductive cough	Pleural friction rub 25% of time; chest examination normal; fever usually present	None
Precordial catch syndrome	Sudden, sharp, nondistressing pain near apex of heart; seen in adolescence	Normal examination	None

SOB, Shortness of breath; *ECG,* electrocardiogram; *WBC,* white blood cell; *ESR,* erythrocyte sedimentation rate; *DOE,* dizziness on exertion; *ICS,* intercostal space; *ABG,* arterial blood gas; URI, upper respiratory tract infection; *GI,* gastrointestinal; *CBC,* complete blood cell count; *CT,* computed tomography.

CHAPTER RESOURCES

Cava J, Saygor P: Chest pain in children and adolescents, *Pediatr Clin North Am* 51:1553, 2004.

Cayley WE: Diagnosing the cause of chest pain, *Am Fam Physician* 72:2012, 2005.

DeVon HA, Ryan CJ: Chest pain and associated symptoms of acute coronary syndromes, *J Cardiovasc Nurs* 20:232, 2005.

Eslick GD, Coulshed DS, Talley NJ: Diagnosis and treatment of noncardiac chest pain, *Natl Clin Pract Gastroenterol Hepatol* 2:10, 2005.

Expert Panel on Detection, Evaluation, and Treatment of High Blood Cholesterol in Adults: Executive summary of the third report of the National Cholesterol Education Program (NCEP) Expert Panel on Detection, Evaluation, and Treatment of High Blood Cholesterol in Adults (Adult Treatment Panel III), *JAMA* 285:2486, 2001.

Grundy SM, Cleeman JI, Merz CNB et al: Implications of recent clinical trials for the National Cholesterol Education Program Adult Treatment Panel III Guidelines, *Circulation* 110:227, 2004.

Kruip MJHA, Leclercq MGL, van der Heul C et al: Diagnostic strategies for excluding pulmonary embolism in clinical outcome studies: a systematic review, *Ann Intern Med* 138:941, 2003.

Lee TH, Goldman L: Evaluation of the patient with acute chest pain, *N Engl J Med* 342:1187, 2000.

Swap CJ, Nagurney JT: Value and limitations of chest pain history in the evaluation of patients with suspected acute coronary syndromes, *JAMA* 294:20, 2005.

Syncope

S yncope is the reversible loss of consciousness and postural tone that results from a sudden decrease in cerebral perfusion. It is distinct from a coma, seizures, shock, vertigo, or other states of altered consciousness. It is a symptom that many adults of any age will experience at least some time during their lives. It is less common in children; fewer than 15% of children between the ages of 8 and 18 have a syncopal event. It is uncommon in children under 6 years of age except when there is a seizure disorder, primary cardiac arrhythmia, or a breath-holding incident.

The causes of syncope can be difficult to determine because patients generally are seen long after the event has occurred. Syncope can be quite benign, such as a vasovagal response, or it can indicate serious disease. However, even benign syncope can place the patient at risk for falls or injury. Cardiogenic syncope has high associated morbidity and mortality, and the emphasis in diagnosis is to rule out the most serious causes through a careful history and physical examination, with a few laboratory and diagnostic tests to establish a possible diagnosis. Box 10-1 describes an evidence-based approach to the diagnosis of syncope.

DIAGNOSTIC REASONING: FOCUSED HISTORY

Is This Really Syncope?

Key Questions
- Did you lose consciousness?
- Did you have any prodromal symptoms?
- What were you doing when the event occurred?

- If you lost consciousness, how long did it last?
- Did your limbs jerk during the event?
- Did anyone see you faint?

Loss of Consciousness
Distinguish syncope from other symptoms. Dizziness, vertigo, and presyncope do not cause loss of consciousness or postural tone.

Prodromal Symptoms
Prodromal symptoms of sweating, vertigo, nausea, and/or yawning are associated with syncope; seizures may be associated with an aura or tongue biting. Aura also suggests migraine etiology.

Prevent Characteristics
Characterize what precipitated the episodes. Loss of consciousness precipitated by pain, exercise, urination, defecation, or stressful events is probably not a seizure. Breath-holding spells are common in children, causing syncope. They are usually precipitated by pain, anger, a sudden startle, or frustration. Syncope occurs with rest or when supine during a seizure or arrhythmia. Syncope that occurs without warning is considered cardiovascular in origin.

Event and Postevent Characteristics
Rhythmic movements of extremities during the event are usually a seizure, although they can occur with syncope. Disorientation after the event, slowness in returning to consciousness, and unconsciousness lasting longer than 5 minutes indicate seizure. Often children with breath-holding spells have associated cyanosis, clonic jerks, opisthotonos, and bradycardia.

Box 10-1	**Evidence-Based Practice: Diagnosing Syncope**

Syncope is a common symptom with no diagnostic gold standard and a range of prognoses. The authors of this guideline undertook an extensive review of the literature to help clinicians maximize the diagnostic yield in the workup of syncope and here report the following key points that assist in the evaluation of syncope:

1. History, physical examination, and electrocardiography (ECG) are the core of syncope workup (combined diagnostic yield, 50%).
2. Neurological testing is rarely helpful unless additional neurological signs or symptoms are present (diagnostic yield of EEG, CT, and Doppler ultrasound, 2% to 6%).
3. Patients in whom heart disease is known or suspected and those with exertional syncope who are at higher risk for adverse outcomes should have cardiac testing, including echocardiography, stress testing, Holter monitoring, or EPS, alone or in combination (diagnostic yield, 5% to 35%).
4. Syncope in the elderly often results from polypharmacy and abnormal physiological responses to daily events.
5. Long-term loop electrocardiography (diagnostic yield, 25% to 35%) and tilt-table testing (diagnostic yield, ≤60%) are most useful in patients with recurrent syncope in whom heart disease is not suspected.
6. Psychiatric evaluation can detect mental disorders associated with syncope in up to 25% of cases.
7. Hospitalization may be indicated for patients at high risk for cardiac syncope or with acute neurological signs.

Data from Linzer M, Yang EH, Estes NA III et al: Diagnosing syncope. Part 1: Value of history, physical examination, and electrocardiography. Clinical Efficacy Assessment Project of the American College of Physicians, *Ann Intern Med* 126(12):989-996, 1997.

Witness

The patient is unconscious when the syncopal event takes place and therefore is a poor historian. A careful history is needed from both the patient and a witness to help in the diagnosis. Adolescents who have hysterical syncope episodes generally have an audience when the event occurs. Often the adolescent is able to describe details of the event that would not be known in an unconscious patient.

Does This Require Immediate Referral?

Key Questions

- Do you have a history of heart disease? What is it?
- Do you have a congenital heart problem?
- Are you having chest pain and/or shortness of breath?
- Did this occur after exercise?

History of Heart Disease/Congenital Heart Problem

The presence of structural heart disease increases the risk of sudden death. Patients with a history of coronary artery disease, congestive heart failure, or ventricular arrhythmia should be hospitalized. Cardiac syncope may be either arrhythmic or mechanical in origin. Cardiac outflow obstruction from aortic or mitral stenosis or a prosthetic valve may cause syncope. Complete heart block is a leading cause of syncope, the result of interruption of atrioventricular conduction. Children who have had cardiac surgery to correct severe congenital heart disease are at risk for arrhythmias.

Chest Pain or Shortness of Breath

Obstructive mechanical blockage may be caused by pulmonary embolism, cardiac ischemia, or myocardial infarction with pump failure.

After Exercise

Syncope that accompanies exercise should be considered of cardiac origin unless proved otherwise. Syncope after exertion in a well-trained athlete who has no heart disease is likely vasovagal in origin.

What Do Associated Symptoms Tell Me?

Key Questions

- What other symptoms did you have?
- Do you have palpitations?
- Have you had headaches?
- Have you had vertigo, dizziness, diplopia, or other visual changes?

Palpitations

Supraventricular or ventricular tachycardias are associated with syncope and sudden death. Ventricular tachycardia with a heart rate of 200 beats per minute may be asymptomatic or cause syncope. Chaotic ventricular activity of ventricular fibrillation is always fatal unless it is reversed with electrical defibrillation.

Headaches

The pain of migraine headaches and the effect of the migraine on the brainstem can cause syncope. Generally the patient has associated symptoms such as vomiting, photophobia, severe headache (often on one side), and a strong family history of migraines. The headache continues after consciousness is regained.

Vertigo, Dizziness, and Diplopia/Visual Symptoms

The presence of vertigo, dizziness, or visual changes may accompany migraine headache. Interruption in cerebral perfusion, such as with a transient ischemic attack, also must be considered.

Is This Neurocardiogenic in Origin?

Key Questions

- Did this occur in response to a specific situation (e.g., stressful event, urination, defecation)?
- What position were you in when you fainted? Were you sitting, standing, or lying flat?
- Are you an athlete? Do you have a history of any heart problems?

Situational Fainting

Vasovagal syncope is the most common type seen in adults and healthy children. It is neurocardiogenic and tends to occur in families. It is often precipitated by emotional stress, fear, extreme fatigue, or injury. It can occur without any obvious antecedent cause. Warm temperature, anxiety, blood drawing, and crowded rooms may cause peripheral vasodilation. Lack of large muscle activity

prevents the venous return that is needed for cardiac filling with consequent bradycardia and fainting. Once supine, venous return to the heart occurs, awakening the patient. Rapid standing will cause recurrence of the episode. Mental alertness is present.

Situational syncope can occur in response to urination, defecation, cough, or emotional stress. Posttussive syncope follows paroxysmal coughing caused by increased intrathoracic pressure, which is then transmitted to the intracranial circulation, increasing intracranial pressure and decreasing cerebral blood flow. Postmicturition syncope, occurring during or after urination, is caused by the release of intravascular pressure on urination, which triggers vasodilation and vagally mediated bradycardia.

Is This Orthostasis?

Key Questions

- What medications are you taking?
- Have you recently started taking blood pressure medicine or increased the dose?
- What other health problems/conditions do you have?

Medications

About 10% of syncopal episodes are caused by prescribed medications (e.g., antidepressants, antiarrhythmics, β-blockers, diuretics), over-the-counter medications, and recreational drugs (e.g., alcohol, cocaine) that produce orthostasis, bradycardia, or prolonged QT interval. Adolescents may use drugs such as amyl nitrite and butyl nitrite as aphrodisiacs and euphoriants. These drugs lead to vasodilation, and syncope may occur.

Children may ingest medications that belong to family members, and a history of such activity must be investigated as a cause of the syncope.

Other Health Problems or Conditions

Diabetes may induce hypoglycemia, causing a gradual syncope. Anemias and chronic gastrointestinal bleeding from an ulcer or another source may cause syncope.

Patients who are pregnant or dehydrated or who have been on prolonged bed rest are at risk for orthostatic hypotension and syncope.

Is This Explained by Other Factors?

Key Questions

- Have you had this before? How often?
- Did it occur with sudden head turning?
- If a child: Has the child had Kawasaki disease?
- Do you have Lyme disease?

Frequent Syncope With No Heart Disease

Psychogenic syncope is often associated with repeated episodes in which unpredictable motor reflexes appear, with a lack of pathological reflexes. Also, blood pressure and pulse rate measurements are normal, and skin and mucous membranes do not change color. Panic attacks, or hyperventilation, are often interpreted as feeling faint, but the patient does not usually appear pale, nor are the symptoms relieved when recumbent.

After Sudden Head Rotation

Carotid sinus hypersensitivity produces a cardioinhibitory response that results in a profound drop in heart rate or may induce an abrupt vasopressor response with a drop in blood pressure.

History of Kawasaki Disease

Syncope can occur in children who have had Kawasaki disease. These children are at risk for coronary heart disease, which may present as chest pain associated with exercise.

Lyme Disease

Lyme disease can cause arrhythmia in the form of heart block, which can result in syncope.

What Other Things Do I Need to Consider?

Key Questions

- Do you have a family history of sudden death?

- Do you have a family history of fainting?
- If a child: Did the mother have systemic lupus erythematosus (SLE) while pregnant?

Family History of Sudden Death

A family history of idiopathic hypertrophic subaortic stenosis is a risk factor for sudden death, and referral is necessary to rule out this condition. A history of a family member who had a myocardial infarction before age 30 is a significant risk factor for sudden death.

Family History of Fainting

Neurocardiogenic syncope is common in families.

Prenatal Systemic Lupus Erythematosus

SLE in a pregnant woman may cause autoimmune injury, resulting in congenital complete atrioventicular block.

DIAGNOSTIC REASONING: FOCUSED PHYSICAL EXAMINATION

Measure Blood Pressure and Pulse Rate

Obtain blood pressure readings in standing, sitting, and supine positions. Orthostatic hypotension is either a decrease in systolic blood pressure of at least 20 mm Hg or symptoms that prevent further standing, such as fainting, weakness, or lightheadedness.

Compare blood pressure readings in the two arms. Unequal measurements may indicate a cardiac cause of the syncope.

Bradycardia of 35 to 40 beats per minute usually does not compromise cerebral blood flow. Rates below this, however, will impair cerebral circulation and function. Tachycardia up to 180 beats per minute also does not usually compromise cerebral circulation.

Observe Hydration Status

Poor hydration status secondary to diuretic use, poor nutrition, or loss of fluids from vomiting and diarrhea may be associated with syncope.

Perform Heart and Lung Examination

Observe for jugular venous distention. Palpate the precordium to assess the point of maximal impulse to estimate the size of the left ventricle. Feel for lifts. Listen for heart rate and murmurs and for radiation of murmurs. Listen for an abnormally loud S_2 or the presence of an S_3. Auscultate for carotid bruits and pericardial rub. Listen to the lungs to assess for rales associated with congestive heart failure.

Perform a Neurological Examination

Begin with a brief mental status examination. Assess cranial nerves, deep tendon reflexes, and motor function. Perform Romberg's test as well as gait and proprioception evaluation. Assess pupillary asymmetry and look for nystagmus (see Chapter 29).

Perform an Abdominal Examination

Auscultate and observe for signs of aortic aneurysm.

Examine Extremities

Observe lower extremities for signs of thrombophlebitis, a source of a pulmonary embolism.

LABORATORY AND DIAGNOSTIC STUDIES

Suspected or Known Cardiac Cause

Electrocardiography

The usefulness of the electrocardiogram usually lies in identifying abnormalities that provide clues to underlying cardiac causes of syncope. These findings include evidence of conduction disorder or signs of coronary artery disease or left ventricular hypertrophy. A 12-lead electrocardiogram is used for the basic evaluation. This electrocardiogram should be first evaluated for rhythm and rate. Hand-measured interval measurement should be made. A Q wave found in the anterolateral lead may indicate abnormal placement of the left coronary artery. A patient with a prolonged QT interval or the presence of Q waves must be referred.

Complete heart block requires immediate referral for pacemaker insertion.

Event Monitoring or Continuous-Loop Monitoring

These measures are used in patients with suspected cardiac arrhythmias as the cause of the syncope. Holter (24 hours) or long-term (weeks, months) event monitoring is used to document electrocardiographic recordings. Holter monitoring is a continuous, 24-hour electrocardiographic recording to evaluate the type and amount of irregular heartbeats during regular activities, exercise, and sleep. The patient keeps a 24-hour diary to record daily activities and any symptoms experienced.

Cardiac event monitoring is a continuous-loop, digital memory recorder worn for extended periods of time (up to 30 days or longer) that saves and records transient events felt by the patient. These monitors are patient activated as symptoms occur.

Doppler Studies

Transcranial Doppler and carotid ultrasonography are used to detect hemodynamically significant stenoses in the major intracranial or extracranial arteries.

Treadmill Testing

Cardiac stress testing is used to evaluate exercise-associated arrhythmias and syncope. It can confirm the presence of coronary artery disease.

Echocardiography

This is used in patients with exercise-induced symptoms to exclude left ventricular outflow tract obstruction.

Electrophysiological Studies

Electrophysiological studies (EPSs) are invasive tests that use electrical stimulation and monitoring to diagnose conduction disorders or the propensity for the development of tachyarrhythmias. Electrodes are threaded through arm or leg veins and placed at strategic positions in the ventricles, atria, or both. The electrodes record electrical signals and allow mapping of electrical impulses. The electrodes also can electrically stimulate the heart at programmed rates to trigger latent ventricular tachycardias.

Suspected Neurological Cause
Baseline Blood Testing
Routine blood tests (electrolyte levels, renal function, blood glucose level, complete blood cell count) rarely yield useful diagnostic information. Most patients with abnormalities in these areas have seizures rather than syncope.

Electroencephalography
Electroencephalography (EEG) may be useful in patients whose history suggests seizure.

Computed Tomography Scanning
Computed tomography (CT) may be useful if the patient has focal neurological findings.

Unexplained Syncope
Toxicology Screen
Toxicology screening is indicated on the basis of the history.

Tilt-Table Testing
Tilt-table testing is used to provoke vasovagal syncope in susceptible persons. Provocative agents such as isoproterenol or nitroglycerin may be used. Using the table, the patient is tilted upright while continuous minute-to-minute blood pressure, heart rate, and oxygen saturation measurements are recorded. Patient symptoms are recorded in each position. Patients with neurocardiogenic syncope develop a sudden drop in heart rate and/or blood pressure after their body has been tilted up for several minutes. If symptoms of lightheadedness or fainting occur during this test, the test is considered positive for neurocardiogenic syncope.

DIFFERENTIAL DIAGNOSIS
Cardiac Causes
Cardiac causes have a higher rate of mortality than do other causes of syncope. Cardiac causes include coronary artery disease, congenital and valvular disease, cardiomyopathy, arrhythmias, and conduction system disorders. Coronary artery disease, congestive heart failure, and ventricular hypertrophy can result in arrhythmias and syncope. Patients with organic heart disease may have chest pain, dyspnea, and syncope with exertion. Patients with arrhythmias may have palpitations or sudden syncope without other physical symptoms. On physical examination, murmurs or carotid bruits may be present. Other findings might include a loud S_2, precordial lift, S_3, pericardial rub, or unequal blood pressure measurements in the two arms. Electrocardiographic testing is indicated; other cardiac testing may be helpful.

Neurocardiogenic Causes
Vasovagal syncope is the most common type in young people, but it may occur at any age. It usually occurs in a standing position and is precipitated by fear, emotional stress, or pain. Autonomic symptoms such as nausea, sweating, blurred or fading vision, epigastric discomfort, lightheadedness, and a feeling of warmth may precede syncope by a few minutes. The syncope occurs secondary to efferent vasopressor reflexes resulting in decreased peripheral vascular resistance. Physical examination is usually negative. Tilt-table testing may be useful in establishing a diagnosis.

Situational syncope is vasovagal syncope with a known precipitant. It is commonly related to conditions that produce a Valsalva maneuver. Micturition, defecation, and cough are types of situational syncope. These stimuli result in autonomic reflexes with a vasopressor response, ultimately leading to transient cerebral hypotension. The physical examination is negative.

Carotid sinus hypersensitivity produces a cardioinhibitory response or vasopressor response that produces syncope with head turning.

Orthostasis
Orthostatic (postural) syncope indicates variable or unstable vasomotor reflexes. A drop in blood pressure when one assumes an upright

position is caused by loss of vasoconstriction reflexes in the lower extremities. Sudden standing or rapid movement after assuming a standing position can trigger syncope; the prevalence of this type of syncope increases with age. The syncope is caused by hypotension that occurs as a blunted baroreceptor response and inability of the cardiovascular system to respond to hypotensive stresses. It may also occur from age-related physiological changes, volume depletion, medication, and autonomic insufficiency. Orthostatic hypotension is produced with testing.

Medication Related

Prescribed medications or recreational drugs may produce syncope that is associated with their use. Medications that can cause syncope include antidepressants, antiarrhythmics, β-blockers, and diuretics. Recreational drugs (e.g., alcohol, cocaine) can produce orthostasis, bradycardia, or prolonged QT interval. Amyl nitrite and butyl nitrite cause vasodilation and syncope.

Physical findings depend on the underlying physical condition of the patient.

Neurological Causes

Neurological causes include transient ischemic attacks, migraines, and seizures. Prodromal symptoms may include vertigo, diplopia, and loss of balance. Syncope results from vertebrobasilar insufficiency. In an acute syncopal attack, circulation is briefly obstructed to the reticular activating system in the brainstem, resulting in loss of consciousness. Neurological findings such as diplopia, pupillary asymmetry, nystagmus, ataxia, and gait instability may be present.

Psychiatric Causes

Syncope of unexplained origin may be psychogenic. Panic and anxiety disorders, somatization, major depression, and substance abuse are the main psychiatric problems associated with syncope. Physical examination is usually negative. Psychiatric evaluation may reveal the underlying disorder.

Unknown Causes

Syncope from unknown causes accounts for about one third of all episodes of syncope. The workup is negative.

DIFFERENTIAL DIAGNOSIS OF *Common Causes of Syncope*

DISORDER	HISTORY	PHYSICAL FINDINGS	DIAGNOSTIC STUDIES
Cardiac Causes			
Organic heart disease	Shortness of breath, chest pain, palpitations, exercise associated	May have bradycardia or tachycardia, cyanosis	Refer
Arrhythmias		Loud S_2, S_3; murmur, lift	Electrocardiogram, Holter, echocardiogram Doppler studies, treadmill
Neurocardiogenic Causes			
Vasovagal	Emotional event, standing for long periods, crowded room, warm environment	None	Tilt-table testing
Situational	Occurs with cough, micturition, defecation, swallowing	None	None
Breath holding	Children 6 mo to 5 yr; associated with anger, pain, brief cry; breath-holding LOC; may have twitching	Cyanosis or pallor	None

Continued

DIFFERENTIAL DIAGNOSIS OF *Common Causes of Syncope—cont'd*

DISORDER	HISTORY	PHYSICAL FINDINGS	DIAGNOSTIC STUDIES
Hyperventilation	Anxiety- or fear-induced event, shortness of breath	None	None
Cough syncope	History of asthma; coughing paroxysm awakens child from sleep, becomes flaccid with clonic muscle spasm, LOC	Wheezes	None
Orthostasis			
Orthostatic hypotension	Position change from lying/sitting to standing, pregnancy, prolonged bed rest	Hypotension on testing orthostatic blood pressure	20 mm Hg drop in systolic pressure on standing
Medication Related			
Prescribed medications	History of antidepressants, antiarrhythmic agents, β-blockers, or diuretics	Depends on underlying condition	None
Drug induced	History of use of illicit drugs	Arrhythmia may be present	Toxicology screen
Neurological Causes			
Migraine	Headache, vomiting, photophobia, positive family history	Usually none; nystagmus, photophobia	None
Seizure	Convulsion, incontinence, postictal phase	Usually none; nystagmus	Electroencephalogram
Psychiatric Causes			
Mental disorder	Symptoms consistent with depression, anxiety, panic	None	Psychiatric evaluation
Hysterical reaction	Adolescent, event occurs with audience present; gentle fall, memory of incident exact	None	None
Unknown causes	No diagnostic characteristics	None	Workup negative

LOC, Loss of consciousness.

CHAPTER RESOURCES

Batra AS, Holn AR: Palpitations, syncope and sudden cardiac death in children: who's at risk? *Pediatr Rev* 24:269, 2003.

Brignole M, Alboni P, Benditt DG et al: Guidelines on management (diagnosis and treatment) of syncope: update 2004. Executive summary, *Eur Heart J* 25:22, 2004.

Kapoor WN: Syncope, *N Engl J Med* 343:1856, 2000.

Kenny RA: Syncope in the elderly: diagnosis, evaluation, and treatment, *J Cardiovasc Electrophysiol* 14:9, 2003.

Lewis D, Dhala A: Syncope in the pediatric patient, *Pediatr Clin North Am* 46:205, 1999.

Miller TH: Evaluation of syncope, *Am Fam Physician* 72:1492, 2005.

Narchi H: The child who passes out, *Pediatr Rev* 21:384, 2000.

Schnipper JL, Kapoor WN: Diagnostic evaluation and management of patients with syncope, *Med Clin North Am* 2:423, 2002.

Taylor B, Green MS: Evaluating and managing syncope, *Clin Rev* 10:55, 2000.

Willis J: Syncope, *Pediatr Rev* 21:201, 2001.

Common Problems of the Respiratory System

V

Dyspnea

Dyspnea, or shortness of breath, is a subjective sensation of air hunger that results in labored breathing. True dyspnea results from three general causes: an increased awareness of normal breathing, such as with hyperventilation; an increase in the work of breathing, such as in airway obstruction or restricted volume; and abnormalities in the ventilatory system, as in neurological disorders, diseases of the muscles, and chest wall abnormalities. In disease states it is usually a result of pulmonary or cardiac pathology. When eliciting the history, it is helpful to determine if this is new-onset acute dyspnea, chronic progressive dyspnea, or chronic recurrent dyspnea. Carefully directed questioning will provide essential clues for identifying the differential diagnoses. In children younger than 3 years, who usually cannot express the sensation, caregivers may observe tachypnea, retractions, stridor, nasal flaring, or feeding difficulty.

DIAGNOSTIC REASONING: FOCUSED HISTORY

Is This an Emergency?

Severe dyspnea is a medical emergency. If not treated immediately, respiratory failure and death may occur. Assess the adequacy of the airway first. Emergency measures should be instituted to establish ventilation. Once the patient is stabilized, search for the underlying cause of the dyspnea.

Key Questions

- Did this occur suddenly, or has it been developing gradually? Over what period of time (hours, days, weeks) has it developed?

- What were you or the child doing just before having difficulty in breathing?
- Do you have other symptoms, such as itching or swelling?

Onset

New-onset acute dyspnea in a patient in acute distress may signal a life-threatening problem. In the patient with no previous history of heart or lung disease, dyspnea may indicate several conditions that require immediate treatment, such as aspiration of a foreign body, anaphylaxis, pulmonary embolism (PE), and pneumonia. A common cause of acute-onset dyspnea is left ventricular dysfunction.

Acute upper or lower airway obstruction in children has the greatest potential to cause serious morbidity or mortality and therefore must initially be ruled out. The most serious problem is hypoxemia caused by the inability to transport oxygen past a blocked upper airway, such as with epiglottitis, croup, or a foreign body.

Acute dyspnea requires that assessment of the airway and ventilatory status with oxygen and cardiac monitoring be initiated immediately. Often this must occur before a definitive diagnostic evaluation has been completed.

Acute epiglottitis in children is caused by *Haemophilus influenzae*. Inflammation of the epiglottis causes edema that obstructs the tracheal airway. The onset is sudden and the course of the disease is rapid. The patient's presenting symptoms usually include drooling, dysphonia, dysphagia, and respiratory distress with inspiratory stridor. The child looks anxious and sits up and forward with the jaw open to assist in air intake.

Status asthmaticus is a progressive bronchospasm from an increase in airflow resistance in children who are having an asthma event that does not respond to pharmacological intervention. Fever may be present, and pulse rate and respirations are increased. The use of accessory respiratory muscles is seen. Wheezing may not be heard because of lack of air movement. The combination of hypoxia, hypercapnia, and acidosis may result in cardiovascular depression and cardiopulmonary arrest.

Foreign Body Aspiration

The adult patient with foreign body aspiration may report that dyspnea occurred while eating solid foods or drinking large amounts of alcohol. Children who put small objects in their mouth are at risk for aspiration of the object into the airway and subsequent airway obstruction. The patient or the care provider gives a history of sudden onset of choking, coughing, or wheezing, without preceding upper respiratory tract infection. Many times the child has been playing on the floor or outside at the time of the onset of symptoms.

Anaphylaxis

Anaphylaxis may follow insect bites or the ingestion of medication or other potential allergens (e.g., shellfish). Primary symptoms include not feeling well, flushing, generalized pruritus, fear, faintness, and sneezing. In severe cases, an allergic response may occur within minutes, followed by death from suffocation caused by edema of the larynx, epiglottis, and pharynx. Shock and cardiac arrhythmia ensue within a short time unless emergency measures are instituted.

The sooner the symptoms occur, the more severe the reaction.

Is the Dyspnea Caused by a Secondary Obstruction in the Lower Respiratory Tract?

Key Questions

- Have you had cough or cold symptoms recently?
- Do you have a history of asthma?
- Is there a family history of asthma?

Cough

Secondary partial airway obstruction caused by small airways disease contributes to hypoxemia via intrapulmonary shunting. The pulmonary obstruction can be intraluminal (distal foreign objects, asthma), intramural (edema, bronchomalacia, bronchiolitis), or extramural (compression from tumor, lymph nodes). The narrowing increases both airway resistance and turbulence of airflow. The imbalance between pulmonary ventilation and perfusion affects oxygen exchange. This causes the patient to work harder to maintain adequate ventilation, resulting in dyspnea.

History of Asthma

Both adults and children may experience airway obstruction caused by reactive airways disease or asthma. Personal or family history of asthma increases the risk of dyspnea from acute bronchospasm.

Is the Dyspnea Caused by Trauma to the Chest?

Key Question

- Have you experienced any trauma to the chest?

Trauma

Limitation of motion of the thoracic cage because of pain and/or trauma may be associated with the development of severe alveolar hypoventilation and subsequent dyspnea.

Pneumothorax occurs most frequently in young persons during strenuous activity. Spontaneous pneumothorax results in sudden loss of lung volume, hypoxia, hypercapnia, and significant shortness of breath. Blunt chest trauma may be caused by a fall or motor vehicle accident.

Is the Dyspnea Caused by a Pulmonary Embolus?

Key Questions

- Have you been confined to bed recently?
- Have you had recent surgery? Have you recently sustained a fracture?
- Are you taking birth control pills? Do you smoke?

- Do you take any medications?
- Are you feeling anxious or scared?

The person with PE is usually in acute distress and reports significant shortness of breath, localized pleuritic chest pain, apprehension, bloody sputum production, diaphoresis, fever, and history of conditions causing risk for emboli. These risk factors include age of greater than 60 years, pulmonary hypertension, congestive heart failure, chronic lung disease, ischemic heart disease, stroke, and cancer. Predisposing factors that can contribute to thrombus formation include (1) venous stasis, (2) hypercoagulability, and (3) endothelial injury with inflammation to the vessel lining. Trauma, muscle spasm, or clot dissolution may cause the thrombus to dislodge, creating an embolus. Emboli circulate in the blood to the right side of the heart and enter the lungs via the pulmonary artery. If the clot is not dissolved within the lungs, it occludes the pulmonary artery and obstructs blood flow and perfusion of the lungs. Patients with suspected PE are referred for emergency pulmonary/vascular consultation.

Confinement, Surgery, and Fracture

PE is most likely to occur in persons with a history of deep vein thrombosis or prolonged immobility. Vascular lung disease is characterized by a decrease in the size of the pulmonary vascular bed. When emboli reach the pulmonary artery, the reduced blood flow through the lungs results in arterial hypoxemia and hypercapnia, which in turn lead to symptoms of dyspnea. Dyspnea resulting from PE is usually accompanied by fever, chest pain, and restlessness.

Trauma to Leg

There is an increased risk of PE in adolescents who have sustained traumatic injury to their lower limbs.

Anxiety

People with PE feel a sense of impending doom. Significant oxygen deprivation may contribute to this symptom.

Oral Contraceptives

The estrogen in oral contraceptives causes increased coagulation of red blood cells, which increases the risk for PE. In addition, the risk of PE increases with the combination of smoking and oral contraceptives, especially in women older than age 35.

Medications

A complete medication history may provide clues to a possible hypercoagulability state. Patients who are taking anticoagulants and perhaps are underdosed may be at risk for PE. Patients taking medication for heart failure, such as digitalis or angiotensin-converting enzyme (ACE) inhibitors, are at risk because of chronic heart failure. In addition, it should be determined if menopausal women are taking hormone replacement therapy because these drugs increase the risk of PE.

Is the Dyspnea Related to a Preexisting Disease?

Key Questions

- Do you have a history of heart problems, lung problems (asthma), or anemia?
- Do you have any numbness or tingling in your body? Where?
- Have you noticed any other symptoms?

Past History of Disease

History of coronary artery disease (CAD), heart failure, valvular heart disease, chronic obstructive pulmonary disease (COPD), or asthma should raise the level of suspicion for recurrence or complications of that disease. Myocardial infarction (MI) may cause sudden dyspnea in persons with or without prior history of CAD. Careful questioning regarding associated symptoms and risk factors may reveal characteristics of probable MI (see Chapter 9).

Progressively increasing shortness of breath is frequently a symptom of worsening COPD. It is often associated with (1) frequent cough that is worse in the morning, (2) sputum production that is clear to yellow in color, (3) decreasing exercise tolerance, and (4) mild to moderate fatigue. Chronic progressive dyspnea in the patient with a history of heart failure or cardiac valve disease is most frequently a symptom of heart failure. Associated symptoms include (1) peripheral edema, (2) ascites, (3) cough possibly with frothy sputum production, (4) chest pain, and (5) fatigue. Orthopnea (difficulty breathing when lying flat) and paroxysmal nocturnal dyspnea (PND) (a sudden onset of shortness of breath when lying flat) are most often associated with heart failure.

In children with heart disease, dyspnea occurs because of insufficient blood being pumped to the lungs as a result of congenital structural anomaly or pump failure or secondary to pulmonary hypertension. Simple respiratory tract infections may cause severe respiratory insufficiency in the child who has cardiopulmonary disease. Associated symptoms include retractions (including abdominal muscles), tachypnea, nasal flaring and grunting, peripheral edema, ascites, cough, and fatigue.

Chronic progressive dyspnea because of lung involvement may also be present in patients with a history of systemic illnesses such as sarcoidosis, rheumatological disease (rheumatoid lungs), cystic fibrosis, or Goodpasture's syndrome—a rare syndrome of progressive glomerulonephritis, hemoptysis, and hemosiderosis.

Periodic recurrent dyspnea is most often the result of bronchospasm and inflamed bronchi caused by asthma. Persons with asthma may be relatively symptom free between episodes and can often identify the cause of their shortness of breath with little prompting. Symptoms are frequently associated with recent respiratory tract infection, exercise, or exposure to allergens. Associated symptoms reported by the patient may include audible wheezes, decreased exercise tolerance, and frequent paroxysmal cough. Most children also have associated wheezing. Wheezing is extremely unusual in the neonatal period and generally signifies a structural or functional congenital abnormality. The symptom implies intrathoracic airway obstruction with one or more of the following causes: intraluminal obstruction, fixed airway narrowing, variable narrowing, or external compression. All of these factors lead to turbulent expiratory flow and audible wheeze.

Hematological diseases can affect the oxygen-carrying capacity of the blood, resulting in tissue hypoxia and a decrease in arterial pH, which stimulates the central nervous system to cause the symptom of dyspnea. Severe anemia from any cause can result in this reaction. Also, whenever the oxygen-carrying capacity of the blood is decreased because of the inability of hemoglobin to bind oxygen, dyspnea can occur. Carbon monoxide poisoning, cyanide poisoning, and methemoglobinemia are examples.

The progressive dyspnea of anemia is usually associated with unusual fatigue, palpitations, lightheadedness, or dizziness.

Hyperventilation

Hyperventilation syndrome, a nonemergent but frightening experience, is usually accompanied by paresthesias around the mouth and of the distal extremities. Anxiety-related dyspnea should not be diagnosed until one has ruled out more serious causes.

When dyspnea is caused by pulmonary or cardiac conditions, the shortness of breath worsens with increasing activity and improves with rest. Dyspnea caused by anxiety does not improve, and may worsen, with rest.

What Factors Precipitate or Aggravate the Dyspnea?

Key Questions

- What activities are associated with shortness of breath?
- Do you take any medication?
- Do you have any known allergies—to trees, dust, pollen, animals? Have you been exposed to these recently?
- Is there anything you can do to help yourself feel less short of breath, such as sit up, stay indoors, lie down, use medication?

Precipitating Factors

Chronic dyspnea of pulmonary origin is most frequently precipitated and aggravated by exposure to smoke. This is true for both progressive and recurrent dyspnea. Progressive dyspnea manifested in COPD is often exacerbated by exertion and is alleviated or improved with rest. As the disease progresses, less and less intense exercise, even talking, can result in increased shortness of breath. In addition, respiratory tract infections are frequent causes of increased shortness of breath for these patients. Exercise-induced asthma will cause dyspnea related to activity and is relieved with rest or use of bronchodilators.

Medication Use

The dyspnea related to asthma is relieved by use of bronchodilator agents and steroids.

Allergies

Exposure to cold and/or allergens, exercise, and viral respiratory tract infections frequently precipitate chronic recurrent dyspnea associated with asthma.

Recumbence, missed medications, high sodium intake, and exertion often precipitate chronic dyspnea associated with heart failure. This applies to both progressive and recurrent chronic dyspnea.

Alleviating Factors

Alleviating factors for dyspnea include sitting upright, taking diuretic medications, using bronchodilators, and resting for a prolonged period.

Is the Dyspnea Caused by a Neuromuscular Problem?

Key Questions

- Are the patient's immunizations up to date?
- If a child: Has the child eaten any honey?
- Do you live on a farm?
- If a child: Is the child at risk for lead poisoning?
- Do you have a headache, muscle weakness, or visual changes?

Neuromuscular Effects

Abnormalities of neural or neuromuscular transmission to the respiratory muscles may result in paresis or paralysis, leading to alveolar hypoventilation. Direct involvement of the respiratory muscles affected by systemic musculoskeletal diseases may lead to reduction of vital capacity and total lung capacity and result in hypercapnic hypoventilation and dyspnea. Examples of neuromus-

cular health problems leading to dyspnea include infections, such as poliomyelitis or tetanus, or a central nervous system insult.

Immunizations

Lack of childhood or adult immunizations for poliomyelitis or tetanus may lead to paralysis or tetany of the respiratory musculature, resulting in dyspnea and subsequent respiratory distress.

Honey

Honey is a common source of contamination of *Clostridium botulinum,* which can cause respiratory distress in infants and small children. The incubation period is only a few hours. Nausea, vomiting, and diarrhea result, followed by cranial nerve involvement, diplopia, weak suck, facial weakness, and absent gag reflex. Generalized hypotonia and weakness then develop and may progress to respiratory failure.

Farm Residence

Organophosphate chemicals that are commonly used as insecticides may cause a myasthenia-like syndrome in children exposed to these toxins. Children residing on farms are most at risk.

Neuromuscular Affects

In children, some causes that affect the primary respiratory center are myasthenia gravis, myopathies, insecticide poisoning, and lead poisoning.

Secondary Causes

Diseases that affect the central nervous system include respiratory distress from meningoencephalitis, seizures, or a central nervous system lesion.

Does the Patient Have Any Pertinent Risk Factors That Will Point Me in the Right Direction?

Key Questions

- Do you smoke? Have you ever smoked? Are you regularly exposed to cigarette smoke?

- What type of work do you do?
- Have you had a recent weight gain?
- Have you ever had eczema?

Risk Factors

Persons at risk for developing dyspnea are those with a history of pulmonary and/or heart disease, cigarette smokers and those persons subjected to passive exposure or second-hand smoke, persons exposed to noxious environmental pollutants, and persons with a predisposition to allergies or asthma.

Work

Occupational exposure to asbestos, silicon, paint and chemical fumes, and coal dust place the patient at risk for lung disease with resultant dyspnea.

Obesity

Physically deconditioned and obese persons report dyspnea on exertion more frequently than their counterparts. Obese persons may have a complaint of dyspnea, especially during exercise. This is caused by an increase in the metabolic requirement for a given amount of work. In addition, the diaphragm moves against increased abdominal pressure, and the chest wall is heavier, resulting in more energy required to maintain ventilation.

Eczema History

Asthma occurs in 20% to 40% of children with a history of atopic dermatitis.

DIAGNOSTIC REASONING: FOCUSED PHYSICAL EXAMINATION

Note General Appearance and Observe Posture

Patients who appear in acute distress with manifestations of severe oxygen deprivation require emergent evaluation and treatment. Assess vital signs immediately. Tachypnea, eupnea, and hypopnea are critical clues to impending respiratory failure. Use of accessory muscles to breathe, posturing, and chest retraction all point to severe dyspnea. The severity of the dyspnea almost always correlates with the severity of the problem.

In such situations consider pulmonary embolism, anaphylaxis, foreign body aspiration, pneumothorax, status asthmaticus, and severe heart failure. Persons presenting with COPD, anemia, mild asthma, and mild heart failure appear less acutely ill.

Determine if the patient has to lean forward or sit up to breathe comfortably. With severe respiratory distress or upper airway obstruction, an infant may adopt a posture of hyperextension of the trunk and neck. A child with epiglottitis prefers to sit up and lean forward.

A child in acute respiratory distress, sitting forward, and perhaps drooling with a muffled voice may have epiglottitis, and immediate assistance should be secured. Do not attempt to lay the child down or inspect the throat because this may occlude the airway.

Assess Level of Consciousness

Diminished level of consciousness, confusion, and restlessness are manifestations of hypoxia in a patient experiencing respiratory problems. Frequently the patient with a PE expresses a sense of impending doom.

An acutely ill child may have an alteration in level of consciousness, restlessness, mouth breathing, and flaring of the nostrils.

Observe Chest Movement

Place the patient in a sitting or side-lying position with the chest exposed. The chest cannot be adequately viewed through clothing. Many respiratory abnormalities are unilateral or localized. Compare findings on one side of the body with those on the other. Also compare front to back. Pneumothorax and PE may cause unequal expansion of the chest.

Inspect the Shape and Symmetry of the Chest

Cardinal features of restrictive pulmonary disease are deformities of the chest wall and reduction in lung volume and pulmonary compliance secondary to pathological changes in the lung parenchyma or pleura. Examples of deformities that cause decreased lung volume include kyphosis, scoliosis, and kyphoscoliosis. Decreased volume necessitates an increase in respiratory rate to maintain a normal volume. The work of breathing must be increased to overcome the reduced compliance.

Kyphoscoliosis is associated with marked structural abnormality of the thoracic cage, leading to abnormal positioning and functioning of the respiratory muscles. The lungs are compressed by the thoracic deformity, leading to a small lung volume. Breathing entails a high work and energy cost, and dyspnea can appear.

An increased anteroposterior (AP) diameter indicates air trapping. This is a frequent finding in persons with COPD. Other musculoskeletal chest abnormalities to note include pectus excavatum, pectus carinatum, severe scoliosis, and kyphoscoliosis. These conditions can contribute to chest infection and respiratory failure because of decreased lung volume and ability to cough. Also, bronchomalacia, a softening of the bronchial tissue, is an abnormality associated with pectus excavatum. Pectus carinatum is associated with chronic lung disease such as asthma or with cystic fibrosis, heart disease, and idiopathic scoliosis. Harrison's sulci are exaggerated grooves running parallel to the subcostal margins, produced by prolonged diaphragmatic traction, and are associated with chronic airway disease or rickets.

In the presence of neuromuscular disease, chest movement in children should be examined in both the supine and sitting positions. Diaphragmatic weakness leads to paradoxical abdominal movements in the supine position, which may be missed if the child is examined only in the sitting position.

Respiratory distress triggered by placing the child in the supine position may be the only subtle abnormality in older children with mediastinal compression of the trachea.

Look for Retractions

In normal breathing, inspiration is the work necessary to overcome the elastic forces of the lung, the tissue viscosity of the lung and chest wall, and airway resistance. When there is a problem with any of these, the accessory muscles (sternocleidomastoid, anterior serratus, and external intercostal muscles) are recruited to help. Contraction of these muscles causes forceful expansion of the thorax, resulting in increased negative pressure that draws in the soft tissues of the chest wall and results in retractions. Retractions begin in lower intercostal spaces and then move up to the higher spaces. In an infant, head-bobbing in time with respiration reflects use of the accessory muscles of respiration.

Observe the Rate, Rhythm, and Depth of Respiration for 1 Full Minute

In children, the respiratory rate should be counted while the child sleeps, if possible.

Tachypnea is an early sign of most pulmonary, parenchymal, cardiac, or systemic causes of respiratory distress. Hyperventilation can occur secondary to acidosis or central nervous system disease. Slow respirations may indicate central nervous system depression, hypoxia, shock, or systemic infection.

Exhaling should take about twice as long as inhaling, but in patients with COPD, it may take up to four times longer. Rhythm should be even, with occasional sighs. Shallow respirations, which are rapid, indicate that restrictive forces must be overcome. Box 11-1 describes abnormal breathing patterns.

Box 11-1 | Abnormal Breathing Patterns

Cheyne-Stokes respirations are manifested by rhythmic increase and decrease in depth, punctuated by regular episodes of apnea. This may be a sign of severe heart failure or neurological disease.

Tachypnea is rapid breathing with no change in depth and can be caused by hypoxia, pain, fever, or anxiety. Consider pulmonary embolism, foreign body aspiration, anaphylaxis, pneumothorax, heart failure, asthma, or pneumonia.

Asymmetrical chest movement with respirations may be observed in lobar pneumonia, pleural effusion, or any condition that affects just one side of the chest.

Use of accessory muscles indicates respiratory distress. Observe for bulging or retraction of the intercostals, sternocleidomastoid, and/or trapezius muscles.

Nasal flaring is an objective manifestation of hypoxia.

Listen for Stridor

Stridor is caused by extrathoracic inspiratory dynamic narrowing of the airway in the oropharynx, glottis, subglottic region, or midtrachea. Any condition that causes further decrease in the lumen of the airway will obstruct airflow and produce stridor. Inspiratory stridor usually indicates a supraglottic obstruction. If the obstruction varies or is extrathoracic (above the vocal cords), inspiration is affected more because the negative intraairway pressure during inspiration tends to collapse the extrathoracic airway. If the obstruction varies and affects the intrathoracic airways, expiration is prolonged because the positive intrathoracic pressure tends to collapse these airways during expiration. Expiratory or biphasic respiratory stridor generally indicates an obstruction at or below the larynx.

With severe narrowing of the air passage, stridor may be audible on both inspiration and expiration but is worse during inspiration. Biphasic or expiratory stridor alone usually indicates a more significant obstruction. Supraglottic stridor is usually quiet and wet and is associated with a muffled voice, dysphasia, and a preference to sit. Subglottic lesions produce a loud stridor, often causing a hoarse voice, barky cough, and possibly facial edema. Inspiratory stridor may be a sign of incomplete obstruction of the airway by a foreign body.

Infants younger than 6 months who present with stridor may have an underlying anatomical abnormality that may be symptomatic secondary to an acute illness. Common anomalies that predispose the infant to upper airway obstruction are anomalous vascular rings, laryngeal webs, laryngomalacia, or tracheomalacia. Stridor in older children may indicate foreign body aspiration, infection, inflammation, trauma, or tumor.

Listen for Audible Wheeze

Expiratory wheezing is a high-pitched musical sound caused by partial airway obstruction. It is commonly associated with disorders of the lower respiratory tract that cause inflammation, infection, or bronchoconstriction such as asthma and bronchitis.

Increased inspiratory effort suggests disease in the upper airways, whereas increased expiratory effort suggests disease in the smaller airways or lower respiratory tract.

Listen for Voice Changes

Voice changes may occur in association with upper airway obstruction. Paralysis of the vocal cords results in dysphonia. Subglottic stenosis results in decreased volume of the voice because a much smaller column of air is making the vocal cords vibrate. Involvement of the supraglottic area, proximal to the vocal cords, can result in a hyponasal or muffled voice (seen in tonsillitis and epiglottitis). A normal voice with stridor may indicate the lesion is subglottic or tracheal (see Chapter 5).

Take Pulse, Temperature, and Blood Pressure

Palpate the radial, femoral, popliteal, and pedal pulses for rate and quality.

Tachycardia increases cardiac output. It occurs either as a result of primary heart disease or as a secondary process in response to oxygen deprivation because of PE, pneumonia, fever, and/or heart failure. Tachycardia and drowsiness may indicate a metabolic acidosis. Bradycardia is usually seen late in respiratory disease.

Tachycardia may occur with an irregular pulse, signaling heart failure from atrial fibrillation and/or heart block. Diminished peripheral pulses indicate possible atherosclerotic vessel disease or decreased cardiac output.

Fever may indicate epiglottitis or any other upper and/or lower respiratory tract infection.

Orthostatic hypotension may be secondary to dehydration associated with pneumonia or status asthmaticus. Anaphylaxis is also manifested by severe hypotension. Pulsus paradoxus, an inspiratory drop in systolic blood pressure of more than 10 mm Hg, is caused by greater inspiratory effort from increased airway resistance. Negative intrathoracic pressure is associated with increased afterload and low systolic blood pressure. In heart failure, decreased stroke volume reduces the systolic blood pressure. Compensatory vasoconstriction maintains a constant diastolic pressure and along with the decreased systolic pressure may produce a decreased pulse pressure.

Inspect the Oral Cavity

First observe the oropharyngeal cavity for any evidence of a foreign body that may be obstructing the airway. Also, evidence of vomitus may indicate possible aspiration. Note the color of the tongue and mucous membranes for signs of central cyanosis.

Inspect the posterior pharynx for peritonsillar cellulitis, retropharyngeal abscess, or other intraoral pathology that might be causing obstruction. Lift the jaw forward. Obstruction of the airway associated with micrognathia, depressed airway reflexes, or an enlarged tongue will diminish with this maneuver because the tongue will be lifted off the posterior pharynx. If epiglottitis is suspected, do not examine the oral cavity.

Inspect the Nose

Assess the patency of the nares. Fifty percent of airway resistance comes from the nose. Check for nasal flaring. An infant who has nasal flaring is using a compensatory mechanism to decrease airway resistance. Noisy, difficult breathing in an infant, especially while feeding, may signal choanal atresia. A deviated septum compromises the patency of one side of the nose when there is mucosal swelling.

Palpate the Neck

Neck masses caused by intraoral, paratracheal, or intrathoracic malignant disease may cause respiratory distress. Inspect the position of the trachea. To assess the trachea for lateral displacement, position your index finger first on the right side of the suprasternal notch and then on the left. If the trachea has shifted to the side, you will feel the wall on one side but only soft tissue on the other. This is most likely to occur with pneumothorax. Observe the neck for jugular venous distention; this is a sign of heart failure.

Examine the Skin and Extremities

Note cyanosis. Bluish color seen in the lips and mucous membranes of the mouth (central cyanosis) is associated with low arterial saturation and may result from inadequate gas exchange in the lungs or from cardiac shunting. Cyanosis implies more than 5 g/100 ml of desaturated hemoglobin, but its absence does not imply that hypoxemia is not present. Dark-skinned patients' mucous membranes may appear gray with central cyanosis. Central cyanosis may also be seen in persons with COPD. Bluish color of extremities (peripheral cyanosis) may be observed in Caucasians and is associated with low venous saturation, resulting from vasoconstriction, vascular occlusion, or reduced cardiac output.

Pallor may be a manifestation of severe anemia.

Note clubbing, which is characterized by the loss of the angle between the skin and nail bed. This is a manifestation of chronic tissue hypoxia that occurs with lung cancer and other chronic lung diseases. It is uncommon in children other than those with cystic fibrosis or cyanotic congenital heart disease. Clubbing develops rapidly with infective endocarditis.

Test for peripheral edema. Edema of the lower extremities may be a sign of increased right-heart filling pressure caused by primary lung disease or left-ventricular failure. Make note of how high the edema extends up the extremity. In children, the location of peripheral edema is age dependent. In young infants, edema occurs as hepatomegaly and periorbital or flank edema. In older children, lower extremity edema can occur.

Note any angioedema. The presence of generalized or local giant urticaria is objective evidence of probable anaphylaxis.

Check skin perfusion by pressing on the skin of a finger or sole of a foot and saying "capillary refill" after removing the pressure. A normal finding is that the color returns to the skin in 2 seconds or before you can finish saying the words.

Feel the skin for diaphoresis. When respiratory muscles are working at their maximum level to overcome increased resistive and elastic forces, the child will sweat, especially on the forehead and above the lip.

Palpate the Chest

Using the palmar surface of the hands, palpate the entire chest for tenderness, depressions, bulges, and crepitus (presence of air in the subcutaneous tissues). Crepitus may indicate a chest injury, pneumothorax, or emphysema.

Pneumothorax, atelectasis, pneumonia, and partial paralysis of the diaphragm will result in reduced expansion of one side of the chest wall, and chest wall motion will be decreased.

Assess for Vocal Fremitus

Fremitus is diminished in pneumothorax, asthma, emphysema, and other conditions that trap air in the lung. Vocal fremitus intensity may be increased in pneumonia, heart failure, and tumor, all conditions that increase the lung density.

Percuss the Chest

Sounds produced by percussion indicate the density of lung tissue (see Chapter 12). In children, transmission of a percussion note and assessment of the quality of transmitted sound are useful to reveal an area of consolidation or effusion that would be difficult to auscultate with an uncooperative child.

Auscultate Breath Sounds

Auscultation of bronchial or bronchovesicular breath sounds over the peripheral lungs may indicate consolidation, which occurs when lungs fill with exudate. Young children normally have bronchovesicular sounds because of the thinness of their chest wall.

If breath sounds are diminished over all lung fields, suspect shallow breathing, lack of air movement, neuromuscular diseases, obesity, or COPD. Breath sounds will be inaudible in areas of pneumothorax.

Abnormal lung sounds are superimposed on normal sounds and can be auscultated over any area of the lung field during inspiration or expiration. Documentation of abnormal lung sounds should include type of sound, location where it is heard, and the phase(s) of respiration in which it is noted. In small children it may be difficult to distinguish upper and lower airway sounds. Listening with the stethoscope over the nose or mouth and then returning to the lungs may help to identify the findings.

Crackles or rales are discontinuous popping sounds heard most often during inspiration.

They are caused by the explosive equalization of gas pressure between two compartments of the lung when a closed section of the airway that separates them suddenly opens. They indicate the presence of fluid, mucus, or pus in the smaller airways. Fine crackles are soft and high pitched. Medium crackles are louder and lower pitched. Coarse crackles are moist and more explosive.

The frequency and timing of crackles are the important parts of assessment. In resolving pneumonia, crackling is heard on inspiration caused by a mix between the aerated and nonaerated alveoli and bronchioles. In airways that are swollen and narrowed, such as in asthma bronchiolitis, generalized medium or coarse crackles are heard throughout both phases of respiration. Early inspiratory crackles are heard in COPD. Mid to late inspiratory crackles are more likely a sign of interstitial lung disease or heart failure. Crackles may be heard over the site of a pulmonary embolus.

Wheezing is frequently described as a whistling sound and can be heard during inspiration, expiration, or both. The sound is high pitched and musical. Wheezing indicates that there is fluid in the large airways such as in severe heart failure or, more often, heralds bronchospasm, as seen in asthma. In addition, localized wheezing may accompany incomplete obstruction of the airway by a foreign body.

A wheeze of fixed pitch occurring with inspiration and expiration suggests a localized abnormality. Wheezes of varying pitch occurring predominantly throughout expiration reflect the narrowing of airways of different calibers.

Rhonchi are continuous, deep-pitched, coarse breath sounds usually heard during expiration. Rhonchi are frequently present when the patient has bronchitis or pneumonia.

Pleural friction rub is a grating or squeaking sound usually heard in the lateral lung fields during inspiration and expiration. It indicates that parietal and visceral pleural linings are inflamed and are rubbing together as may occur with pneumonia, pleural effusion, pleuritis, and tumors. It is often accompanied by limited chest expansion because of pain.

If abnormal lung sounds are detected, additional auscultation for bronchophony, egophony, and whispered pectoriloquy is indicated. Consolidation will produce positive findings for each of these tests. To test for bronchophony, instruct the patient to say "ninety-nine." The words are heard louder and clearer than usual. In egophony, instruct the patient to say "ee." This sound is transmitted as "ay" if consolidation is present. To test whispered pectoriloquy, instruct the patient to whisper a sentence. Whispered sounds are louder and clearer than normal.

Auscultate Heart Sounds

In COPD, lung hyperinflation may muffle heart sounds. Poor tissue oxygenation may result in tachycardia. In children, muffled heart sounds may indicate pericarditis.

In heart failure, S_1 and S_2 may equal rapid pulse rate or may indicate a pulse deficit. An S_3 (ventricular gallop) is an early sign of heart failure and is heard best at the apex of the heart. S_4 (atrial gallop) typically indicates a stressed heart and heart failure in children. In adults it may be the result of hypertension, MI, or CAD causing heart failure. A summation gallop may also occur with heart failure; this is the result of S_3, S_4, and rapid rate.

Listen for the presence of any murmurs and note their location, grade of loudness, timing, or radiation. Incompetent heart valves may be the cause of heart failure.

LABORATORY AND DIAGNOSTIC STUDIES

Diagnostic tests are indicated in almost all initial evaluations of the patient presenting with shortness of breath. Posteroanterior (PA) and lateral chest radiographs, hemoglobin level, and spirometry are useful preliminary tests.

Transcutaneous Pulse Oximetry (Paco₂)

Oximetry measures the fraction of oxygen carried in hemoglobin and provides non-invasive information about the delivery of oxygen from the atmosphere to the pulmonary capillaries. A PaO_2 in healthy adults ranges from 80 to 103 mm Hg, and more than 95%

saturation of hemoglobin is considered normal. In children, a pulse oximetry reading of 95% to 98% is normal, 90% to 95% is mild hypoxia, 85% to 90% is moderate hypoxemia, and less than 85% is severe hypoxemia.

Chest Radiography

Chest radiographs are essential in the diagnosis of dyspnea and may show pneumothorax, pneumonia, malignant disease, pleural disease, foreign body, or pulmonary edema. They may also provide clues to other causes of dyspnea such as cardiomegaly, deformities of the chest bones and musculature, and the position of the diaphragm. When a foreign body is suspected, both inspiratory and expiratory chest films may be helpful.

Electrocardiography

An electrocardiogram (ECG) may provide important information about myocardial ischemia, arrhythmias, pericarditis, or the presence of pulmonary disease. Cardiopulmonary exercise testing may be done if the severity of the dyspnea is disproportionate to objective tests, there are coexisting cardiac and pulmonary causes, or deconditioning, obesity, or psychological factors are suspected.

Echocardiography

An echocardiogram is performed when cardiac disease is suspected; this test can define the cause of dyspnea related to heart chamber size, valves, pericardial disease, and ventricular function.

Hemoglobin and Hematocrit

Significantly decreased hemoglobin and hematocrit levels suggest anemia as a possible cause of dyspnea. Erythrocytosis may indicate chronic hypoxia resulting from a number of causes, including COPD.

Spirometry

Spirometry is indicated if the dyspnea is related to obstructive or restrictive lung disease. Spirometry measures forced vital capacity (FVC), 1-second forced expiratory volume (FEV_1), the FEV_1/FVC ratio, and the peak expiratory flow rate (PEFR). In obstructive lung disease (i.e., asthma and

COPD), the FEV_1 and the FEV_1/FVC ratio are less than predicted. In restrictive lung disease (i.e., pneumonia, pneumothorax, pleural effusion), the FVC is reduced and the ratio is normal or elevated.

Additional Testing

Additional diagnostic tests may be indicated after the initial data gathering and can include the following:

- Computed tomography (CT) provides more detailed assessment of mass lesions.
- Pulmonary angiography confirms PE.
- Complete blood cell count with differential is used to determine the presence of bacterial infection.
- Blood urea nitrogen and creatinine levels help assess renal function. Renal insufficiency frequently presents with dyspnea as a result of the combined effects of volume overload and anemia.
- Arterial blood gases (ABGs) should be determined in an acutely ill patient with dyspnea and tachypnea.
- If sputum is present, a sputum culture should be obtained to determine the presence of an infectious agent.

DIFFERENTIAL DIAGNOSIS

When patients report severe dyspnea and manifest significant oxygen deprivation, emergent assessment and referral are indicated. The following health problems may be the cause of the emergent situation.

EMERGENT CONDITIONS MANIFESTED BY DYSPNEA

Pulmonary Embolus

A patient reporting severe dyspnea, cough, fever, hemoptysis, chest pain, history of deep vein thrombosis, and/or history of recent immobilization should be evaluated for possible PE (see Chapter 9).

Foreign Body Aspiration

Foreign body aspiration occurs most frequently in children and the elderly. If the event was witnessed, history of aspiration is usually clear. If the person is found after the event, the history may not be as revealing.

Generally, the onset of cough is sudden and unexpected. If the foreign body is obstructing the airway, the patient is in acute respiratory distress and immediate intubation or bronchoscopy is indicated to remove the foreign body and open the airway. Partial obstruction of the airway may cause stridor, cyanosis, labored respirations, and/or wheezing. Lateral neck and chest radiographs may reveal the location and size of the obstructing object (see Chapter 12).

Anaphylaxis

Anaphylaxis is an emergent situation. History may include history of insect bite, drug ingestion, recent meal containing shellfish, or exposure to known allergens. Early symptoms include pruritic rash, feeling of warmth, wheezing, fatigue, lightheadedness, and increasing dyspnea. On examination, persons in anaphylaxis manifest angioedema, tachypnea, clammy skin, hypotension, wheezes, and tachycardia. Immediate treatment and support of ventilation may be necessary.

Pneumothorax

History of blunt chest trauma often seen after a motor vehicle accident or a fall may cause pneumothorax, hemothorax, or pulmonary contusion. Cystic fibrosis may cause a spontaneous pneumothorax from rupture of subpleural blebs located at the apex of the upper lobe or in the superior segment of the lower lobe. Spontaneous pneumothorax may also occur in males, with the highest incidence between ages 15 and 30 in tall, thin individuals. There is sudden severe chest pain and dyspnea aggravated by normal respiratory movement. Absent or decreased breath sounds are found on the side of the pneumothorax. Chest radiography may be diagnostic.

Croup

Croup, or laryngotracheobronchitis, is a viral infection that is usually preceded by symptoms of an upper respiratory tract infection. The illness is usually gradual in onset and includes a hoarse, seal-bark cough and fever. The degree of respiratory distress can be variable.

Acute Epiglottitis

Acute epiglottitis is a serious, life-threatening bacterial infection of the epiglottis caused primarily by *H. influenzae*. It typically has a rapid onset with stridor, high fever, drooling, muffled voice, and sore throat. A child will appear anxious and may be sitting forward. Parents should be asked if a child has received an *H. influenzae* B, or HiB, immunization. This condition is rare in children who have been immunized.

Bacterial Tracheitis

Bacterial tracheitis is usually a secondary infection caused by *Staphylococcus aureus* or *H. influenzae* that inflames the trachea after an antecedent viral infection. It is a subglottic lesion and mimics croup; however, a high fever and toxic appearance are present. Frequently there is a copious amount of purulent sputum present.

Status Asthmaticus

Acute bronchoconstriction in a patient with asthma can develop as a result of a respiratory tract infection, exposure to allergens, inhalation of fumes, airway irritants, and environmental factors. Airway obstruction is caused not only by bronchial smooth muscle constriction but also by mucosal edema and excessive mucus production. Predominant symptoms include breathlessness, wheezing, and coughing. Absence of wheezing in a child with asthma may indicate severe airway obstruction with poor air exchange.

Botulism

Botulism is poisoning that may occur after ingestion of the toxin in inadequately cooked or improperly canned food. Infant botulism is caused by ingestion of the spores of *C. botulinum* rather than the exotoxin. It occurs before the first year of life, and honey has been implicated in 20% of patients. Symptoms occur 1 to 2 days after ingestion of contaminated food. Weakness and respiratory dyspnea and failure often accompany visual problems. Infant botulism begins with constipation, and the infant becomes weaker and listless. Respiratory arrest may be sudden.

NONEMERGENT CONDITIONS MANIFESTED BY DYSPNEA

Chronic progressive dyspnea is most often caused by chronic pulmonary disease, heart failure, and obesity. It is seen less often in severe anemia and carcinoma of the pulmonary system. These patients report gradual onset of shortness of breath over days or weeks.

Chronic Obstructive Pulmonary Disease

COPD is associated with frequent cough that is worse in the morning, sputum production that is clear to yellow in color, decreasing exercise tolerance, and mild to moderate fatigue. History of smoking is present in most instances. Exposure to asbestos, coal dust, and other significant environmental pollutants may also be reported. Objective manifestations of COPD include rapid, shallow respirations, reddish complexion, increased AP diameter, use of accessory muscles to breathe, pursed-lip breathing, decreased tactile fremitus, decreased respiratory excursion bilaterally, hyperresonant lungs, distant breath sounds, prolonged expiration, occasional wheezes, and muffled heart sounds. Chest radiography, pulmonary function tests, and possible exercise tests are indicated to confirm the diagnosis of COPD.

Heart Failure

Persons reporting history of heart disease or heart valve disease, dyspnea, orthopnea, PND, peripheral edema, weight gain, cough with frothy sputum, fatigue, and palpitations must be further assessed for acute heart failure. Physical examination findings may include altered level of consciousness, anxiety, jugular venous distention, tachypnea, rales, rhonchi, tachycardia, displaced point of maximum impulse, S_3, S_4, and possible ascites. Symptoms in children also include sweating on the forehead or upper lip. An ECG and chest radiograph will show increased heart size, oximetry will reveal a decreased arterial P_{O_2}, and an echocardiogram will display a significantly reduced ejection fraction.

Anemia

Patients reporting dyspnea (especially on exertion), fatigue, lightheadedness, palpitations, and possible history of chronic disease should have blood tests to measure the oxygen-carrying capacity of their blood (hemoglobin and hematocrit levels). Hematological diseases affect the oxygen-carrying capacity of the blood, with resulting tissue hypoxia. A decrease in arterial pH stimulates the central nervous system and dyspnea is seen. Objective signs of anemia include tachycardia and pallor.

Poor Physical Conditioning

Poor physical conditioning can cause the patient to experience shortness of breath with exertion. Associated symptoms may include cardiac palpitations and history of excessive weight and sedentary lifestyle. The physical examination is often normal except for tachycardia and possible obesity. Exercise stress tests may be done for an adult with cardiovascular risk factors or a history of cardiovascular disease.

Asthma

Asthma is the most frequent cause of recurrent dyspnea. Persons usually report a history of asthma and possibly allergies, and may be taking prescribed inhaled bronchodilators and/or inhaled steroids. Paroxysmal cough and audible wheeze often accompany dyspnea. They may report recent respiratory tract infection, exposure to known allergens, or strenuous exercise. Objective manifestation on physical examination includes restlessness, tachypnea, use of accessory muscles to breathe, intercostal retraction, decreased vocal fremitus, decreased breath sounds, and inspiratory and possible expiratory wheezes. Pulse oximetry and spirometry testing will provide confirming evidence of asthma. ABGs are indicated in the patient manifesting acute O_2 deprivation, and chest radiographs are indicated if a lower respiratory tract infection is suspected. If the patient does not have a history of asthma and the spirometry test result is normal, a methacholine challenge test may be diagnostic.

The lessening or absence of wheezes in a person with asthma may indicate mucus plugging and an impending episode of status asthmaticus.

Pneumonia

Pneumonia is usually associated with dyspnea, pleuritic chest pain, cough with greenish or rusty-colored sputum, fever, and chills. In children, irritability, feeding problems, and lack of playfulness may also be seen. Objective manifestations of pneumonia include fever, tachycardia, tachypnea, inspiratory crackles, asynchronous breathing, vocal fremitus, dull percussion sound over area of consolidation, and bronchophony. Pneumonia can be confirmed by chest radiography and sputum cultures.

Hyperventilation Syndrome

Hyperventilation syndrome is a common cause of recurrent faintness without actual loss of consciousness. Dyspnea, lightheadedness, palpitations, and paresthesias (perioral and extremities) occur. Restlessness, anxiety, and a normal cardiovascular examination are present. Recumbency does not relieve the symptoms. Chest radiography is normal.

Laryngomalacia

Laryngomalacia is the most common cause of persistent stridor in infancy. Onset of the stridor is almost always within the first 4 weeks of life, commonly in the first week (with preterm neonates who were on ventilation at high risk). Occasionally parents become aware of the condition when a respiratory tract infection is present. Stridor is predominantly inspiratory, and the sound may change with change in position of the infant. The cry and cough are normal. Direct visualization of the larynx is performed for diagnosis.

Vascular Ring

Tracheal compression from vascular anomalies may cause stridor and dyspnea in infants. The main symptom is soft inspiratory stridor with expiratory wheeze. Frequently a brassy cough and difficulty in swallowing may be present. Barium swallow followed by echocardiography is done to establish the diagnosis.

DIFFERENTIAL DIAGNOSIS OF *Emergent Conditions Manifested by Dyspnea*

CONDITION	HISTORY	PHYSICAL FINDINGS	DIAGNOSTIC STUDIES
Pulmonary embolus	Acute-onset dyspnea, cough, mild to severe chest pain, sense of impending doom; hemoptysis; history of DVT, recent surgery, oral contraceptive, smoker, hypercoagulability states	Restlessness, fever, tachycardia, tachypnea, diminished breath sounds, crackles, wheezing, pleural friction rub	ABGs, chest radiograph, ECG, ventilation/perfusion scans
Foreign body aspiration	Acute-onset dyspnea; history of eating or drinking large amounts of alcohol; in children, history of putting small objects in mouth; possible cough	Apnea or tachypnea, restlessness, suprasternal retractions, intoxication, inspiratory stridor, localized wheeze	Lateral neck radiograph, chest radiograph, bronchoscopy
Anaphylaxis	Acute-onset dyspnea; history of insect sting, ingestion of drug, or allergen	Angioedema, tachypnea, clammy skin, hypotension, bilateral wheezes, tachycardia	None; emergency measures necessary
Pneumothorax	Acute-onset dyspnea; sharp, tearing chest pain; pain may radiate to ipsilateral shoulder	Tachycardia, diminished breath sounds, decreased tactile fremitus, hyperresonance of lung area affected; possible hypertension and tracheal shift	Chest radiograph, ABGs
Croup	History of upper respiratory tract infection	Hoarse, seal-bark cough, fever (variable)	None initially; if respiratory distress increases, pulse oximeter and referral
Acute epiglottitis	Positional sitting forward; sore throat, anxious, toxic child	High fever, drooling, stridor, muffled voice	Admit; life threatening
Bacterial tracheitis	Recent viral infection	Fever, stridor, purulent sputum	Radiography of airway, WBC increased, tracheal culture
Status asthmaticus	Recent URI, exposure to allergens, breathlessness	Wheezing, coughing, tachycardia, tachypnea	Peak flows, chest radiograph, ABGs
Botulism	Honey ingestion in infant, contaminated food ingestion	Hypoventilation, drooling, weak cry, ptosis, ophthalmoplegia, loss of head control	Pulmonary function testing, chest radiograph, fluoroscopy, stool culture

ABG, Arterial blood gas; *ECG*, electrocardiogram; *DVT*, deep vein thrombosis.

DIFFERENTIAL DIAGNOSIS OF *Nonemergent Conditions Manifested by Dyspnea*

CONDITION	HISTORY	PHYSICAL FINDINGS	DIAGNOSTIC STUDIES
Pneumonia	Dyspnea, cough, sputum production (green, rust, or red), pleuritic chest pain, chills; in infants and children: irritability and feeding problems	Fever, tachycardia, tachypnea, inspiratory crackles, asynchronous breathing, vocal fremitus, percussion dull or flat over area of consolidation, bronchophony, egophony	Chest radiograph, sputum cultures, ABGs, WBC

Continued

DIFFERENTIAL DIAGNOSIS OF *Nonemergent Conditions Manifested by Dyspnea—cont'd*

CONDITION	HISTORY	PHYSICAL FINDINGS	DIAGNOSTIC STUDIES
Hyperventilation syndrome	Dyspnea, lightheadedness, palpitations, paresthesias (perioral and extremities)	Restlessness, anxiety, normal CV examination	Chest radiograph
Laryngomalacia	Neonate, infant: history of stridor, history of URI	Inspiratory stridor; normal cough, cry	Refer for visualization of larynx
Vascular ring	Infant: dyspnea, brassy cough, difficulty swallowing	Inspiratory stridor with expiratory wheeze	Barium swallow, echocardiography
Heart failure	Chronic progressive dyspnea, cough, frothy sputum, fatigue, lightheadedness, syncope, weight gain, ankle swelling, palpitations, PND, orthopnea, history of heart disease; in children: chronic progressive dyspnea, sweating above lip and forehead, especially while eating	Altered level of consciousness, restlessness, jugular venous distention, tachypnea, use of accessory muscles to breathe, rales, rhonchi, wheezes, tachycardia, decreased peripheral pulses, cool extremities, displaced PMI, S_3, S_4, ascites, liver enlargement	ECG, chest radiograph, ABGs, echocardiogram
Anemia	Dyspnea on exertion, fatigue, palpitations, lightheadedness, history of chronic disease	Pallor, tachypnea, cool dry skin of extremities, possible orthostatic hypotension	CBC, iron studies
Poor physical conditioning	Dyspnea on exertion, weight gain, palpitation on exertion, sedentary lifestyle, cigarette smoker	Overweight, tachycardia	Cardiac stress test
Asthma	Dyspnea, paroxysmal cough, audible wheeze, history of asthma or allergies	Restlessness, tachypnea, use of accessory muscles to breathe, intercostal retractions, decreased vocal fremitus, decreased breath sounds, inspiratory and possibly expiratory wheezes	Spirometry, chest radiograph, ABGs
COPD	Chronic progressive dyspnea, dyspnea on exertion, persistent cough, minimal sputum, easy fatigue, history of smoking	Rapid shallow respirations, reddish complexion, increased AP diameter of thorax, use of accessory muscles to breathe, pursed-lip breathing, decreased tactile fremitus, decreased respiratory excursion bilaterally, lungs hyperresonant, distant breath sounds, prolonged expiration, occasional wheezes, possible tachycardia, muffled heart sounds	Chest radiograph, pulmonary function tests, exercise tests, ABGs

ABGs, Arterial blood gases; *WBC,* white blood cell; *CV,* cerebrovascular; *URI,* upper respiratory tract infection; *PND,* paroxysmal nocturnal dyspnea; *PMI,* point of maximal impulse; *ECG,* electrocardiogram; *COPD,* chronic obstructive pulmonary disease; *AP,* anteroposterior.

CHAPTER RESOURCES

Evans SE, Scanlon PD: Current practice in pulmonary function testing, *Mayo Clinic Proceedings* 78:758, 2003.

Karnani NG, Reisfield GM, Wilson GR: Evaluation of chronic dyspnea, *Am Fam Physician* 71:8, 2005.

Leung AKC, Kellner JD, Johnson DW: Viral croup: a current perspective, *J Pediatr Health Care* 18:297, 2004.

Meek PM: Measurement of dyspnea in chronic obstructive pulmonary disease: what is the tool telling you? *Chron Respir Dis* 1:1, 2004.

Malhotra A: Viral croup, *Pediatr Rev* 22:5, 2001.

Owens S: Exercise intolerance, *Pediatr Rev* 21:6, 2000.

Schwartzstein RM: Evaluation of the patient with chronic dyspnea: clinical application of pathophysiologic principles, *Prim Care Case Rev* 3:201, 2000.

Werner HA: Status asthmaticus in children: a review, *Chest* 119:1913, 2001.

Zoorob R, Campbell J: Acute dyspnea in the office, *Am Fam Physician* 68:1803, 2003.

Cough

Cough is one of the most common symptoms for which patients seek health care. Cough occurs when inspiration is followed by an explosive expiration. Coughing promotes clearance of secretions and foreign bodies from the airways. Cough is usually the result of a reflex initiated by stimulation of the sensory nerve endings beneath and between the epithelium of the larynx and tracheobronchial tree. A cough arises from the stimulation of the cough reflex in the upper respiratory tract by postnasal drip, clearing of the throat, or both. The reflex stimulation follows the vagus nerve to the "cough center," which is located in the medulla oblongata of the brainstem. However, other anatomical locations may be stimulated and initiate the cough reflex, including the pleura, pericardium, ear canals, esophagus, and stomach. The cough reflex is absent in very young infants. Effective coughing may also be impossible in emaciated persons, in persons whose respiratory musculature is weak or paralyzed, and in those with massive ascites.

Although most coughs are a symptom of minor upper respiratory tract infections such as the common cold, a persistent cough can greatly affect a patient's quality of life and ability to sleep. Keep in mind, however, that a cough in a patient in acute distress may signal a life-threatening problem (such as foreign body aspiration with occlusion of airway), severe asthma, escalating heart failure, or pneumonia.

DIAGNOSTIC REASONING: FOCUSED HISTORY

What Type of Cough Is This?

Key Question
- How long have you had a cough?

Duration

Cough can be characterized by the following three categories of duration: (1) acute, less than 3 weeks; (2) subacute, lasting 3 to 8 weeks; and (3) chronic, lasting more than 8 weeks. A cough of recent onset is most often the result of viral or bacterial infection in the respiratory system. Allergies can also precipitate acute onset of cough in both children and adults. Coughs of longer duration (>3 weeks) are more likely caused by chronic lung or heart disease, such as chronic obstructive pulmonary disease (COPD), cystic fibrosis, chronic bronchitis, asthma, postnasal drainage, heart failure, pertussis, and chronic sinusitis. Gastroesophageal reflux disease (GERD) and a foreign body in the ear canal should also be considered in both adults and children.

Is This Cough Related to a Life-Threatening Condition?

Key Questions
- Are you short of breath?
- Do you have a history of heart failure?
- Do you have a history of asthma?
- If a child: Have you noticed the child putting small objects in his or her mouth?

Shortness of Breath

Cough associated with shortness of breath (SOB) usually suggests a physical obstruction of the airway caused by a foreign body or the effects of acute asthma. Persons with heart failure report orthopnea, paroxysmal nocturnal dyspnea (PND), cough with possible frothy sputum, possible weight gain with swollen feet and ankles, and often a history of heart disease. Cardiac failure of any kind results in decreased lung compliance and cough.

History of Asthma

Acute exacerbation of asthma is characterized by an irritating nonproductive cough that can progress to tachypnea, dyspnea, wheezing, grunting, cyanosis, fatigue, and finally respiratory and cardiac failure. Viral infection, especially respiratory syncytial virus (RSV), parainfluenza viruses, and rhinoviruses, are the most important triggers of asthma in children.

Foreign Body

Consider a foreign body aspiration in any child. A child who has aspirated a foreign body can have a varied presentation; generally, the onset of cough is sudden and unexpected. A brief period of severe coughing, gagging, and choking occurs; then a quiet period ensues of no coughing. This can last for hours, days, or even months. A foreign body in the lower airway can produce either emphysema caused by a ball-valve phenomenon or complete distal atelectasis because of absorption of the trapped gas. A mobile foreign body in the lower airway can also produce a paroxysmal cough, with cyanotic episodes and stridor as a result of proximal migration and subglottic impaction.

A foreign body in the esophagus can also produce airway obstruction and cough as well as dysphasia to solid foods because the posterior trachea is compliant and adjacent to the anterior esophagus. Coins are the most frequently found foreign bodies.

What Do I Need to Know if the Cough Is Acute (<3 Weeks' Duration)?

Key Questions

- Do you have nasal congestion or a sore throat?
- Do you have or have you had a fever? Do you have chills?
- Do you have a headache?

Nasal Congestion

Nasal congestion occurs as a result of a cascade of events. First, the offending organism invades the epithelial cells of the upper respiratory tract. Inflammatory mediators are released, resulting in altered vascular permeability, edema, and nasal stuffiness. Stimulation of cholinergic nerves in the nose and upper respiratory tract leads to increased mucus production (rhinorrhea) and occasionally to bronchoconstriction, which causes cough. It is hypothesized that cellular damage to the nasopharynx is probably what causes the sore and scratchy throat.

Runny nose with cough and mild fever followed by a persistent cough for more than 1 week with clear to off-white mucus greater in the morning suggests bronchitis.

Nasal congestion or a sensation of postnasal discharge, especially associated with facial pain or pressure, suggests sinusitis. A history of bloody nasal discharge may also be present.

Infants with nasal congestion 3 days to 8 weeks after birth who have a cough but are afebrile may have *Chlamydia trachomatis,* contracted from the mother during childbirth. Older children, adolescents, and adults with a sore throat, fever, headache, and malaise progressing to a cough may have mycoplasmal pneumonia.

Fever

In adults, a temperature that is less than 38.3° C (101° F), small amounts of clear to yellow sputum production, nasal congestion, sore throat, and generalized malaise most frequently accompany acute cough with a viral etiology. Acute cough of a more serious nature (e.g., bacterial pneumonia) is usually accompanied by a temperature of greater than 38.3° C (>101° F), chest pain, SOB, and purulent or dark sputum. Acute cough resulting from noninfectious processes (heart failure or pulmonary embolism) lacks the signs of infectious disease such as fever, chills, and purulent sputum.

Viral infection is the most common cause of a low-grade fever in a child who has nasal congestion and little interruption of appetite and activity. An acute cough associated with a persistent fever, loss of appetite, and ill appearance indicates a more serious illness, such as bacterial pneumonia.

Headache

Headache pain may signal sinusitis as the cause of the cough (see Chapter 2).

What Does the Nature of the Sputum Tell Me?

Key Questions

- Do you cough up sputum?
- Does it have an odor?
- How much have you coughed up?
- What color is the sputum?

The presence of sputum and its characteristics are not helpful in distinguishing bacterial from viral infections. Malodorous sputum suggests anaerobic infection of the lungs and sinuses. Very thick, tenacious, dark sputum is characteristic of bronchiectasis. Cloudy, thick sputum suggests lower respiratory tract infection but may also reflect an increase in the number of eosinophils from an asthmatic process. Viral bronchitis rarely causes more than 2 tablespoons of mucopurulent sputum per day. Bacterial bronchitis, however, is frequently associated with purulent sputum, often more than 2 tablespoons per day. Clear, mucoid sputum indicates allergic disorder. Hemoptysis, uncommon in children, usually indicates a more serious disease, such as bacterial pneumonia, an acute inflammatory bronchitis, cystic fibrosis, tumor, or a foreign body.

Children tend to swallow rather than expectorate sputum. Occasionally emesis will have mucus in it and can be used to identify the sputum. A child with a persistent cough and purulent sputum is likely to have an infectious lung disease.

What Does the Nature of the Cough Tell Me?

Key Questions

- Is the cough getting worse or more frequent?
- What time of day is the cough most bothersome?
- If a child: Did the child have an episode of severe cough, gagging, and choking a few weeks ago?
- What type of work do you do?
- What does the cough sound like?

Severity and Progression of Cough

A cough in children or adults that becomes progressively worse may indicate pertussis. Pertussis has three stages. The first stage presents with a mild cough, rhinorrhea, conjunctivitis, and low-grade fever for 1 to 2 weeks. In the next stage, the cough becomes severe and comes in short paroxysms. There is a "whoop" on the inspiration effort at the end of the paroxysm. In the convalescent stage, the coughing and paroxysmal whooping decrease, but the cough may persist in a milder form for 3 months.

Young infants and older adults with pertussis do not "whoop."

A cough in children that begins with a history of mild upper respiratory tract illness followed in 2 to 3 days with a cough that is brassy in sound may indicate croup. The cough is usually worse at night. Symptoms escalate as compromise of the upper airway continues from the viral agent (usually parainfluenza). Obstruction increases, stridor becomes continuous, and there is nasal flaring and suprasternal, infrasternal, and intracostal retraction. The child is agitated and sits up. In most children recovery occurs within a few hours. However, any intensification of symptoms of respiratory obstruction requires hospitalization.

Persistent paroxysmal coughing is often associated with asthma.

Timing of Cough

Coughs that awaken persons at night are frequently associated with respiratory problems in which bronchial irritation is a factor, such as asthma or chronic bronchitis, or with nonrespiratory conditions, such as GERD or heart failure. A hallmark of asthma is coughing at night, usually between midnight and 2:00 AM. This is because of the low level of glucocortisol in the body at this time. A severe cough in the early morning indicates postnasal drip, cystic fibrosis, or bronchiectasis. Secretions accumulate through the night, and fits of coughing are followed by bronchorrhea. Cough that is worse at night indicates croup, postnasal drip, lower respiratory tract infection, and allergic reaction. A cough that disappears with sleep is a habit cough.

History of Choking Episode

Consider foreign body aspiration in any child with a cough lasting longer than 3 weeks. Frequently the caregivers report an episode of severe coughing and choking occurring 1 to 3 weeks before with a period of absence of cough (because the level of obstruction is in a lobar or segmental bronchus) and then sudden recurrence of coughing. This period of absence can last for hours, days, or even months. The cough may reappear when irritation of the foreign body or reaction to the foreign body occurs.

Occupation

An occupational and hobby review is warranted. Asbestos or coal dust exposure increases a person's risk of lung disease, including lung cancer. Aerosol sprays, insecticides, chemical exposures, and sawdust can cause cough.

Nature of the Cough

A throat-clearing cough is indicative of postnasal drip caused by irritation of the cough receptors in the pharynx, which are sensitive to mechanical stimulation such as secretions. A dry, brassy cough indicates pharyngeal or tracheal irritation, allergy, or habit. A loose or moist cough may indicate lung disease such as cystic fibrosis or asthma.

A paroxysmal cough is seen with asthma, pertussis, and cystic fibrosis and occasionally after inhalation of a foreign body. A barking, croupy cough indicates an irritation in the glottic and subglottic area. A sudden short burst of a cough in infants, called a staccato cough, is indicative of *Chlamydia trachomatis*. A harsh, dry cough caused by airway compression from enlarged nodes in the perihilar or paratracheal region seems to occur with tuberculosis (TB) or fungal infection.

A loud, bizarre cough that seems to be attention seeking may have a psychogenic origin. The cough usually is vibrating, throaty, and dry. The severity can range from occasional clearing of the throat to spells lasting several minutes. The cough usually follows a respiratory tract infection. The cough disappears with sleep or when the child is distracted. School absences are common.

Is the Cough Related to Any Event That Would Help Me Narrow Down the Cause?

Key Questions

- Does eating affect your cough?
- Does your cough get worse during certain times of the year?
- Does exercise affect your cough?

Eating

Inhalation into the tracheobronchial tree may occur as a result of lack of esophageal motility, GERD with regurgitation into the pharynx, or central nervous system and neuromuscular disorders. Difficulty with sucking and swallowing or coughing and choking during eating are highly suggestive of an underlying disorder such as congenital malformations, congenital heart disease, or pneumonia.

In the adult, GERD probably causes cough through direct stimulation of cough receptors with acid or through inflammation from aspiration of stomach contents into the airway.

Season

Chronic cough during winter months suggests viral infections. Exacerbation of cough during spring, summer, and fall is suggestive of allergic disease with increased pollen counts. Croup occurs most commonly in the fall from the parainfluenza virus type 1. Smaller peaks of croup are seen with influenza B outbreaks in the winter months. RSV is common in infants during the winter months. In the warmer months, parainfluenza type 3 is the agent frequently isolated.

Exercise

The hyperpnea of exercise causes bronchospasm because of heat loss from the airway surface and is more pronounced in cold dry air. Asthma attacks are frequently exercise related, as is cough resulting from heart disease or airway compression.

Is This Something That Is Going Around?

Key Questions

- Is anyone else at home ill?
- Is anyone else ill in day care, school, or the workplace?

Exposure to respiratory viruses is very common in day care, school, and the workplace. Viruses that cause the common cold are shed in nasal secretions. Contacts acquire the virus by being sneezed on or by touching a sneezed-on object and then touching their own nose or conjunctivae. The incubation period is 2 to 5 days. *Mycoplasma* pneumonia tends to spread through school/households slowly as the incubation period is 21 days.

Is There Anything That Would Lead Me to Suspect Allergies or Reactive Airway Disease?

Key Questions

- Does anyone in your family have allergies or asthma?
- Is there anything you do or take that stops the cough?
- Do you have pets?

Family History

Allergy-prone individuals are at increased risk for coughs associated with postnasal drip and asthma. Allergy-prone adults and children are those persons with personal or family history of atopic dermatitis, asthma, and allergic rhinitis. Pets residing in the household are frequently the source of the allergen, especially cats and dogs.

Environmental Exposure

Frequently persons notice that the cough occurs after exposure to certain environmental irritants, such as smoke, pollen, dust, or animals. The cough may resolve spontaneously with withdrawal from these irritants. Ingestion of antihistamines or inhalation of bronchodilators may relieve a cough associated with allergies or asthma.

Smoke Exposure

Chronic cough is not uncommon in persons who smoke. Smoke exposure can trigger cough in persons with allergies or asthma.

Getting Better or Worse

A change in the chronic cough of a smoker may indicate the development of a new and serious underlying problem such as pneumonia or lung cancer.

Does the Patient Have Any Risk Factors for Systemic Disease That May Present With Cough?

Key Questions

- Do you have any chronic health problems?
- Do you have human immunodeficiency virus (HIV) infection, heart disease, or high blood pressure?
- Are you receiving treatment for cancer?
- Have you ever been exposed to TB?

Chronic Health Problems

Chronic lung and heart disease may present with cough, indicating an exacerbation and/or complication of the disease. In addition, information about chronic health problems may indicate which medications patients take, placing them at risk for cough. Angiotensin-converting enzyme (ACE) inhibitors may be given to treat hypertension or heart failure. Consider exacerbation of heart failure or consider an ACE inhibitor–induced dry, hacking cough, which can be eliminated by stopping the medication. In addition, a medication history may reveal use of drugs that treat or cause immunocompromise.

Immunocompromise

Cancer therapy, HIV, and administration of steroids should raise suspicion of immunocompromise. Adults and children who are immunocompromised are at high risk for infectious lung problems.

Tuberculosis

Inquiry should be made about potential exposure to TB. Family history of TB, incarceration, international travel, and inner city habitation put persons at risk for TB.

DIAGNOSTIC REASONING: FOCUSED PHYSICAL EXAMINATION

Note General Appearance

When a patient appears to be in acute distress with manifestations of oxygen deprivation, dehydration, and fever, think first of bacterial pneumonia. If a patient has significant oxygen deprivation that is not accompanied by fever, consider foreign body aspiration, acute heart failure, or pulmonary embolism.

The setting in which the patient is encountered will influence your response to the situation of acute distress. In most instances, oxygen is started immediately. If obstruction by a foreign body is strongly suspected, emergency personnel should be summoned for removal of the object if you are unable to accomplish this. Emergency chest radiographs may be needed to look for pulmonary infiltrates, and pulse oximetry may be ordered to assess oxygen saturation. Adults and children in acute respiratory distress require specialized care by health care professionals, and their assistance should be requested immediately.

Persons with viral respiratory tract infections or chronic cough from postnasal drainage, GERD, and chronic bronchitis appear less acutely ill and are able to participate in the interview process without difficulty. Those whose cough is caused by bronchospasm may exhibit varying degrees of distress.

Assess Mental Status

Diminished level of consciousness, confusion, and restlessness are likely manifestations of hypoxia in the patient experiencing respiratory problems. Frequently the patient with a pulmonary embolus expresses a sense of impending doom.

Restlessness and agitation in the child may indicate hypoxemia. A lethargic and somnolent child may have CO_2 retention.

Take Vital Signs

An elevated pulse rate and temperature may signal bacterial or viral infection.

Respiratory rate is the best indicator of pulmonary function in young infants. The respiratory rate and tidal volume together produce adequate alveolar ventilation. For any given level of alveolar ventilation, there is an optimum respiratory rate at which the muscular work of breathing is at a minimum. Airway resistance increases at higher flow rates. In children with decreased compliance (e.g., pneumonia, pulmonary edema), respirations are very rapid and shallow. Children with increased airway resistance (e.g., asthma) have respirations that are relatively slow and deep to minimize the high-resistance work. The most reliable and reproducible respiratory rate is the sleeping respiratory rate.

Weigh the Patient

Children with a cough from a chronic disease may present with failure to thrive.

Examine the Head and Neck

Erythema of upper respiratory tract mucous membranes, accompanied by enlarged anterior cervical nodes, is a common finding in an upper respiratory tract infection.

Observe the neck for jugular venous distention; this may be a sign of heart failure.

The ororespiratory reflex is mediated by Arnold's nerve, the auricular branch of cranial nerve X, and is a rare cause of chronic cough. Careful examination of the ears with removal of cerumen and any hairs in contact with the tympanic membrane (TM) or the opposite wall of the external auditory canal should be done.

A cobblestoning of the posterior pharynx is caused by lymphoid hyperplasia secondary to chronic stimulation by postnasal drip.

Inspect the Chest for Shape, Symmetry, and Use of Accessory Muscles

To inspect the chest, have the patient assume a sitting position. Note if the patient has to lean forward or sit up to breathe comfortably. Also observe the patient in a supine position to note if cough or respiratory symptoms change with position. Some respiratory abnormalities are unilateral or localized, such as pulmonary embolus. Compare findings on one side of the body with those on the other. Also compare front to back.

Upper airway obstruction causes supra-sternal and supraclavicular retractions. Inter-costal retractions and subcostal retractions occur with lower airway obstructive disease. Severe obstruction of either upper or lower airways causes retractions of all the accessory muscles. Retractions occur when an increase in the work of breathing requires an increase in the negative pressure within the chest. Remember that the pediatric airway is much smaller in diameter than that of the adult, and because resistance to flow is related inversely to the fourth power of the radius, decreased diameter of this airway causes enormous increases in resistance. The chest wall is pliable and the softest parts of the thorax are pulled inward on inspiration, causing retractions of the intracostal, supra-sternal, and infrasternal spaces. The degree of retraction is proportional to the negative pressure generated within the thorax and therefore correlates with the severity of the problem.

Normally, the anteroposterior (AP) diameter is approximately one third to one half of the lateral diameter. If the AP diameter is equal to the lateral diameter, the condition known as barrel chest is evident and indicates probable COPD. Children with chronic cough because of cystic fibrosis or severe asthma may have an increase in the AP diameter. In children up to 6 months of age, the head circumference is larger than the chest circumference. After 6 months of age, the chest circumference is larger than the head circumference (see Chapter 11).

Observe Respirations
Next, observe the rate, rhythm, and depth of the patient's breathing. The normal respiratory rate in adults is 12 to 20 breaths per minute; in the elderly, it is 16 to 25 breaths per minute. Children younger than 12 years may have respiratory rates up to 30 to 40 breaths per minute. The only way the infant or child can increase oxygen uptake is to increase the ventilation rate. The depth and pattern of respiration change: the infant has more shallow and more frequent breaths.

Exhalation normally lasts about twice as long as inhalation, but in patients with COPD it may take up to four times longer.

Note any abnormal breathing patterns (see Box 11-1).

Listen to the Cough
Note whether the cough is dry or moist. Listen also for the quality of the cough, such as whooping or honking.

Palpate the Chest
Palpate the entire chest for tenderness, depressions, bulges, and crepitus. Assess for chest symmetry by measuring diaphragmatic expansion and chest excursion. As the patient takes a deep breath, each hand should move the same distance out from the spine. With COPD, less movement will be seen. Pneumonia and partial paralysis of the diaphragm will result in a reduction in expansion of one side of the chest wall.

Assess for vocal fremitus (the vibrations transmitted to the chest wall during speech) by placing the ball of the hand lightly on the chest and asking the patient to repeat the words "ninety-nine." Evaluate the intensity of the vibration over all lung fields, comparing side to side. Dense tissue conducts sound better than does air; thus conditions such as pneumonia, heart failure, and tumors may increase fremitus. Fremitus is diminished in pneumothorax, asthma, and emphysema.

Percuss the Chest
Percuss systematically at 3- to 5-cm intervals, starting just above the scapulae and moving downward from side to side. Note any differences in volume and pitch. Resonance is a long, low-pitched sound that can normally be heard over most lung fields. Hyperresonance is an abnormally long, low-pitched sound that may signal emphysema or pneumothorax. Dullness or flatness may be heard with pleural effusion, pneumonia, or large tumors.

Auscultate Breath Sounds
Instruct the patient to breathe through the mouth slowly and deeply. Determine the presence, type, and location of both normal and abnormal breath sounds (see Chapter 11).

Most children know what a stethoscope is, and you should use this to your advantage.

Infants see the shiny parts; have older children listen to their own chests. Some clinicians begin by listening to the child's leg or hand first. Ensure that the stethoscope is warm before you place it on the chest. Infants are in good position when supine, toddlers should be on the parent's lap, and older children should be sitting or standing.

Auscultate Heart Sounds

Note the location of normal and abnormal heart sounds, the location of their greatest intensity, and the heart rate and rhythm. Also note any murmurs and their location, grade, and radiation. Incompetent heart valves may be the cause of heart failure. In COPD, lung hyperinflation may muffle heart sounds. Poor tissue oxygenation or fever may result in tachycardia.

Examine the Skin and Extremities

Note the presence of cyanosis of the oral cavity (central cyanosis). It is associated with low arterial saturation and may result from inadequate gas exchange in the lungs or from cardiac shunting. Mucous membranes in dark-skinned patients may appear gray with central cyanosis. This may also be seen in persons with COPD. Bluish color of the extremities (peripheral cyanosis) may be observed in Caucasians and is associated with low venous saturation, resulting in vasoconstriction, vascular occlusion, or reduced cardiac output.

Clubbing is a loss of the angle between the skin and nail bed. This is a manifestation of chronic tissue hypoxia, which occurs with chronic lung disease. Edema of the lower extremities may be a sign of increased right-heart filling pressure, caused by primary lung disease or left ventricular failure.

Examine the Abdomen

Epigastric tenderness to palpation may be elicited in the patient with GERD, or the abdominal examination may be entirely normal. In addition, if heart failure is the cause of cough, ascites or hepatojugular reflex may be present. To test for hepatojugular reflex, position the patient so that the jugular pulsation is evident in the neck. Exert firm and sustained pressure with the hand over the patient's right upper quadrant for 30 to 60 seconds. An increase in the jugular venous pressure of more than 1 cm during this maneuver is abnormal.

LABORATORY AND DIAGNOSTIC STUDIES

Some authorities suggest all patients with a cough lasting longer than 3 weeks have a chest radiograph. If the radiograph is abnormal and consistent with infectious or noninfectious inflammatory disease or malignancy, the health care provider should order expectorated sputum studies, computed tomography (CT) scan of the lungs, or bronchoscopy. If the history and physical examination and radiography suggest heart failure, an ECG, echocardiogram, or both may be indicated (see Chapter 9).

If the patient's history and physical examination strongly suggest a specific etiology (i.e., postnasal drip, asthma, GERD), proceed to those treatments initially. Keep in mind that there may be more than one cause for the cough. For those patients whose history and physical examination suggest chronic symptoms, sinus radiography or CT scan of the sinuses may be indicated. Also consider allergy testing for those individuals whose history indicates allergens may precipitate the syndrome.

In those situations in which investigation of signs and symptoms leads to probable asthma or if no likely cause is identified, a spirometry test (see Chapter 11) should be performed. If the test is normal but asthma is still suspected, a methacholine challenge test may be done. This test is performed in the laboratory and involves administering methacholine chloride by nebulizer and then repeating the spirometry test. If the patient's cough is likely related to reactive airways disease, the patient exhibits a 20% decrease in FEV_1.

Complete Blood Cell Count

A complete blood cell count may provide evidence of acute infection with an elevated white blood cell count. Eosinophilia indicates atopy.

Esophageal Probe

GERD is best diagnosed with 24-hour esophageal pH probe monitoring. A barium swallow is less sensitive, and a gastroscopy will verify ulcerative disease but not mild reflux.

Sputum Culture

Sputum culture is important for the diagnosis of a specific infectious agent in the pulmonary system. A sputum specimen must originate from deep within the bronchi. Coughing usually enables the patient to produce a satisfactory specimen. Examination includes macroscopic appearance, cellular composition, and bacterial count.

Sweat Test

A result of >60 mEq/L of chloride is considered diagnostic of cystic fibrosis.

Tuberculin Skin Testing

The Mantoux test is used to detect TB. A Mantoux test result is considered positive at three different levels (≥5, ≥10, and ≥15 mm) of induration (diameter transverse to the long axis of the arm measured and recorded), depending on the individual's degree of risk for TB. In adults, a diameter of less than 5 mm is considered negative, a 5- to 9-mm diameter is considered a weak positive, a 10- to 14-mm diameter is considered an intermediate positive, and a ≥15-mm diameter is considered a strong positive. In a child who has no known risk factors for TB, only a large reaction (≥15 mm) is considered to be positive. If a child is very young (<4 years old), has other medical risk factors, or has some environmental exposure to TB, then an intermediate reaction (≥10 mm) is considered to be positive. If a child is at high risk (e.g., a child who lives in a household with someone who has TB), then a small reaction (≥5 mm) is considered to be positive.

Nasal Swab for Pertussis

Nasopharyngeal (NP) secretions for culture should be obtained using a calcium alginate or Dacron-tipped swab. The swab is inserted into the posterior nasopharynx and gently rotated for a minimum of 15 seconds and optimally for 1 minute. Throat swabs are not acceptable for the diagnosis of pertussis.

DIFFERENTIAL DIAGNOSIS

Life-threatening causes of cough must be initially considered when arriving at a differential diagnosis. Conditions that present with cough as a symptom have been discussed in Chapters 9 and 11 and include pulmonary embolus, heart failure, bacterial tracheitis, foreign body aspiration, and asthma. The reader is encouraged to review these conditions associated with cough.

Common Cold (Nasopharyngitis)

The common cold is a self-limiting viral infection of the upper respiratory tract that is generally caused by a rhinovirus. The virus invades the mucous membranes of the upper respiratory tract and causes swelling and hypersecretion of mucus. Associated symptoms include a low-grade fever, mild sore throat, and rhinorrhea of clear to yellow mucus. Hypersecretion of mucus causes coughing, especially at night when secretions pool in the nasopharyngeal cavity. Physical examination findings may include red and swollen nasal mucosa with secretions present, mild pharyngeal erythema, and enlarged cervical lymph nodes. Other physical examination findings are negative. The patient is advised to return if the cough persists for more than 3 weeks or if symptoms develop such as temperature of more than 38.3° C (101° F), chest pain, or SOB.

Chronic Obstructive Pulmonary Disease Exacerbation

COPD is a condition primarily consisting of emphysema and chronic bronchitis. It is almost always a condition of heavy smokers. Acute exacerbations of COPD include three clinical findings: worsening dyspnea, increase in sputum purulence, and increase in sputum volume. Patients will have a chronic cough, associated with barrel chest, tachypnea, and distant breath sounds on physical examination. Chest radiography will show hyperexpansion of the lungs, and spirometry will indicate airflow obstruction when emphysema is present. Acute COPD exacerbations may also be associated with an upper respiratory tract infection, fever without a known cause, increased wheezing or cough, and a 20% increase in respiratory rate and heart rate above baseline.

Bordetella pertussis Infection

Pertussis (whooping cough) is an acute infection of the respiratory tract caused by *Bordetella pertussis*. It is a condition primarily seen in children under the age of 2 and in persons who have not had adequate diphtheria and tetanus toxoids and pertussis (DTP) vaccination. Pertussis infection has occurred among adolescents who become susceptible approximately 6 to 10 years after childhood vaccination. It begins with a prodromal stage of malaise, cough, coryza, and anorexia. The cough then becomes more severe and ends in a high-pitched inspiratory "whoop." Vomiting and cyanosis may also be present. Physical examination may be within normal limits. Pertussis is associated with extremely high white blood cell counts.

Pneumonia

Pneumonia is usually associated with dyspnea, pleuritic chest pain, cough with greenish or rusty-colored sputum, fever, and chills. Infants and young children will not produce sputum. Anorexia, malaise, and posttussive vomiting are seen. Objective manifestations of pneumonia include fever, tachycardia and tachypnea, inspiratory crackles, asynchronous breathing and vocal fremitus, dull percussion sound over area of consolidation, and bronchophony. Pneumonia can be confirmed by chest radiography, complete blood cell count, and sputum and nasal cultures.

Fever is frequently absent in the elderly with pneumonia, and thus a new onset of cough, especially when accompanied by either tachypnea or altered mental status, should suggest pneumonia.

The majority of pediatric pulmonary infections are viral and usually caused by RSV, parainfluenza viruses, or influenza viruses. In the infant and young child, acute nonbacterial pneumonia presents after a 1- to 2-day history of coryza, decreased appetite, and low-grade fever. Increasing fretfulness, respiratory congestion, vomiting, cough, and fever may occur. Objective manifestations include tachypnea, tachycardia, nasal flaring, and retractions.

Mycoplasma Pneumonia

Mycoplasma pneumonia is the most common cause of infection of the lower respiratory tract in children and young adults. There is a slow onset of symptoms with fever (39° C or 102.2° F), a cough that is usually dry at the onset, headache, malaise, and sore throat. The child does not look particularly ill, but on auscultation rales and rhonchi are frequently present. The white blood cell count is usually normal, and cold agglutinin titer may be elevated during the acute presentation in more than half of patients with this infection. A titer of 1:32 or higher supports the diagnosis.

Chlamydial Pneumonia

Chlamydial pneumonia is a pulmonary disease caused by *C. trachomatis* transmitted during delivery. It also occurs in young adults. In infants 3 to 11 weeks of age, it is one of the most common causes of interstitial pneumonitis and presents with tachypnea and a characteristic staccato cough in an afebrile child. In adults, infection is associated with upper respiratory tract symptoms followed by fever and a nonproductive cough. Fine rales, usually without wheezes, are heard on auscultation. Chest radiographs show hyperinflated lungs with diffuse interstitial or alveolar infiltrates.

Bronchiolitis

RSV is mainly responsible for bronchiolitis in children less than 2 years old. The infection is associated with 1 to 2 days of fever, rhinorrhea, and cough, followed by wheezing, tachypnea, tachycardia, and respiratory distress. Nasal flaring and retractions with accessory muscle use are seen, along with shallow, rapid respirations. Cough increases as inflammation increases. The infant appears lethargic and has circumoral cyanosis. Wheezes are predominant, with a long expiratory phase. Crackles and rhonchi may also be heard diffusely throughout the lung fields. The chest radiograph shows hyperinflation with mild interstitial infiltrates. Viral isolates from sputum, throat swabs, or nasal washings are used for diagnosis.

Acute Bronchitis

Inflammation of the large airways causes bronchitis that begins with a dry, nonproductive cough usually seen in winter. Continued cough and nasal congestion produce a productive cough and fever. Chest pain may accompany the cough. Lung auscultation reveals diffuse rhonchi on expiration. White blood cell count is normal or mildly elevated.

Croup (Acute Laryngotracheobronchitis)

Inflammation or edema of the subglottic area causes obstruction of the airways of the larynx, trachea, or bronchi. Parainfluenza virus causes most inflammation. Generally the onset occurs after a few days of an upper respiratory tract infection. Hoarseness, inspiratory stridor, and a characteristic barking cough are heard and are usually worse at night. A low-grade fever may be present. Inspiratory stridor, suprasternal and intercostal retractions, and an increased respiratory rate are seen. Lateral neck radiographs in croup show a normal epiglottis, subglottic narrowing, and ballooning of the hypopharynx. The posteroanterior neck view shows a steeple sign (narrowing of the air column at the top).

Subacute and Chronic Cough
Postnasal Drainage Syndrome

Postnasal drainage syndrome is the most common cause of chronic cough. The cough results from stimulation of the afferent limb of the cough reflex in the upper respiratory tract. Causes of postnasal drip include allergic response, secondary infection after an upper respiratory tract illness, environmental irritants, vasomotor rhinitis, or sinusitis. Both children and adults report dry cough, throat clearing, sensation of something in the back of the throat, and nasal congestion. Physical examination may reveal mucus in the posterior pharynx or a cobblestone appearance of the posterior pharynx. Sinus radiographs, CT scan of the sinuses, and allergy testing may be indicated if this syndrome is suspected to be the cause of cough.

Asthma

Asthma is the most common cause of chronic cough in children. It initially produces a dry cough, commonly worse at night, characteristically exercise related, and often triggered by respiratory tract infections. Physical examination findings depend on the severity of the disease. Prolonged expiratory phase of respiration may be heard. Lungs may have crackles that clear with coughing, and overt or latent wheeze may be produced with forced expiration. Use of neck muscles to facilitate inspiration (called tracheal tugging or chin lag) may be seen. A chest radiograph may show hyperinflation during acute attacks. Pulmonary function testing with and without an aerosolized sympathomimetic bronchodilator is positive.

Gastroesophageal Reflux Disease

GERD should be considered when patients report heartburn, a sour taste in the mouth, or a history of esophagitis. Often persons with GERD are cigarette smokers, overuse alcohol, and are overweight. Microaspiration into the airways or reflux of acid into the esophagus occurs. Young infants may also experience reflux with their cough, usually worsening after feeding, which may be the only symptom. A recurrent, effortless vomiting with failure to gain weight and irritability may also occur. The physical examination of persons with GERD is most often normal. The diagnostic test of most significance is esophageal pH monitoring; values outside the normal physiological range indicate reflux.

Chronic Bronchitis

Chronic bronchitis should be considered when the patient expectorates sputum on most days during a period spanning at least 3 consecutive months and such periods have occurred for more than 2 successive years. In addition, exposure to smoke, irritating dust, or fumes is highly likely. Cigarette smoking as well as fumes and dust stimulate the afferent limb of the cough reflex as irritants, inducing inflammatory changes in the mucosa of the respiratory tract, causing hypersecretion of mucus and slowing of mucociliary clearance.

Persons with chronic bronchitis exhibit a rasping, hacking cough, possible rhonchi that clear with coughing, resonant to dull chest, possible barrel chest, prolonged expiration, and possible wheezing. Chest radiography and pulmonary function tests are indicated.

Angiotensin-Converting Enzyme Inhibitor–Induced Cough

This cough occurs hours to months after beginning an ACE inhibitor. Persons report a nonproductive cough associated with an irritating, tickling, or scratching sensation in the throat. Physical examination is normal. The cough resolves within days to weeks after the drug is discontinued.

Bronchogenic Carcinoma

Hemoptysis reported by a cigarette smoker as well as weight loss and/or shortness of breath are frequent health concerns reported by a patient with bronchogenic cancer. Physical findings may include enlarged supraclavicular nodes, dull chest percussion over the tumor, and increased breath sounds distal to the tumor. Hemoptysis should be evaluated with a chest radiograph and a CT scan if indicated.

Cystic Fibrosis

A chronic cough is associated with cystic fibrosis. The cough is productive, and the child has signs of failure to thrive with poor weight gain. The child may have a family history of the disease. The cough is initially dry and hacking but eventually becomes loose and productive of purulent material. Physical examination often shows an increased anteroposterior diameter of the chest. Scattered or localized coarse rales and rhonchi are audible. Digital clubbing is often present. Sweat chloride test is positive.

Foreign Body Aspiration

Foreign body aspiration occurs most frequently in children and the elderly. A child or adult who aspirates a foreign body can have a varied presentation. Generally the onset of cough is sudden and unexpected. A brief period of severe coughing, gagging, and choking occurs. If the foreign body does not completely obstruct the airway, an asymptomatic period ensues. This period can last for hours, days, or even months. A foreign body in the lower airway can present with emphysema because of the ball-valve phenomenon or can occur as a complete distal atelectasis created by absorption of the trapped gas. A mobile foreign body in the lower airway can also produce a paroxysmal cough, with cyanotic episodes and stridor because of proximal migration and subglottic impaction. A foreign body in the esophagus can also cause airway obstruction and cough as well as dysphagia for solid foods because the posterior trachea is compliant and opposed to the anterior esophagus. Coins are the most frequent culprit.

Allergic Rhinitis

Upper airway allergy and vasomotor rhinitis can cause a reflex cough secondary to post-nasal drip and irritation of the cough receptors. Such a cough is generally seasonal in nature, with a history of sneezing. Allergic shiners, allergic salute, and eczema may be present. Rhinorrhea with clear, watery drainage is seen. Skin testing for allergies is positive.

Chronic Sinusitis

Chronic sinusitis produces a recurrent cough that is especially worse at night because of trickling of infected mucus from the nasopharynx down the posterior pharyngeal wall. Involvement is usually in the maxillary sinuses. History reveals cold-like symptoms that become persistent or recurrent. Noisy breathing and snoring with sleep may also be present. Physical examination reveals clear to mucopurulent secretions in the posterior throat. Purulent rhinorrhea may be present. Sinus tenderness is less frequently present than in acute sinusitis. A radiograph using the Waters view of the head is positive.

Tuberculosis

Brassy cough is the most common symptom of tuberculosis but is often ascribed to smoking, a recent cold, or a bout of influenza several weeks before. At first, it is minimally productive of yellow or green mucus, usually on arising in the morning. As the disease progresses, the cough becomes more productive. In adults, a multinodular infiltrate above or behind the clavicle (the most characteristic location) suggests recurrence of an old TB infection. In younger persons in whom recent infection is more common, infiltration may be found in any part of the lung, and unilateral pleural effusion is often seen. In sputum examination, the finding of acid-fast bacilli (AFB) in a sputum smear is strong presumptive evidence of TB. A definitive diagnosis is made only on results of a culture.

Smoking

Smoking is more prevalent in female adolescents, and many smoke in closed rooms, increasing their respiratory irritation. History of a mildly productive hacking cough may be indicative of smoking. Infants exposed to passive cigarette smoke inhalation have increased bronchial reactivity. Physical examination may reveal yellow stains on the fingers, teeth, or tongue. Mild chronic conjunctivitis may also be present. Chest radiography may be positive with interstitial markings.

Psychogenic Origin

Psychogenic or habit cough is a rare cause of cough and can be misdiagnosed in a patient with postnasal drip syndrome. School-age children or adolescents with a history of a loud, brassy, disturbing cough that is non-productive and explosive may indicate a psychogenic etiology. The child usually has missed many school days. The cough is not heard while sleeping, and the child is afebrile with no weight loss. The physical examination is negative.

DIFFERENTIAL DIAGNOSIS OF *Common Causes of Recent Onset of Cough*

CONDITION	HISTORY	PHYSICAL FINDINGS	DIAGNOSTIC STUDIES
Nasopharyngitis	Acute-onset, low-grade fever, rhinorrhea, cough especially at night	Nasal mucosa red and swollen, pharynx mildly red; otherwise negative	None
COPD exacerbation	Worsening dyspnea, increased wheezing or coughing, smoker	Purulent sputum, fever, and increased respiratory and heart rates	Chest radiograph, spirometry
Pertussis	Persistent hacking cough; may have inspiratory whoop, vomiting	Fever absent, coryza	Nasopharyngeal aspirate positive, chest radiograph to rule out pneumonia
Pneumonia*	Noisy cough, dyspnea, pleuritic chest pain, sputum production (yellow, green, red color), chills; in children also see poor feeding and irritability	Fever, tachycardia, tachypnea, inspiratory crackles, asynchronous breathing, vocal fremitus, percussion dull or flat over area of consolidation, bronchophony, egophony	Chest radiograph, CBC, sputum and nasal cultures, O_2 saturation
Viral URI	Cough, nasal congestion, sore throat, fever, chills, myalgias	Fever, pharyngitis, enlarged anterior cervical lymph nodes, normal TMs, nasal mucosa erythema, normal chest examination	None
Mycoplasmal pneumonia	Child or young adult: dry cough, headache, malaise, sore throat	Fever, rales and rhonchi on auscultation	Cold agglutinin, chest radiograph

Continued

DIFFERENTIAL DIAGNOSIS OF *Common Causes of Recent Onset of Cough* —*cont'd*

CONDITION	HISTORY	PHYSICAL FINDINGS	DIAGNOSTIC STUDIES
Chlamydial pneumonia	Paroxysmal staccato cough in infant 4-12 weeks	Afebrile, conjunctivitis in 50% of infants, tachypnea of 40-80 breaths/min, crackles, no wheezing	Radiograph shows hyperexpansion of lungs with diffuse interstitial infiltrates
Bronchiolitis (RSV)*	Grunting, sneezing, cough, anoxia, exposure to passive smoke	Fever, wheezing on auscultation, prolonged expiratory phase, tachypnea of 60-80 breaths/min, tachycardia >200 beats/min	WBC 5000-24,000/mm^3 with increased PMNs; chest radiograph shows hyperinflation; infants less than 2 months, refer; progressive respiratory distress, refer
Acute bronchitis	Duration <3 months, winter months, URI for 3-4 days; loose, hacking cough that becomes productive, afebrile	Coarse, fine crackles on auscultation; low-grade fever or afebrile	Chest radiograph negative
Croup (acute laryngotracheobronchitis)*	History of URI; brassy, barking cough usually at night	Low-grade fever, inspiratory stridor, flaring of nares, prolonged expiratory phase, may see retraction of accessory muscles, breath sounds diminished	None

*Because of the possible rapid changes in condition in infants and children, nonemergent causes of cough may become emergent.
COPD, Chronic obstructive pulmonary disease; *PMNs*, polymorphonuclear neutrophils; *RSV*, respiratory syncytial virus; *TM*, tympanic membrane; *URI*, upper respiratory infection.

DIFFERENTIAL DIAGNOSIS OF *Common Causes of Chronic Cough*

CONDITION	HISTORY	PHYSICAL FINDINGS	DIAGNOSTIC STUDIES
Postnasal drainage	Cough, sore throat	Mucoid secretions in posterior pharynx, cobblestone appearance of posterior pharynx, tenderness to palpation of sinuses, normal chest examination	Sinus radiographs, sinus CT scan, allergy testing
Asthma	Dry, hacking cough, especially at night, and with feeding and laughter	End-expiratory wheeze, prolonged expiratory phase	Pulmonary function testing
GERD	Cough worse at night, sour taste in mouth, heartburn, history of esophagitis, cigarette smoker, alcohol abuse, overweight; in children 0-18 months: failure to thrive, dysphagia, cough after eating and lying down, vomiting	Normal chest examination, normal upper respiratory tract examination, possible epigastric pain with palpation or normal abdominal examination	Esophageal pH monitoring, blood count for anemia, radiograph for aspiration pneumonia

Continued

DIFFERENTIAL DIAGNOSIS OF *Common Causes of Chronic Cough—cont'd*

CONDITION	HISTORY	PHYSICAL FINDINGS	DIAGNOSTIC STUDIES
Chronic bronchitis	Cough, mild dyspnea, history of COPD, history of cigarette smoking, yellow sputum	Hacking, rasping cough; normal breath sounds or rhonchi that clear with coughing; resonant to dull chest, possible barrel chest, prolonged expiration, possible wheezing	Chest radiograph, pulmonary function tests
ACEI-induced cough	Begins hours to months after starting ACEI; nonproductive, dry cough; scratching sensation in throat	Normal examination	Trial off ACEI
Bronchogenic carcinoma	Cough with hemoptysis; history of cigarette smoking, weight loss, shortness of breath	Enlarged supraclavicular nodes, dull chest percussion over tumor, increased breath sounds distal to tumor	Chest radiograph, CT scan of chest
Cystic fibrosis	Failure to thrive, chronic cough, bulky stools, family history	Nasal polyps, clubbing of fingernails, sputum	Sweat test positive
Foreign body in ear canal	Cough	Cerumen in ears, hairs in contact with TM or opposite wall of external auditory canal	None
Foreign body aspiration	History of environmental hazard, choking episode	Asymmetrical physical findings of decreased breath sounds, wheezing	Asymmetrical radiograph with forced expiratory view
Allergic rhinitis	History of sneezing, cough	Allergic shiners, allergic salute, rhinorrhea clear and watery	Chest radiograph negative, allergy testing positive
Chronic sinusitis	Rhinorrhea >7-10 days	Mucopurulent rhinorrhea	Waters radiograph
Mycoplasmal pneumonia	School-age child, gradual onset, headache, malaise, sore throat, hacking cough	Reddened pharynx, slightly enlarged lymph nodes, rales often fine and crackling	Radiograph shows interstitial pneumonia; cold agglutinins positive, ESR elevated
Tuberculosis	History of exposure, high-risk group, weakness, malaise, weight loss	Brassy cough, weight loss, may have fever, night sweats	Mantoux test, chest radiograph shows abnormalities in apical and hyaline, sputum culture positive for *M. tuberculosis*
Smoking (passive/active)	History of smoking or being around a smoker	Yellow teeth, fingers; odor of smoke, productive sputum	Radiograph may be positive with interstitial markings
Psychogenic origin	School age or adolescent; dry, hacking cough present only during waking hours	None	As indicated to rule out other causes

ACEI, Angiotensin-converting enzyme inhibitor; *ESR,* erythrocyte sedimentation rate; *GERD,* gastroesophageal reflux disease.

CHAPTER RESOURCES

Chang AB, Asher MI: A review of cough in children, *J Asthma* 38:299, 2001.

de Jongste JC, Shields MD: Cough 2: chronic cough in children, *Thorax* 58:998, 2004.

Irwin RS, Madison JM: The diagnosis and treatment of cough, *N Engl J Med* 342:1715, 2000.

Malhotra A: Influenza and respiratory syncytial virus. Update on infection, management and prevention, *Pediatr Clin North Am* 47:353, vi, 2000.

Morton RL, Sheikh S, Corbett ML et al: Evaluation of the wheezy infant, *Ann Allergy Asthma Immunol* 86:251, 2001.

Snow V, Lascher S, Mottur-Pilson C: Evidence base for management of acute exacerbations of chronic obstructive pulmonary disease, *Ann Intern Med* 134:595, 2001.

Tierney LM, McPhee SJ, Papadakis MA: *Current medical diagnosis and treatment*, ed 44, New York, 2005, McGraw-Hill.

Valente J: Diagnosing persistent childhood cough, *Practitioner* 245:337, 2001.

VI

Common Problems of the Abdomen and Gastrointestinal System

Abdominal Pain

Abdominal pain is a subjective feeling of discomfort in the abdomen that can be caused by a variety of problems. The goal of initial clinical assessment is to distinguish acute life-threatening conditions from chronic/recurrent or acute mild, self-limiting conditions. Assessment is complicated by the dynamic rather than static nature of acute abdominal pain, which can produce a changing clinical picture, often over a short period of time. In addition, both children and older adults tend to deviate from the usual and anticipated clinical pattern of abdominal pain.

The following three processes can produce abdominal pain: (1) tension in the gastrointestinal (GI) tract wall from muscle contraction or distention; (2) ischemia; and (3) inflammation of the peritoneum. Pain can also be referred from within or outside the abdomen.

Colic is a type of tension pain. It is associated with forceful peristaltic contractions and is the most characteristic type of pain arising from the viscera. Colicky pain can be produced by an irritant substance, from infection with a virus or bacteria, or by the body's attempt to force its luminal contents through an obstruction. Another type of tension pain is caused by acute stretching of the capsule of an organ, such as the liver, spleen, or kidney. The patient with this visceral pain is restless, moves about, and has difficulty getting comfortable.

Ischemia produces an intense, continuous pain. The most common cause of intestinal ischemic pain is strangulation of the bowel from obstruction.

Inflammation of the peritoneum usually begins at the serosa covering the affected and inflamed organ, causing visceral peritonitis. The pain is a poorly localized aching. As the inflammatory process spreads to the adjacent parietal peritoneum, it produces localized parietal peritonitis. The pain of parietal peritonitis is more severe and is perceived in the area of the abdomen corresponding to the inflammation. The patient with parietal pain usually lies still and does not want to move.

Pain may be referred from within the abdomen or from other parts of the body (Box 13-1).

Referral of pain occurs because tissues supplied by the same or adjacent neural segments have the same common pathways inside the central nervous system. Thus stimulation of these neural segments produces the sensation of pain. For example, nerves that supply the appendix are derived from the same source as those that supply the small intestine, resulting in the onset of appendicitis pain in the epigastric area.

Abdominal pain in adults can be classified as acute, chronic, or recurrent. The term "acute abdomen" refers to any acute condition within the abdomen that requires immediate surgical attention. Not all acute abdominal pain, however, requires surgical intervention. Acute abdominal pain refers to a relatively sudden onset of pain that is severe or increasing in severity and has been present for a short duration. Chronic pain is characterized by its persistent duration or recurrence. Recurrent episodes of pain may be either acute or chronic in nature.

In adults, acute pain requiring surgical intervention is commonly caused by appendicitis, perforated peptic ulcer, intestinal obstruction, peritonitis, perforate diverticulitis, ectopic pregnancy, or dissection of aortic aneurysm. Common causes of acute pain not requiring surgical intervention include cholelithiasis, gastroenteritis, peptic gastroduodenal syndrome, pancreatitis, pelvic inflammatory disease (PID), or urinary tract infection (UTI).

Box 13-1	Some Causes of Pain Perceived in Anatomical Regions

Right Upper Quadrant		**Left Upper Quadrant**
Duodenal ulcer		Ruptured spleen
Hepatitis		Gastric ulcer
Hepatomegaly		Aortic aneurysm
Pneumonia		Perforated colon
Cholecystitis	**Periumbilical**	Pneumonia
	Intestinal obstruction	
Right Lower Quadrant	Acute pancreatitis	**Left Lower Quadrant**
Appendicitis	Early appendicitis	Sigmoid diverticulitis
Salpingitis	Mesenteric thrombosis	Salpingitis
Ovarian cyst	Aortic aneurysm	Ovarian cyst
Ruptured ectopic pregnancy	Diverticulitis	Ruptured ectopic pregnancy
Renal/ureteral stone		Renal/ureteral stone
Strangulated hernia		Strangulated hernia
Meckel's diverticulitis		Perforated colon
Regional ileitis		Regional ileitis
Perforated cecum		Ulcerative colitis

Modified from Judge R, Zuidema G, Fitzgerald F: *Clinical diagnosis*, ed 5, Boston, 1988, Little, Brown.

Chronic or recurrent pain can be caused by GI disorders such as irritable bowel syndrome (IBS), diverticulitis, or esophagitis; pelvic disorders such as dysmenorrhea or uterine fibroids; genitourinary disorders such as recurrent UTI or chronic prostatitis; or conditions outside the abdomen such as costochondritis, hip disease, or hernia.

In children, abdominal pain can be classified as acute or recurrent. Common causes of acute pain include appendicitis, food poisoning, UTI, viral gastroenteritis, and bacterial enterocolitis. Recurrent abdominal pain (RAP) is defined as more than three episodes of pain in 3 months in children older than 3 years. It affects 10% to 15% of children between the ages of 3 and 14; of these children, 90% will not have an organic etiology.

DIAGNOSTIC REASONING: FOCUSED HISTORY

Is This an Acute Condition?

Key Questions
- How long ago did your pain start?
- Was the onset sudden or gradual?
- How severe is the pain (on a scale of 1 to 10)?

- If a child: What is the child's level of activity?
- Does the pain wake you up from sleep?
- What has been the course of the pain since it started? Is it getting worse or better?
- When was your last bowel movement?
- Have you ever had this pain before?

Onset/Duration
Acute onset of pain that is getting progressively worse may signal a surgical emergency. In general, patients who present with severe pain 6 to 24 hours from the onset probably have an acute surgical condition. Acute abdominal pain may signal a few potentially life-threatening conditions that must be considered first. **The following are possible surgical emergencies that require immediate evaluation and intervention:**
- Perforation: look for signs and symptoms of peritonitis (Box 13-2)
- Ectopic pregnancy: in any woman of childbearing age
- Obstruction: in the elderly
- Ruptured abdominal aortic aneurysm: when back pain is present
- Intussusception: in infants
- Malrotation: in infants usually less than 1 month old

Box 13-2	**Features of Peritonitis**

*P*ain: front, back, sides, shoulders
*E*lectrolytes fall; shock ensues
*R*igidity or rebound of anterior abdominal wall
*I*mmobile abdomen and patient
*T*enderness with involuntary guarding
*O*bstruction
*N*ausea and vomiting
*I*ncreasing pulse rate, decreasing blood pressure
*T*emperature falls and then rises; tachypnea
*I*ncreasing girth of abdomen
*S*ilent abdomen (no bowel sounds)

Modified from Shipman JJ: *Mnemonics and tactics in surgery and medicine,* ed 2, Chicago, 1984, Mosby.

Pain of sudden onset is more likely associated with colic, perforation, or acute ischemia (torsion, volvulus). Slower onset of pain generally is associated with inflammatory conditions, such as appendicitis, pancreatitis, and cholecystitis.

Acute pain that comes and goes may be related to intestinal peristalsis. The onset of pain in relation to food ingestion provides diagnostic clues: pain occurring several hours after a meal suggests a duodenal ulcer (pain with stomach empty), whereas pain immediately after eating occurs with esophagitis.

In children, RAP occurs in attacks lasting less than 1 hour and rarely longer than 3 hours and frequently interferes with daily routines. Between episodes, the pain resolves completely. When interviewing a child, remember that he or she may not be old enough to have a clear sense of time.

Severity and Progression

Severity is the most difficult symptom to evaluate because of its subjective quality. It is helpful to use a 1-to-10 scale in adults. Children may respond to the use of the pain faces or the Oucher Pain Scale (Figure 13-1).

Determine if the pain is an acute episode or if it is chronic or recurrent. Acute abdominal pain requires immediate attention, as it may signal an acute surgical condition in the abdomen. Chronic or recurrent episodes of pain can be handled in a more temperate manner.

Pain that is steady, severe, and progressive is worrisome. Pain that causes one to awake from sleep is serious. A sudden pain severe enough to cause fainting suggests perforated ulcer, ruptured aneurysm, or ectopic pregnancy. A severe knifelike pain usually indicates an emergency. Tearing pain is characteristic of an aortic aneurysm. Appendicitis is often described as an ache. Colicky pain that becomes steady can indicate appendicitis or strangulating intestinal obstruction.

Children are poor historians regarding the severity of pain. The caregiver should indicate how severe the child's pain is by a description of the activity level of the child. In general, avoidance of favorite activities indicates an organic problem, as does avoidance of motion. Organic disease awakens the child from sleep.

Last Bowel Movement

Obstipation (the absence of stools) occurs with complete obstruction, but diarrhea may be present with partial obstruction. Lack of a bowel movement for 3 days may signal constipation. Children can have sudden onset of constipation that can cause severe abdominal pain.

Previous Pain

Chronic pain may result when a potential surgical event is partially controlled but is not totally resolved. Chronic pain that has been present for longer than 1 year generally is not caused by a neoplasm; consider instead IBS or colorectal, endometrial, or inflammatory causes.

Recurrent attacks of acute pain may be caused by inflammation and exacerbation of a chronic condition, such as functional colonic pain, IBS, cholecystitis, chronic pancreatitis, diverticulitis, or ulcer disease. Acute pain may also be caused by recurrent infection, such as pyelonephritis or cystitis. Urinary tract stones can also cause acute attacks of recurrent pain.

Will the Location of Pain Give Me Any Clues?

Key Questions

- Where is the pain? Point to it.
- Does it travel (radiate) anywhere?

FIGURE 13-1 The Oucher Pain Scale illustrated with African American, Caucasian, and Hispanic children to best fit the child's cultural identity. The African American child version of the Oucher was developed and copyrighted in 1990 by Mary J. Denyes, PhD, RN, FAAN (Wayne State University), and Antonia Villarruel, PhD, RN, FAAN (University of Michigan), at the Children's Hospital of Michigan. Cornelia P. Porter, PhD, RN, and Charlotta Marshall, MSN, RN, contributed to the development of this scale. The Caucasian child version of the Oucher was developed and copyrighted in 1983 by Judith E. Beyer, PhD, RN, currently at the University of Missouri—Kansas City School of Nursing. Photographs were taken by Lynn Julaino, RN, BSN, at Martha Jefferson Hospital in Charlottesville, Va. The Hispanic child version of the Oucher was developed and copyrighted in 1990 by Antonia M. Villarruel, PhD, RN (University of Michigan), and Mary J. Denyes, PhD, RN (Wayne State University). Photographs were taken at Children's Hospital of Michigan in Detroit.

Location of the Pain

The viscera is innervated bilaterally so that pain is perceived in the midline. It is often described as a deep, dull, diffuse pain. Visceral pain originates from epigastric, periumbilical, and hypogastric causes; from intraabdominal extraperitoneal organs (pancreas, kidneys, ureters, great vessels, pelvic organs); or from a referred source.

Parietal (also known as peritoneal or somatic) pain is more localized and is described as a sharp pain. Peritoneal pain originates from intraabdominal and intraperitoneal organs.

Inflammation (for example, with appendicitis) can produce either visceral or parietal peritonitis. Initially the inflammation is limited to the serosa covering an inflamed organ. The pain is visceral and is felt diffusely. As the inflammation progresses to the adjacent parietal peritoneum, it produces a more severe localized pain that is perceived in the corresponding area of the abdomen. Children have a poor ability to localize pain and in general are not helpful in the majority of cases.

The Apley rule states that the further the localization of pain from the umbilicus, the more likely it is that there is an underlying organic disorder.

When the peritoneal cavity is flooded suddenly by blood, pus, or gastric fluid, the pain is frequently reported as "all over the abdomen" at first. However, the maximum intensity of pain at the onset is likely to be in the upper abdomen with gastric problems and in the lower abdomen with tubal and appendix rupture. Irritating fluid from a perforated duodenal ulcer produces pain in the right hypochondrium, lumbar, and iliac regions.

Pain arising from the small intestine is always felt in the epigastric and umbilical areas of the abdomen. The ninth and eleventh thoracic nerves supply the small intestine via the common mesentery nerve. Appendicular nerves are derived from the same source as those that supply the small intestine, resulting in onset of pain in the epigastric area with appendicitis.

Table 13-1 describes the structures involved in specific pain locations.

Radiation of Pain

Radiation of pain can help in diagnosis. Pain that radiates will do so to the area of distribution of the nerves coming from that segment of the spinal cord that supplies the affected area. Biliary colic pain is frequently referred to the region just under the right scapula (eighth dorsal segment), whereas renal colic in males is frequently felt in the testicle of the same side. Pain from a ruptured spleen is often referred to the top of the left shoulder.

What Do the Pain Characteristics Tell Me?

Key Questions

- Describe the pain (e.g., burning, sharp, achy, crampy).
- What makes it worse or better?

Character of Pain

Colicky or cramping pain occurs with obstruction of a hollow viscus that produces distention. Generally there are pain-free intervals when the pain is much less intense but still present, although it is subtle. During the painful episodes, the patient is exceedingly agitated and restless, and often pale and diaphoretic. The pain from obstruction of the small intestine is rhythmic, peristaltic pain with intermittent cramping. When the obstruction site is in the proximal small intestine rather than in the more distal portion, the paroxysms of cramping occur with greater frequency.

Steady pain is associated with perforation, ischemia, inflammation, and blood in the peritoneal cavity. Burning pain is characteristic

Table 13-1	**Pain Location and Involved Structures**
PAIN LOCATION	**STRUCTURES**
Epigastric	Esophagus, stomach, duodenum, liver, gallbladder, pancreas, spleen
Upper abdominal	Esophagus, stomach, duodenum, pancreas, liver, gallbladder, or thorax
Right upper quadrant	Usually esophagus, stomach, duodenum, pancreas, liver, gallbladder, or thorax; often indicates acute cholecystitis
Left upper quadrant	Spleen
Periumbilical	Jejunum, midgut, ileum, appendix, ascending colon; pain caused by inflammation, ischemic spasm, or abnormal distention
Lower abdominal	Colon, sigmoid colon, rectum, and genitourinary structures—bladder, uterus, prostate
Right lower quadrant	Commonly caused by pelvic inflammatory disease, appendicitis, ectopic pregnancy, or ovarian cyst; establish date of last normal menstrual period
Left lower quadrant	Sigmoid colon
Flanks	Kidney(s)
Localized	Occurs from local inflammation of skin or peritoneum, as with appendicitis; lateralized pain occurs in paired organs—kidneys, ureters, fallopian tubes, gonads
Generalized	Produced by diffuse inflammation of gastrointestinal tract, peritoneum, or abdomen wall

of esophagitis. Pain from a duodenal ulcer has been described as burning or "gnawing." Pain of pancreatic origin is steady, epigastric, and prostrating. Pricking, itching, or burning pain comes from superficial causes such as herpes zoster. Dull, aching pain indicates deeper pain. In children, abdominal pain is generally characterized as colicky or inflammatory.

Remember, however, that despite descriptions of characteristic or typical abdominal pain, presentation in children and the elderly is often atypical and may not fit any pattern.

Precipitating or Aggravating Factors

Lying down or bending forward often produces pain from esophagitis. Alcohol may aggravate gastritis or an ulcer.

Pain that is made worse by deep inspiration and is stopped or diminished by a respiratory pause indicates pleuritic origin. If the cause is peritonitis, intraperitoneal abscess, or abdominal distention from intestinal obstruction, pain will increase on deep inspiration. Biliary colic is made worse by forced inspiration. The pain from biliary colic often causes inhibition of movement of the diaphragm.

The patient with visceral pain is restless, moves about, and has difficulty getting comfortable. The patient with parietal pain usually lies still and does not want to move. Children with inflammatory pain secondary to peritoneal irritation usually appear quiet and motionless because movement exacerbates the pain.

Relieving Factors

Food or antacids may relieve pain caused by an ulcer or gastritis. Both colicky pain and inflammatory pain are alleviated significantly with analgesics. However, the pain of a vascular accident will not respond to analgesics.

Are There Any Precipitating Events That Will Help Narrow My Diagnosis?

Key Questions

- Is the pain related to any other activity (e.g., eating, lying down)?
- Can you identify any trigger?

Relation to Other Events

Pain that is relieved by defecation, flatus, laxatives, or diet changes implicates the intestine. Pain associated with meals implicates the GI tract.

Pain with sexual activity (dyspareunia) suggests a pelvic origin. Pain that occurs with position changes may be referred from the spine, hips, sacroiliac joint, pelvic bones, or abdominal musculature. Exertional pain may be of cardiac origin.

What Does the Presence of Vomiting and Diarrhea Tell Me?

Key Questions

- Are you vomiting? What does the vomitus look like?
- What do your stools look like?
- How frequent are your stools?

Vomiting

Vomiting that precedes the onset of abdominal pain is unlikely to signal a problem requiring surgery. Vomiting suggests that the pain is visceral in origin. Anorexia is a nonspecific symptom, but its absence makes serious disease less likely.

Vomiting associated with an acute condition of the abdomen may be from one of the following three causes:

- Severe irritation of the nerves of the peritoneum or mesentery: sudden stimulation of many sympathetic nerves causes vomiting to occur early and to be persistent.
- Obstruction of an involuntary muscular tube: obstruction of any of the muscular tubes causes peristaltic contraction and consequent stretching of the muscle wall, which results in vomiting. The area behind the obstruction becomes dilated, and as each peristaltic wave occurs, the tension and stretching of the muscular fibers are temporarily increased; therefore the pain of colic usually occurs in spasms. Vomiting usually occurs at the height of the pain.
- The action of absorbed toxins on the medullary centers: the chemoreceptor trigger zone is stimulated by drugs such as cardiac glycosides, ergot alkaloids, and morphine or by uremia, diabetic ketoacidosis, and general anesthetics. Impulses to

the medullary vomiting center then activate the vomiting process.

Pain With Vomiting

In sudden and severe stimulation of the peritoneum or mesentery, vomiting comes soon after the pain. In acute obstruction of the urethra or bile duct, vomiting is early, sudden, and intense. In intestinal obstruction, the timing of the vomiting indicates how high in the gut the obstruction is. If the duodenum is obstructed, vomiting occurs with the onset of pain. Obstruction of the large bowel has very late or infrequent vomiting.

Vomiting is not usually seen in ectopic pregnancy, gastric or duodenal perforation, or intussusception. Vomiting occurring before pain indicates gastroenteritis. With appendicitis, pain almost always precedes the vomiting.

Vomitus Appearance

Clear vomitus suggests gastric fluid; bile-colored vomitus is from upper GI contents. Feculent vomitus occurs with distal intestinal obstruction. Patients with gastric outlet obstruction vomit fluid that contains food particles if the patient has eaten recently, but later the vomitus becomes clear. Infants with duodenal atresia will vomit bilious fluid, but in pyloric stenosis no bile is seen.

Stool Characteristics

Diarrhea is associated with inflammatory bowel disease, diverticulitis, or early obstruction. The presence of blood in the stool suggests that the pain originates in the intestinal tract. Blood may indicate neoplasm, intussusception, or inflammatory lesions.

Diarrhea may precede perforation of the appendix as a result of irritation of the sigmoid colon by an inflammatory mass. Some patients will complain of gas stoppage symptoms: the sensation of fullness that suggests the need for a bowel movement. With appendicitis, the patient may attempt to defecate but without relief.

In children, mild diarrhea associated with the onset of pain suggests acute gastroenteritis but may also occur with early appendicitis. A low-lying appendix, close to the sigmoid colon and rectum, may induce an inflammatory process of the muscle wall of the

sigmoid colon. Any distention of the sigmoid by fluid or gas signals the child to pass gas and small amounts of stool. The cycle repeats a few minutes later. In gastroenteritis, typically the child will have large liquid stools. Children can also have abdominal pain from chronic constipation. Constipation that precedes pain suggests disease of the colon or rectum.

Are There Any Clues to Implicate a Particular Organ System?

If the patient gives a positive response to the following history questions, refer to the topic or chapter indicated for additional discussion. Pain that is not abdominal in origin may be referred to or perceived to be in the abdomen. Accompanying symptoms of headache, sore throat, and general aches and pains suggest a viral, flulike cause.

Key Questions

Cardiovascular system (Chapter 9):
■ Does the pain occur with exertion or at rest?
■ Do you have any chest pain, palpitations, fast heartbeat, or pain that goes to the arm or jaw?

Referred pain from the chest is not uncommon. Pain on exertion signals coronary artery disease and angina. Right upper quadrant pain can be caused by congestive heart failure. Myocardial infarction and pericarditis can also cause abdominal pain.

Key Questions

Gastrointestinal system (Chapters 14 and 15):
■ Do you have any GI symptoms (e.g., gas, diarrhea, constipation, vomiting, heartburn)?
■ Have you had any changes in your bowel habits, stools, or eating pattern?
■ Is the pain relieved by defecation, burping?

Gas, bloating, diarrhea, constipation, and rectal bleeding may occur with pain that is intestinal in origin. Heartburn and dysphagia are characteristic of esophagitis. Changes in bowel habits may signal obstruction or neoplasm. Constipation alternating with diarrhea is characteristic of IBS. The patient may also complain of distention, bloating, belching, gas, and mucus in the stools.

Pain relieved by defecation or the passage of gas suggests IBS or gas entrapment in the large intestine. Pain relieved by burping suggests distention of the stomach by gas.

Key Questions

Genitourinary system (Chapters 17 to 23):
- When was your last menstrual period (LMP)? Was it normal for you? Could you be pregnant?
- Do you have any vaginal symptoms or problems, such as unusual discharge, unusual bleeding, or pain with sexual intercourse?
- Do you have any menstrual irregularity or unusual bleeding? (Sexual history may provide information relevant to the possibility of sexually transmitted infections [STIs], pelvic inflammatory disease [PID], and pregnancy.)
- Do you have any urinary symptoms (frequency, urgency, dysuria, blood in urine, change in urine color)?
- Do you have pain in the back (flank)? Point to it.

Menstrual irregularities, vaginal discharge, unusual bleeding, or dyspareunia indicate a pelvic origin of the pain. Sexually active adolescent girls are at the highest risk for contracting PID. Patients with PID may complain of both vaginal discharge and abnormal vaginal bleeding, although pain is often the only presenting symptom. The pain is usually severe and progressive. Pain just before the onset of menses may indicate endometriosis. Pain related to ovulation (mittelschmerz) occurs mid-cycle. In women of childbearing age, always consider ectopic pregnancy. Regard women of childbearing age as pregnant until pregnancy is ruled out.

Urinary symptoms (dysuria, hematuria, hesitancy, or frequency) point to a urinary tract cause of the pain. Flank pain is usually associated with renal calculi or pyelonephritis. Upper abdominal pain that radiates to the groin signals ureterolithiasis.

Key Questions

Musculoskeletal system (Chapters 26 and 27):
- Does the pain occur with change in position or movement?
- Do you have any joint pain, heat, swelling, noises, or limitation in range of motion?
- Do you have any difficulty walking?

Pain produced by musculoskeletal problems and referred to the abdomen may be provoked by position changes or walking. Costochondritis can produce pain with vigorous respiration. Symptoms of joint involvement point to either a local cause with referred pain or a systemic cause such as rheumatoid arthritis.

Key Questions

Respiratory system (Chapters 11 and 12):
- Do you have a cough or difficulty breathing?
- Do you have any shortness of breath?

Pneumonia, especially of a lower lobe, is a common cause of pain perceived in the abdomen, especially in children. Pleurisy can produce pain on deep inspiration. Persistent coughing can produce musculoskeletal soreness that may be referred to the abdomen.

Is the Pain Psychogenic Organic, or Functional?

Key Questions
- Do you feel unhappy, sad, depressed?
- Are you able to eat, sleep, engage in usual activities?
- Have you had recent problems with diarrhea or constipation?
- How is your energy level?
- Have you ever been diagnosed with or treated for a mental health or psychiatric problem?

Abdominal pain can be functional or psychogenic in origin and presents somewhat differently from organic pain (Table 13-2). The presence of vegetative symptoms suggests depression (see Chapter 32).

What Else Do I Need to Consider?

Key Questions
- What medications are you taking? Why are you taking them?

Table 13-2	Organic Versus Functional Pain	
HISTORY	**ORGANIC PAIN**	**FUNCTIONAL PAIN**
Pain character	Acute, persistent pain increasing in intensity	Less likely to change or get more severe
Pain localization	Sharply localized	Various locations
Pain in relation to sleep	Awakens at night	Does not affect sleep
Pain in relation to umbilicus	Farther away	At umbilicus
Associated symptoms	Fever, anorexia, vomiting, weight loss, anemia, elevated ESR	Headache, dizziness, and multiple system complaints
Psychological stress	None reported	Present

- Have you had any operations? What were they?
- Have you recently had an involuntary weight loss?
- Have you been camping?
- If a child: Is the child in a day care setting?

Medications

Gastrointestinal distress is a common adverse reaction to many medications. Erythromycin and tetracycline are commonly associated with abdominal pain.

Surgery

Prior surgery can produce adhesions that cause intestinal obstruction. Adhesion of organs to the abdominal wall can also produce pain. Prior appendectomy does not preclude appendicitis; the stump may become inflamed.

Involuntary Weight Loss

Involuntary weight loss raises the index of suspicion for colon cancer. Identify other factors that would lead you to suspect neoplasms, such as a recent change in bowel habits in the middle-age patient, family history of colorectal or gynecological cancer, and the presence of blood in the stool.

Camping or Day Care

Ingestion of untreated water can result in intestinal parasites. Transmission of intestinal parasites is also common in day care settings. Intestinal parasites may cause only abdominal pain in children; therefore stools should be evaluated for ova and parasites.

DIAGNOSTIC REASONING: FOCUSED PHYSICAL EXAMINATION

Note General Appearance

Patients with visceral pain are restless, move about, and have difficulty getting comfortable. These are patients with colicky type pain, often indicative of biliary obstruction, ureterolithiasis, obstruction, gastroenteritis, or early peritonitis.

Patients with parietal pain usually lie still and do not want to move. These are patients with localized peritonitis indicative of appendicitis, rupture, or perforation.

In children, note whether the child looks sick (see Chapter 32, Yale Observation Scale). Children may react to pain differently than adults. With peritoneal irritation, they are typically quiet and motionless with their knees flexed and drawn up. Children who are septic or have serious diseases such as perforation or intussusception generally lie still and look lethargic, withdrawn, and apprehensive. A child with colicky pain frequently writhes in discomfort, occasionally rocking in a rhythmic fashion.

Assess Vital Signs

In patients who are tachycardic and tachypneic, suspect a serious thoracic, intraabdominal, or pelvic disorder that is producing an acute condition in the abdomen. Shallow respirations may indicate pneumonia or pleurisy with referred pain. Orthostatic hypotension, an unusually low blood pressure, or a "normal" blood pressure in someone who is usually hypertensive may indicate an acute abdominal condition.

The presence of a fever suggests an acute inflammatory condition. A temperature of greater than 39.4° C (102.9° F) is associated more with pulmonary and renal infection than with an abdominal problem and may indicate pneumonia or pyelonephritis.

In adults, look for documented recent involuntary weight loss, which may indicate a neoplasm. Weigh a child to determine weight loss and dehydration status.

Observe Abdominal Musculature

A rigid abdomen characterizes peritoneal irritation, whereas a soft abdomen suggests otherwise. A rigid abdomen may signal an acute condition of the abdomen that requires surgical intervention.

Note Coloring of Abdominal Skin

Ecchymosis around the umbilicus (Cullen's sign) is associated with hemoperitoneum caused by either pancreatitis or ruptured ectopic pregnancy. Ecchymosis of the flanks (Grey Turner's sign) is associated with hemoperitoneum and pancreatitis. Look for skin rashes of viral exanthema.

In children, a rash (palpable purpura) located on the lower extremities, buttocks, and arms indicates Henoch-Schönlein purpura (a syndrome of purpura with urticaria, erythema, arthritis, and GI symptoms).

Note Abdominal Distention

Generalized symmetrical distention may occur as the result of obesity, enlarged organs, fluid, or gas. Distention from the umbilicus to the symphysis can be caused by ovarian tumor, pregnancy, uterine fibroids, carcinoma, pancreatic cyst, or gastric dilation. Asymmetrical distention or protrusion may indicate hernia, tumor, cysts, bowel obstruction, or enlargement of abdominal organs. Remember the "Fs of distention": fat, fluid, feces, fetus, flatus, fibroid, full bladder, false pregnancy, fatal tumor.

To determine distention in children, stoop down by the child's side and view across the abdomen. The skin is tense and taut with a distended abdomen, and if the umbilicus is everted, ascites is often present. Superficial abdominal veins are often distended in children with peritonitis. The healthy child will usually have a flat abdominal profile. A flat abdomen is a straight line from the xiphoid to pelvis with no scaphoiding. A scaphoid abdomen may occur with marked dehydration or high intestinal obstruction.

Auscultate Bowel Sounds

If bowel sounds are absent, suspect peritonitis or ileus. Hyperactive bowel sounds suggest gastroenteritis, early pyloric or intestinal obstruction, or GI bleeding. High-pitched tinkling bowel sounds may indicate obstruction.

In children, use of the stethoscope can be helpful in palpation to determine abdominal pain. Begin listening to the chest; the child accepts this as painless. Then gently move the stethoscope down to the belly, slightly increasing the pressure, watching the child's face and feeling the resistance when painful.

Percuss for Tones and Guarding

In percussion, look for unexpected dullness. Guarding with percussion suggests peritoneal irritation. Tenderness can be elicited with gentle tapping. Tenderness is usually local and only rarely referred.

Palpate Abdomen

Start with gentle palpation and palpate the area of pain last. Testing for rebound tenderness should be performed gently. Tenderness, guarding, and rebound tenderness suggest peritoneal irritation. The most reliable clinical indicator of parietal peritonitis is involuntary guarding, which must be distinguished from voluntary guarding because of pain or fear of worsening pain as a result of the examination. Guarding is determined with gentle palpation of the abdomen, not by deep palpation of the underlying organs.

You can induce guarding by having the patient place the chin on the chest or cross the arms on the chest and sit up. Palpate the painful area again. Note that intraperitoneal pain is made less severe by induced guarding.

If the severity of pain is not decreased by induced guarding, consider other causes such as functional pain or abdominal wall pain.

Palpate for the liver, gallbladder, spleen, kidneys, aorta, and bladder to detect organ tenderness or involvement. Abrupt cessation of inspiration on palpation of the gallbladder (Murphy's sign) indicates acute cholecystitis.

Palpate for Masses

Palpation of a mass may indicate neoplasm, obstruction, hernia, or the presence of feces in the colon. Anatomical structures may be mistaken for an abdominal mass. A mass in the upper abdomen that pulsates laterally suggests an abdominal aortic aneurysm.

A sausage-shaped mass may be felt in the upper mid-abdomen in 85% to 95% of infants with intussusception. An olive-shaped mass may be palpable in the right upper quadrant with pyloric stenosis.

Palpate the Groin

The groin must be examined in everyone who has abdominal pain to exclude an incarcerated hernia/ovary or torsion of the ovary or testicle (see Chapter 20 for testicular evaluation).

Palpate for Hernias

Palpate for inguinal, incisional, femoral, and umbilical hernias. Uncomplicated hernias will reduce; strangulated ones will not. Bowel sounds will be present in uncomplicated hernias.

Percuss for Flank Tenderness

The use of direct or indirect percussion over the costovertebral angle may elicit tenderness if the kidney is involved. Flank pain, especially with the occurrence of hematuria, may indicate a kidney stone.

Test for Peritoneal Irritation

Several maneuvers can be used to test for peritoneal irritation.

- **Obturator muscle test.** Perform this test when you suspect a ruptured appendix or pelvic abscess because these conditions can cause irritation of the obturator muscle. Pain in the hypogastric region is a positive

sign, indicating obturator muscle irritation. With the patient supine, flex the right leg at the hips and knee to 90 degrees. Hold the leg just above the knee, grasp the ankle, and rotate the leg laterally and medially.

- **Iliopsoas muscle test.** Perform this test when you suspect appendicitis because an inflamed appendix may cause irritation of the lateral iliopsoas muscle. Pain in the lower quadrant is a positive test. With the patient supine, place your hand over the lower thigh and have the patient raise the leg, flexing at the hip while you push downward against the leg.
- **Markle's (heel jar) test.** Perform this test if you suspect appendicitis. The patient stands with straightened knees, and then raises up on the toes. The patient then relaxes and allows the heels to hit the floor, thus jarring the body. The maneuver will cause abdominal pain if positive.
- **Rovsing's test.** Perform this test if you suspect appendicitis. Press on the left lower quadrant. If pain in the right lower quadrant is intensified, the test is positive.

Perform a Pelvic Examination in Women

Perform a pelvic examination in women to rule out sexually transmitted infection (STI), pelvic inflammatory disease (PID), ovarian pain, ectopic pregnancy, and uterine fibroids. Vaginal discharge may or may not be present with STI or PID. Bleeding may accompany ectopic pregnancy.

Cervical motion tenderness (CMT) is the hallmark of PID. CMT plus adnexal pain (often bilateral) in the presence of abdominal pain and lower abdominal tenderness are criteria for a presumptive diagnosis of PID.

Adnexal tenderness in the region of pain may signal ectopic pregnancy. An adnexal mass may or may not be palpable, and its presence is not diagnostic. Vague adnexal tenderness may be present with STI. Bilateral, inflammatory ovarian pain and tenderness are usually related to salpingitis (PID), appendicitis, or peritonitis. A functional cyst may produce unilateral tenderness. Uterine fibroids may be palpable as masses in the uterus, or the entire uterus may be enlarged.

Perform Genital and Prostate Examinations in Men

Perform a genital and prostate examination in men to rule out STIs and prostatitis. Look for penile discharge as an indicator of STI and perhaps prostatitis. A tender prostate signals prostatitis. In acute prostatitis, make sure the examination is gentle; vigorous examination or massage of the prostate can cause bacterial release and produce septicemia (see Chapter 19).

Perform Digital Rectal Examination

Look for frank blood and test for occult blood. The presence of blood may indicate an acute process or carcinoma. Palpate for masses, polyps, and lesions. Occasionally patients with a rectocecal appendix and appendicitis may have a tender, localized mass on rectal examination, even though the abdominal examination is normal.

Check Peripheral Pulses

Diminished femoral pulses in the presence of a pulsatile abdominal mass suggest ruptured abdominal aortic aneurysm.

Perform a Generalized Examination as Indicated

Because abdominal pain may be referred from other areas, examine the lungs, cardiovascular system, head and neck structures, and musculoskeletal system. Palpate for regional lymphadenopathy.

LABORATORY AND DIAGNOSTIC STUDIES

Complete Blood Cell Count With Differential

An elevated white blood cell (WBC) count greater than 12,000/microliter indicates an inflammatory or infectious condition. The WBC count is the total number of WBCs in a cubic millimeter of blood. This is an absolute number. The other measure of WBCs is the relative percentage of each of the types. Neutrophils are the body's first defense against bacterial infection and severe stress. Normally the circulating neutrophils are in a mature form. The mature forms are known as "segs" because the nuclei of the cells are segmented. Immature forms are known as "bands" because the nuclei of the cells are not in segments but are still in a band. An increased need for neutrophils will cause an increase in both the segs (mature cells) and the bands (immature cells). Infection causes both leukocytosis (an increase in the absolute number of WBCs) and an increase in neutrophils, both mature (segs) and immature (bands). This is also called a "shift to the left." When laboratory reports were written by hand, the bands were written first on the left-hand side of the page. Thus a "shift to the left" means that the bands have increased, which is seen as an increase in the relative percent.

Qualitative Urine/Serum hCG Tests

Qualitative urine/serum human chorionic gonadotropin (hCG) tests are monoclonal antibody tests using radioimmunoassay (RIA) to determine or exclude pregnancy. The serum hCG test is more sensitive than the urine hCG test. The serum test can be performed in about 2 hours, and hCG can be detected as early as 6 days after conception. The result is reported as either negative or positive. Because the β-subunits are measured, it is highly specific and does not cross-react with luteinizing hormone.

Depending on the specific test used, urine testing can detect pregnancy from before a missed period to several days after a missed period. The results are obtained in minutes. A positive test (usually a color change) indicates pregnancy.

Quantitative Serum hCG

Quantitative serum hCG is a fluorometric enzyme immunoassay that is highly specific for the β-receptors of hCG, with almost no cross-reactivity with other hormones. Results are provided as values. The reference ranges for determining an abnormal pregnancy are as follows.

Not significant:	0 to 5.0 mIU/ml
Borderline significance:	5.0 to 25 mIU/ml
Evaluate with serial determinations:	>25 mIU/ml

Use this test if you are concerned about ectopic pregnancy. Ectopic pregnancy causes an increase in hCG levels at the same rate as a normal pregnancy, up to a certain point. In ectopic pregnancy, that point is usually less than 4 to 6 weeks, at which time the hCG levels plateau or begin to fall. Therefore serial determinations are more useful than a single determination.

Erythrocyte Sedimentation Rate

The erythrocyte sedimentation rate (ESR) measures the speed with which red blood cells (RBCs) settle in a tube of anticoagulated blood. The results are expressed as millimeters per hour (mm/hr). An increase in plasma globulins or fibrinogen causes the cells to stick together and to fall faster than normal. Cells that are smaller than normal also fall faster, whereas cells that are larger than normal fall more slowly. A marked increase in ESR during pregnancy is expected because there is an increase in the number of plasma globulins and in the fibrinogen level during pregnancy. Inflammation or tissue injury also causes an increase in the number of globulins and fibrinogens and causes an increased sedimentation rate. However, the test is nonspecific; although it shows inflammation, it does not show the source. The ESR is often elevated as a result of PID, infectious states, or AIDS.

Cardiac Enzymes

Creatinine kinase MB (CK-MB) isoenzyme, L-lactate dehydrogenase (LDH) levels, and troponin I (Tn-I) are used in diagnosing myocardial infarction (see Chapter 9).

Urinalysis

Evaluation of kidney infection and determination of the presence of a kidney stone, renal failure, or a systemic disease process are done with a urinalysis (U/A). Microscopic hematuria suggests urinary tract infection or stone. Glycosuria and ketonuria suggest metabolic disturbances. A positive nitrite test on a U/A dipstick indicates the presence of bacteria, which can be seen on microscopic examination. The finding of 20 or more bacteria/high-powered field (HPF) indicates a urinary tract infection. The presence of greater than 0 to 1 RBCs/HPF or greater than 0 to 4 WBCs/HPF on microscopic examination also suggests urinary tract infection. RBCs may also be present as a contaminant with vaginal bleeding. The presence of red cell casts suggests kidney disease or renal infarction. White cell casts indicate pyelonephritis.

Urine for Culture and Sensitivity

If you suspect urinary tract infection, obtain a urine test for culture and sensitivity (C & S).

Culture for Sexually Transmitted Infection

Perform a culture for STI. Collect a specimen of vaginal or penile discharge on a sterile swab and place in the medium provided for gonorrhea, chlamydia, or mycoplasma. For penile discharge, use a sterile urethral swab to collect a specimen from the anterior urethra by gentle insertion and scraping of the mucosa (see Chapter 20).

DNA Probe

DNA probes to test for infectious organisms are available for *Chlamydia, Neisseria gonorrhoeae, Trichomonas vaginalis, Gardnerella vaginalis,* and *Candida* species. Obtain a sample of vaginal or penile discharge with a sterile swab and place it in the medium provided. This test involves the construction of a nucleic acid sequence (called a probe) that will match a sequence in the DNA or RNA of the target tissue. The results are rapid and sensitive.

Potassium Hydroxide (KOH) Test

The KOH test involves direct microscopic examination of material on a slide to determine whether fungus is present. Place a specimen of vaginal or penile discharge on a glass slide, apply a drop of aqueous 10% KOH, and put a coverslip in place. The KOH dissolves epithelial cells and debris and facilitates visualization of the mycelia of a fungus. The presence of fishy odor (the "whiff test") suggests bacterial vaginosis. View under the microscope for the presence of mycelial fragments, hyphae, and budding yeast cells (see Chapter 21).

Saline Wet Prep

In a female with vaginal discharge, this test can demonstrate the presence of *Trichomonas vaginalis* or *Gardnerella* organisms by microscopic examination. Place a specimen of vaginal discharge on a slide and add a drop of normal saline. Place a coverslip on the slide. The presence of trichomonads indicates *T. vaginalis*. The presence of bacteria-filled epithelial cells (clue cells) indicates bacterial vaginosis (*Gardnerella*) (see Chapter 21).

Gram Stain

Place a smear of vaginal or cervical discharge on a glass slide for Gram staining. Gram-positive organisms stain purple, whereas gram-negative organisms stain red. *N. gonorrhoeae* is a gram-negative organism.

Fecal Occult Blood Test (FOBT)

Perform the fecal occult blood test (FOBT) to rule out GI bleeding. The test is positive if a stool smear on a prepared card turns color (usually blue or green) when a solution is applied. A three-sample series provides more reliable results.

Fecal Immunochemical Test (FIT)

Also called immunochemical FOBT (iFOBT), FIT uses antibodies to human globin to detect a specific portion of a human blood protein. FIT does not react with non-human hemoglobin or peroxidase, so food restrictions before the test are not necessary. Immunochemical FOBTs are also more specific for lower gastrointestinal tract bleeding as they target the globin portion of hemoglobin, which does not survive passage through the upper gastrointestinal tract. This test is done essentially the same way as conventional FOBT, but is more specific and reduces the number of false positive results. Vitamins or foods do not affect the fecal immunochemical test, and some forms require only one or two stool specimens.

Electrocardiogram

An electrocardiogram (ECG) can add objective data to the diagnostic process if you suspect the pain is of cardiac origin. ST segment elevation or depression indicates the presence of injured myocardium. T wave inversion will demonstrate the presence of ischemia. The appearance of both strongly supports ischemia but is not diagnostic of coronary artery disease (CAD). Arterial spasm, pericarditis, and electrolyte imbalance can also cause these variations from normal (see Chapter 9).

Radiography

Abdominal radiographs are of limited value in evaluating abdominal pain. An anteroposterior radiograph of the abdomen shows the kidneys, ureters, and bladder (KUB) and adjacent structures. It can be used to exclude free air (perforation) and obstruction (e.g., renal calculi). A chest radiograph can reveal the presence of pneumonia or air under the diaphragm.

Abdominal/Pelvic Ultrasound

Abdominal ultrasound is useful if you are considering an ectopic pregnancy, abdominal aortic aneurysm, or acute cholecystitis.

Computed Tomography

Computed tomography (CT) scanning is appropriate if you suspect retroperitoneal bleeding or a pelvic abscess.

Non–Contrast-Enhanced Helical Computed Tomography

This sensitive and specific radiological test is used to definitively diagnose urolithiasis. It is the best imaging study for diagnosing suspected appendicitis.

Other Tests as Indicated for Gastrointestinal Tract

Consider flexible sigmoidoscopy, proctoscopy, colonoscopy, upper GI series, or lower GI series if you suspect pain that is GI in origin.

DIFFERENTIAL DIAGNOSIS

When there is no worrisome history or no physical findings, use the specific history questions as the "best test" to point you in the right direction. Then determine if the clinical findings are consistent. Review the history to see evolution over time, especially of an acute condition.

Box 13-3	Indicators of Abdominal Emergencies

Subjective Findings	Objective Findings
Progressive intractable vomiting	Involuntary guarding
Lightheadedness on standing	Progressive abdomen distention
Acute onset of pain	Orthostatic hypotension
Pain that progresses in intensity over hours	Fever
	Leukocytosis and granulocytosis
	Decreased urine output

Identify physical findings that are worrisome as well, such as lower abdominal pain beginning at older age, involuntary weight loss, abnormal bleeding in a perimenopausal or postmenopausal woman, palpable abdominal or pelvic mass, or stool that is positive for occult blood.

Look initially for surgical problems. Serial abdominal examinations are the best indicator of progression of an abdominal problem. Try to identify what organ seems to be involved and remember that extraabdominal systems can cause abdominal pain (e.g., pneumonia). Try to determine if the pain is organic or functional in origin. Remember that common causes of acute pain differ from common causes of chronic pain. Box 13-3 lists indicators of abdominal emergencies.

ACUTE CONDITIONS THAT CAUSE ABDOMINAL PAIN

Appendicitis

The incidence of appendicitis peaks at age 10 to 20 years, although it can occur at any age. The patient complains of sudden onset of colicky pain that progresses to a constant pain. The pain may begin in the epigastrium or periumbilicus and later localize to the right lower quadrant (RLQ). The pain worsens with movement or coughing. Vomiting after the onset of pain sometimes occurs. On physical examination, the patient will be lying still and will demonstrate involuntary guarding. Classically, tenderness occurs in the RLQ. The other tests for peritoneal irritation will be positive. Rebound tenderness will be present. Variation in presentation is common, particularly with infants, children, and the elderly. Diagnostic testing includes complete blood cell count (CBC) with differential to confirm or rule out infection and the use of either ultrasonography, CT scan, or laparoscopy (Box 13-4).

Ectopic Pregnancy

Ectopic pregnancy can occur in any sexually active woman of childbearing age, especially those with a history of irregular menses. The patient experiences a sudden onset of spotting and persistent cramping in the lower

Box 13-4	Evidence-Based Practice: Clinical Diagnosis of Appendicitis

Historical symptoms that increase the likelihood of appendicitis are right lower quadrant pain, initial periumbilical pain with migration to the right lower quadrant, and the presence of pain before vomiting.

On physical examination, the presence of rigidity, a positive psoas sign, fever, or rebound tenderness increases the likelihood of appendicitis. Conversely, the absence of right lower quadrant pain, the absence of the migration of the pain, and the presence of similar pain previously are historical findings that make appendicitis less likely. On physical examination, the lack of right lower quadrant pain, rigidity, or guarding makes appendicitis less likely. No finding effectively rules out appendicitis.

Although the precision and accuracy of combinations of these findings have not been reported, history and physical examination are at least as accurate as other modalities in diagnosing or excluding appendicitis.

From Wagner JM, McKinney WP, Carpenter JL: Does this patient have appendicitis? *JAMA* 276:1589, 1996.

quadrant that begins shortly after a missed period. On examination the patient shows signs of hemorrhage, shock, and lower abdominal peritoneal irritation that may be lateralized. On pelvic examination, the uterus is enlarged but smaller than anticipated from dates provided. The cervix is tender to motion, and a tender adnexal mass may be palpable. Diagnosis is confirmed by positive hCG test results and ultrasound. Serial quantitative serum hCG levels may be useful. **A ruptured ectopic pregnancy is a surgical emergency.**

Peptic Ulcer Perforation

The patient complains of sudden onset of severe, intense, steady epigastric pain that radiates to the sides, back, or right shoulder. The patient may give a history of burning, gnawing pain that worsens with an empty stomach. The patient lies as still as possible. Epigastric tenderness will be present with palpation or percussion. Rebound tenderness is intense. The abdominal muscles are rigid, and bowel sounds may be absent. Diagnosis is confirmed by upright or lateral decubitus radiographs, showing air under the diaphragm or in the peritoneal cavity. Perforation is a surgical emergency.

Dissection of Aortic Aneurysm

This condition occurs more frequently in males and persons older than 50 years, especially those with a history of uncontrolled hypertension. The patient experiences the sudden onset of excruciating pain that may be felt in the chest or abdomen and may radiate to the legs and back. The patient will appear shocky. Vital signs will reflect impending shock, and there may be a deficit or difference in femoral pulses. Diagnosis can be made by CT or magnetic resonance imaging (MRI). Additional tests include electrocardiography and cardiac enzymes. This is a surgical emergency with a high death rate.

Myocardial Infarction

In patients older than 50 years, acute MI may present with abdominal pain and gastrointestinal symptoms rather than the classic chest pain. If there is no other explanation for the pain, consider a cardiac origin.

Peritonitis

The most common cause of peritonitis is perforation of the GI tract. It occurs more often in the elderly. The patient experiences the sudden onset of severe pain that is diffuse and worsens with movement or coughing. On examination the patient will be guarding and have rebound tenderness. Bowel sounds will be decreased or absent. Diagnosis includes CBC with differential and abdominal radiographs.

Acute Pancreatitis

Acute pancreatitis is more common in patients with cholelithiasis or a history of alcohol abuse. The pain is steady and boring in quality and is unrelieved by change of position. It is located in the left upper quadrant (LUQ) and radiates to the back. The patient may also experience nausea, vomiting, and diaphoresis and will appear acutely ill. Abdominal distention, decreased bowel sounds, and diffuse rebound tenderness will be present on physical examination. The upper abdomen may show muscle rigidity. Examination of the lungs may reveal limited diaphragmatic excursion. Diagnostic testing includes CBC with differential, ultrasonography, radiography, and serum amylase and lipase levels.

Mesenteric Adenitis

Adenovirus-induced (commonly *Yersinia*) adenopathy of the mesenteric lymph nodes may result in fever and RLQ abdominal pain that mimics appendicitis. This condition is difficult to diagnose, but the WBC count is elevated and an abdominal radiograph will show abnormalities of the terminal ileus.

Cholecystitis/Lithiasis

Cholecystitis/lithiasis occurs more often in adults than in children and more often in females than in males. The pain is colicky in nature and progresses to a constant pain. The patient complains of pain in the right upper quadrant (RUQ), which may radiate to the right scapular area. The typical pain of cholelithiasis is constant, progressively rising to a plateau and falling gradually. The patient may also experience nausea and vomiting and give a history of dark urine and/or light stools.

On physical examination, the patient will be tender to palpation or percussion in the RUQ. The gallbladder is palpable in about half of cases of cholecystitis. Painful splinting of respiration during deep inspiration (Murphy's sign) is frequently present with cholecystitis. Diagnostic testing includes CBC with differential, ultrasonography, radiography, and serum amylase and lipase levels.

Ureterolithiasis

The patient complains of the sudden onset of excruciating intermittent colicky pain that may progress to a constant pain. The pain is in the lower abdomen and flank and radiates to the groin. The patient may also experience nausea, vomiting, abdominal distention, chills, and fever. There is costovertebral angle (CVA) tenderness on examination along with increased sensitivity in the lumbar and groin areas. Hematuria and increased frequency of urination may be present. Urinalysis should be performed. Urine pH and the presence of crystals may help identify stone composition. Definitive diagnostic testing is via non–contrast-enhanced helical CT.

Urinary Tract Infection/Pyelonephritis

Abdominal pain associated with UTI or pyelonephritis is common in children and may be the only presenting complaint. Urinalysis and culture and sensitivity are done to confirm the diagnosis.

Pelvic Inflammatory Disease/Salpingitis

PID occurs most commonly in women younger than 35 who are sexually active and have more than one sexual partner. Infection results from organisms transmitted via intercourse, through childbirth, or with abortion. PID is most often caused by *Chlamydia trachomatis* and *Neisseria gonorrhoeae*. Infection begins intravaginally in most cases and then spreads upward, causing salpingitis. The tubal infection produces an exudate, and, as it spreads, peritonitis can result. Onset is usually shortly after menses. Patients have lower abdominal pain that becomes progressively more severe. On examination, abdominal tenderness, CMT, and adnexal tenderness

(usually bilateral) are present. With peritonitis, patients may also have guarding and rebound tenderness. Patients may also have a fever, irregular bleeding, vaginal discharge, or vomiting. WBC count and ESR are usually elevated. Cultures and Gram staining can assist with diagnosis.

Obstruction

Obstruction occurs most often in the newborn, the elderly, and those with recent GI surgery. The patient presents with a sudden onset of crampy pain, usually in the umbilical area of the epigastrium. Vomiting occurs early with small intestinal obstruction and late with large bowel obstruction. Obstipation (the absence of stools) occurs with complete obstruction, but diarrhea may be present with partial obstruction. Hyperactive, high-pitched bowel sounds may be present in small bowel obstruction. A mass may be palpable in lower obstruction. Abdominal distention may be present. The rectum will be empty on digital examination. Diagnosis is confirmed with abdominal radiographs (supine and sitting).

Ileus

Ileus is associated with intraperitoneal or retroperitoneal infection, metabolic disturbances, and intraabdominal surgery. The patient experiences abdominal distention, vomiting, obstipation, and cramps. On auscultation, there is minimal or absent peristalsis. Abdominal radiographs show gaseous distention of isolated segments of both the small and large intestines.

Intussusception

Bowel obstruction in children ages 2 months to 2 years usually occurs in the ileocecal region and classically presents with vomiting, colicky abdominal pain with drawing up of the legs, and eventual currant jelly stools. The onset is dramatic. The child is asleep or awake when suddenly he or she cries out with severe pain. The child twists and squirms; nothing gives any relief until, almost suddenly, there is a lull with absence of pain followed by a similar painful episode. The abdomen has a sausage-shaped mass that can be felt in the RUQ. The stool tests positive for blood.

Malrotation/Volvulus

Improper rotation and fixation of the duodenum and colon can cause an artery to obstruct, and the patient experiences ischemic necrosis. This disorder of the embryonic gut is usually seen in the first month of life. The infant presents with bilious emesis followed by abdominal distention and GI bleeding. Shock occurs from progression of the ischemia.

Henoch-Schönlein Purpura

In Henoch-Schönlein purpura, crampy, acute abdominal pain and bleeding are secondary to edema and hemorrhage of the intestinal wall. This disease is an immunoglobulin A (IgA)–mediated vasculitis that affects very small vessels. A urticarial rash occurring on the buttocks and lower extremities progresses to papular purpuric lesions. The laboratory findings show an elevated WBC count but a normal platelet count. A mild increase in ESR, an increase in IgA concentration, and negative antinuclear antibodies (ANA) are also found.

Incarcerated Hernia

Incarcerated hernia occurs more commonly in the elderly. The patient complains of a constant severe pain in the RLQ or left lower quadrant (LLQ) that worsens with coughing or straining. Physical examination reveals a hernia or mass that is nonreducible. Diagnosis is confirmed by upper GI series or radiography. Surgical intervention is indicated.

Pneumonia

Pneumonia is a frequently overlooked cause of abdominal pain in children. The pain is referred from right lower lobe pneumonia because of associated phrenic nerve irritation, which may cause muscular spasm, ileus, and pain referred to the RLQ. The WBC count in pneumonia is typically higher than that in early appendicitis.

CHRONIC CONDITIONS THAT CAUSE LOWER ABDOMINAL PAIN

Irritable Bowel Syndrome

IBS begins in adolescent and young adult years. It produces crampy hypogastric pain that is of variable, infrequent duration. The pain is associated with bowel function, gas, bloating, and distention. Relief is often obtained with the passage of flatus or feces. The patient has a normal abdominal examination and the stool is negative for blood. Consider a proctosigmoidoscopy or barium enema (BE) if onset is at middle age or older, the stool is positive for blood, there is a family history of colorectal cancer or polyps, or the patient fails to improve after 6 to 8 weeks of therapy.

Lactose Intolerance

Lactose intolerance produces crampy pain and diarrhea after the consumption of milk or milk product foods (see Chapter 14). It is caused by a deficiency in lactase, an enzyme that decreases in activity with increasing age. It is more common in Asians, Native Americans, and African Americans.

Diverticular Disease

Diverticular disease causes localized abdominal pain and tenderness. The patient will have a fever, elevated ESR, and leukocytosis. Perform a BE or proctoscopy/colonoscopy if there is rectal bleeding.

Simple Constipation

In adults, constipation is associated with infrequency or difficulty passing dry, hard stools and abdominal bloating.

Children with constipation frequently complain of abdominal pain. The pain is usually colicky in nature but may be dull and steady. The pain varies and is not persistent or progressively worsening. Mild, poorly localized periumbilical tenderness and perhaps guarding are reported. A fecal mass may be palpable.

Habitual Constipation

With habitual constipation, the patient presents with a lifelong history of constipation with onset as a young adult, has a normal physical examination, and does not have occult blood in the stool. Diet, activity, and bowel habits are often causally associated factors. Consider a proctoscopy or BE if you suspect a metabolic or systemic cause, the stool is heme positive, or the patient is middle-age or older or fails to respond to treatment.

Dysmenorrhea

Dysmenorrhea, a typically lower abdominal pain or cramping, occurs with menstruation. Dysmenorrhea can be classified as primary (no organic cause) or secondary (pathological cause). In primary dysmenorrhea, the onset is usually soon after menarche and gradually diminishes with age. The woman will have a normal pelvic examination. Secondary dysmenorrhea is associated with specific conditions and disorders such as endometriosis, PID, cervical stenosis, and uterine fibroids. Obtain a gynecological (GYN) consult and/or pelvic ultrasound for secondary dysmenorrhea, dysmenorrhea with increasing severity, or abnormal findings on pelvic examination.

Uterine Fibroids

Fibroids produce pain related to the menstrual cycle and intercourse. The woman may experience dysfunctional uterine bleeding. On examination, palpable myomas are often present. Suspect this cause when there is no suspicion of other pelvic disorder. Order a pelvic ultrasound if ovarian or uterine neoplasm cannot be excluded. Obtain a gynecological consult for abnormal bleeding or severe symptoms.

Hernia

A hernia is a loop of intestine that has prolapsed through the inguinal wall or canal or through the abdominal musculature. The patient complains of intermittent localized pain that may be exacerbated with exertion or lifting. A physical examination will document the hernia, especially when the patient is instructed in maneuvers or positions to increase intraabdominal pressure. Consider proctoscopy or BE if you suspect strangulation or bowel obstruction.

Ovarian Cysts

Ovarian cysts occur most commonly in young women and produce adnexal pain. The cysts may be palpable, late-cycle (corpus luteum) cysts. A pelvic ultrasound is indicated. Ovarian cysts can become quite large before producing symptoms.

Abdominal Wall Disorder

With abdominal wall disorder, the patient may present with a history of trauma. Ecchymosis or swelling may be visible. The patient may complain of pain with rectus muscle stress. GI and genitourinary symptoms are absent. A hernia may be palpable. Obtain a CT scan if internal disease cannot be excluded.

CHRONIC CONDITIONS THAT CAUSE UPPER ABDOMINAL PAIN

Esophagitis/Gastroesophageal Reflux Disease (GERD)

With gastroesophageal reflux disease (GERD), the patient complains of a burning, gnawing pain in the mid-epigastrium ("heartburn") that worsens with recumbency. Regurgitation of gastric contents or water brash (hypersalivation secondary to acid stimulation of the lower esophagus) may also be a complaint. The pain typically occurs after eating or when lying down and may be relieved with antacids. The physical examination is negative. Consider an upper GI series, radiography, or endoscopy if symptoms are severe or the patient does not respond to therapy.

Peptic Ulcer

The patient complains of a burning or gnawing pain that occurs most often with an empty stomach, stress, and alcohol intake. The pain is relieved by food intake. Some patients describe the pain as a soreness, empty feeling, or hunger. Typical pain is steady, mild, or severe and located in the epigastrium. Complaints may be atypical in children and minimal in the elderly. There may be epigastric tenderness on palpation. Endoscopy, upper GI series, and gastric analysis can be used for diagnosis.

Gastritis

Gastritis pain is a constant burning pain in the epigastric area that may be accompanied by nausea, vomiting, diarrhea, or fever. Alcohol, nonsteroidal anti-inflammatory drugs, and salicylates make the pain worse. Physical examination results are negative. No diagnostic testing is necessary if the patient responds to therapy.

Gastroenteritis

Gastroenteritis may occur at any age and produces a diffuse, crampy pain that is accompanied by nausea, vomiting, diarrhea, and fever. Hyperactive bowel sounds will be heard on auscultation. The condition usually resolves on its own, and no diagnostic testing is needed.

Functional Dyspepsia

Functional dyspepsia refers to GI symptoms in which a pathological condition is not present or does not entirely explain the clinical presentation, although altered physiological activity may be present. The patient has vague complaints of indigestion, heartburn, gaseousness, or fullness. The patient also complains of belching, abdominal distention, and occasionally nausea. The physical examination results are negative. Perform a CBC and fecal testing for occult blood. Consider an upper and lower GI series if the patient also has dysphagia, weight loss, vomiting, or a change in the pattern of the symptoms.

Recurrent Abdominal Pain

RAP usually presents in children 5 to 10 years of age—rarely after age 14. The patient complains of dull, colicky periumbilical pain that is intermittent, occurs daily, and lasts from 1 to 3 hours with complete recovery between episodes. The pain does not awaken the child from sleep but may interfere with the ability to fall asleep. The child may have a low-grade fever, pallor, headache, and constipation. A history of stress associated with school social activities, parental conflicts, or loss is frequently elicited. Physical examination results are essentially negative. Initial laboratory tests are CBC, ESR, urinalysis, fecal blood testing, and stool for ova and parasites (O & P).

DIFFERENTIAL DIAGNOSIS OF *Common Causes of Acute Abdominal Pain*

CONDITION	HISTORY	PHYSICAL FINDINGS	DIAGNOSTIC STUDIES
Appendicitis	Age 10-20 years, although it can occur at any age; patient complains of sudden onset of colicky pain that progresses to constant pain; pain may begin in epigastrium or periumbilicus and then later localizes in RLQ; pain worsens with movement or coughing; vomiting after onset of pain is sometimes present	Patient lying still; involuntary guarding; tenderness in RLQ; other tests for peritoneal irritation positive; rebound tenderness; variation in presentation common, particularly with infants, children, and elderly	CBC with differential, ultrasonography, CT scan, laparoscopy
Ectopic pregnancy	Women of childbearing age; sudden onset of spotting and persistent cramping in lower quadrant that begins shortly after missed period	Signs of hemorrhage, shock, and lower abdominal peritoneal irritation that may be lateralized; enlarged uterus; cervical motion tenderness; tender adnexal mass	Positive hCG, ultrasound; ruptured ectopic pregnancy is surgical emergency
Peptic ulcer perforation	Sudden onset of severe intense, steady epigastric pain that radiates to sides, back, or right shoulder; history of burning, gnawing pain that worsens with empty stomach	Patient lying still; epigastric tenderness; rebound tenderness; abdominal muscles rigid; bowel sounds may be absent	Diagnosis confirmed by upright or lateral decubitus radiograph showing air under diaphragm or in peritoneal cavity; perforation is surgical emergency

Continued

DIFFERENTIAL DIAGNOSIS OF *Common Causes of Acute Abdominal Pain* —*cont'd*

CONDITION	HISTORY	PHYSICAL FINDINGS	DIAGNOSTIC STUDIES
Dissection of aortic aneurysm	More frequent in elderly, especially if hypertensive; sudden onset of excruciating pain that may be felt in chest or abdomen and may radiate to legs and back	Patient appears shocky, vital signs reflect impending shock; deficit or difference in femoral pulses	CT or MRI; additional tests include ECG and cardiac enzymes; surgical emergency
Myocardial infarction	Over age 50; upper or diffuse abdominal pain; may be accompanied by nausea, vomiting, dyspepsia	Hypertension or hypotension, cardiac arrhythmia, paradoxical S_2	Serial ECGs, serial cardiac enzymes
Peritonitis	Occurs more often in elderly; sudden onset of severe pain that is diffuse and worsens with movement or coughing	Guarding; rebound tenderness; bowel sounds decreased or absent	CBC with differential, abdominal radiographs
Acute pancreatitis	History of cholelithiasis or alcohol abuse; pain is steady and boring in quality and is unrelieved by change of position; located in LUQ and radiates to back; nausea, vomiting, and diaphoresis	Patient appears acutely ill; abdominal distention, decreased bowel sounds, diffuse rebound tenderness; upper abdomen may show muscle rigidity; may have limited diaphragmatic excursion of lungs	CBC with differential, ultrasonography, x-rays, serum amylase and lipase levels
Mesenteric adenitis	Fever, pain in RLQ, other symptoms suggestive of appendicitis	Pain on palpation in RLQ; there may be pharyngitis, cervical adenopathy	CBC with differential; adenovirus found in tissue of surgical specimen
Cholecystitis/lithiasis	Appears in adults more than in children, females more than males; colicky pain with progression to constant pain; pain in RUQ that may radiate to right scapular area; pain of cholelithiasis is constant, progressively rising to plateau and falling gradually; nausea, vomiting, history of dark urine and/or light stools	Tender to palpation or percussion in RUQ; gallbladder palpable in about half cases of cholecystitis; positive Murphy's sign	CBC with differential, ultrasonography, radiographs, serum amylase and lipase levels
Ureterolithiasis	Sudden onset, excruciating intermittent colicky pain that may progress to constant pain; pain in lower abdomen and flank and radiates to groin; nausea, vomiting, abdominal distention, chills, and fever; increased frequency of urination	CVA tenderness; increased sensitivity in lumbar and groin areas; hematuria	Urinalysis, non–contrast-enhanced helical CT

Continued

DIFFERENTIAL DIAGNOSIS OF *Common Causes of Acute Abdominal Pain* —cont'd

CONDITION	HISTORY	PHYSICAL FINDINGS	DIAGNOSTIC STUDIES
Urinary tract infection (UTI)/pyelonephritis	Urinary symptoms with UTI, back pain with pyelonephritis; infants present with fever, failure to thrive, irritability; toddlers complain of pain in abdomen; may not complain of dysuria or frequency	Altered voiding pattern, malodorous urine, fever	Urinalysis and culture
Pelvic inflammatory disease	Lower abdominal pain that becomes progressively more severe; may have irregular bleeding, vaginal discharge, and vomiting; most common in sexually active women	Abdominal tenderness, CMT and adnexal tenderness (usually bilateral); with peritonitis may also have guarding and rebound tenderness; fever and vaginal discharge common	WBC and ESR are usually elevated; cultures and Gram staining
Obstruction	Sudden onset of crampy pain usually in umbilical area of epigastrium; vomiting occurs early with small intestinal obstruction and late with large bowel obstruction; obstipation or diarrhea	Hyperactive, high-pitched bowel sounds; fecal mass may be palpated; abdominal distention; empty rectum on digital examination	Diagnosis confirmed with abdominal radiographs (supine and sitting)
Ileus	Abdominal distention, vomiting, obstipation, and cramps	Minimal or absent peristalsis on auscultation	Gaseous distention of isolated segments of both small and large intestines shown on radiographs
Intussusception	Sudden-onset pain in infant; occurs with sudden relief, then pain again	Fever, vomiting, currant jelly stools	Abdominal films
Malrotation/volvulus	Seen in infants up to 1 month old; irritability, pain	Bilious emesis, abdominal distention	Abdominal films
Henoch-Schönlein purpura	Seen in children 2-8 years old	Rash on lower extremities/ buttocks; arthralgias; hematuria	CBC, ESR, serum IgA
Incarcerated hernia	More common in elderly; constant severe pain in RLQ or LLQ that worsens with coughing or straining	Hernia or mass that is nonreducible	Upper gastrointestinal series or radiograph
Pneumonia	Children 2-5 years of age may present only with abdominal pain and fever	Tachypnea, retractions, pallor, nasal flaring, crackles	CBC, chest radiograph

DIFFERENTIAL DIAGNOSIS OF *Common Causes of Chronic Lower Abdominal Pain*

CONDITION	HISTORY	PHYSICAL FINDINGS	DIAGNOSTIC STUDIES
Irritable bowel syndrome (IBS)	Begins in adolescence, young adult years; hypogastric pain; crampy, variable infrequent duration; associated with bowel function; associated with gas, bloating, distention; relief with passage of flatus, feces	Normal examination; heme-negative stool	Proctosigmoidoscopy, barium enema if onset middle age/older, stool positive for blood, family history of colorectal cancer or polyps, failure to improve after 6-8 weeks of therapy
Lactose intolerance	Crampy pain after eating milk or milk products	Negative physical examination	Trial elimination of offending foods
Diverticular disease	Localized pain; older patient	Abdominal tenderness; fever	Barium enema, elevated ESR, proctoscopy/colonoscopy if rectal bleeding
Simple constipation	Colicky or dull and steady pain that does not progress and worsen	Fecal mass palpable, stool in rectum	None
Habitual constipation	Lifelong history; younger patient	Normal examination; heme-negative stool	Proctoscopy, barium enema if metabolic or systemic cause suspected, heme-positive stool, onset in middle age or beyond, failure to respond to treatment
Dysmenorrhea	Typical premenstrual pain onset soon after menarche, gradually diminishing with age	Normal pelvic examination	GYN consult; pelvic USG if secondary dysmenorrhea, increasing disability, or abnormal pelvic examination
Uterine fibroids	Pain related to menses, intercourse	Palpable myomas; no suspicion of other pelvic disorder	Pelvic USG if ovarian or uterine neoplasm cannot be excluded; GYN consult if abnormal bleeding or severe symptoms
Hernia	Localized pain that increases with exertion or lifting	Physical examination documents hernia	Proctoscopy, barium enema if suspect strangulation or bowel obstruction
Ovarian cyst(s)	Young woman	Adnexal pain and palpable ovarian cysts, especially in late cycle (corpus luteum)	Pelvic USG
Abdominal wall disorder	History of trauma	Visible ecchymosis or swelling; palpable hernia pain with rectus muscle stress; no GI/genitourinary symptoms	CT scan if internal disease cannot be excluded

DIFFERENTIAL DIAGNOSIS OF *Common Causes of Chronic Upper Abdominal Pain*

CONDITION	HISTORY	PHYSICAL FINDINGS	DIAGNOSTIC STUDIES
Esophagitis/GERD	Burning, gnawing pain in mid-epigastrium that worsens with recumbency; water brash; pain occurs after eating and may be relieved with antacids; in infant: failure to thrive, irritability, postprandial spitting and vomiting	Physical examination negative; in infants: weight loss, in some cases aspiration pneumonia	Upper gastrointestinal series, radiography, or endoscopy if symptoms are severe or do not respond to therapy
Peptic ulcer	Burning or gnawing pain; soreness, empty feeling, or hunger; occurs most often with empty stomach, stress, and alcohol, and relieved by food intake; pain steady, mild, or severe and located in epigastrium; may be atypical in children and minimal in elderly	May be epigastric tenderness on palpation	Endoscopy, upper gastrointestinal series, gastric analysis
Gastritis	Constant burning pain in epigastric area that may be accompanied by nausea, vomiting, diarrhea, or fever; alcohol, NSAIDs, and salicylates make pain worse	Physical examination negative	No diagnostic testing necessary if patient responds to therapy
Gastroenteritis	Occurs at any age and produces diffuse crampy pain accompanied by nausea, vomiting, diarrhea, and fever	Hyperactive bowel sounds will be heard on auscultation; dehydration if severe	No diagnostic testing needed
Functional dyspepsia	Vague complaints of indigestion, heartburn, gaseousness, or fullness; belching, abdominal distention, and occasionally nausea	Physical examination negative	CBC, FOBT or FITA; may consider upper and lower gastrointestinal series if patient also has dysphagia, weight loss, vomiting, or change in pattern of symptoms
Recurrent abdominal pain (RAP)	Children 5-10 years old; history of environmental or psychological stress	Physical examination negative	CBC, urinalysis, ESR, FOBT or FIT, stool for O & P

CHAPTER RESOURCES

Aschcraft K: Consultation with the specialist: acute abdominal pain, *Pediatr Rev* 21:363, 2000.

Fass R, Longstreth GF, Pimentel M et al: Evidence- and consensus-based practice guidelines for the diagnosis of irritable bowel syndrome, *Arch Intern Med* 161(17):2081, 2001.

Leung A, Sigalet D: Acute abdominal pain in children, *Am Fam Physician* 67:11, 2003.

Levy J: Gastroesophageal reflux and other causes of abdominal pain, *Pediatr Ann* 30:42, 2001.

Matthews PJ, Aziz Q: Functional abdominal pain, *Postgrad Med* 81:448, 2005.

McCollough M, Sharieff G: Abdominal surgical emergencies in infants and young children, *Emerg Med Clin North Am* 21:909, 2003.

Munoz A, Katerndahl DA: Diagnosis and management of acute pancreatitis, *Am Fam Physician* 62:164, 2000.

Old JL, Dusing RW, Yap W et al: Imaging for suspected appendicitis, *Am Fam Physician* 71(1):71, 2005.

Rothrock SG, Pagane J: Acute appendicitis in children: emergency department diagnosis and management, *Ann Emerg Med* 36:39, 2001.

Sachs CJ: Abdominal pain: a rational approach, *Consultant* November:1433, 2005.

Tay JI, Moore J, Walker JJ: Ectopic pregnancy, *West J Med* 173(2):131, 2000.

Wagner JM, McKinney WP, Carpenter JL: Does this patient have appendicitis? *JAMA* 276:1589, 1996.

Zeiter DK, Hyams JS: Recurrent abdominal pain in children, *Pediatr Clin North Am* 49:53, 2002.

14

Diarrhea

Next to respiratory disease, acute gastroenteritis is the most common illness in families in the United States. Most cases are of viral origin and are self-limiting. In children, 50% are of viral origin, approximately 25% are of bacterial origin, and approximately 25% are of undetermined cause. Diarrhea can be classified according to its pathophysiological pattern (osmotic, secretory, exudative, or motile), its cause (infectious or noninfectious), or its duration (acute or chronic).

Osmotic or malabsorptive diarrhea occurs when nonabsorbable water-soluble solutes remain in the bowel and retain water. This can occur through damage to the intestinal microvillus membrane. The result is malabsorption of luminal solutes with osmotic loss of free water into the gut lumen. This is the most common cause of chronic diarrhea in children. Lactose intolerance is an example of this kind of diarrhea. Ingestion of large amounts of sugar substitutes in diet foods, drinks, candies, and chewing gum can cause osmotic diarrhea through a combination of slow absorption and rapid small bowel motility.

Secretory diarrhea occurs when the balance between fluid secretion and absorption across the intestinal mucosa is altered. When there is a change in this balance produced by physiological causes, diarrhea occurs. The loss of water and electrolytes can be rapid and massive. Traveler's diarrhea and diarrhea caused by *Vibrio cholerae* are examples.

Exudative diarrhea occurs in the presence of mucosal inflammation or ulceration, which results in an outpouring of plasma, serum proteins, blood, and mucus. The consequence is an increase in fecal bulk and fluidity. Many mucosal diseases such as regional enteritis, ulcerative colitis, and carcinoma can cause this exudative enteropathy.

Diarrhea from abnormal intestinal motility (either increased or decreased) results in alteration in contact between luminal contents and the mucosal surface. Examples include irritable bowel syndrome (IBS) and laxative use.

Infectious bacteria may be caused by viral, bacterial, or parasitic agents.

DIAGNOSTIC REASONING: FOCUSED HISTORY

What Does This Patient Mean by "Diarrhea"?

Key Questions
- How frequent is the stool?
- What is the volume of stools?
- Are the stools formed or liquid?
- At what intervals does the diarrhea occur?

Frequency of Stools
In the United States, typical bowel frequency ranges from 1 to 3 times a day to 2 or 3 times per week and varies considerably from person to person. Changes in stool frequency, consistency, or volume may indicate disease.

Stool Volume and Consistency
Processes involving the small bowel tend to produce large-volume watery stools that are relatively infrequent. Large bowel involvement, usually resulting from a bacterially induced inflammatory process, tends to produce more frequent and less watery stools.

Intervals

A history of acute diarrhea followed by continuous or intermittent episodes of loose stools suggests malabsorption commonly caused by lactase deficiency exacerbated by the ingestion of lactose in milk or milk products. Intermittent diarrhea alternating with constipation suggests IBS.

Proximal Colon Symptoms

Proximal colon symptoms include large-volume, less-frequent, more-homogeneous stools, without urgency or tenesmus (painful defecation), and suggest food intolerance or infectious or inflammatory disease.

Distal Colon Symptoms

Symptoms of small volume, frequency, urgency, tenesmus, incontinence, and mucus suggest proctocolitis, colon cancer, diverticular disease, or IBS.

If This Is an Infant, Is There a Risk of Dehydration?

Key Questions

- How many wet diapers has the child produced in the past 24 hours?
- Does the infant seem thirsty?
- Does the child have tears when crying?

Wet Diapers

Dehydration in infants and young children can occur quickly and with fatal consequences, especially in infants. Diagnosis and treatment must be done in a timely manner. A general rule of thumb to determine signs of dehydration in infants is fewer than six wet diapers per 24 hours or a period of longer than 4 hours without urination.

Thirst

Infants demonstrate their thirst with irritability, crying, and eagerness to drink fluid that is offered to them. Test for thirst by offering fluids either in a bottle or on a spoon. The child with mild dehydration will exhibit increased thirst; the moderately dehydrated child will be very thirsty; and, with severe dehydration, the child will continue to be very thirsty. If left untreated, a child may become stuporous and unresponsive and therefore may be unable to manifest thirst.

Tears

In mild dehydration, tears are present; in moderate dehydration, tears may or may not be present; and in severe dehydration, no tears are present.

If This Is an Adult, Is There Risk for Dehydration?

Key Questions

- How many times have you urinated in the past 24 hours?
- Are you thirsty?
- Do you have a dry mouth or dry eyes?

Dehydration

Symptoms of dehydration in an adult are more related to the rate of fluid loss than to the absolute degree of fluid loss. The degree of dehydration can be estimated by symptoms of thirst, dry mouth, or dry eyes, and by frequency and volume of urination. Patients may also experience weakness.

Is This an Acute or Chronic Problem?

Key Questions

- How long have you had diarrhea?
- Have you had this problem before?

Acute Diarrhea in Adults

An acute onset of diarrhea in a previously healthy patient without signs or symptoms or other organ involvement suggests an infectious cause. Acute diarrhea in adults is commonly viral in origin. The viral illnesses are self-limited, and an aggressive diagnostic workup is not indicated. Acute diarrhea in adults usually has an abrupt onset and lasts less than 2 weeks. Most of the disorders cause some combination of abdominal pain, diarrhea, nausea, vomiting, fever, and tenesmus.

Acute Diarrhea in Children

Acute diarrhea in children is characterized by loose or liquid stools. A large quantity of fluid and electrolytes that become pooled in the intestinal lumen is lost as stool is expelled. The number of stools is usually increased, but this is not an essential manifestation. Severe or protracted diarrhea may lead to metabolic acidosis, dehydration, azotemia, and oliguria. Diarrhea in the neonate and young infant is considered more serious than that in the older child because of lower tolerance to associated fluid shifts and the greater likelihood of associated infection or congenital anomaly.

Chronic Diarrhea in Adults

Diarrhea is chronic when it lasts more than 2 weeks. Unless the diarrhea is bloody or the patient has a systemic illness, the most common causes of chronic diarrhea are parasites, medications, IBS, lactose intolerance, and inflammatory bowel disease.

Chronic Diarrhea in Children

Chronic diarrhea in children is defined as diarrhea for longer than 3 weeks. The major causes of the diarrhea change with age. In the infant, formula protein intolerance is the most common cause. Toddler's diarrhea (irritable colon of infancy), protracted enteritis following a viral infection, and *Giardia* are the common causes in the toddler. In children and adolescents, malabsorption disorders are the most common causes. The diarrhea is the result of the ingestion of solutes that cannot be digested or absorbed, such as lactose products or excessive intake of sorbitol. Another cause of diarrhea in this age-group is inflammatory bowel disease (ulcerative colitis and Crohn's disease).

Does the Presence or Absence of Blood Help Me Narrow the Cause?

Key Questions

■ Is there any noticeable blood in the stool or tissue? How much?
■ What color is the blood?
■ What color are the stools?

Blood in the Stools

Bright red blood limited to small spots on the toilet tissue suggests that the source of bleeding is from hemorrhoids and not from a diarrheal process higher in the gastrointestinal tract. Because diarrhea and repeated cleansing of the rectum produce local irritation, minor bleeding from hemorrhoids is not uncommon and must be distinguished from true blood in the stool. Reports of blood in the stool in acute diarrhea are suggestive of a bacterial pathogen, notably *Shigella*. The blood is red.

In infants and children, blood in the stool is most commonly caused by cow's milk intolerance or anal fissures. In the newborn, blood in stools may be a result of hemorrhagic disease of the newborn, thought to be caused by a lack of vitamin K. Premature infants or infants who are of low birth weight are at risk for necrotizing enterocolitis presenting with red or maroon stools (hematochezia) as well as vomiting and abdominal distention.

In adults and children, chronic bloody diarrhea may indicate inflammatory bowel disease, dysentery, colitis, or an invasive organism. Blood that is red usually indicates lower gastrointestinal tract bleeding, whereas dark or black, tarry stools (melena) typically indicate upper gastrointestinal tract bleeding. However, bleeding from the small bowel or right colon can also produce melena.

Color of Stools

Some patients believe they have blood in their stool based on stool color. Sources of black stools are blood, iron, charcoal, bismuth, licorice, huckleberries, and lead. Sources of red or pink stools include blood, food (beets, cranberries, tomatoes, peppers), food coloring (breakfast cereals, Jell-O-water), and drugs (anticoagulants, salicylates, rifampin, pyridium pamoate, diazepam syrup, phenolphthalein in alkaline stool). Green-black stools may be caused by grape-flavored drinks and iron. Dark gray stools occur with cocoa and chocolate ingestion. Pale gray or white stools may be caused by cholestasis, obstructive jaundice, malabsorption, excessive milk ingestion, and antacid ingestion. Green stools are produced by bile salts and chlorophyll-containing vegetables such as spinach.

What Does the Presence or Absence of Pain Tell Me?

Key Questions

- Are you having any abdominal pain or gas with the diarrhea?
- Where is the pain?
- What does the pain feel like?
- Is the pain constant or does it come and go?
- Does the pain awaken you at night?
- Does the pain interfere with your activities (e.g., work, sleep, eating)?

Occurrence of Pain

Diarrhea with abdominal pain and flatulent stools is characteristic of a malabsorptive process. Most self-limiting viral diarrheas cause some combination of abdominal pain, diarrhea, nausea, vomiting, fever, and tenesmus.

Abdominal pain is common when diarrhea is caused by infective bacteria in the colon, such as ingestion associated with food poisoning. *Giardia lamblia,* introduced through the ingestion of contaminated water or by the orofecal route, produces crampy abdominal pain and is frequently seen in children and diapered infants in day care where handwashing may not be done between diapering.

Location of Pain

Generalized abdominal pain is produced by diffuse inflammation of the gastrointestinal tract as occurs with inflammatory bowel disease or abdominal cramping from infective diarrhea. The pain from ulcerative colitis may be perceived over the entire abdomen or localized to the lower quadrants. The pain associated with IBS is usually confined to the lower quadrants or over the sigmoid colon. Large intestine pain is felt in the lower abdominal quadrants, whereas small intestine pain is felt in the epigastric and umbilical areas.

Severity of Pain

Self-limited diarrhea usually presents with cramping but not severe abdominal pain. Other causes of abdominal pain should be investigated (see Chapter 13).

Sleep Related

Persistent diarrhea that awakens the patient from sleep usually indicates a serious organic disease, such as diabetes enteropathy or human immunodeficiency virus (HIV) enteropathy. The symptoms associated with IBS occur during the waking hours.

What Do Associated Symptoms Tell Me?

Key Questions

- Do you have any fever? Did you measure your temperature? What was the highest temperature?
- Do you have any vomiting?
- What occurred first: the diarrhea or the vomiting?

Fever

Patients often report having a "fever" when they have symptoms such as facial flushing, shaking chills, headache, malaise or muscle aches, or a sensation of warmth. These symptoms are usually not validated by measuring body temperature with a thermometer. Fever is a cardinal manifestation of disease. Gastrointestinal tract and respiratory tract infections are responsible for 80% of febrile illnesses.

Vomiting

Vomiting is often present early in the course of viral gastroenteritis (especially the Norwalk virus), food poisoning, and foodborne bacterial infection. Vomiting is one of the main causes of dehydration in acute diarrhea. Also, small bowel processes commonly associated with viral agents cause delayed gastric emptying and luminal distention, which often induces vomiting before the onset of diarrhea.

Occurrence of Vomiting and Diarrhea

When diarrhea occurs before the vomiting, suspect a bacterial etiology.

Could This Be Caused by Exposure to Others or to Contaminated Food?

Key Questions

■ If a child: Does the child attend day care?
■ If a child: Are any of the other children in day care ill?
■ Have you been around others who have similar symptoms?

Day Care Attendance

Children who attend day care are at greater risk to acquire many bacterial infections as the causes are transmitted through orofecal contamination and diapering.

Others With Similar Symptoms

It is common for food-borne infections to be acquired at social gatherings in which food is served; in this case, others at the gathering may become ill with similar symptoms. However, patients may not always know if others became ill, especially when the onset of diarrhea occurs 1 to 2 hours after food ingestion.

Could This Be the Result of Exposure to Animals?

Key Questions

■ What pets do you have?
■ Have you had contact with or have you handled dogs, cats, or turtles?

Exposure to Infectious Agents Through Animal Contact

Campylobacter jejuni infection can be acquired from infected dogs or cats. Infected turtles are a source of *Salmonella*.

Could This Be Caused by Exposure to Contaminated Water?

Key Question

■ Have you traveled recently? Where?

Recent Travel

Travel outside of the United States carries the potential to acquire enterotoxigenic *Escherichia coli* or, less commonly, *G. lamblia,*

Salmonella, Shigella, C. jejuni, or *Entamoeba histolytica.* Camping exposes individuals to *Giardia* and *Campylobacter* through untreated water. Outbreaks of diarrhea caused by *Cryptosporidium* have been linked to contaminated water in urban areas of the U.S.

Could Sexual Activities Explain the Diarrhea?

Key Question

■ Do your sexual practices include anal sex?

Suspect *Shigella* infection in patients who engage in anal sex, particularly homosexual males. Accompanying pain, tenesmus, and the passage of mucus suggest the presence of proctitis.

Could This Be the Result of an Immune Problem?

Key Questions

■ Have you been diagnosed with an immune system problem?
■ Do you have frequent colds or other illnesses?
■ Are you receiving chemotherapy?

Immunocompromised Host

Immmunoglobulin A (IgA) and immunoglobulin G (IgG) deficiencies are frequent causes of chronic diarrhea in children. Patients with a compromised immune system from acquired immunodeficiency syndrome (AIDS) or chemotherapy often develop enteropathy.

Could This Be Caused by Medications?

Key Questions

■ Have you taken any antibiotics recently? Which one(s)?
■ What prescription medications are you currently taking?
■ What over-the-counter medications/preparations are you currently using?

Recent Treatment With Antibiotics

Pseudomembranous enterocolitis caused by *Clostridium difficile* has been reported in persons who have been recently treated with antibiotics, most commonly ampicillin, clindamycin, or cephalosporins. Pseudomembranous enterocolitis is a very serious disorder that can lead to paralytic ileus. More often, antibiotics disturb the normal flora of the gut, leading to diarrhea.

Medications

Diarrhea can be caused by antacids that contain magnesium, antibiotics, methyldopa, digitalis, β-blockers, systemic antiinflammatory agents, colchicine, quinidine, phenothiazine, high-dose salicylates, and laxatives.

Could This Be Related to a Surgical Procedure?

Key Question

■ Have you had surgery recently?

Recent Gastrointestinal Surgery

Gastrointestinal surgery can result in dumping syndrome after the ingestion of meals. Inadequate mixing and digestion take place in the stomach, resulting in rapid transit and diarrhea. Anatomical derangement from surgery can also cause stagnant loops of bowel. This stagnation leads to bacterial overgrowth and results in diarrhea. Extensive bowel resection can produce short bowel syndrome, which results in diarrhea from malabsorption.

Is This Diet Related?

Key Questions

■ How much apple juice or how many sodas do you drink in a day?
■ Do you drink milk or eat milk products?
■ Do you eat wheat products?
■ What have you had to eat in the past 3 days?

Excessive Intake of High-Carbohydrate Fluids

The ingestion of large amounts of apple juice and nonabsorbable fillers such as sorbitol may lead to malabsorptive diarrhea. Bacterial contamination of nonpasteurized apple juice can cause diarrhea.

Lactose Intolerance

The ingestion of specific disaccharides, such as lactose, produces a malabsorptive osmotic diarrhea.

Cow's Milk Protein/Soy Protein Hypersensitivity

Diarrhea, vomiting, colic, occult or grossly bloody stools, and white blood cells within the stools that begin within 2 to 3 weeks after starting either cow's milk or soy formulas may be caused by protein hypersensitivity.

Celiac Sprue (Gluten Enteropathy)

Gluten enteropathy is manifested by increasing frequency, looseness, paleness, and bulkiness of stool within 3 to 6 months of dietary intake of wheat, rye, barley, or oat products. Patients have a hypersensitivity reaction to the protein in these grains.

Starvation Stools

The history of this condition includes diarrhea that persists for 2 to 3 weeks. Stools are loose because the liquid low-fiber diet used to ease the symptoms of acute diarrhea is continued for too long. Health care providers may neglect to tell patients or parents to resume a regular diet once acute diarrhea begins to resolve. New guidelines recommend refeeding soon after rehydration has been achieved.

Could This Be Caused by Food Preparation Problems?

Key Questions

■ Have you recently eaten raw or undercooked poultry, shellfish, or beef?
■ Have you recently ingested unpasteurized milk?
■ Do you prepare poultry and/or beef on the same surface as other foods?
■ Is anyone else you know ill with similar symptoms?

Dietary Exposure to Infectious Agents

Undercooked poultry is a potential cause of *Salmonella* or *C. jejuni* diarrhea. Undercooked beef and unpasteurized milk are food sources that contain *E. coli* 0157:H7. Raw shellfish is a potential for source of Norwalk virus. Food can be contaminated through bacteria that remain on incompletely cleaned food preparation surfaces.

Other Ill Persons

Food poisoning should be considered if diarrhea develops in two or more persons after ingestion of the same food. Such multiple occurrences suggest ingestion of infected food or toxic substances (e.g., lead, mercury).

Is There Any Family Predisposition that May Point to a Cause?

Key Questions

- Have you or anyone in your family been diagnosed with cystic fibrosis?
- Does anyone in your family have a history of chronic diarrhea, ulcerative colitis, or inflammatory bowel disease?

Family History of Cystic Fibrosis

Cystic fibrosis is the most common genetic disease in Caucasians. It has an autosomal recessive mode of inheritance. The condition leads to fat malabsorption and produces fatty, foul-smelling diarrhea.

Family History of Diarrheal Illnesses

Inflammatory bowel disease is genetically linked.

DIAGNOSTIC REASONING: FOCUSED PHYSICAL EXAMINATION

Inspect General Appearance

Observe the patient's general appearance. Diarrhea should be considered a symptom in all instances, and principal attention should be directed to determination and correction of the cause.

Assess Hydration Status

Assessment of hydration status is the most important aspect of physical examination in the child. Dehydration in otherwise healthy adults is uncommon unless the diarrhea is very severe (Table 14-1). Hydration is also an important consideration in older adults and the chronically ill and in those persons who cannot replace fluid losses with oral intake. In the presence of hypernatremia, the state of dehydration may be found to be greater than suggested by physical examination because extracellular fluid volume

Table 14-1	**Determining Hydration Status**		
SIGNS/SYMPTOMS	MILD DEHYDRATION	MODERATE DEHYDRATION	SEVERE DEHYDRATION
Estimated fluid deficit (% of body weight)*	<5	>6-9	>10
Estimated fluid deficit (ml/kg)	30-50	60-90	>100
Thirst	Increased	Marked increase	Very marked increase
Blood pressure	Normal	Postural drop only	Low or absent (peripherally)
Pulse (peripheral)	Normal	Rapid	Rapid, thready
Heart rate	Mildly elevated	Elevated	Greatly elevated
Mucous membranes	Thick saliva	Dry	Very dry
Eyes	Normal	Sunken	Deeply sunken
Tears when crying	Present	Absent	Absent
Skin turgor	Normal	Tenting	None
Fontanel	Normal	Sunken	Very sunken
Urine output	Mildly decreased	Decreased	Markedly decreased or absent
Affect/sensorium	Normal	Restlessness/ irritability	Lethargy/coma

*Percent body weight loss = [(normal weight − present weight)/normal weight] × 100.

tends to be preserved at the expense of intracellular volume.

Indicators of Hydration Status
Mucous Membranes
The earliest clinical sign of dehydration is dryness of mucous membranes. Hyperventilation with mouth-breathing may dry the mucous membranes of the mouth in the absence of dehydration. Recent vomiting makes the mucous membranes appear moist. The patient may also have halitosis.

Tissue Turgor
Turgor reflects the amount of fluid in the interstitial spaces and is best assessed on the thigh, chest, and abdomen. Abdominal testing alone may be misleading because distention may mask the loss of turgor. Obese children may not appear to have loss of skin turgor because of the elasticity of their skin.

Fontanel
The fontanel, if still open, is best assessed with the child in an upright position. The normal fontanel may feel tense in the infant who is supine. In the crying child, physiological bulging occurs only during expiration; this bulging disappears when the child relaxes or inspires. The fontanel will be sunken in a dehydrated state.

Peripheral Perfusion
Blanching of the nail bed with pressure and quick refill of capillary blood are normal. In dehydration, it takes longer for the blood to reappear in the tissue.

Urine Output/Specific Gravity
In a mildly dehydrated child, the output decreases with a slight increase in specific gravity. In a moderately dehydrated child, the urinary output is decreased and the specific gravity is increased. In a severely dehydrated child, the urinary output is decreased to oliguria and the specific gravity is markedly increased, up to 1.030.

Take Temperature
An elevated temperature increases insensible water loss and may lead to more rapid dehydration. The presence of a fever in a patient with acute diarrhea indicates viral or bacterial infection. Fever in a patient with chronic diarrhea points to inflammatory causes.

The generally accepted normal basal body temperature is 37° C (98.6° F) determined orally or 0.6° C (1° F) higher determined rectally. Fever is generally accepted as any oral temperature above 37.8° C (100° F).

Weigh Patient and Note Persistent or Involuntary Weight Loss
Lactose intolerance, cystic fibrosis, intestinal malabsorption, infectious diarrhea, and inflammatory bowel disease can cause weight loss to occur. Persons with these conditions have adequate or even increased food intake, but they cannot absorb sufficient nutrients to sustain normal nutrition. In children, this can cause failure to thrive and interruption of growth. In adults, colonic neoplasm can cause partial obstruction and diarrhea, and weight loss may be evident.

Observe Abdominal Contour
Abdominal distention may be associated with an ileus as in enteritis or with gaseous dilation resulting from malabsorption. A scaphoid abdomen may be seen in children with severe dehydration.

Auscultate the Abdomen
The major objective is to detect the presence of bowel sounds anywhere in the abdomen. Listen in all four quadrants. The absence of bowel sounds is established only after 5 minutes of continuous listening. Bowel sounds that are high pitched are heard with peristaltic rushes found in enteritis and secretory diarrhea. Bowel sounds are diminished or absent with necrotizing enterocolitis.

Palpate the Abdomen for Tenderness
Peritonitis may cause diarrhea as a result of inflammation and local enteric irritation. Signs of peritoneal irritation include a rigid abdomen, rebound tenderness (Blumberg's sign), and positive signs on the following tests: iliopsoas muscle test, obturator muscle test, and heel jar test (Markle's sign) (see

Chapter 13). Tenderness is uncommon in self-limiting diarrhea. Localized right lower quadrant tenderness in a "sick" patient with acute diarrhea may indicate appendicitis, Crohn's disease, right-sided diverticulitis, or carcinoma. Localized left lower quadrant tenderness suggests diverticulitis, fecal impaction, colon cancer, and various causes of proctocolitis. Localized pain in chronic diarrhea can also occur with IBS.

Perform a Digital Rectal Examination

Look for fissures and lacerations and feel for impacted stool. Impacted stool may be felt as a puttylike mass that fills the rectum and extends upward. Also obtain a stool sample for occult blood testing and for laboratory studies. Observe stool on finger for color and the presence of blood.

Palpate Lymph Nodes

Evidence of systemic disease should be assessed. Chronic diarrhea in patients who have lymphadenopathy is associated with lymphoma and AIDS.

LABORATORY AND DIAGNOSTIC STUDIES

Laboratory or diagnostic studies are not necessary if the patient appears to have a viral or toxigenic bacterial infection because the disease is usually mild and self-limiting. Reserve stool cultures and examine for ova and parasites in patients who appear relatively ill, with signs of invasive diarrhea or persistent diarrhea, or who have a history of suspected parasite infection.

Fecal Leukocytes

Fecal leukocyte detection is an easy and inexpensive test that is 75% specific for bacterial diarrhea. Leukocytes are found in inflammatory diarrheal disease and are present in bacterial infections that invade the intestinal wall (*E. coli, Shigella,* and *Salmonella*). Leukocytes are also present in diarrhea from ulcerative colitis and Crohn's disease as well as antibiotic-related diarrhea. They are not seen in viral gastroenteritis, parasitic diarrhea, *Salmonella* carrier states,

or enterotoxigenic bacterial diarrheas. Obtain a small fleck of mucus or stool. Do not allow the specimen to dry. Place the specimen on a slide, add two drops of Löffler's alkaline methylene blue stain, and wait 2 minutes. Microscopic white and red blood cells indicate the presence of *Shigella,* enterohemorrhagic *E. coli,* enteropathogenic *E. coli, Campylobacter, C. difficile,* or other inflammatory or invasive diarrhea.

Fecal Occult Blood Testing

Fecal occult blood testing (FOBT) is used to test for occult blood in the stool. A stool sample is placed on a filter paper, and an activating solution is applied. A positive test is indicated by the appearance of a color (usually blue or green). A positive result indicates the presence of occult blood. Red blood cells often appear in diarrhea caused by enteropathic bacteria or protozoa. A 3-day series of stool samples is used to screen for colon cancer and is recommended annually in adults ages 50 and older.

Fecal Immunochemical Test (FIT)

Also called immunochemical FOBT (iFOBT), FIT uses antibodies to human globin to detect a specific portion of a human blood protein. FIT does not react with non–human hemoglobin or peroxidase, so food restrictions before the test are not necessary. Immunochemical FOBTs are also more specific for lower gastrointestinal tract bleeding as they target the globin portion of hemoglobin, which does not survive passage through the upper gastrointestinal tract. This test is done essentially the same way as conventional FOBT, but is more specific and reduces the number of false positive results. Vitamins or foods do not affect the fecal immunochemical test, and some forms require only one or two stool specimens.

Fecal Fat

A 72-hour fecal fat analysis is done by instructing the patient to have a daily dietary intake of 100 g of fat for 3 days before and during a 72-hour period of stool collection. In children, a fat retention coefficient is determined. An abnormal result is greater than

6 g/day in the stool on a 80- to 100-g diet of fat and indicates a malabsorption syndrome.

D-Xylose Absorption Test

The D-xylose absorption test is used to determine whether diarrhea is caused by malabsorption or maldigestion. Blood is taken before the patient ingests the D-xylose. The patient is then asked to drink a fluid containing 25 g of D-xylose. Repeat venipuncture to obtain blood is performed in exactly 2 hours for adults and 1 hour for children. Urine is collected approximately 5 hours after ingestion of the fluid. Blood and urine levels are subsequently evaluated. An abnormal result is found if less than 4.5 g of the D-xylose is excreted in a 5-hour urine collection and blood levels are less than 25 to 40 mg/dl in adults (30 mg/dl in children). The abnormal result indicates the diarrhea is caused by malabsorption.

Stool pH

The pH of the stool specimen is determined by using litmus strips. A pH value of 5.5 indicates lactose or other carbohydrate malabsorption. Normal stool pH is neutral or weakly alkaline.

Wet Mount

Wet mounts are useful to assess for trophozoites, cysts, ova, and certain helminth larvae. Obtain a sample of feces on a wooden applicator stick, mix with a drop of saline, and add iodine contrast to view and examine under a microscope. *V. cholerae* can be identified by using dark-field microscopy. The characteristic darting motility of vibrios can be recognized in fresh wet preparations.

C. difficile Toxin Assay

This assay detects *C. difficile* toxin in the stool, which is diagnostic of clostridial enterocolitis. The clostridial bacterium releases a toxin that causes necrosis of the colonic epithelium.

Stool Culture

Stool culture is used to detect common bacteria such as *Enterococcus, E. coli, Proteus, Pseudomonas, Staphylococcus aureus, Can-* *dida albicans, Bacteroides,* and *Clostridia.* Special enriching techniques or media are necessary to look for some agents. Pathogenic bacteria are *Salmonella, Shigella, Campylobacter, Yersinia,* pathogenic *E. coli, Staphylococcus,* and *C. difficile.*

Stool for Ova and Parasites

Stool can be tested for the presence of ova and parasites (O & P). Fresh stool is required to preserve the trophozoites of some parasites. Common parasites are *Ascaris* (hookworm) and *Strongyloides* (tapeworm).

Giardia Antigen Test

Giardia antigen test is a solid phase immunoassay used for the detection of *Giardia* specific antigen 65. Only one stool specimen is required and the test result is available within 1 day.

Indirect Hemagglutinin Assay

The indirect hemagglutinin assay (IHA) detects antibodies to *E. histolytica.* A positive titer is greater than 1:128.

Complete Blood Cell Count With Differential

A CBC with differential should be obtained in severely ill or dehydrated patients to screen for infection. Infection is indicated with increased leukocytes. Microcytic hypochromic anemia (mean corpuscular hemoglobin concentration [MCHC], <30 g/dl; mean corpuscular volume [MCV], >85 fl) may indicate the presence of chronic disease. Most bloody diarrhea produces an elevated platelet count as an acute-phase reactant in an inflammatory process. In hemolytic uremic syndrome (HUS), the platelet count may be normal or low.

Peripheral Blood Smear

A peripheral blood smear is an examination of the cellular contents of the blood under a microscope using a variety of stains. Hemoglobin can be roughly estimated by the depth of staining present. This quantitative analysis assists in characterizing a number of conditions, including hemolytic anemia associated with HUS. In HUS, the peripheral smear shows characteristic schistocytes.

Blood Urea Nitrogen and Creatinine

The blood urea nitrogen (BUN) and creatinine tests are indicated in severely ill or dehydrated patients to ascertain adequate kidney functioning. Dehydration is a cause of prerenal failure. HUS will cause impaired renal function.

Endoscopic Studies

Further endoscopic diagnostic studies such as flexible sigmoidoscopy or colonoscopy should be considered when the cause of diarrhea is not determined or when the diarrhea lasts for longer than 1 month.

DIFFERENTIAL DIAGNOSIS

Acute Diarrhea

Viral Gastroenteritis

Viral gastroenteritis presents with explosive onset of diarrhea, vomiting, low-grade fever, anorexia, and myalgia. Symptoms last for 1 week or less. Norwalk virus is a major causative agent and is usually seen in school-age children and adults. Rotavirus is the most common cause of diarrhea in children ages 6 to 24 months and is usually seen in the winter.

Shigella

Shigella presents with acute diarrhea that contains mucus and blood. The patient has up to 7 days of watery diarrhea; then toxins are produced that result in ulceration, mucosal irritability, and frequent bowel movements. Stools are yellow or green and contain undigested food, mucus, and blood. Leukocytes and red blood cells are seen in the stools. It is the second most common cause of diarrhea in children ages 6 to 10 years old and is common in day care settings. Upper respiratory tract infection symptoms may also be present.

Food Poisoning With *Staphylococcus* or *Bacillus aureus*

Staphylococcus or *Bacillus aureus* food poisoning causes explosive diarrhea 2 to 6 hours after eating. High attack rates are seen among persons eating contaminated food (improperly stored meats or custard-filled pastries). Cramping and vomiting in addition to

diarrhea are present. There usually is no fever. The diarrhea lasts 18 to 24 hours, and the person recovers quickly. However, the condition could be life threatening in the elderly and in persons with other serious illness.

Food Poisoning With *Clostridium perfringens*

C. perfringens causes severe diarrhea 8 to 20 hours after eating. The patient complains of crampy abdominal pain and diarrhea. The stool is watery and nonbloody. Nausea, vomiting, and fever may be present but are less common. The diarrhea usually lasts for less than 3 days.

Salmonella

Salmonella causes severe diarrhea with fever. It is seen 20 times more often in patients with AIDS, sickle cell disease, or reticuloendothelial dysfunction. The incubation period is 3 to 40 days with insidious or abrupt onset. The patient has fever, anorexia, and weight loss. Gastrointestinal symptoms occur first, followed by fever, abdominal cramps, and vomiting. Stools are green, loose, and slimy and have the odor of spoiled eggs. Rarely is blood present.

Campylobacter

Campylobacter infection causes fever, headache, and myalgia for 12 to 24 hours; then diarrhea develops. Roughly two thirds of patients have watery diarrhea and one third have bloody dysentery. The incubation period is 2 to 5 days. The patient has abdominal cramping, pain, and fever, and the diarrhea contains mucus and blood. The condition may mimic appendicitis because of mesenteric lymphadenitis. Toxic megacolon and colonic hemorrhages can occur, especially if antimotility agents have been used.

Vibrio cholerae

V. cholerae causes severe watery diarrhea without a preceding illness. It usually occurs in epidemics. The onset is acute, usually 8 to 18 hours after the ingestion of contaminated seafood, water, or food prepared in contaminated water. Diarrhea resolves in 3 to 5 days. The essential element in cholera is the speed at which fluid is lost. This quick loss of fluid and dehydration can lead to death within hours. Red and white blood cells are not seen on stool examination.

Enterotoxic *E. coli*

E. coli causes moderate amounts of nonbloody diarrhea. This develops acutely 8 to 18 hours after the ingestion of contaminated food/water and typically lasts for 24 to 48 hours. The patient experiences cramping and abdominal pain with the diarrhea. The organism (gram-negative rod) is transmitted via the fecal-oral route. It is spread through contaminated water or incompletely cooked food that was cleaned in contaminated water, or through incompletely cooked beef, especially ground hamburger meat. Enterotoxigenic *E. coli* is the leading cause of traveler's diarrhea. The diagnosis can be confirmed with fecal leukocytes or stool culture.

Entamoeba histolytica

A patient with diarrhea caused by this parasite presents with large amounts of bloody diarrhea and abdominal cramping and vomiting that develop acutely 12 to 24 hours after the ingestion of contaminated food or water. The diagnosis is confirmed through an IHA. Antibodies to *E. histolytica* are formed; a positive titer is greater than 1:128.

Antibiotic Induced

This condition produces a mild, watery diarrhea and is caused by taking antibiotics, especially ampicillin, tetracycline, lincomycin, clindamycin, and chloramphenicol. The patient often complains of crampy abdominal pain. Diagnosis is made through history and clinical findings.

Pseudomembranous Colitis

Pseudomembranous colitis is most often caused by *C. difficile*. This diarrhea is induced by antibiotics, most commonly ampicillin, clindamycin, or cephalosporins. An acute inflammatory bowel disorder occurs with symptoms that range from transient mild diarrhea to active colitis with bloody diarrhea, abdominal pain, fever, and leukocytosis. Symptoms usually begin during a course of

antibiotic therapy but may begin 1 to 10 days after treatment is completed. The diagnosis is established with sigmoidoscopy or colonoscopy. The diagnosis is confirmed with *C. difficile* toxin assay or stool culture.

Necrotizing Enterocolitis

Necrotizing enterocolitis is an inflammatory bowel condition that occurs in newborns. The patient is usually a premature or low–birth-weight infant who presents with feeding intolerance, vomiting, abdominal distention, lethargy, and loose, bloody stools containing mucus. It is the most common cause of death in the second week of life for low–birth-weight infants. Radiography shows pneumatosis intestinalis, indicating air within the subserosal bowel wall, which is the radiological hallmark used to confirm the diagnosis.

Hemorrhagic Disease of the Newborn

Hemorrhagic disease of the newborn is due to a deficiency in coagulation factors dependent on vitamin K. Most newborns do not have adequate levels of vitamin K, but bleeding problems develop in only a few. Gastrointestinal bleeding occurs 2 to 3 days postnatally. Laboratory studies typically show markedly elevated prothrombin time (PT) and partial thromboplastin time (PTT) and depressed levels of vitamin K–dependent factors. The routine use of prophylactic vitamin K prevents most cases.

Hemolytic Uremic Syndrome

HUS is seen in children and is usually preceded by a gastrointestinal illness. The leading bacterial cause of HUS in the United States is now *E. coli* 0157:H7. The patient presents with a history of bloody diarrhea, fever, and irritability. Initially, laboratory blood values are essentially normal except that the platelet count is normal or low. The stool culture is negative. A peripheral blood smear reveals schistocytes, confirming the diagnosis. Fragmented red blood cells are often seen on the peripheral smear before complications of renal involvement occur. The child may have a sudden onset of acute renal failure. Renal function test results will be altered.

Chronic Diarrhea
Irritable Bowel Syndrome
IBS is characterized by alternating periods of constipation and diarrhea. Patients often have mucus in their stools. It is commonly seen in young and middle-age women with a history of intermittent diarrhea. Patients often present with complaints of constipation rather than diarrhea. The patient complains of abdominal pain in the left lower quadrant, although it can occur anywhere. The pain seldom occurs at night, does not awaken the patient, and is commonly present in the morning. The patient may have rectal urgency and abdominal distention. There is no weight loss, the patient is afebrile, and the colon may be tender on palpation. IBS is a diagnosis of exclusion, and sigmoidoscopy or proctoscopy is used to rule out other disorders.

Ulcerative Colitis
Ulcerative colitis is an inflammatory bowel disease that causes proctitis with rectal bleeding, tenesmus, and the passage of mucopus. Abdominal cramping is common, but abdominal pain and tenderness are not common. The greater the extent of colon involvement, the more likely it is that the patient has diarrhea.

Crohn's Disease
Crohn's disease is an inflammatory bowel disease that presents with abdominal cramping, tenderness, rectal bleeding, and diarrhea. The disease may produce chronic, bloody diarrhea and cause failure to thrive in children. The patient may have a fever. Weight loss is common because of malabsorption or a reduced intake of food used to minimize postprandial symptoms. Diagnosis is made through colonoscopy and biopsy.

Carbohydrate Malabsorption and Lactose Intolerance
Malabsorption and/or lactose intolerance causes the patient to experience diarrhea, bloating, and increased flatus. The ingestion of specific disaccharides, such as lactose or sorbitol, exacerbates the episodes of diarrhea.

A trial of elimination of offending foods often confirms the clinical diagnosis.

Fat Malabsorption
Fat malabsorption is seen with patients who have cystic fibrosis or vitamin A, D, or K deficiency. Patients with cystic fibrosis have foul, pale, bulky diarrhea that is greasy, oily, and consistent with steatorrhea. The diarrhea usually precedes lung involvement. Laboratory testing for fat malabsorption includes a 72-hour fecal fat analysis.

Toddler's Diarrhea
Toddler's diarrhea is described as the occurrence of abnormal amounts of formless stools with mucus in children ages 1 to 3 years. Symptoms rarely persist beyond age 4 to 5 years. The diarrhea is chronic and nonspecific, with three or four stools per day, some containing mucus. Physical examination and growth are within normal limits for the child's age. This is a diagnosis of exclusion, and other causes of chronic diarrhea must first be ruled out.

Celiac Sprue/Protein Hypersensitivity
This diarrhea causes increasing stool frequency, looseness, paleness, and bulkiness 3 to 6 months after dietary intake of wheat, rye, and other grains. Patients have a hypersensitivity reaction to the protein in wheat, rye, barley, and oats. Children appear lethargic, irritable, and anorexic.

Giardia
Giardia is the leading parasitic cause of chronic diarrhea in children in the United States and can be contracted through travel both in and outside of the country. Patients experience watery, foul-smelling diarrhea, abdominal pain, distention, and gas.

Cryptosporidium and *Isospora belli*
These parasites produce recurrent episodes of nonbloody diarrhea with varying amounts of water. The volume can be massive. The organisms are transmitted via the fecal-oral route and are spread through the ingestion of contaminated water or direct oroanal contact.

Postgastrectomy Dumping Syndrome

This syndrome occurs after gastrointestinal surgery. The condition can occur whenever the pyloric mechanism is disrupted by pyloroplasty, gastroduodenostomy, or gastrojejunostomy. The diarrhea occurs after meals because of increased transit of food through the colon. Patients may experience associated symptoms, including diaphoresis and tachycardia.

Diabetic Enteropathy

Diabetic enteropathy occurs in patients with diabetes. Patients may experience nocturnal diarrhea, postprandial vomiting, and fatty stools from malabsorption. The condition is a diagnosis of exclusion in diabetic persons.

HIV Enteropathy

HIV enteropathy has an insidious onset and is recurrent. Patients have large amounts of nonbloody diarrhea and mild to moderate nausea and vomiting. It is caused by direct infection of mucosa and neuronal cells in the gastrointestinal system. Patients will demonstrate other HIV-related symptoms and lymphadenopathy.

Medication Induced

Diarrhea can occur as a result of taking prescription or over-the-counter drugs; the most common ones are antacids that contain magnesium, antibiotics, methyldopa, digitalis, β-blockers, systemic anti-inflammatory agents, colchicine, quinidine, phenothiazine, high-dose salicylates, and laxatives.

DIFFERENTIAL DIAGNOSIS OF *Common Causes of Acute Diarrhea*

CONDITION	HISTORY	PHYSICAL FINDINGS	DIAGNOSTIC STUDIES
Viral gastroenteritis (e.g., Norwalk or rotavirus viral agents)	Abrupt onset 6-12 hr after exposure; nonbloody, watery diarrhea; lasts <1 wk; nausea/vomiting, fever, abdominal pain, tenesmus	In children may see severe dehydration; hyperactive bowel sounds, diffuse pain on abdominal palpation	None
Shigella (gram-negative rod; fecal-oral transmission; common in day care setting; common in gay bowel syndrome)	Acute onset 12-24 hr after exposure; lasts 3-7 days; large amounts of bloody diarrhea with abdominal cramping and vomiting	Lower abdominal tenderness, hyperactive bowel sounds, no peritoneal irritation	Fecal leukocytes, positive stool culture
S. aureus food poisoning (gram-positive cocci; from improperly stored meats or custard-filled pies)	Acute onset 2-6 hr after ingestion; lasts 18-24 hr; large amounts of watery, nonbloody diarrhea; cramping and vomiting	Hyperactive bowel sounds	Fecal leukocytes, negative stool culture
Clostridium perfringens food poisoning (gram-positive rod; from contaminated food)	Acute onset 8-20 hr after ingestion; lasts 12-24 hr; large amounts of watery, nonbloody diarrhea; abdominal pain and cramping	Hyperactive bowel sounds, diffuse pain on abdominal palpation	Fecal leukocytes, negative anaerobic cultures of stool
Salmonella food poisoning (gram-negative bacilli; ingestion of contaminated food, poultry, eggs)	Acute onset 12-24 hr after ingestion; lasts 2-5 days; moderate to large amounts of nonbloody diarrhea; abdominal cramping and vomiting	Fever of 38.3-38.9° C (101-102° F) common; hyperactive bowel sounds, diffuse abdominal pain	Fecal leukocytes, positive stool culture, WBC count normal

Continued

DIFFERENTIAL DIAGNOSIS OF *Common Causes of Acute Diarrhea—cont'd*

CONDITION	HISTORY	PHYSICAL FINDINGS	DIAGNOSTIC STUDIES
Campylobacter jejuni (gram-negative rod; fecal-oral transmission; household pet)	Acute onset 3-5 days after exposure; lasts 3-7 days; moderate amounts of bloody diarrhea	Fever, lower quadrant abdominal pain	Fecal leukocytes, positive stool culture
Vibrio cholerae (gram-negative rod; fecal-oral transmission; ingestion of contaminated water, seafood, or food)	Acute onset 8-24 hr after ingestion of contaminated food; lasts 3-5 days; large amounts of nonbloody, watery, painless diarrhea; can be mild or fulminate	Cyanotic, scaphoid abdomen, poor skin turgor, thready peripheral pulses, voice faint	Fecal leukocytes, negative stool culture
Enterotoxic *E. coli* (gram-negative rod; fecal-oral transmission; ingestion of contaminated water or food)	Acute onset 8-18 hr after ingestion of contaminated food/water; lasts 24-48 hr; moderate amounts of nonbloody diarrhea; pain, cramping, abdominal pain; adults in United States generally do not develop illness from enterotoxic *E. coli*	No fever; dehydration is major complication	Fecal leukocytes, positive stool culture
Entamoeba histolytica parasite (cysts in food and water, from feces)	Acute onset 12-24 hr after ingestion of contaminated food or water; large amounts of bloody diarrhea; abdominal cramping and vomiting	Right lower quadrant abdominal pain; in small number of cases hepatic abscess forms	IHA: antibodies to *E. histolytica*; positive titer is >1:128
Antibiotic-induced (begins after taking antibiotics)	Mild, watery diarrhea; crampy abdominal pain	Diffuse abdominal pain on palpation, fever absent	Usually not needed
Pseudomembranous colitis (*Clostridium difficile* antibiotic induced)	Induced by antibiotics, most commonly ampicillin, clindamycin, or cephalosporins; symptoms range from transient mild diarrhea to active colitis with bloody diarrhea, abdominal pain, fever	Lower quadrant tenderness, fever	CBC: leukocytes; sigmoidoscopy/colonoscopy; *C. difficile* toxin assay or stool culture; *C. difficile* toxin
Hemolytic uremic syndrome (HUS) (primary cause of HUS in United States is *E. coli* O157:H7)	Children <4 yr with history of gastroenteritis; history of bloody diarrhea, fever, and irritability	Fever, irritability; may have oliguria or anuria	CBC, platelet count, renal function tests, peripheral blood smear; negative stool culture
Necrotizing enterocolitis	Premature or low–birth-weight infant who presents with feeding intolerance	Vomiting, abdominal distention, lethargy, loose, bloody, mucousy stools	Refer
Hemorrhagic disease of the newborn	Gastrointestinal bleeding 2-3 days postnatal; history of lack of vitamin K injection; history of mother on anticonvulsants prenatally	Bruising, ecchymoses, mild to moderate bleeding	Laboratory studies typically show markedly elevated PT and PTT with depressed levels of vitamin K–dependent factors

DIFFERENTIAL DIAGNOSIS OF *Common Causes of Chronic Diarrhea*

CONDITION	HISTORY	PHYSICAL FINDINGS	DIAGNOSTIC STUDIES
Irritable bowel syndrome (IBS)	Intermittent diarrhea alternating with constipation; mucus with stool; seldom occurs at night or awakens patient; commonly present in morning; may have rectal urgency; episodes usually triggered by stress or ingestion of food; affects women 3 times as often as men	Tender colon on palpation; may have abdominal distention; no weight loss; afebrile	Diagnosis of exclusion; sigmoidoscopy, proctoscopy
Ulcerative colitis (distal colon is most severely affected and rectum is involved)	History of severe diarrhea with gross blood in stools, no growth retardation; few complaints of pain; age of onset second and third decades with small peak during adolescence; positive family history	Overt rectal bleeding; initially no fever, weight loss, or pain on palpation of abdomen; moderate colitis: weight loss, fever, abdominal tenderness	CBC shows leukocytosis or anemia, ESR elevated; stool cultures to rule out other causes of diarrhea; colonoscopy
Crohn's disease (associated with uveitis, erythema nodosum)	History of chronic bloody diarrhea with abdominal cramping, tenderness, and rectal bleeding; in children a history of growth retardation, weight loss, moderate diarrhea, abdominal pain, and anorexia	Weight loss, rare gross rectal bleeding, fistulas common	Colonoscopy with biopsies
Carbohydrate malabsorption	Bloating, flatus, diarrhea exacerbated by ingestion of certain disaccharides (e.g., lactose, milk, milk products); may follow viral gastroenteritis	Diffuse abdominal pain	Trial elimination of offending foods
Fat malabsorption	Greasy, fatty, malodorous stools; associated with deficiencies of vitamins K, A, and D; cystic fibrosis	Rectal prolapse, poor weight gain, abdominal distention	73-hr fecal fats, sweat test
Toddler's diarrhea	3-4 stools/day; some contain mucus; rare past 4-5 yr of age	Physical examination and growth normal	Clinical diagnosis
Celiac sprue/protein hypersensitivity (reaction to protein in wheat, rye, barley, and oats)	Increased stool frequency, looseness, paleness, and bulkiness of stool within 3-6 mo of dietary onset; children are lethargic, irritable, and anorectic; peak frequency 9-18 mo	Failure to thrive, abdominal distention, irritability, muscle wasting	Clinical findings, improvement on gluten-free diet, CBC, anemia, folate deficiency, radiography, biopsy

Continued

DIFFERENTIAL DIAGNOSIS OF *Common Causes of Chronic Diarrhea—cont'd*

CONDITION	HISTORY	PHYSICAL FINDINGS	DIAGNOSTIC STUDIES
Giardia parasite (primary cause of chronic diarrhea in children)	Watery, foul diarrhea; common in day care, among travelers, and in male homosexuals	Low-grade fever, weight loss; chronic form: fatigue, growth retardation, steatorrhea	*Giardia* antigen test
Cryptosporidium species/*Isospora belli* protozoan parasites (fecal-oral transmission; ingestion of contaminated water or direct oral-anal contact)	Recurrent episodes; variable amounts watery, nonbloody diarrhea; amounts can be massive	Weight loss, severe right upper quadrant abdominal pain with biliary tract involvement	Stool for O & P
Postgastrectomy dumping syndrome	Following GI surgery, diarrhea occurs after meals; diarrhea occurs after meals because of increased transit of food through colon	Diaphoresis and tachycardia	Upper GI series
Diabetic enteropathy	Nocturnal diarrhea, postprandial vomiting, fatty stools from malabsorption	Findings associated with diabetes	Diagnosis of exclusion in diabetic persons
HIV enteropathy (direct infection of mucosa and neuronal cells in gastrointestinal system)	Insidious onset, recurrent large amounts of nonbloody diarrhea, mild to moderate nausea/vomiting	Findings associated with HIV infection	Testing for HIV
Medication induced	Mild to moderately severe nonwatery, nonbloody diarrhea	No specific findings related to diarrhea	Usually none needed

CHAPTER RESOURCES

American Academy of Pediatrics: The use and misuse of fruit juice in pediatrics, *Pediatrics* 107:1210, 2001.

Armon K et al: An evidence and consensus based guideline for acute diarrhoea management, *Arch Dis Child* 85:132, 2001.

Carollo AA, Schiller LR: Chronic diarrhea: differential diagnosis and initial management, *Consultant* December:1604, 2005.

Casper C: Detecting and treating foodborne infections, *The Clinical Advisor* February:24, 2005.

Corrigan JJ: Hemolytic uremic syndrome, *Pediatr Rev* 22:365, 2001.

Dennehy PH: Acute diarrheal disease in children: epidemiology, prevention, and treatment, *Infect Dis Clin North Am* 19(3):585, 2005.

Goodgame RW: Viral causes of diarrhea, *Gastroenterol Clin North Am* 30:779, 2001.

Keating J: Chronic diarrhea, *Pediatr Rev* 26:5, 2005.

Practice parameter: The management of acute gastro-enteritis in young children, *Pediatrics* 97:424, 1996.

Ramaswamy K: Infectious diarrhea in children, *Gastroenterol Clin North Am* 30:611, 2001.

Tobillo ET, Schwartz SM: Acute diarrhea, *Adv Nurse Pract* 6:38, 1998.

Turgeon DK: Laboratory approaches to infectious diarrhea, *Gastroenterol Clin North Am* 30:693, 2001.

Constipation

Constipation is a common symptom and is a subjective interpretation of a disturbance of bowel function. There is lack of general agreement on the norms for stool frequency, size, or consistency, with considerable uncertainty on how much deviation is required to warrant the label of constipation. Generally, constipation refers to a failure to completely evacuate the lower colon. This is associated with difficulty in defecating, infrequent bowel movements, straining, abdominal pain, and pain on defecating. It can also refer to hardness of stool or a feeling of incomplete evacuation. Obstipation refers to intractable constipation or the regular passage of hard stools at 3- to 5-day intervals.

There are five areas in the defecation process where interference can cause a disturbance in motility and lead to clinical problems: (1) the peristaltic reflex, (2) the spinal arc, (3) relaxation of the anal sphincter, (4) contraction of the voluntary muscle associated with defecation, and (5) the autonomic and cortical control of defecation. Both functional and organic disturbances can cause constipation.

Acute constipation refers to a sudden change for that individual, suggesting an organic cause such as mechanical obstruction, adynamic ileus, or traumatic interruption of the nervous system from medications or following anesthesia. Persistent constipation occurs when the condition lasts for weeks or occurs intermittently with increasing frequency or severity. Partial obstruction or local anorectal conditions may be the cause.

Chronic constipation occurs as the result of disruption of the storage, transport, and evacuation mechanisms of the colon. Functional causes are the most common and include poor bowel habits; inadequate intake of dietary fiber, bulk, and fluids; and anal fissure pain. Genetic predisposition to constipation seems to exist.

DIAGNOSTIC REASONING: FOCUSED HISTORY

Is This Really Constipation?

Key Questions
- How many stools are there per day?
- What is the consistency of the stool?

Frequency of Stool
Stool frequency is the easiest parameter to quantify. In the general adult population, the "normal" frequency of bowel movements ranges from 3 to 12 per week. Fewer than three bowel movements per week is considered to be constipation.

Infants and children have decreasing stool frequency with age, from more than 4 stools per day during the first week of life to 1.2 per day at age 4. Infants who have fewer number of stools than average seem to constitute a disproportionate percentage of those who develop frank constipation.

Alternating episodes of constipation and diarrhea are characteristic of irritable bowel syndrome (IBS). Patients may describe their constipation stools as hard, round balls.

Stool Consistency
Stools that are hard and dry are an additional parameter to consider in assessing constipation. Stools that are marginally frequent but are soft and moist may not indicate constipation, whereas this same number of stools that are hard and dry would indicate constipation.

Is the Constipation Acute or Chronic?

Key Questions

- When did the constipation start?
- How long have you been constipated? Is this an individual episode or is it chronic?
- At what age did the constipation first begin?

Onset and Duration

Recent onset usually reflects changes in lifestyle or physical health such as dietary changes, activity changes, new medications, partially obstructing lesions, or recent illness. Chronic constipation or constipation of long duration is usually associated either with functional causes such as lack of dietary fiber and bulk or with concurrent systemic disorders such as diabetes mellitus (DM) or hypothyroidism.

Age of Onset

New-onset constipation in adults older than age 40 is suspicious for colon lesions. Constipation in the newborn is likely to have an anatomical cause. In infants, the cause is likely inadequate fluid and fiber in the diet. In children, the cause is likely to be diet as well as developmental and psychological factors. In adults, the cause is usually related to dietary and bowel habits.

If the Constipation Is Acute, What Conditions Should I Consider?

Key Questions

- Have you been ill recently? Have you had a fever?
- Do you have any chronic health problems?

Recent Illness

Dehydration and fever cause hardening of the stools by diminishing intestinal secretions and increasing water absorption from the colon. A transient period of constipation is common during an acute febrile illness. Also, reflex ileus is sometimes seen with pneumonia.

Chronic Illness

Hardened stools are found in patients with renal acidosis and diabetes insipidus. Infants and children with hypotonia of the abdominal and intestinal musculature from neurological conditions may be predisposed to constipation.

Medical disease can cause constipation because of neurological gut dysfunction, myopathies, endocrine disorders, and electrolyte abnormalities. Constipation in infants may be an early symptom of congenital hypothyroidism.

If the Constipation Is Chronic or Recurrent, What Should I Consider?

Key Questions

- What do you usually eat in a day?
- How many glasses of liquid do you drink each day?
- What are your usual bowel habits?
- How active are you?
- What medications are you taking?
- Do you use laxatives? How often do you take laxatives? How long have you used laxatives?

Dietary Pattern

A 3-day dietary history is more accurate than a 24-hour recall, although a 24-hour recall can provide a reasonable picture of the patient's dietary habits. Diets that lack roughage result in lack of fecal bulk, causing an inadequate stimulus for peristaltic movement. Diets that are high in protein result in complete digestion of the protein, leaving little residue to stimulate movement. Diets high in calcium content lead to the formation of calcium caseinate in the stools, which does not stimulate peristalsis. Teenagers often drink several quarts of milk per day, causing constipation. Inadequate fluid intake (less than six 8-ounce glasses per day) contributes to dry, hard, and infrequent stools.

Bowel Habits

Postponing a bowel movement because of time constraints or other reasons suppresses the normal gastrocolic reflex and can produce constipation.

Activity Level

Constipation is a common problem in individuals with a sedentary lifestyle. The lack of physical activity reduces the peristaltic reflex.

Medications

Medications that commonly cause or contribute to constipation include narcotics, imipramine, diuretics, calcium channel blockers, anticholinergics, psychotropic agents, antacids, decongestants, anticonvulsants, iron, bismuth, and lead.

Use of Enemas, Laxatives, and Suppositories

Use of stimulants to empty the colon removes the peristalsis stimulus for 2 to 3 days. Diarrhea is usually followed by infrequent stools for several days. Chronic use of stimulants can produce chronic atonic constipation.

How Can I Further Narrow the Causes?

Key Questions

- What does your stool look like? Is the stool size large or small? What is the general shape of the stool (e.g., small, round, ribbonlike)?
- Is the stool formed or liquid?
- Have you had any involuntary loss of stool?
- Does the constipation alternate with periods of diarrhea?

Size or Caliber of Stool

Infrequent passage of small, hard stools may indicate congenital aganglionic megacolon. Very large stools may indicate functional constipation, with the size of the stools a function of the size of the colon. Ribbonlike stools suggest a motility disorder such as IBS. They can also be caused by narrowing of the distal or sigmoid colon from an organic lesion. A progressive decrease in the caliber of stool suggests an organic lesion. Stools with a toothpaste-like caliber suggest fecal impaction. Constipation can also be the result of dietary habits and may be seen in teenagers who drink several quarts of milk per day.

Consistency of Stool

Dry, hard stools suggest a lack of sufficient dietary fluids or fiber. Liquid stool and fecal incontinence, particularly in the elderly, may represent stool impaction and overflow. Overflow incontinence in children may indicate constipation from a fecal impaction.

Alternating Constipation and Diarrhea

Alternating episodes are characteristic of IBS. Patients often describe the stool during the constipation episodes as hard and pellet-like.

What Else Do I Need to Consider?

Key Questions

- Do you have the urge to defecate?
- Do you have any urinary tract symptoms?
- Do you have any nausea or vomiting?
- Is there any pain with defecation?
- Is there any bleeding with defecation? How much?
- What color are your stools? Are the stools very dark colored or black?

Urge to Defecate

Children with Hirschsprung's disease (aganglionic megacolon) do not have an urge to defecate because the stool accumulates proximal to the lower portion of the rectum where the proprioceptors for defecation are located. Evidence of stiffening, squeezing, and crying indicates stool is being propelled to the rectum. Adults who overuse laxatives or other stimulants also may not experience the urge to defecate.

Associated Urinary Tract Problems

Voiding problems may indicate an abdominal mass. Day and night enuresis is seen in some children with encopresis (fecal soiling). Rarely does a neurological lesion produce fecal incontinence without a disturbance in bladder control.

Vomiting

Bilious vomiting may indicate intestinal obstruction in the newborn. Vomiting associated with pain in adults may indicate obstruction.

Pain

Chronic recurrent abdominal pain is commonly present in constipation. Pain is intermittent and may be localized to the periumbilical region. Crampy lower abdominal pain is usually caused by bowel distention, which can result from IBS, intermittent obstruction, or adhesions. Noncrampy dull pain in the left abdomen is associated with diverticulosis. Pain on defecation may indicate an anal or a rectal lesion such as hemorrhoids or anal fissures.

Bleeding

Bright red blood in the stool indicates hemorrhoids, fissure, or possible rectal mass. Black stools may indicate bleeding from a site in the upper gastrointestinal tract because blood mixed with gastric acid makes the stools appear black. Brisk bleeding is uncommon with hemorrhoids and requires immediate thorough investigation.

Color

Red stools may be the result of using laxatives of vegetable origin. A black or very dark brown color may be caused by drugs such as iron and bismuth, both of which contribute to constipation.

If This Is a Child, Is There Anything Else I Need to Consider?

Key Questions

- Is there fecal soiling of underpants?
- Is there crying with defecation?
- If an infant: Is there a history of delayed passage of meconium stool?
- Has the child begun to drink milk?
- Has the child recently started toilet training?
- Does the child have urinary frequency?

Crying With Defecation

Small children with constipation will cry with movement when a fissure is present. With large hard stools, the child will not want to defecate because of the pain and will do stool-holding mannerisms such as sitting and standing still.

Fecal Soiling of Underpants

Repeated fecal soiling from involuntary passage of small amounts of feces into the underpants of children older than age 4 is consistent with encopresis from functional megacolon secondary to chronic constipation. The constipation is usually secondary to painful defecation, with a resultant anal fissure. Coercive bowel training, fear of the toilet, or reactive voluntary withholding of bowel movements can also cause this condition.

History of Delayed Passage of Meconium Stool

Such a history may indicate congenital aganglionic megacolon (Hirschsprung's disease).

Change in Diet

Cow's milk is a common cause of constipation in young children who have been on breast milk or formula.

Toilet Training

Some children develop stool withholding when toilet training is initiated.

History of Urinary Frequency

Urinary frequency, enuresis, and urinary tract infections may be the result of constipation. Fecal soiling may cause urinary tract infection by the ascending of the fecal flora. Further, an enlarged dilated rectum may push on the bladder, causing frequent need to urinate.

Is There a Family History or Genetic Predisposition?

Key Question

- Is there a family history of constipation or IBS?

Genetic predisposition to constipation seems to exist. It is common for more than one family member to have a history of chronic constipation or IBS.

DIAGNOSTIC REASONING: FOCUSED PHYSICAL EXAMINATION

Plot Growth Curve in Children

Slow growth may indicate congenital aganglionic megacolon. Also incorrect formula mixing, underfeeding, starvation, and anorexia nervosa may first be recognized by a complaint of constipation.

Perform Abdominal Examination

Observe abdominal contour, looking for distention. Abdominal distention is frequently not marked in patients with functional constipation but may be present with other causes. Auscultate for bowel sounds. Silent or abnormal bowel sounds may also indicate an organic cause such as obstruction. On palpation, stool may be felt as mobile, nontender masses in the left lower quadrant (LLQ). Firm, rubbery masses of stool palpable in the right lower quadrant in newborns may indicate meconium ileus. Palpable abdominal masses or organomegaly point to an organic cause. Note tenderness, which may indicate an organic cause, although a tender bowel may be palpable in IBS. Inspect the sacral region of the back. The presence of dimpling could indicate a spinal deformity contributing to the constipation.

Look for hernias. Large abdominal wall hernias may interfere with the ability to generate the intraabdominal pressure that is required to initiate defecation.

Perform Digital Rectal Examination

On perianal inspection, look for skin excoriation, skin tags, fissures, strictures, tears, or hemorrhoids, any of which may cause painful defecation. Early fissures have the appearance of superficial erosions. More advanced lesions are linear or elliptical breaks in the skin. Long-standing fissures are deep and indurated. Internal fissures are seen when the anal sphincter relaxes as the examining finger is withdrawn. To examine for a fissure in a child, place the infant/child in the knee-chest position and spread the buttocks to reveal the mucocutaneous junction of the anus.

Look for rectal prolapse and feel for a rectocele, which might interfere with defe-

Table 15-1	Superficial and Deep Tendon Reflexes and Spinal Level Tested
REFLEX	**SPINAL LEVEL TESTED**
Superficial	
Upper abdominal	T7, T8, T9
Lower abdominal	T10, T11
Cremasteric	T12, L1, L2
Deep	
Biceps	C5, C6
Brachioradial	C5, C6
Triceps	C6, C7, C8
Patellar	L2, L3, L4
Achilles	S1, S2

cation. A normal anal sphincter with an empty rectal ampulla may indicate Hirschsprung's disease. In functional constipation, expect to find a large dilated rectum full of stool. Sphincter tone is increased in functional problems and strictures but is decreased in neurological diseases. The presence of a mass in the rectum indicates an impaction or obstructive lesion. A pilonidal dimple is seen with spinal bifida occulta.

Perform a Focused Neurological Examination

Test relevant deep tendon and superficial reflexes. Interruption of T12-S3 nerves causes loss of voluntary control of defecation (Table 15-1).

LABORATORY AND DIAGNOSTIC STUDIES

Fecal Occult Blood Test (FOBT)

A positive FOBT indicates blood in the stool, which may be the result of ulcerative or malignant lesions. The sensitivity of this test in detecting colorectal cancers and adenomas ranges from 50% to 90%. It is an inexpensive and noninvasive method to screen for bleeding lesions. A stool sample is placed on filter paper, and an activating solution is applied. A positive test is indicated by the appearance of a color (usually blue or green). Serial testing (3 days) is done using stool cards at home that are returned by mail for analysis. Annual FOBT, beginning at age 50 years, is one of the recommended screening tests for colon cancer. Box 15-1 describes the current recommendations.

Fecal Immunochemical Test (FIT)

Also called immunochemical FOBT (iFOBT), FIT can be used as an alternative to FOBT. FIT uses antibodies to human globin to detect a specific portion of a human blood protein. FIT does not react with non–human hemoglobin or peroxidase, so food restrictions before the test are not necessary. Immunochemical FOBTs are also more specific for lower gastrointestinal tract bleeding as they target the globin portion of hemoglobin, which does not survive passage through the upper gastrointestinal tract. This test is done essentially the same way as conventional FOBT, but is more specific and reduces the number of false positive results. Vitamins or foods do not affect the fecal immunochemical test, and some forms require only one or two stool specimens.

Complete Blood Cell Count

Obtain a complete blood cell count (CBC) when you suspect bleeding. Hematocrit and hemoglobin levels will be below the expected reference range with a bleeding lesion.

Serum Electrolytes

Severely ill patients may develop hypokalemia and hypercalcemia, which are causes of constipation. Patients on thiazide diuretics may develop hypokalemia and subsequent constipation.

Serum Thyroid-Stimulating Hormone

An elevated thyroid-stimulating hormone (TSH) level may suggest hypothyroidism, which can be a cause of constipation. Screen for elevated TSH level in persons with other symptoms suggestive of hypothyroidism, such as sparse, coarse, dry hair; hirsutism; dry skin; or hoarse speech.

Urinalysis

A urinalysis and culture should be done if a child has an associated rectosigmoid impaction because of encopresis.

Anoscopy

Anoscopy is indicated if digital rectal examination detects hemorrhoids, fissures, strictures, or masses in the anus or rectum. It

---

Box 15-1	**Evidence-Based Practice: Screening for Colon Cancer**

Options for average-risk screening (age 50 years or older with no additional risk factors for colorectal cancer) for colon cancer include the following:
• Annual fecal occult blood test (FOBT) or fecal immunochemical test (FIT)
• Flexible sigmoidoscopy every 5 years
• Annual FOBT/FIT plus flexible sigmoidoscopy every 5 years
• Double-contrast barium enema every 5 to 10 years
• Colonoscopy every 10 years

Currently there is no consensus on which of these options to recommend—each has risks and benefits. The preferred screening strategy, according to the American College of Gastroenterology, is colonoscopy every 10 years in the average-risk patient. Colonoscopy improves the detection rate of precancerous and cancerous lesions in both the distal and proximal colon. The 10-year interval improves compliance. Recent reports documenting higher than anticipated numbers of proximal neoplasms in those patients without distal colon pathology support the use of colonoscopy as the screening procedure. However, colonoscopy has a higher risk of complications and costs substantially more than any of the other options. The Agency for Healthcare Research and Quality recommends sigmoidoscopy every 5 years and annual fecal blood testing as the two most cost-effective strategies.

Data from Rex DK, Johnson DA, Lieberman DA et al: Colorectal cancer prevention 2000: screening recommendations of the American College of Gastroenterology, *Am J Gastroenterol* 95:868, 2000; Khandker RK, Dulski JD, Kilpatrick JB et al: A decision model and cost-effectiveness analysis of colorectal cancer screening and surveillance guidelines for average-risk adults, *Int J Technol Assess Health Care* 16(3):799, 2000.

enables a view of the immediate internal anal canal that is not possible on manual digital rectal examination. A hand-held anoscope is warmed, lubricated, and slowly eased into the anus while the patient bears down to relax the external sphincter muscle. A light source is necessary; a head lamp is preferable. Anoscopy may not be possible initially with a fissure or abscess because of the pain. However, it should be performed on a follow-up visit to detect inflammatory bowel disorder or rectal cancer.

Flexible Sigmoidoscopy and Colonoscopy

These tests are indicated for patients in whom conservative treatment fails, for persons older than age 50 or with new-onset constipation, and for persons with anemia or fecal occult blood.

Barium Enema

This contrast technique can be used to detect diverticula, polyps, and masses. It is also used to determine the extent of dilated bowel in megacolon. The barium enema in children is usually reserved to rule out Hirschsprung's disease. A barium enema is contraindicated if enterocolitis is suspected.

Colon Transit Studies

Colon transit studies are useful for patients with severe chronic constipation that responds poorly to treatment.

DIFFERENTIAL DIAGNOSIS

Despite the high prevalence of constipation, only a small number of adults or children with constipation have a significant abnormality. In otherwise healthy individuals, first consider functional causes, particularly dietary, fluid, bowel, and laxative habits. In adults, depression may be associated with constipation.

Simple Constipation

Typically individuals with simple constipation report a diet low in fiber and bulk and/or inadequate fluid intake. A sedentary lifestyle is common. They also often report pain before and with bowel movements because of the hard, dry nature of the stools. Patients may

also complain of loss of appetite. The physical examination of the abdomen and rectum is normal. You may feel fecal masses in the colon and rectum. No diagnostic workup is needed unless the patient does not respond to therapy.

Functional Constipation

Functional constipation is seen in children who have large, hard stools that become difficult or painful to pass. The resulting fecal retention sets up a cycle in which the sensitivity of the defecation reflex and the effectiveness of peristalsis lessen. Watery stool from the proximal colon soils the underwear. On physical examination, stool is present in the left lower quadrant and the rectum is dilated and filled with packed stool. The external sphincter is intact.

Irritable Bowel Syndrome

IBS is common in adults, with onset usually in young adulthood. The presenting complaint may be either diarrhea or constipation. Alternating episodes of each is characteristic of IBS. Mucus in the stools is common. Abdominal pain often occurs, usually in the left lower quadrant, and the bowel may be tender to palpation. A tender bowel may be palpable (see also Chapter 14).

Fecal Impaction

Fecal impaction is common in older adults and in those who are confined to bed. The passage of hard stools at 3- to 5-day intervals may occur. Some persons with impaction have continuous diarrhea-like passage of stools and may experience incontinence. Stools may be of small caliber, sometimes described as toothpaste-like. On rectal examination, large quantities of hard feces will be palpable in the rectal ampulla. On abdominal examination, feces-filled bowel may be palpable.

Idiopathic Slow Transit

This condition is most common in older persons, especially those who are less active and have inadequate dietary fiber and fluid intake. These patients experience decreased stool frequency; stools are typically dry and hard.

Hirschsprung's Disease (Aganglionic Megacolon)

Hirschsprung's disease is present from birth and is usually detected in young children. Delayed passage of a meconium stool may indicate Hirschsprung's disease in infants. Children with Hirschsprung's disease do not have an urge to defecate because the stools accumulate proximal to the lower portion of the rectum where the proprioceptors for defecation are located. Evidence of stiffening, squeezing, and crying indicates stool is being propelled to the rectum. On examination the rectal ampulla is empty.

Secondary Constipation From Anorectal Lesion

Because defecation is painful with an anorectal lesion, the patient suppresses it. With the eventual passage of hard stools, the patient may report blood on the surface of the stool, on the toilet paper, or in the toilet. On digital rectal examination, look for hemorrhoids (very rare in children), fissures, tears, or abrasions.

Drug Induced

Drug-induced constipation is consistent with a history of chronic laxative use or taking those medications that can produce constipation. It occurs most often in older persons. Abdominal and rectal examinations are usually normal.

Tumors

Tumors are uncommon in children, and the frequency increases over the age of 40. Constipation occurs in less than one third of persons with colon cancer; diarrhea is more common. Onset is recent, and there may be progressive narrowing of stool caliber. Colicky abdominal pain and distention may occur in persons with bowel tumors. Persons with rectosigmoid tumors may complain of rectal discomfort, stool leakage, urgency, and tenesmus. Stool may test positive for occult blood. An abdominal mass may be palpable. Suspect right-sided lesions in elderly patients who present with constipation, anemia, anorexia, and weight loss.

DIFFERENTIAL DIAGNOSIS OF *Common Causes of Constipation*

CONDITION	HISTORY	PHYSICAL FINDINGS	DIAGNOSTIC STUDIES
Simple constipation	Low dietary fiber and bulk; inadequate fluid intake; physical inactivity; pain before and with bowel movements; anorexia	Normal abdominal and rectal examination; may feel fecal masses in colon and rectum	None if resolved; consider sigmoidoscopy if not resolved
Functional constipation	Preschool and school-age children; history of abdominal pain and stool soiling	Palpable stool in LLQ; large dilated rectum with packed stool; external sphincter intact	Abdominal radiography, unprepped barium radiography
Irritable bowel syndrome (IBS)	Onset in young adulthood; alternating diarrhea and constipation; mucus in stools	May have tender, palpable colon	Sigmoidoscopy if indicated
Obstipation/impaction	Passage of hard stool at 3- to 5-day intervals; diarrhea, small caliber stools; common in those confined to bed	Hard feces in rectal ampulla; may have palpable feces-filled bowel	Sigmoidoscopy if indicated

Continued

DIFFERENTIAL DIAGNOSIS OF *Common Causes of Constipation—cont'd*

CONDITION	HISTORY	PHYSICAL FINDINGS	DIAGNOSTIC STUDIES
Slow transit	Common in older adults; physical inactivity; decreased stool frequency; stool dry and hard	Normal abdominal and rectal examination	FOBT or FIT to rule out tumors
Hirschsprung's disease	Delayed passage of meconium at birth; no urge to defecate	Empty rectal ampulla on examination	Colonoscopy
Anorectal lesions	Rectal pain on defecation; history of hemorrhoids; blood on stool, on toilet tissue, or in toilet	On rectal examination: hemorrhoids, fissures, tears, abrasions; increased sphincter tone	Anoscopy
Drug induced	History of chronic laxative use; history of taking medications that produce constipation	Normal rectal and abdominal examinations	None if resolved; consider sigmoidoscopy, barium enema if not resolved
Tumors	Diarrhea more common than constipation; recent onset: pain and abdominal distention, stool leakage, urgency; late onset: weight loss, anorexia; increased incidence over age 40; uncommon in children	May have palpable abdominal mass or organomegaly	CBC, FOBT or FIT, sigmoidoscopy, colonoscopy, barium enema

CHAPTER RESOURCES

[No authors listed]: Constipation, *Postgrad Med* 109:193, 2001.

Arce DA, Ermocilla CA, Costa H: Evaluation of constipation, *Am Fam Physician* 65(11):2284, 2002.

Basson MD: Constipation, eMedicine, last updated Feb 3, 2006; available at http://www.emedicine.com/med/topic2833.htm.

Borum ML: Constipation: evaluation and management, *Prim Care* 28:577, 2001.

Coughlin E: Assessment and management of pediatric constipation in primary care, *Pediatr Nurs* 29(4):296, 2004.

Hsieh C: Treatment of constipation in older adults, *Am Fam Physician* 72(11):2277, 2005.

Rao SS: Constipation: evaluation and treatment, *Gastroenterol Clin North Am* 32(2):659, 2003.

Rao SS, Ozturk R, Laine L: Clinical utility of diagnostic tests for constipation in adults: a systematic review, *Am J Gastroenterol* 100(7):1605, 2005.

Wald A: Constipation, *Med Clin North Am* 84:1231, 2000.

Youssef NN: Adolescent constipation: evaluation and management, *Adolesc Med Clin* 15(1):37, 2004.

Youssef NN, Di Lorenzo C: Childhood constipation: evaluation and treatment, *J Clin Gastroenterol* 33:199, 2001.

Rectal Pain, Itching, and Bleeding

Anorectal problems can cause significant discomfort and anxiety. Because patients are often embarrassed by pain or problems in the anal area, they may delay seeking care and present with a more advanced disease or condition. Anorectal disorders can range from minor problems to those with significant morbidity. Rectal bleeding in children can be frightening for caretakers.

Rectal complaints include pain, irritation, discomfort, itching, soreness in the anal area, or bleeding. Tenesmus is painful sphincter contraction that may be caused by anorectal infection. Rectal pain can be caused by tears, infection, or hemorrhoids. Itching can be caused by inflammation from hemorrhoids or parasites or by hypersensitivity to substances in the environment. Because colorectal cancer is common in adults and may be present with a benign condition, a high index of suspicion for cancer should be maintained when investigating all anorectal symptoms.

The anatomy of the anorectal area is important in describing the occurrence of various disorders. The anus is the most distal portion of the gastrointestinal tract and is approximately 4 cm long. Its distal end is lined by stratified squamous epithelium while the proximal component is lined by simple columnar epithelium. The two components are divided by the dentate line—the line where the distal end and the columns and crypts of Morgagni meet. The dentate line is also known as the anorectal junction, which also denotes the boundary between the somatic (sensory) and the visceral nerve supply. Above (proximal to) the dentate line, the rectum is supplied by stretch nerve fibers but not pain nerve fibers. Below the dentate line, the area is extremely sensitive. The columns of Morgagni are longitudinal columns of mucosa located in the proximal anus; they

fuse in a ring distally to form the anal papillae at the level of the dentate line. The crypts are the invaginations of the columns of Morgagni. From four to eight anal glands drain into the crypts of Morgagni at the level of the dentate line. Most rectal abscesses and fistulas originate in these glands. Figure 16-1 shows the anatomy of the anus and rectum.

DIAGNOSTIC REASONING: FOCUSED HISTORY

Might This Condition Require Immediate Hospitalization or Referral?

Key Questions
- Are you receiving anticoagulation therapy? Have you had bleeding?
- Do you have a bleeding disorder?
- Is the patient an infant?
- Do you have HIV/AIDS?
- Are you on chemotherapy?
- Is there purulent discharge?

Coagulopathy With Bleeding
Bleeding in anorectal problems is usually self-limiting and, if not a problem, resolves spontaneously or with local pressure. However, a bleeding internal hemorrhoid in a patient with a coagulopathy indicates the need for hospitalization. Newborns with melena (black, tarry stool) and/or hematemesis may have a vitamin K deficiency. Infants who present with rectal bleeding could have necrotizing enterocolitis (NEC), which is life threatening.

Immunocompromised With an Infection
Because of the acute infectious process, a perirectal abscess may require hospitalization,

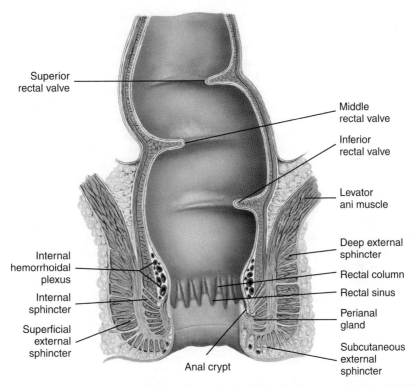

FIGURE 16-1 Anatomy of the anus and rectum.(From Seidel HM et al: *Mosby's guide to physical examination,* ed 6, St Louis, 2006, Elsevier.)

especially in a person who is immunocompromised because the infection is more likely to spread systematically. Individuals who are immunocompromised are at risk for the development of proctitis, especially by herpes simplex.

What Do the Presenting Symptoms Tell Me?

Key Questions

- Have you had any bleeding? How much bleeding has there been? When does it bleed? Describe the color of the blood.
- If a child: How old is this patient?
- Have you had pain? When does it occur? Describe the pain.
- Specifically, do you have pain on defecation? If a child: Does the child cry on defecation?
- Have you had itching? When does it itch?

- Can you feel a lump?
- Have you had any stains on your underwear? Describe the stains (e.g., blood, stool, pus).
- Have you had diarrhea?
- Have you been constipated?

Bleeding

Bleeding associated with defecation is characteristic of hemorrhoids and fissures. Bleeding from hemorrhoids typically occurs after defecation and is noted on the toilet paper ("wipe hematochezia") or coating the stool. The blood is bright red and may vary from a few spots on the toilet paper to a thin stream or coating on the stool. Bleeding with fissures occurs with defecation and is accompanied by pain. Spontaneous rectal bleeding can occur with proctitis. Condyloma acuminata may grow to a size sufficient to occlude the rectal opening and will bleed on defecation. Significant pathological conditions such as carcinomas and polyps can bleed intermittently.

Blood that is black and tarry and has an aroma is from the upper gastrointestinal (GI) tract and is called melena. Melena stools should be differentiated in patients who have dark stools. Stools with melena will test positive for blood. When blood is bright red, the source is usually in the more distal GI tract or the rectum. Melena is seen in children with Meckel's diverticulum.

Some foods such as fruit juices and drinks, food coloring, and beets affect the stools, making the stools appear reddish. Foods such as spinach, blueberries, and grape juice may cause the stools to be dark. Iron supplementation also may affect the color of the stools, making them appear dark.

A loose stool that has blood that is bright red and mixed with mucus may indicate chronic ulcerative colitis. Currant jelly–like coloring of the stool in young children often is a sign of intussusception, which is potentially life-threatening.

Age of the Child With Bleeding

Premature Infants. All premature infants with lower GI bleeding must be referred and evaluated for NEC.

Newborns. The most common cause of blood in the stools is from swallowing maternal blood during delivery. Newborns who have not received vitamin K and have a prolonged prothrombin time may have hemorrhagic disease of the newborn.

Neonatal stress can cause gastritis and gastroduodenal ulceration. Another cause of neonatal rectal bleeding may be gastroduodenal ulceration from sepsis.

Infants Younger Than 6 Months. Nonspecific colitis or allergic colitis due to milk allergy can cause blood-streaked stools. Bacterial etiologies may occur (see Chapter 14).

Age 6 Months to 5 Years. Intussusception is seen in children less than 1 year old and may cause currant jelly stools (see Chapter 13). Meckel's diverticulum that ulcerates because of acid secretion onto the gastric mucosa

can cause painless, sometimes significant, bleeding resulting in black or maroon stools. Henoch-Schönlein purpura may first manifest as lower GI bleeding (see Chapter 14).

Juvenile colonic polyps are seen in children ages 2 to 5 years. These are benign hamartomatous lesions. Bleeding occurs with defecation because of the sloughing of the polyps.

Anal tears resulting from constipation and stool holding can cause bleeding as well as pain. Blood may be visible on the stool or in the underwear (see Chapter 15).

Age 5 to 18 Years. Ulcerative colitis presents in children as acute bloody diarrhea, cramping, and tenesmus. The child may have skin lesions, arthralgia, and growth retardation. Crohn's disease may present with bloody diarrhea, abdominal pain, and fever. In mild stages, rectal bleeding may be minor with only small amounts of blood. Blood increases with proximity of the lesion to the anus (see Chapter 14).

Pain

Pain with defecation is characteristic of anal fissures. The pain may be so severe that the patient avoids defecating to avoid the pain. Children will cry with defecation. The pain may last for several hours and then subside until the next bowel movement. Patients with anal fissures complain of cutting or tearing anal pain during defecation and of gnawing, throbbing discomfort after defecation.

Hemorrhoids rarely cause severe pain unless they are ulcerated or thrombosed. Thrombosed hemorrhoids cause an inflammatory reaction by activating tissue thromboplastin within the hemorrhoidal blood vessels. Internal hemorrhoids, because they start above the dentate line, are not painful even if prolapsed or thrombosed.

Anorectal pain that begins gradually and becomes excruciating over a few days may indicate infection. A localized area of tenderness could signal an abscess. Patients with a recoil abscess or fistula complain of a throbbing, continuous, progressive pain. Pain may also occur with proctitis as a result of the infectious and inflammatory processes. The pain is not limited to defecation.

Proctalgia fugax is a unique anal pain. Patients with proctalgia fugax experience severe episodes of spasmlike pain that often occur at night. Proctalgia fugax may occur only once a year or may be experienced in waves of three or four times per week. Each episode lasts only minutes.

Tenesmus

Tenesmus is common with anal fissures, as the tear and inflammation involve the internal sphincter. On defecation, the sphincter may go into spasm. The patient experiences a tearing pain.

Itching

Itching is common with both hemorrhoids and fissures. Both external hemorrhoids that are covered by skin and fissures that involve breaks in the skin stimulate cutaneous sensation and lead to pain and itching.

Intense itching is a hallmark of pruritus ani, which occurs from hypersensitivity caused by irritating soap, lubricants, fragrance, or dyes present in toilet paper. Itching, particularly at night, can also be caused by pinworms.

Mass

The sensation of a mass or lump may indicate hemorrhoids or anal fissures. When the supportive tissues around the anal canal deteriorate, veins in the anorectal mucosa become tortuous and dilated and then bulge and descend into the anal canal. Both external and internal hemorrhoids can protrude and then regress spontaneously or be reduced manually. The patient may feel them as a bulge or lump.

With chronic anal fissures, the anal papillae hypertrophy and a skin tag ("sentinel pile") may form, which the patient may feel as a mass or lump.

Condyloma, molluscum contagiosum, and malignant lesions can also produce the sensation of a lump or mass.

Fecal Soiling

Fecal soiling is common with hemorrhoids. Mucous discharge with internal hemorrhoids is less common. Fecal soiling is also common with chronic constipation in children.

Some stool discharges around the feces that are in the rectum.

Diarrhea

Explosive diarrhea may be a contributing cause of anal fissures. Diarrhea can also cause irritation and excoriation, producing symptoms of itching, bleeding, and soreness.

Constipation

Constipation may be a cause or result of anal fissure. Hard, dry stool can tear the rectal mucosa and produce an anal fissure. The pain associated with defecation because of a fissure may result in constipation because the patient avoids defecating.

Could This Be Caused by Sexual Practices?

Key Questions

- How many sexual partners do you have?
- Do your sexual practices include anal intercourse?
- Do you insert any objects into your rectum?

Multiple Sexual Partners

Multiple sexual partners place the individual at risk for the development of condyloma acuminata and viral or bacterial proctitis. HIV infection is possible and places the individual at risk for the development of proctitis.

Anal Intercourse

Anal intercourse predisposes individuals to anal fissure as a result of rectal trauma. The transmission of bacterial or viral organisms can result in condyloma acuminata or proctitis.

Foreign Bodies

The insertion of objects into the rectum can cause anal tears and fissures.

Could This Be the Result of Sexual Abuse?

Key Questions

- Have you had unwanted sexual contact? If a child: You might ask, "Has anyone touched your private parts?"
- Do you think the child has been abused?

Sexual Contact

Unwanted sexual contact that includes anal contact or intercourse may cause anal fissures as a result of rectal trauma. The transmission of bacterial or viral organisms can result in the development of condyloma acuminata or proctitis.

A Child's Reporting

Children who have been abused try to tell about the abuse in some way. Subtle indications that are not proof but may indicate abuse include a preschooler's regression to earlier safer times: for example, thumb sucking, clinging behavior, bedwetting, fear of sleeping in one's own room, and expressing feelings through art, especially drawing. Children draw what they see. Ask the child to talk about what he or she has drawn. School-age children develop physical symptoms from abuse (e.g., sore throat, stomach pains). The child's play may portray intercourse and may include violence toward animals. The child may appear to lack concentration, but in fact all energy is being focused into keeping a secret. Some children overcompensate, getting straight A's so that no one will suspect. Failure to thrive and undereating may be other behaviors that raise suspicion of abuse.

A Parent's Reporting

When a stranger sexually assaults a child, most parents bring the child into an emergency facility or clinic for immediate investigation. Abuse by a friend or family member is less overt and is often detected only when a primary care provider is alert to a suspicious history or physical findings. In some cases, a parent may voice concerns about the possibility of abuse or report that the child has told them of the incident.

A child who has been sexually abused must be referred to Children's Protective Services and to a health care provider who is an expert in the area of child abuse.

Do Risk Factors Point to a Likely Condition?

Key Questions

■ Do you strain to have a bowel movement?

■ How often do you move your bowels? How often do you experience constipation? Are your stools hard and dry?
■ What is your occupation? Does it require sitting for long periods?
■ Describe your personal hygiene practices.
■ For women: Determine the number of pregnancies and childbirth history.
■ Do you have HIV/AIDS or are you on chemotherapy?
■ Do you have diabetes?
■ Note patient's gender.
■ Do you have a family history of familial adenomatous polyposis (FAP), hereditary nonpolyposis colon cancer, or Gardner's syndrome?

Straining at Stool

Straining during bowel movements predisposes individuals to the development of hemorrhoids and anal fissures, especially in the presence of chronic constipation. Hemorrhoids develop secondary to the pressure. Fissures develop as a result of traumatic laceration from a hard or large stool.

Chronic Constipation

Chronic constipation predisposes an individual to hemorrhoids and anal fissures as a result of straining.

Prolonged Sitting

Occupations that require prolonged periods of sitting predispose to the development of hemorrhoids, pruritus ani, and pilonidal cysts.

Poor Hygiene

Inadequate hygiene practices are a risk factor for the development of pruritus ani and pinworms. Improper cleaning can result in excessive moisture around the canal, which causes breakdown of the epidermal layer of skin. Organisms and parasites can invade the damaged skin.

Excessive Hygiene

Another risk factor in the development of pruritus ani is overzealous cleansing. Pruritus ani can result from excessive use of chemical irritants such as soap or from excessive rubbing.

Pregnancy and Childbirth

The increased pressure and trauma from pregnancy and childbirth predispose women to the development of hemorrhoids.

Diabetes Mellitus

Diabetes mellitus places the individual at risk for the development of pruritus ani with secondary yeast infections.

Gender

Many more males than females experience pruritus ani; the reason for this is not clear.

Family History

FAP or hereditary nonpolyposis colon cancer places the patient at higher risk for colorectal cancer. Gardner's syndrome is characterized by polyps, primarily of the colon, that are associated with benign tumors of the skin and bone. The polyps of Gardner's syndrome may become malignant in individuals who also have an inherited FAP. There is genetic screening for members of families with FAP.

DIAGNOSTIC REASONING: FOCUSED PHYSICAL EXAMINATION

Obtain Vital Signs

Infants who present with rectal bleeding should first be assessed to determine if they are hemodynamically stable. A smaller blood volume makes blood loss more significant. Children maintain blood pressure with tachycardia and vasoconstriction, and when this compensation is exhausted, severe shock develops rapidly.

Inspect the Perirectal Area

Look for scars, warts, petechiae, bruising, and skin tags. Midline skin tags immediately anterior to the anus that have been present from birth are seen in some children. Skin tags may also develop when tears or hemorrhoidal bleeding resolves. Hemorrhoids are very uncommon in children, and their presence should heighten suspicion of sexual abuse. Perirectal erythema is common with streptococcal cellulitis, and you may occasionally see vesicles surrounding the anus. Perianal ulceration can be seen with Crohn's disease.

Perform a Digital Rectal Examination

A thorough gentle digital rectal examination is essential. Look for skin excoriation, skin tags, fissures, strictures, tears, or hemorrhoids, any of which may cause painful defecation. The knee-chest position affords the best visualization in both adults and children. A side-lying position can also be used. Spread the buttocks to reveal the mucocutaneous junction of the anus, and carefully inspect the rectum first in the resting position and then as the patient bears down. As the patient bears down, an additional 1 to 2 cm of anorectal tissue is palpable.

Look for inflammation, swelling, and erythema that characterize inflammation or infection. These signs may be present with a fissure, fistula, abscess, or proctitis.

Note any lesions or discharge. Condyloma acuminata present as warty growths that are pink or white with a papilliform surface. In anal regions, they tend to grow in radial rows around the anal orifice, forming a confluent mass that can obscure the anal opening. Examination of the entire genital region, including the anal canal, is important because they can extend 1 or 2 cm above the dentate line. Purulent discharge may be present with proctitis or an infected fissure or fistula. An external mass, verrucous growths, polyps, or ulcers may indicate malignancy.

Look carefully around the periphery to see small longitudinal ulcers or tears that characterize anal fissures. Early fissures have the appearance of superficial erosions. More advanced lesions are linear or elliptical breaks in the skin. Long-standing fissures are deep and indurated. Internal fissures are seen when the anal sphincter relaxes as the examining finger is withdrawn. A sentinel tag may be visible.

External hemorrhoids, if present, will be visible as bluish swellings. Internal hemorrhoids may or may not become present as the patient bears down.

Palpate for tenderness. Hemorrhoids are generally not tender. Pain from an abscess, fissure, or fistula may preclude digital examination.

Palpate for the presence of a mass. Masses from anal or colorectal cancer are usually painless and may be so soft that they are easily missed on palpation.

Feel for foreign bodies, which might be present as the result of insertion of objects. Foreign bodies can also be present as a result of ingestion; for example, children may eat chicken bones or small objects.

Perform Anoscopy

Anoscopy is essential in the evaluation of all patients with rectal pain. It enables a view of the immediate internal anal canal that is not possible on manual digital rectal examination. A hand-held anoscope warmed and lubricated is eased slowly into the anus while the patient bears down to relax the external sphincter. A light source is necessary; a head lamp is preferable. Anoscopy may not be possible initially with a fissure or abscess because of the pain. However, it should be performed on a follow-up visit to detect inflammatory bowel disorder or rectal cancer.

LABORATORY AND DIAGNOSTIC STUDIES

Fecal Occult Blood Testing (FOBT)

FOBT should be performed on all patients with rectal pain. A positive test indicates blood in the stool that may be the result of ulcerative or malignant lesions. A stool sample is placed on a piece of filter paper, and an activating solution is applied. A positive test is indicated by the appearance of a color (usually blue or green). The sensitivity of this test in detecting colorectal cancers and adenomas ranges from 50% to 90%. It is an inexpensive and noninvasive method to screen for bleeding lesions. Serial testing (three samples) can be performed through the use of stool cards at home that are returned by mail for analysis.

Fecal Immunochemical Test (FIT)

Also called immunochemical FOBT (iFOBT), FIT uses antibodies to human globin to detect a specific portion of a human blood protein. FIT does not react with non-human hemoglobin or peroxidase, so food restrictions before the test are not necessary. Immuno-chemical FOBTs are also more specific for lower gastrointestinal tract bleeding as they target the globin portion of hemoglobin, which does not survive passage through the upper gastrointestinal tract. This test is done essentially the same way as conventional FOBT, but is more specific and reduces the number of false positive results. Vitamins or foods do not affect the fecal immunochem-ical test, and some forms require only one or two stool specimens.

Flexible Sigmoidoscopy/Colonoscopy

Flexible sigmoidoscopy or colonoscopy should be performed when you suspect inflammatory bowel disease, polyps, or car-cinoma. Colonoscopy is particularly impor-tant for adult patients older than 50 and for those with a history of familial polyposis or hereditary nonpolyposis colon cancer.

Gram Stain Rectal Discharge

Place a smear of rectal discharge on a glass slide for Gram staining. Gram-positive organ-isms stain purple, whereas gram-negative organisms stain red. *Neisseria gonorrhoeae,* a common cause of rectal discharge in proc-titis, is a gram-negative organism.

Cultures for Infectious Organisms

When discharge or lesions are present, col-lect a specimen to culture for *N. gonorrhoeae* or herpes. Collect the specimen on a sterile swab and place in the medium provided. Bacterial culture confirms the identity of the causative organism and its sensitivity to antibiotics. A swab specimen of the perianal cellulitis usually yields a heavy growth of group A *Streptococcus*. Viral culture is also used for the diagnosis of herpes. Results may take from 1 to 7 days, with maximum sen-sitivity achieved at 5 to 7 days. The herpes culture will probably not identify the caus-ative agent if the specimen is taken from a lesion that is 5 or more days old.

Herpesvirus Antigen Detection Test

This test detects antigens on the surface of cells infected with the herpesvirus. Cells from a fresh sore are scraped off and then smeared onto a microscope slide. This test may be done in addition to or in place of a viral culture.

Molecular Testing for Infectious Organisms

Molecular testing using a sample of the rectal discharge provides rapid, sensitive, and specific results. A number of products are available. Follow manufacturer's directions to collect and transport the sample.

DNA probes and nucleic acid amplification tests (NAATs) are available to test for *Chlamydia trachomatis* and *N. gonorrhoeae.* Single or dual organism tests are available.

Serology for Syphilis

Serological tests are used for screening and diagnosing syphilis and are recommended if other sexually transmitted infections (STIs) are found or suspected. The screening tests are nontreponemal and include VDRL (Venereal Disease Research Laboratory), RPR (rapid plasma reagin), and enzyme immunoassay (EIA) tests. Diagnostic tests are *Treponema pallidum* specific and include FTA-ABS (fluorescent treponemal antibody absorption test) and TPPA (*Treponema pallidum* particle agglutination assay).

Alum-Precipitated Toxoid Test

This test is performed to distinguish maternal blood ingestion in newborns. The neonate's gastric contents are mixed with 1% NaH. A brown or rusty color indicates that the infant swallowed maternal blood.

Technetium 99m Scan

This scan is used to identify Meckel's diverticulum that is bleeding.

Microscopic Examination of Stool

Stool examination should be considered in patients with symptoms of enterocolitis to rule out infection from common causes. Fecal leukocyte detection is an easy and inexpensive test that is 75% specific for bacterial diarrhea. Leukocytes are found in inflammatory diarrheal disease and are present in bacterial infections that invade the intestinal wall (*Escherichia coli, Shigella,* and *Salmonella*). Microscopic white blood cells and red blood cells indicate the presence of *Shigella,* enterohemorrhagic *E. coli,* enteropathogenic *E. coli, Campylobacter, Clostridium difficile,* or other inflammatory or invasive diarrhea. Leukocytes are also present in diarrhea from ulcerative colitis and Crohn's disease, as well as antibiotic-related diarrhea. They are not seen in viral gastroenteritis, parasitic diarrhea, *Salmonella* carrier states, or enterotoxigenic bacterial diarrheas. Obtain a small fleck of mucus or stool. Do not allow the specimen to dry. Place the specimen on a slide with two drops of Löffler's alkaline methylene blue stain and wait 2 minutes before viewing under the microscope.

Stool for Ova and Parasites

Stool examination for ova and parasites (O & P) should also be considered in patients with symptoms of enterocolitis. Stool can be tested for the presence of parasites. Fresh stool is required to preserve the trophozoites of some parasites. Use this test in patients with symptoms of diarrhea to rule out infection from *Campylobacter, Shigella, Giardia,* and *Cryptosporidium.* Usually three serial samples are obtained.

Scotch Tape Test

Use this test when you suspect pinworms, which occur most commonly in children. Instruct the adult to apply adhesive cellophane tape to the perianal region early in the morning on awakening. The tape is then brought in. Place it on a glass slide and examine under a microscope for the presence of eggs. Parents may also be able to see the worms in the external anus of the child at night with a flashlight. The female worm is about 10 mm long.

DIFFERENTIAL DIAGNOSIS
Pain
Anal Fissure

Anal fissures are longitudinal ulcers that extend from just below the dentate line to the anal verge. They occur most often in the posterior midline. Acute fissures are cracks in the epithelium, but chronic fissures may result in the formation of a skin tag at the outermost edge that is visible on examination. In the chronic stage, fissures can suppurate and extend into the surrounding tissue, causing perirectal abscess.

Patients with anal fissures complain of cutting or tearing anal pain during defecation and of gnawing, throbbing discomfort after defecation. Digital and visual examinations reveal the presence of the fissure. Early fissures have the appearance of superficial erosions. More advanced lesions are linear or elliptical breaks in the skin. Long-standing fissures are deep and indurated. Internal fissures are seen when the anal sphincter relaxes as the examining finger is withdrawn. A sentinel tag may be visible at the anal verge.

Risk factors for the development of fissure include straining at stool, chronic constipation, and anal intercourse. Anal fissures are the most common cause of constipation or rectal bleeding in children up to 2 years old.

Perirectal Abscess/Fistula

The most common source of infection is the anal glands, located at the base of the anal crypts at the level of the dentate line. Infection may also result from fissure, Crohn's disease, trauma, or anal surgery.

Acute infection presents as an abscess, and chronic infection results in a fistula. The patient complains of swelling, throbbing, and continuous progressive pain. On examination, erythema and swelling in the perirectal region of ischiorectal fossa are found. Pain may preclude examination.

Proctalgia Fugax

Proctalgia fugax is fleeting pain in the anus. It is sudden and severe, lasting several seconds or minutes and then disappearing completely. The spasmlike pain often occurs at night. Proctalgia fugax may occur only once a year or may be experienced in waves of three or four times per week. Each episode is transient, but the pain is excruciating and may be accompanied by sweating, pallor, and tachycardia. Patients experience urgency to defecate, yet pass no stool. No specific cause

has been found, but proctalgia fugax may be associated with spastic contractions of the rectum or the muscular pelvic floor in irritable bowel syndrome. A few patients report attacks after sexual activity. Other unproven associations are food allergies, especially to artificial sweeteners or caffeine.

Proctitis/Proctocolitis

Anorectal infection is common in individuals who engage in anal intercourse, both heterosexuals and homosexuals. Most causes of proctitis are sexually transmitted through the anal sphincter via direct invasion of the infectious agent through the mucous membrane.

Proctitis is characterized by anorectal pain, mucopurulent or bloody discharge, tenesmus, and constipation. Proctitis that is caused by an STI may be associated with intense pain. On examination, inflamed mucopurulent mucosa is present. The most common pathogens are *N. gonorrhoeae, Chlamydia, Treponema pallidum,* and herpesvirus. Herpes simplex infection can occur above or below the anal sphincter. Herpes simplex infection is common in immunocompromised individuals. Proctitis can also occur with ulcerative colitis and Crohn's disease or with patients who have an intact rectum with a colostomy or ileostomy in place. Immunocompromised patients are at greater risk for proctitis.

Proctocolitis implies involvement beyond the rectum to include the sigmoid colon. The causes may include those of proctitis but are usually due to *Shigella, Campylobacter,* or *Giardia.* Symptoms of proctocolitis include those of proctitis but may also include diarrhea, fever, and abdominal cramping. On examination, an inflamed mucopurulent rectal mucosa is visible. Gram stain, serology to rule out syphilis, cultures, and molecular testing for infectious organisms assist in diagnosis.

Pilonidal Disease

Pilonidal disease refers to an abscess or draining sinus that occurs from subcutaneous infection in the sacrococcygeal area. Hairs penetrate the subcutaneous tissue, instigate a foreign body reaction, and produce the formation of a cyst or a sinus. Infection by skin organisms occurs, causing rupture of the sinus into the surrounding adipose tissue. The most common manifestation of pilonidal disease is a painful fluctuant mass in the sacrococcygeal region. Pilonidal disease may present as an abscess; as an acute, recurrent, or chronic pilonidal sinus; or as a perianal pilonidal sinus. Pilonidal disease occurs most often in hirsute young males. Risk factors include a sedentary lifestyle, prolonged sitting, obesity, poor hygiene, and increased sweating.

Perianal Streptococcal Cellulitis

Separation of the buttocks reveals erythema and occasionally vesicles surrounding the anus. The patient usually has a history of group A β-hemolytic streptococcal (GABHS) infection. Pain, erythema, proctitis, and blood-streaked stools are common.

Itching

Pruritus Ani

Pruritus ani is a symptom complex consisting of discomfort and itching. It is more common in men than women and is most often idiopathic. Discomfort is exacerbated by friction or a warm, moist, perineal environment. Poor anal hygiene or, conversely, overcleansing is often a contributing factor.

Examination may reveal mild erythema and excoriation of the perirectal skin. In later stages, the skin may be red, raw, oozing, or pale and lichenified with exaggerated skin markings.

Pinworms

Pinworms are nematodes that infect the intestine and cause perianal irritation. The pinworm eggs are ingested and migrate to the duodenum, where they hatch and mature and then travel to the cecum. The adult females emerge at night through the anus, deposit eggs in the perianal region, and die. The eggs stick to the skin and cause perianal pruritus and scratching. The worms may be visible at night, and the ova may be visible under the microscope.

Bleeding

Hemorrhoids

Hemorrhoids are dilated veins located beneath the lining of the anal canal. Internal hemorrhoids are located in the upper anal canal proximal to the dentate line and are covered by rectal mucosa and supported by longitudinal muscle fibers. External hemorrhoids are located in the lower anal canal distal to the dentate line, are covered by skin, and lack muscle support.

Internal hemorrhoids are graded by size (Table 16-1) and most often present with painless rectal bleeding; the blood is bright red and varies in quantity from a few drops coating the stool to a spattering at the end of defecation. Patients also report a dull aching and itching with prolapse. Itching occurs only with chronic prolapse.

External hemorrhoids can also cause itching but produce pain only when they become thrombosed. With thrombosis, patients report an acute onset of constant burning and throbbing pain and a new rectal lump.

External hemorrhoids are visible on examination as bluish skin-covered lumps at the anal verge. Internal hemorrhoids may become visible when the patient bears down. Risk factors for the development of hemorrhoids include pregnancy, childbirth, straining during defecation, and occupations requiring prolonged sitting.

Table 16-1	Classification of Internal Hemorrhoids	
GRADE	DESCRIPTION	SYMPTOMS
1	Do not prolapse	Minimal bleeding or discomfort
2	Prolapse with straining, reduce spontaneously	Bleeding, aching, pruritus when prolapsed
3	Prolapse with straining, require manual reduction	Bleeding, aching, pruritus when prolapsed
4	Cannot be reduced, or manual reduction ineffective	Bleeding, aching, pruritus when prolapsed

Modified from Metcalf A: Anorectal disorders. Five common causes of pain, itching, and bleeding, *Postgrad Med* 98(5):81, 1995.

Condyloma Acuminata

Genital warts are a common STI caused by the human papillomavirus (HPV). Patients with small lesions usually have few symptoms. When the lesions become large, patients experience bleeding, discharge, itching, and pain. On examination, warts are pink or white with a papilliform surface. They may obscure the anal opening. Examination of the entire genital region, including the anal canal, is important because they can extend 1 or 2 cm above the dentate line.

Cancer of the Anus and Rectum

Anal or colorectal cancer can cause many different symptoms or be an incidental finding on rectal examination. Pain is usually absent, and rectal bleeding is inconsistent. The patient may have the sensation of a mass or lump. An external or internal mass may be palpable. Some lesions are so soft that they are missed on palpation. Anal cancer can take several forms, such as ulcers, polyps, or verrucous growths.

Ingestion of Maternal Blood

Newborns may swallow water and maternal blood, and this can appear as upper GI bleeding. To differentiate mother's from baby's blood, perform an alum-precipitated toxoid (APT) test; fetal blood remains pink, whereas maternal blood turns yellow-brown. Diagnosis is best made with an APT test.

Allergic Colitis

Allergic colitis of infancy is a diagnosis of exclusion. It is seen in infants 3 weeks to 10 months old. The infant presents with loose bowel movements that are streaked with blood and mucus. The infant is otherwise healthy with normal growth. History may show early introduction of milk or a recent gastroenteritis. Laboratory studies are performed to rule out other causes such as diarrheal disease and include stool studies for leukocytes, culture, eosinophils, and complete blood cell count. All milk and soy products are eliminated from the infant's diet. If the mother is breastfeeding, milk and soy products are eliminated from her diet. Generally the infant outgrows the problem by the age of 1 year.

Necrotizing Enterocolitis

This inflammation of the bowel may involve only the innermost lining or the entire thickness of the bowel and varying amounts of the bowel. It is seen in premature infants who have fragile and immature colons, but it may also be seen in newborns. The usual presentation may include abdominal distention, lethargy, and bloody stools; however, the signs range from feeding intolerance to sepsis. **This is a life-threatening condition and needs immediate referral.**

Meckel's Diverticulum

Meckel's diverticulum is a congenital abnormality that affects approximately 2% of the population, most of whom are asymptomatic. The diverticulum is thought to be what is left of the fetus's umbilical cord and intestines that were not fully reabsorbed and may contain gastric or pancreatic tissue. Painless rectal bleeding is the usual chief complaint of symptomatic cases in children younger than 2 years.

Intussusception

Intussusception is a telescoping of the intestines. It occurs most commonly in infants between 5 and 9 months of age. The infant experiences severe colicky pains. The child may become pale and limp, and then after the attack, which usually lasts for a few minutes, the child calms down and appears well. The child may vomit. The stools may contain blood and mucus typically described as currant jelly in color. **Referral is necessary to prevent strangulation of the bowel.**

Juvenile Polyps

Benign inflammatory polyps of the colon are found in children between the ages of 2 and 8 years. The patient experiences painless bleeding that occurs during or immediately after defecation. There is no risk for malignancy from these polyps. Colonoscopy is used to diagnosis the condition.

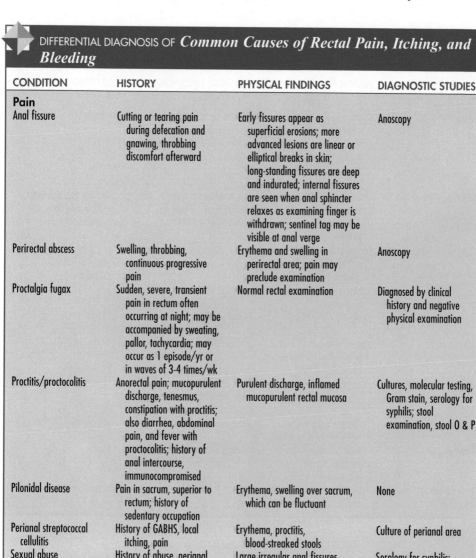

DIFFERENTIAL DIAGNOSIS OF *Common Causes of Rectal Pain, Itching, and Bleeding*

CONDITION	HISTORY	PHYSICAL FINDINGS	DIAGNOSTIC STUDIES
Pain			
Anal fissure	Cutting or tearing pain during defecation and gnawing, throbbing discomfort afterward	Early fissures appear as superficial erosions; more advanced lesions are linear or elliptical breaks in skin; long-standing fissures are deep and indurated; internal fissures are seen when anal sphincter relaxes as examining finger is withdrawn; sentinel tag may be visible at anal verge	Anoscopy
Perirectal abscess	Swelling, throbbing, continuous progressive pain	Erythema and swelling in perirectal area; pain may preclude examination	Anoscopy
Proctalgia fugax	Sudden, severe, transient pain in rectum often occurring at night; may be accompanied by sweating, pallor, tachycardia; may occur as 1 episode/yr or in waves of 3-4 times/wk	Normal rectal examination	Diagnosed by clinical history and negative physical examination
Proctitis/proctocolitis	Anorectal pain; mucopurulent discharge, tenesmus, constipation with proctitis; also diarrhea, abdominal pain, and fever with proctocolitis; history of anal intercourse, immunocompromised	Purulent discharge, inflamed mucopurulent rectal mucosa	Cultures, molecular testing, Gram stain, serology for syphilis; stool examination, stool O & P
Pilonidal disease	Pain in sacrum, superior to rectum; history of sedentary occupation	Erythema, swelling over sacrum, which can be fluctuant	None
Perianal streptococcal cellulitis	History of GABHS, local itching, pain	Erythema, proctitis, blood-streaked stools	Culture of perianal area
Sexual abuse	History of abuse, perianal pain, itching	Large irregular anal fissures, bruising, rectal tone decreased, warts, presence of semen	Serology for syphilis; culture (gonorrhea, *T. vaginalis*, herpes); molecular testing, (herpes, chlamydia, gonorrhea)
Itching			
Pruritus ani	Discomfort and itching exacerbated by friction; history of poor anal hygiene or overcleansing	Mild erythema and excoriation over perirectal skin; in later stages: red, raw, oozing, pale lichenified perirectal skin	
Pinworms	Itching, especially at night	Visualize white-yellow worms 8-13 mm in length at night with flashlight	Scotch tape test positive for eggs

Continued

DIFFERENTIAL DIAGNOSIS OF *Common Causes of Rectal Pain, Itching, and Bleeding—cont'd*

CONDITION	HISTORY	PHYSICAL FINDINGS	DIAGNOSTIC STUDIES
Bleeding			
Hemorrhoids	Bright red rectal bleeding with defecation or blood on stool; burning or itching; straining at stool; prolonged sitting; pregnancy and childbirth	External hemorrhoids: bluish, skin-covered lumps; internal hemorrhoids: may be visible when patient bears down	FOBT or FIT
Condyloma acuminata	Few symptoms with small lesions; bleeding, discharge, itching, and pain with large lesions	Pink or white warty lesions with papilliform surface; may extend into anal canal	Serology to distinguish from condyloma lata caused by syphilis
Cancer of rectum, anus	Feeling of lump; usually painless; may or may not bleed; may have family history of polyposis syndromes	Polyp, internal or external mass, ulcers, verrucous growths	Anoscopy, flexible sigmoidoscopy, colonoscopy
Ingestion of maternal blood	Newborn	Hematemesis	APT test
Allergic colitis	Infant 0-6 mo, milk formula or breastfed mother who has intake of milk	Blood-streaked stools	None
NEC	Preterm, newborn infant	Ileus, abdominal distention, gastrointestinal bleeding, bilious vomiting	Immediate referral
Meckel's diverticulitis	Preschool child, painless gastrointestinal bleeding	Black or maroon stools	Technetium 99m scan and referral
Intussusception	Colicky abdominal pain, vomiting, currant jelly stools	Sausage-shaped mass may be felt in abdomen	Refer
Juvenile polyps	Painless bleeding with stool, ages 2-5 yr	None	Colonoscopy

CHAPTER RESOURCES

Billingham RP, Isler JT, Kimmins MH et al: The diagnosis and management of common anorectal disorders, *Curr Problems Surg* 41(7):586, 2004.

Di Lorenzo C: Pediatric anorectal disorders, *Gastroenterol Clin North Am* 30:269, 2001.

Kong AP, Stamos MJ: Anorectal complaints: office diagnosis and treatment, part 1, *Consultant* June:731, 2005.

Kong AP, Stamos MJ: Anorectal complaints: office diagnosis and treatment, part 1, *Consultant* June:735, 2005.

Lawrence W, Wright J, Cheng T: Causes of rectal bleeding in children, *Pediatr Rev* 22:11, 2001.

Mazza L, Formento E, Fronda G: Anorectal and perineal pain: new pathophysiological hypothesis, *Tech Coloproctol* 8:77, 2004.

Pfenninger JL, Zainea GG: Common anorectal conditions, part I: symptoms and complaints, *Am Fam Physician* 63:2391, 2001.

Pfenninger JL, Zainea GG: Common anorectal conditions, part II: lesions, *Am Fam Physician* 64:77, 2001.

Wald A: Functional anorectal and pelvic pain, *Gastroenterol Clin North Am* 30:243, 2001.

Watson AJ, Loudon M: Diagnosing minor anorectal conditions, *Practitioner* 245:790, 2001.

VII

Common Problems of the Genitourinary System

CHAPTER 17

Urinary Incontinence

Urinary incontinence is the involuntary leakage of urine. It occurs as a result of pathological, anatomical, psychological, or physiological factors that produce obstruction, bladder irritability, or interference with neurological functioning. Environmental factors such as decreased mobility or inaccessibility of toilet facilities may also produce periodic incontinence.

Urinary incontinence is a common problem, particularly in older adults. It is so common in older women that some think of it as "normal." The prevalence in U.S. women is 26% during reproductive years and 30% to 40% in postmenopausal years. In noninstitutionalized elderly women, the prevalence is 15% to 30%, and in men it is 8% to 22%. In elderly persons in nursing homes, the rate rises to almost 50%.

Urinary incontinence in adults is categorized according to the underlying anatomical or physiological impairment—specifically, stress incontinence, urge incontinence (overactive bladder), overflow incontinence, and incontinence from reversible causes.

Stress incontinence is leakage of urine during activities that increase abdominal pressure, such as coughing, sneezing, laughing, or other physical activities. It occurs most often in females and is caused by hypermotility at the base of the bladder and urethra associated with pelvic floor relaxation or intrinsic urethral weakness.

Urge incontinence is an abrupt and strong desire to void with the inability to delay urination and is caused by bladder hyperactivity or hypersensitive bladder. Detrusor muscle overactivity occurs when pathological brain disorders interfere with central inhibitory centers and fail to prevent detrusor muscle contractions.

Overflow incontinence occurs with overdistention of the bladder caused by an underactive or acontractile detrusor muscle; by sphincter-detrusor dyssynergia, which is loss of the synergistic urinary sphincter relaxation that normally occurs with bladder detrusor muscle contraction; or from bladder outlet or urethral obstruction. Sphincter weakness can occur from damage to the urethra or its innervation or from pelvic floor muscle relaxation. Incontinence from reversible factors originates outside of the lower urinary tract and is caused by mental status impairment, immobility, or medication. Some sources term this "functional" or "transient" incontinence.

A final category of incontinence is called mixed incontinence. This occurs when the incontinence is produced as the result of several anatomical, physiological, or functional factors. Involuntary discharge of urine in children is abnormal beyond the age of 4 years for daytime wetting and beyond the age of 6 for nighttime wetting. Daytime wetting constitutes diurnal enuresis; nighttime wetting is known as nocturnal or sleep enuresis. In children, enuresis may be organic or nonorganic; nonorganic enuresis can be primary or secondary. Primary nonorganic enuresis occurs in 75% to 90% of children. This enuresis is defined as wetting that has continued since infancy without an established pattern of dryness. Secondary nonorganic enuresis occurs in 10% to 25% of children and is defined as recurrence of wetting after continence has been established for at least 6 months. The possibility of abnormal urinary anatomy is high in young children who present with urinary tract symptoms.

DIAGNOSTIC REASONING: FOCUSED HISTORY
Adults

Could This Be the Result of Reversible Factors? (Box 17-1)

Key Questions
- What medications are you taking?
- Do you have any of the following urinary tract symptoms: urgency, frequency, burning, pain, blood in urine, flank pain?
- Do you have vaginal dryness or itching?
- Do you have pain/discomfort with sexual activity?
- Have you had changes in bowel function?
- When was your last bowel movement?
- Are you feeling depressed or "blue"?
- Are you aware of incontinence?
- How mobile are you?
- Are you able to get to the toilet easily?
- Do you have any chronic health problems?

Medications
Hypnotic-sedatives, diuretics, anticholinergic agents, adrenergic agents, and calcium channel blockers can cause incontinence. α-Adrenergic agonists and β-adrenergic agonists increase sphincter tone and may cause

Box 17-1	**Reversible Factors That Can Cause Urinary Incontinence in Adults**

D Delirium, dementia, depression
I Infection
A Atrophic vaginitis/urethritis
P Pharmaceuticals
E Endocrine/excess urine production
R Restricted mobility, retention
S Stool impaction

Modified from Resnick NM: Initial evaluation of the incontinent patient, *J Am Geriatr Soc* 38(3):311, 1990.

retention. Anticholinergics, prostaglandin inhibitors, calcium channel blockers, and narcotic analgesics decrease detrusor tone. Diuretics can cause incontinence because of increased production of urine, and central nervous system (CNS) depressants such as hypnotic-sedatives can interfere with functional ability.

Box 17-2 lists categories of medications and their mechanism of action in urinary incontinence.

Urinary Tract Infection, Vaginal Dryness, and Dyspareunia
Urinary tract infection (UTI) and atrophic vaginitis can cause incontinence through local irritation and loss of muscle tone.

Bowel Function
Fecal impaction can cause incontinence through mechanical obstruction of the urethra.

Mental Status, Mobility, and Chronic Health Problems
Excessive urine production may be a problem if mobility is restricted, health is poor, or orientation is variable. Chronic health problems, psychological factors, and restricted mobility can result in incontinence because of loss of functional ability and/or mentation.

What Do the Presenting Symptoms Tell Me?

Key Questions
- What is the primary symptom (e.g., urgency, dribbling, lack of sensation, nocturia, abdominal discomfort, leakage with laughing, coughing, or sneezing)?
- How frequently do you urinate?
- How much urine is voided each time?
- Do you have difficulty starting to urinate?
- Does your urine stream start and stop while you are urinating?

Primary Symptom
Urgency is the primary symptom of detrusor instability. Dribbling indicates overflow incontinence, and sphincter weakness usually increases with postural changes. Men often

Box 17-2	Medications That Can Cause or Contribute to Urinary Incontinence	

Medication Category	Type of Incontinence	Mechanism of Action
Anticholinergics	Overflow	Decreased bladder contractions with retention
Antidepressants	Overflow	Decreased bladder contractions with retention
Antipsychotics	Overflow	Decreased bladder contractions with retention
Sedative-hypnotics	Overflow	Decreased bladder contractions with retention
Antihistamines	Overflow	Decreased bladder contractions with retention
Narcotics	Overflow	Decreased bladder contractions with retention
Alcohol	Overflow	Decreased bladder contractions with retention
Calcium channel blockers	Overflow	Decreased bladder contractions with retention
β-Adrenergic agonists	Overflow	Decreased bladder contractions with retention
α-Adrenergic agonists	Overflow	Sphincter contraction with outflow obstruction
α-Adrenergic antagonists	Stress	Sphincter relaxation with urinary leakage
Diuretics	Urge	Contractions stimulated by high urine flow
Caffeine	Urge	Diuretic effect
Sedative-hypnotics	Urge	Depressed CNS inhibition of micturition
Alcohol	Urge	Diuretic effect and depressed CNS inhibition

Adapted from Weiss BD: Diagnostic evaluation of urinary incontinence in geriatric patients, *Am Fam Physician* 57:2675, 2688, 1998.

complain of nocturia and dribbling with overflow incontinence. Abdominal discomfort often occurs with overflow incontinence because of bladder distention. Incontinence with increase in intraabdominal pressure is usually stress incontinence but can also be the result of detrusor overactivity and bladder irritability.

Frequency of Voiding

Increase in frequency of voiding occurs with detrusor instability or hyperactivity and may occur with some transient causes such as use of diuretics or large-volume fluid intake. Decreased frequency is common in overflow incontinence.

Amount of Urine Lost With Each Episode

Involuntary loss of small amounts of urine occurs with stress incontinence and overflow incontinence.

Character of Stream

Voiding a small-caliber or intermittent stream or difficulty in starting the stream indicates obstructive uropathy. In males, this may be secondary to an enlarged prostate.

Are There Any Other Symptoms That Will Point Me in the Right Direction?

Key Questions

- How much fluid do you drink in a day?
- How much caffeine and alcohol do you drink?
- What time of day do you drink fluids?
- How thirsty are you?
- Have you lost or gained weight recently?

Fluid Intake

A significant increase in the amount of fluid intake or an unusually large volume may indicate diabetes mellitus (DM). Caffeine and alcohol can act as diuretics and may be a cause of reversible incontinence. Caffeine can also be a bladder irritant and either produce or exacerbate urge incontinence. A large volume of fluid intake may produce enuresis secondary to a large urine volume, particularly if fluids are consumed in the evening before bedtime.

Thirst

Unusual thirst accompanied by an unusually large intake of fluid may indicate DM.

Weight Loss or Gain

Weight loss may indicate a chronic health problem, tumor, or dementia. Weight gain may indicate congestive heart failure, DM, or loss of mobility.

Children

Is This Primary or Secondary Enuresis?

Key Question

- Has the child ever had consistent dryness for at least 6 months?

Primary enuresis occurs when a child has never achieved consistent dryness. Secondary enuresis is involuntary voiding of urine in a child who has had a period of dryness of more than 6 months. Secondary enuresis is often indicative of some other form of voiding dysfunction or significant underlying pathology. In children, daytime urinary incontinence beyond the age of 4 years may indicate congenital abnormalities in the urinary tract or nervous system.

Is This Organic Enuresis?

Key Questions

- Does the child have pain on urination?
- Does the child have intermittent daytime wetness?
- Does the child seem very thirsty and urinate a lot?
- Has the child had nervous system trauma?
- Does the child have constipation or encopresis?
- Does the child have constant wetness or dribbling throughout the day?
- Does the child have an abnormal stream, such as dribbling or hesitancy?
- Has the child had a change in gait?
- Has the child had a lumbar puncture recently?
- Does the child snore or have apnea at night?
- Does the child complain of rectal itching at night?

Organic explanations of enuresis focus primarily on the genitourinary and nervous systems.

Genitourinary System

Fifteen percent of children with a UTI present with enuresis. It is unclear whether UTI causes the enuresis or vice versa. A wet perineum predisposes to ascending infection, and prompt treatment of the infection cures the enuresis in about one third of the cases. Asymptomatic bacteremia in school children is associated with enuresis.

Fecal retention that is chronic or intermittent is responsible for production of "functional" bladder neck obstruction. Displacement of the bladder and posterior urethra by the full rectum in the fixed and limited space of the bony pelvis causes detrusor perineal dyssynergism, which is thought to be the mechanism responsible for urinary stasis and interference with micturition produced by constipation.

Abnormal daytime voiding suggests urological abnormality. Dribbling suggests the presence of an ectopic ureter. Chronic leakage of urine in females may indicate an ectopic ureter that terminates in the vagina. Partial distal urethral obstruction can cause straining to urinate. Polyuria from a glucose-induced osmotic diuresis can be seen in patients with DM. Renal tubules lose their ability to concentrate urine, resulting in the production of large volumes of very dilute urine.

Nervous System

Lumbosacral disorders affect bladder innervation and may cause enuresis. Head injury or brain tumor can cause polyuria and polydipsia. If the kidneys are unable to concentrate urine because of deficiency in the hypothalamic production of antidiuretic hormone (ADH), central diabetes insipidus (DI) develops, while renal unresponsiveness to ADH causes nephrogenic DI.

Interference with the nerve supply to the bladder causes a neurogenic bladder and obstruction. This can be functional, resulting from an imbalance between detrusor muscle contraction and urethral sphincter relaxation. It can also be congenital or acquired, such as with meningomyelocele or spinal cord injury.

Sleep apnea interferes with the child's ability to wake appropriately in response to stimuli to void.

Other

Pinworms (*Enterobius vermicularis*) primarily inhabit the cecum and lower bowel and are the most common cause of rectal itching in children. Pinworms have been implicated in incontinence in children, although the reason is not clear.

What Risk Factors Does This Child Have for Nonorganic Enuresis?

Key Questions

- Is the child a boy or a girl?
- Is there a history of bedwetting in the family?
- Is the child a twin?
- Has the child been institutionalized?
- What is the child's birth order?
- Does the child have sickle cell disease?
- What is the child's daily fluid intake?

Gender

Boys are more likely to have nocturnal enuresis. Girls are more likely to have diurnal enuresis related to UTI.

Family History

Children with nonorganic enuresis often have a very strong family history of fathers who had nocturnal enuresis as a child.

Twin/Birth Order

Nocturnal enuresis is most common in the firstborn and in twins.

Institutionalization

Institutionalized children have a greater tendency to enuresis because of developmental delay.

Sickle Cell Disease

Children with sickle cell anemia may have a concentrating defect and excrete low specific gravity urine in large volumes, which may make the child wet the bed.

Fluid Intake

A large volume of fluid intake may produce enuresis secondary to a large urine volume, particularly if the fluids are consumed in the evening before bedtime.

DIAGNOSTIC REASONING: FOCUSED PHYSICAL EXAMINATION

Perform Mental Status Examination

Assess orientation and cognitive function. In adults, incontinence can occur as the result of disorientation, delirium, or dementia.

In children, secondary enuresis can be caused by the presence of stress factors during the developmental period from 2 to 4 years of age. Separation from family, death of a parent, birth of a sibling, a move, marital conflict, and other stress-related causes may produce transient and intermittent enuresis.

Observe Gait

The urinary bladder receives extensive autonomic as well as somatic innervation. Lesions at all levels of the neuraxis from the cortex to peripheral nerves produce abnormalities of micturition.

Take Vital Signs

Blood pressure readings in children are important to rule out nephrotic causes of enuresis. When chronic renal failure is the result of an inadequate amount of normally functioning renal tissue, the clinical presentation may be enuresis. Fever in infants without any other signs is likely caused by UTI.

Examine the Abdomen

Palpate for masses, suprapubic tenderness, or fullness. Palpate the bladder. Abdominal distention or palpable bladder is suggestive of urinary retention and overflow incontinence.

Examine Genitalia in Males

Look for abnormalities of the foreskin, glans, meatus, penis, and perineal skin that might contribute to or produce incontinence.

Perform Pelvic Examination in Females

Note signs of pelvic prolapse (cystocele, rectocele). Palpate for pelvic mass and perivaginal muscle tone. Note condition of the vaginal mucosa and look for atrophic vaginitis. Vaginitis can cause urinary incontinence in children and adults, whereas atrophic vaginitis will produce incontinence only in adults.

Observe for evidence of sexual abuse such as abrasions, tears, or bruising. Urethral irritation, especially if discharge is present, may suggest sexual abuse in children.

Perform Provocative Stress Testing

During the pelvic examination, ask the patient to relax and then cough vigorously (or perform a Valsalva maneuver); watch for urine loss from the urethra. A positive test indicates stress incontinence.

Perform Digital Rectal Examination

Assess for perineal sensation, resting and active sphincter tone, rectal mass, fecal impaction, and fissures. A lax sphincter suggests spinal cord involvement.

In men, assess consistency and contour of the prostate. Prostate enlargement or masses suggest the possibility of overflow incontinence from obstruction.

Conduct a Neurological Examination

Assess the intactness of the neurological system. Note focal deficits, test deep tendon reflexes, and test for sensation in the perineal and perirectal areas. Assess nerve roots S2 to S4. Test for muscle tone and strength. Deficits may point to a neurological cause for the incontinence.

Examine and Palpate the Spine in Children

Look for an undetected birth defect that may be causing a neurological disturbance. A spinal dimple or hair tuft may alert you to a potential problem.

Perform Musculoskeletal Examination

Assess mobility, strength, and functional ability. In many older adults, the inability to get to a toilet causes incontinence.

An easy assessment of mobility is the timed get-up-and-go test. Time the patient getting up from a chair, walking 10 feet, and sitting back down. Although the time required to perform this test will vary, a mobile, independent, older adult can perform this activity in about 10 seconds.

Additional Procedures
Postvoid Residual (PVR)

Have the patient void without straining and then catheterize. A residual volume greater than 100 ml suggests either bladder weakness (stress incontinence) or outlet obstruction (overflow incontinence).

Observe Voiding

Note hesitancy, dribbling, interrupted stream, decreased force, and caliber of stream. These symptoms suggest outlet obstruction and overflow incontinence.

LABORATORY AND DIAGNOSTIC STUDIES
Urinalysis (U/A)

Dipstick U/A can rule out or point to infection or systemic disease as a cause of the incontinence. Note hematuria, pyuria, bacturia, or the presence of leukocyte esterase or nitrites as indicators of UTI. Glycosuria or proteinuria suggests DM or renal disease.

Specific Gravity

A specific gravity greater than 1.015 rules out diabetes insipidus as the cause of incontinence.

Urine Culture

A culture can be used to determine the organism(s) producing a UTI and can confirm the diagnosis.

Urine Cytology

Urine for cytology is indicated if microscopic or gross painless hematuria is present in the absence of infection.

Bladder Diary

A 24-hour bladder diary (3-day voiding diary for children) can provide an accurate record of urine output, average voided volume, frequency of voiding, frequency and nature of incontinent episodes, and type of volume of fluid intake. Patients or parents can catch and measure urine output in a measuring cup.

Blood Urea Nitrogen and Creatinine

Use these indicators of renal function if you suspect obstruction or urinary retention.

Vaginal Specimen Microscopy, Molecular Testing, or Culture

These tests can confirm vaginal infection. See Chapter 21 for the procedures for these tests.

Office Cystometrography

Have the patient void and empty the bladder. Have men lie supine and place women in the dorsal lithotomy position. Insert a sterile 12 to 14 French (nonballooned) catheter and empty the bladder. (Measure the postvoid residual and collect urine for U/A at that time.) Insert a 50-ml syringe with plunger removed into the end of the catheter and position it about 15 cm above the urethra. Fill the syringe by pouring sterile water into it in 25- to 50-ml increments. Record cumulative total fluid instillation in the bladder and note the volume at which the patient first reports the urge to void. Continue adding fluid slowly until the fluid level in the syringe rises, indicating an increase in intrabladder pressure and contraction of the detrusor muscle. The rise may be gradual or sudden. Detrusor contraction at less than 300 to 350 ml of bladder volume indicates detrusor instability (urge incontinence). Have the patient void at the end of the procedure. The amount instilled minus the amount voided will also provide a measure of postvoid residual.

Complete Urodynamic Testing

Complete urodynamic testing includes cystometrography, perineal electromyelography, and voiding cystourethrography (VCUG). It is indicated when a presumptive diagnosis cannot be made and when surgical repair of stress incontinence is a consideration.

Cystoscopy and Contrast Radiography

These procedures are indicated for detection of neoplasms or stones.

Ultrasound

Ultrasonography may be useful in determining the presence of an obstruction.

DIFFERENTIAL DIAGNOSIS

Incontinence From Anatomical Causes

Stress Incontinence

Stress incontinence is associated with activities that increase intraabdominal pressure, such as coughing, sneezing, running, or laughing. The underlying abnormality is typically urethral hypermotility as a result of inadequate pelvic support of the bladder neck (urethrovesical junction). Normally increased intraabdominal pressure is transmitted evenly across the bladder neck and body. When adequate support is lacking, an increase in intraabdominal pressure displaces the bladder neck outside the abdominal cavity. The subsequent disproportionate increase in bladder pressure as compared to urethral pressure results in urine loss. Poor urethral sphincter function also contributes to stress incontinence. The amount of urine lost with each episode is small. The patient usually has a history of childbirth. On examination, pelvic floor relaxation may be evident with the presence of a cystocele and/or rectocele. The urethral sphincter may appear lax, and there is loss of urine with provocative testing. Atrophic vaginitis is a common finding in postmenopausal women. U/A and culture may be performed to rule out infections or urinary tract problems. Postvoid residual is normal.

Urge Incontinence

Urge incontinence is characterized by an uncontrolled urge to void, secondary to detrusor muscle irritability or hyperactivity or to a hypersensitive bladder. Most cases result from an idiopathic inability to suppress detrusor contraction. The urine volume lost is large. Physical examination results are usually normal. Postvoid residual is normal. Diagnostic testing includes U/A and culture to rule out infection and determination of blood urea nitrogen and creatinine levels to rule out nephropathy. On office cystometrography, the urine volume is less than 300 to 350 ml before the urge to void occurs.

Complete urodynamic testing can confirm the diagnosis.

Overflow Incontinence

Overflow incontinence occurs in the presence of obstruction or interruption in the nervous system. It is a result of overdistention of the bladder from an underactive or acontractile detrusor muscle, from sphincter-detrusor dyssynergia (loss of the synergistic urinary sphincter relaxation that normally occurs with bladder detrusor muscle contraction), or from bladder outlet or urethral obstruction. Sphincter weakness can occur from damage to the urethra or its innervation or from pelvic floor muscle relaxation.

Overflow incontinence is small-volume incontinence, with symptoms of dribbling and hesitancy. In men, symptoms of an enlarged prostate may be present (i.e., nocturia, dribbling, hesitancy, and decreased force and caliber of stream). On examination, look for distended bladder, prostate hypertrophy, evidence of spinal cord disease, or diabetic neuropathy. Postvoid residual is more than 100 ml. Diagnostic testing includes U/A and urine culture as well as determination of blood urea nitrogen and creatinine levels.

Interference with the nerve supply to the bladder can result in neurogenic bladder, obstruction, and consequent overflow incontinence, caused by an imbalance between detrusor muscle contraction and urethral sphincter relaxation. Functional incontinence can also be congenital or acquired, such as with meningomyelocele or spinal cord injury, or can be a surgical complication from radical prostatectomy. On examination, the anal sphincter may be lax. Neurological testing may reveal deficits.

Incontinence From Reversible Factors

Medications

Sedatives, hypnotics, diuretics, anticholinergic agents, α-adrenergic agents, and calcium channel blockers can cause incontinence. α-Adrenergic agonists and β-adrenergic agonists increase sphincter tone and may cause retention; they can also cause urge incontinence. Anticholinergics, prostaglandin inhibitors, calcium channel blockers, and narcotic analgesics decrease detrusor tone and can produce incontinence. Diuretics can cause incontinence because of increased production of urine, and CNS depressants such as hypnotic-sedatives can interfere with functional ability.

Urinary Tract Infection

The patient with UTI has symptoms of lower or upper tract infection, such as burning, dysuria, frequency, urgency, flank pain, and fever. The urine may have a foul odor. The patient may exhibit suprapubic or costovertebral angle (CVA) tenderness. In infants, a fever with no localizing signs frequently indicates UTI. Urine analysis and culture can confirm the diagnosis of a lower UTI (see Chapter 18).

Vaginitis

Vaginitis produces incontinence as a result of local irritation. Atrophic vaginitis indicates a loss of estrogen and a concomitant loss of the vesicourethral angle, which predisposes women to stress incontinence. Provocative stress testing can demonstrate stress incontinence. Microscopy, molecular testing, or culture can confirm vaginal infection (see Chapter 21).

Constipation and Fecal Impaction

Constipation or fecal impaction can produce obstructive overflow incontinence by mechanical pressure on the urethra. The patient may experience abdominal pain and fecal soiling. On examination, stool may be felt in the colon and/or ampulla.

Change in Mental or Functional Status

Depression, dementia, or confusion can all produce incontinence (see Chapter 30). Restricted mobility can result in incontinence because of loss of functional ability.

Diabetes Insipidus

In DI, the kidneys are unable to concentrate urine because of a deficiency in the hypothalamic production of ADH (central DI) or a renal unresponsiveness to ADH (nephrogenic DI). The result is polyuria, which may cause incontinence. The patient also exhibits polydipsia. Urine specific gravity will be less than 1.015.

Diabetes Mellitus

DM often presents with excessive fluid intake and urination. The excess fluid volume can result in incontinence, particularly in older adults with chronic health problems, restricted mobility, or compromise in mental or functional health. Urinalysis can screen for glycosuria. Follow-up testing should check fasting blood glucose levels and hemoglobin A_{1c} measurement.

Mixed Incontinence

Patients who experience incontinence as the result of several anatomical, physiological, or functional factors are considered to have mixed incontinence.

Enuresis From Organic Causes

Genitourinary Causes

Genitourinary disorders that can produce enuresis include UTI, ectopic ureter, or urethral obstruction. Physical examination is usually normal. Fever and abdominal tenderness may be present with a UTI. Anatomical genitourinary abnormalities may signal an ectopic ureter. Diagnostic testing includes urinalysis, urine culture, and specific gravity to rule out infection and DM. Referral for further evaluation may be necessary.

Neurological Causes

Nervous system involvement can also produce enuresis. Lumbosacral disorders affect bladder innervation and may cause enuresis. Head injury or brain tumor can cause polyuria and polydipsia. Interference with the nerve supply to the bladder causes neurogenic bladder and obstruction, which can result in enuresis. Interference in innervation can occur from congenital or acquired causes. Sleep apnea interferes with the child's ability to wake appropriately in response to stimuli to void. Diagnostic testing includes urinalysis, urine culture, and specific gravity

to rule out infection and DM. Referral for further evaluation may be necessary.

Enuresis From Nonorganic Causes

Primary Enuresis

Primary enuresis occurs when a child has never achieved consistent dryness. The normal developmental patterns of micturition follow a characteristic pattern in children but at an individual rate. The usual progression depends on the maturation of the CNS; generally, the following stages are seen:

- **Birth to 6 months:** Bladder emptying is an uninhibited reflex action.
- **6 to 12 months:** Bladder emptying is less frequent because of CNS inhibition of reflex action.
- **1 to 2 years:** Child consciously perceives bladder fullness; CNS inhibition increases.
- **3 to 5 years:** At age 5 years, most children are aware of bladder fullness; they develop the ability to inhibit the need to void both voluntarily and unconsciously.

Primary enuresis may represent a developmental delay or maturational lag. Often there is a family history of enuresis. The enuresis usually is only nocturnal. The incidence is higher in boys than in girls and usually resolves as the child matures. Physical examination is normal. Diagnostic testing includes urinalysis, urine culture, and specific gravity to rule out other causes.

Developmental (Secondary) Enuresis

Developmental enuresis, which is secondary, may be related to changes or stresses in a child's life. It can also occur as the result of genital trauma, infection, distended colon, or fecal impaction. The enuresis occurs in a child who has had a period of dryness of more than 6 months. Diagnostic testing includes urinalysis, urine culture, and specific gravity to rule out other causes.

Small Bladder

An anatomically small bladder can also produce enuresis. The child voids frequently but not in excessive volume. Physical examination is normal. Diagnostic testing includes urinalysis, urine culture, and specific gravity to rule out other causes.

Sickle Cell Anemia

Children with sickle cell anemia have a concentrating defect and may experience enuresis because of volume excess. Physical examination findings are consistent with the sickle cell disorder. Diagnostic testing includes urinalysis, urine culture, and specific gravity.

DIFFERENTIAL DIAGNOSIS OF *Common Causes of Urinary Incontinence*

CONDITION	HISTORY	PHYSICAL FINDINGS	DIAGNOSTIC STUDIES
Incontinence From Anatomical Causes			
Stress incontinence	Small-volume incontinence with coughing, sneezing, laughing, running; history of prior pelvic surgery	Pelvic floor relaxation; cystocele, rectocele; lax urethral sphincter; loss of urine with provocative testing; atrophic vaginitis	U/A and culture; PVR normal
Urge incontinence	Uncontrolled urge to void; large-volume incontinence; history of CNS disorders, such as stroke, multiple sclerosis, parkinsonism	Normal examination	U/A and culture; PVR normal; office cystometrography: <300-350-ml volume; BUN, creatinine, urodynamic testing
Overflow incontinence	Small-volume incontinence, dribbling, hesitancy; in men symptoms of enlarged prostate: nocturia, dribbling, hesitancy, decreased force and caliber of stream; in neurogenic bladder: history of bowel problems, spinal cord injury, or multiple sclerosis	Distended bladder; prostate hypertrophy, stool in rectum; fecal impaction; in neurogenic bladder: evidence of spinal cord disease or diabetic neuropathy; lax sphincter; gait disturbance	U/A and culture; PVR >100 ml; BUN, creatinine; in neurogenic bladder, refer for testing
Incontinence From Reversible Factors			
Medications	Hypnotics, diuretics, anticholinergic agents, α-adrenergic agents, calcium channel blockers	Normal except for findings related to other physical conditions	U/A to rule out urinary tract problems; blood chemistry to rule out systemic problem
Urinary tract infection (UTI)	Dysuria, urgency, daytime accidents	Frequency, odor, fever	U/A and culture
Vaginitis	Itching, odor	Discharge, atrophic vaginitis, evidence of sexual abuse	Gram stain, KOH, culture
Constipation/fecal impaction	Abdominal pain	Soiling; stool felt in colon and/or ampulla	None
Change in mental or functional status	Change in mental status; impaired mobility; new environment	Impaired mental status; impaired mobility	U/A and culture; blood chemistry
Diabetes insipidus (DI)	History of trauma to head; thirst, frequency	Weight loss	U/A specific gravity >1.015
Diabetes mellitus (DM)	Thirsty, increased frequency	Weight loss	U/A; serum glucose

Continued

DIFFERENTIAL DIAGNOSIS OF *Common Causes of Urinary Incontinence* *—cont'd*

CONDITION	HISTORY	PHYSICAL FINDINGS	DIAGNOSTIC STUDIES
Enuresis From Organic Causes			
Genitourinary causes	UTI history; dribbling; urine leakage	Fever, abdominal tenderness; anatomical abnormalities (ectopic ureter); examination may be normal	U/A and culture; specific gravity; referral for testing
Neurological causes	Head injury; spinal cord injury; polydipsia, polyuria; sleep apnea	Lax sphincter, spinal tuft, neurological deficits; altered gait; examination may be normal	U/A and culture; specific gravity; referral for evaluation
Enuresis From Nonorganic Causes			
Primary enuresis	Child has never been dry; may have family history	Normal examination; developmental delay	U/A and culture; specific gravity to rule out other causes
Developmental (secondary) enuresis	Child has been dry for 6 mo in a row; changes or stresses in child's life	Examine for genital trauma or abuse, infection, distended colon, fecal impaction	U/A and culture; specific gravity to rule out other causes; screen for glycosuria
Small bladder	Void frequently, not in excessive volume	None	Bladder capacity = child's age + 2, for children <11 yr
Sickle cell anemia	Family history	Findings related to sickle cell disease	U/A and culture; specific gravity

CHAPTER RESOURCES

Alper B, Curry S: Urinary tract infection in children, *Am Fam Physican* 72(12):2483, 2005.

Burkhart KS: Urinary incontinence in women: assessment and management in the primary care setting, *Nurse Pract Forum* 11:192, 2000.

Culligan P, Heit M: Urinary incontinence in women: evaluation and management, *Am Fam Physician* 62:2433, 2447, 2452, 2000.

Eslami MS, Friedman JL: Urinary incontinence: is there effective therapy? *Consultant* June:905, 2004.

Hay-Smith EJ, Bo Berghmans LC, Hendriks HJ et al: Pelvic floor muscle training for urinary incontinence in women, *Cochrane Database Syst Rev* (1):CD001407, 2001.

Ma JF, Shortliffe LM: Urinary tract infection in children: etiology and epidemiology, *Urol Clin North Am* 31(3):517, 2004.

Vapnek JM: Urinary incontinence: screening and treatment of urinary dysfunction, *Geriatrics* 56:25, 2001.

Zorc J, Kiddoo D, Shaw K: Diagnosis and management of pediatric urinary tract infections, *Clin Microbiol Rev* 18(2):417, 2005.

18

Urinary Problems in Females and Children

Common urinary complaints from females include changes in usual urination patterns (frequency, urgency, nocturia, incontinence), changes in urine appearance (color, cloudiness), and pain (dysuria, flank pain, or suprapubic pain).

Urinary problems in females may be caused by infection, inflammation, calculi (stones), congenital malformation, or trauma. The majority of urinary tract infections (UTIs) are caused by gram-negative bacteria, predominantly *Escherichia coli*. The sexually transmitted pathogens *Chlamydia trachomatis, Neisseria gonorrhoeae,* and herpes simplex are common causes of urethritis. Vaginitis may also cause urinary symptoms in women. Urinary stones may occur anywhere in the urinary tract and are common causes of pain, bleeding, obstruction, and secondary infection.

UTI in children is the second most common clinical disease of childhood, following respiratory tract disorders. The symptoms of urinary tract disorder may be vague or absent, making the diagnosis easily overlooked. Infection may be present without symptoms, with symptoms that are obviously related to the urinary system, or with symptoms that may divert attention to another organ system problem. Abdominal masses in the newborn are most frequently caused by renal enlargement, specifically dysplastic kidney and/or congenital hydronephrosis. Vesicoureteral reflux (VUR) is the major structural abnormality associated with UTI and renal damage.

Trauma to the urinary tract may be caused by penetrating, blunt, or crushing injuries or by surgery or instrumentation. Hematuria, oliguria, and pain are the most common symptoms.

DIAGNOSTIC REASONING: FOCUSED HISTORY

Are There Systemic or Upper Urinary Tract Symptoms Present?

Key Questions
- Have you had a fever or chills?
- Have you had nausea or vomiting?
- Have you had acute pain in the abdomen or back?
- Are you positive for HIV infection or receiving chemotherapy?
- In an infant: Has the infant been irritable or had anorexia or lethargy?

Fever and Chills

The presence of fever and chills suggests a systemic inflammatory response and indicates an acute condition that should be aggressively treated. Suspect pyelonephritis or lithiasis of the upper urinary system. UTI is the most common bacterial infection in febrile infants and children who present without an obvious source of infection.

Nausea and Vomiting

Nausea and vomiting often accompany upper UTI, pyelonephritis, or lithiasis. Like fever and chills, these symptoms suggest a systemic inflammatory response and indicate that the patient may be acutely ill. In newborns and infants, nonspecific symptoms, such as vomiting, diarrhea, and feeding difficulties, may indicate UTI.

Acute Pain

Acute pain in the back or abdomen suggests upper UTI and pyelonephritis. Flank pain occurs with stretching of the renal capsule, associated with parenchymal swelling, and may indicate infection, obstruction, or primary renal disease.

Urinary tract stones may produce localized back pain or excruciating pain that often radiates to the thigh.

Immunocompromised Patients

Immunocompromised patients are susceptible to overwhelming infections by both common and atypical organisms, and aggressive investigation is warranted.

Irritable Infant

UTI in neonates and infants is manifested in subtle ways, such as irritability, anorexia, and weight loss. Some infants with UTI present with bacteremia.

Is There Hematuria?

Key Questions

- Have you had blood in your urine? When in the stream does it occur?
- Do you have pain with urination?
- Do you have bleeding without urination?
- Have you done any strenuous exercise recently?

Hematuria

Red-to-brown discoloration is commonly caused by infection, trauma, or urinary tract stones. It can also be caused by parenchymal renal disease, systemic disease, medications, or coagulopathies.

Pyelonephritis or urinary tract stones are common causes of gross (macroscopic) hematuria. Neoplasm, trauma, and some medications can also produce gross hematuria. Gross hematuria occurs in 60% to 90% of bladder tumors. Both bladder and renal neoplasms are less common in women than in men. Hematuria can be produced by local irritation in cystitis. Qualitative and quantitative platelet disorders and hemophilia can cause both gross and microscopic bleeding. Urinary frequency or urgency, dysuria, or suprapubic pain suggests that the origin of hematuria is confined to the lower urinary tract.

Initial hematuria (at the beginning of urination) suggests the urethra is the source, whereas terminal hematuria (at the end of urination) suggests posterior urethra or bladder base involvement. Total hematuria means red blood cells are dispersed throughout the urinary stream, characterizing origination in the kidney, ureter, or bladder.

Pain

Hematuria without pain is usually caused by renal disease or tumor of the bladder or kidney. Other causes of painless hematuria include stones, polycystic kidney disease, renal cysts, sickle cell disease, and hydronephrosis. When discomfort such as renal colic accompanies hematuria, suspect an ureteral stone. Hematuria with dysuria suggests bladder infection or lithiasis.

Bleeding Without Urination

Bladder lesions may produce bleeding independent of micturition.

Strenuous Exercise

Transient hematuria is frequent after strenuous exercise, and the amount of bleeding is proportional to the amount of exercise and the trauma sustained by the urinary tract. Exercise-related hematuria is caused by direct trauma to the kidneys and bladder, as well as by ischemic injury. It is caused by the shifting of blood flow from the renal circulation to the heart, lung, and skeletal muscles during periods of high oxygen demand.

Can the Symptoms Be Localized to the Lower Urinary Tract?

Key Questions

- What are your primary symptoms (e.g., pain, frequency, urgency, small amounts of urine, nausea, nocturia, itching)?
- Have you had any suprapubic pain?
- Do you have involuntary urination?

Primary Symptoms

Dysuria suggests inflammation of the bladder neck or urethra, usually caused by bacterial infection or irritation, that injures the bladder mucosa, leading to inflammatory changes, infiltration, and edema. These changes can result in urgency and frequency, from mild stretching of the bladder to a loss of bladder elasticity.

Dysuria is the cardinal symptom of uncomplicated lower urinary tract infection (acute bacterial cystitis). In children, it may also be the first indication of an anatomical lesion such as obstruction of the urinary tract or VUR. Other common symptoms include frequency, mild nausea, nocturia, urgency, and voiding small amounts. Fever is notably absent. Infants may have strong-smelling urine and continuously damp diapers.

Dysuria also suggests urethritis, especially if accompanied by vaginal discharge. External dysuria, a burning sensation as the urine passes the inflamed labia, suggests vulvovaginitis. Patients with vulvovaginitis may also complain of discharge, odor, or itching. Women who have active herpes lesions may also experience external dysuria. Young children with pinworms (*Enterobius vermicularis*) may have dysuria and vaginitis because of the abrasions that result from periurethral and perivaginal itching and scratching.

Interstitial cystitis produces diminished bladder capacity along with symptoms of frequent painful urination. Hematuria may be present. Increased frequency can also occur as a result of stones or tumor.

Suprapubic Discomfort and Urinary Incontinence

Discomfort in the suprapubic area is indicative of bladder involvement and urinary incontinence and is characteristic of bladder neck irritability caused by inflammation. Local causes of incontinence can also include pelvic relaxation and impaired bladder muscle activity. Preschool-age children with UTIs frequently have enuresis (see Chapter 17).

Could This Be the Result of Trauma?

Key Questions
- Have you had any recent injury?
- Have you been hit recently?

- If a child: Have you noticed the child putting foreign objects in his or her genital tract?

Recent Injury
Injury or a blow to the flank area can produce hematuria, originating from the kidney. Straddle injury may result in abrasions and local inflammation, causing pain on urination. About 5% of childhood trauma involves the kidney, making it a relatively uncommon event. About 10% of the injured kidneys have underlying abnormalities, such as hydronephrosis or a horseshoe shape, making them more vulnerable to injury.

Trauma
A victim of domestic violence may present with blood in the urine secondary to trauma. Trauma may or may not be associated with pain. Active children may not remember trauma to the area.

Foreign Objects
Children have a propensity to put foreign objects in any orifice. Placing foreign objects in the vagina may cause dysuria and pyuria.

Could This Be Genitourinary in Origin?

Key Questions
- Are you sexually active? How frequently do you engage in sexual activity?
- Have you had a new sexual partner recently?
- How many sexual partners do you have?
- Does your sexual partner have any symptoms?
- Do you use a diaphragm?
- Do you have any vaginal discharge?
- If a postmenopausal woman: Are you on hormone replacement therapy?

Sexual Activity
Factors that contribute to the development of acute bacterial cystitis include frequent sexual intercourse, use of a diaphragm, and use of spermicidal gel for contraception. Urethritis is associated with a history of a new sexual partner, a partner with urethritis,

and multiple sexual partners. Masturbation may also cause dysuria in girls, as a result of either local irritation or the introduction of organisms that produce a lower UTI.

Organisms from sexually transmitted infections can cause urethritis when they are present in large numbers in the urethra. A local inflammatory response results. *C. trachomatis* is the most common pathogen, although *N. gonorrhoeae*, *Trichomonas vaginalis*, and herpes simplex can also cause urethritis. Active herpes lesions can also produce dysuria as the urine passes across the inflamed external mucosa.

Diaphragm Use
Some women who use a diaphragm experience mechanical compression of the urethra, with subsequent urine retention that predisposes them to the development of cystitis.

Vaginal Discharge and Hormone Therapy
Vaginal infections are a common cause of dysuria, particularly in college-age women. Atrophic vaginitis can also cause dysuria. Postmenopausal women who are not on hormone therapy are more likely to have atrophic vaginitis.

Are There Any Specific Risk Factors to Point Me in the Right Direction?

Key Questions
- Have you had this or similar problems before? If yes, when and how many times?
- Have you had recent catheterization or urinary tract procedures performed?
- Is there a family history of kidney or urinary problems?
- Do you have diabetes?
- How much spicy food, caffeinated beverages/food, carbonated beverages, or alcohol do you consume?
- How much water do you drink?
- Do you suppress the urge to urinate (postpone urination)?
- Do you use bubble baths, shampoos, feminine hygiene products, powders, and soaps?
- Do you have constipation?

History of Similar Problems
Patients with previous urinary problems are at risk for chronic relapsing conditions, such as unresolved infections, resistant strains of organisms, or reinfection.

Recent Instrumentation
Recent instrumentation in the urinary tract places the patient at risk for infections.

Family History of Urinary Problems
A family history of renal or urinary tract problems places the patient at increased risk for urinary tract disorders. A family history of deafness or renal insufficiency suggests hereditary nephritis or Alport's syndrome.

History of Diabetes Mellitus
Diabetes mellitus is associated with recurrent bacterial cystitis.

Types of Food Consumed
Dysuria without pyuria can be caused by chemical irritants, such as spicy foods, caffeine, carbonation, and alcohol.

Decreased Fluid Intake
Decreased fluid intake with concentrated urine produces an irritant effect on bladder mucosa and may be a cause of dysuria without pyuria. It can also predispose to the development of bacterial cystitis.

Urge to Urinate
Women who ignore the urge to urinate or who postpone urination are predisposed to the development of bacterial cystitis. Urine in the bladder for a prolonged period promotes bacterial growth.

Girls who have a history of squatting or leg crossing to stop urination may have a UTI. Uncontrolled bladder contractions against a closed bladder sphincter cause the behavior. These children may develop vesicoureteral reflux and infection.

Bubble Bath and Hygiene Products
Common chemical irritants can cause dysuria without infection. The most common irritant, particularly in children, is found in bubble baths.

Constipation

Mechanical factors related to compression of the bladder and bladder neck by a hard mass of stool from constipation may cause UTI. There is also a relationship between constipation and dysfunctional voiding accompanied by incomplete bladder emptying.

What Else Could This Be?

Key Questions

- Have you had recent treatment for a sexually transmitted infection?
- Have you been diagnosed with, but not treated for, a sexually transmitted infection?
- Have you had excessive urination?
- Have you had a sore throat or been treated for strep throat recently?

Sexually Transmitted Infections

Because vaginitis may cause urinary tract symptoms in females, a sexually transmitted vaginitis may be producing symptoms. Recent treatment for a sexually transmitted infection may indicate treatment failure, a coinfection that was not covered by the prescribed drug, or a reinfection (see Chapter 21).

Excessive Urination

The presence of polyuria suggests diabetes mellitus or diabetes insipidus. Women with diabetes mellitus are also prone to development of UTIs.

Recent Streptococcal Infection

Poststreptococcal glomerulonephritis may develop after a 1- to 3-week latency period following pharyngeal or skin infections with certain strains of group A β-hemolytic *Streptococcus*. The peak incidence is at age 7.

DIAGNOSTIC REASONING: FOCUSED PHYSICAL EXAMINATION

Note General Appearance

A patient who appears ill or who is pacing in pain is likely to have an upper urinary tract problem such as pyelonephritis or urolithiasis. Patients with lower urinary tract problems usually do not present with signs of systemic involvement, are free of fever, and generally appear well. Neonates present with malaise, irritability, and difficulty feeding. Toddlers and preschoolers appear ill with nausea, vomiting, and diarrhea.

Obtain Vital Signs, Height, and Weight

Failure to thrive is a common presenting sign of urinary tract disease in neonates or young children. Hypertension is seen in patients with nephritis.

Examine the Skin

Neonates with UTI may present with jaundice.

Palpate and Percuss for Flank Pain and at the Costovertebral Angle Bilaterally

Pain that is reproducible is indicative of renal capsule distention and characterizes acute pyelonephritis or acute ureteral obstruction.

Palpate and Percuss the Abdomen

Polycystic kidneys may produce abdominal distention. A flank mass may indicate a hydronephrotic kidney. Pain in the lower quadrant indicates lower ureter involvement. Suprapubic tenderness is characteristic of lower UTI. Perform deep palpation to identify kidneys or other abdominal masses. Normal kidneys are usually not easily palpated. A distended bladder rises above the symphysis pubis and is characteristic of residual urine resulting from incomplete bladder emptying. Palpation of an enlarged bladder may cause pain. In hypertensive patients, auscultate at the subcostal anterior abdomen for bruits that could indicate a renovascular cause of hypertension.

Inspect the Perirectal Area

Inspect the skin and hair for inflammation or lesions, parasites, or dermatitis. Note inflammation, presence of lesions, or vaginal discharge. Observe for the presence of labial adhesions that might predispose the child to perineal bacterial colonization. Note personal hygiene. External excoriation could be the cause of burning or pain on urination. Note if there are any abrasions, tears, or bruising present, which might indicate trauma and/or sexual abuse.

Perform a Pelvic Examination if Indicated

A pelvic examination is essential if you suspect vaginitis or vulvovaginitis as a cause of the urinary tract symptom(s). On external examination, observe for bladder or uterine prolapse. On internal examination, note vaginal color, moistness, rugation, and characteristics of discharge. Pale, dry mucosa with lack of rugation characterizes atrophic vaginitis in a mature woman. Vaginal discharge not characteristic of physiological discharge suggests a vaginal infection. For discussion of vulvovaginitis, see Chapter 21. Determine rectal tone. An atonic anal sphincter suggests a neurogenic bladder. Rectal examination for fecal impaction is indicated if the history suggests significant constipation or encopresis.

LABORATORY AND DIAGNOSTIC STUDIES

The extent of diagnostic investigation is determined by the history and the findings of the examination. The symptoms reported by the patient are taken into account when ordering diagnostic tests to corroborate or verify the diagnosis. General screening tests can be used to provide additional data for patients with urinary tract problems.

Urine should be freshly voided and usually taken midstream. If not examined immediately, the specimen should be refrigerated because cells begin to disintegrate after 1 to 2 hours.

Urine Dipstick

Reagent strips can be used to screen urine in the clinical setting.

Specific Gravity

Urine specific gravity depends on the patient's hydration. The urine pH also depends on the level of hydration, as well as acid-base status, time of urine collection, diet, and drugs that may affect the urine pH.

Leukocyte Esterase

The leukocyte esterase strip is calibrated to turn purple in 60 seconds, indicating 5 or more white blood cells in the urine. A positive test is indicative of urethritis (75% to 90% sensitivity, 95% specificity). Urine that tests positive for leukocyte esterase should be cultured for bacteria. Vaginal infection with *Trichomonas* can produce false positive results; diets high in vitamin C can produce false negative results.

Nitrite

The nitrite strip is calibrated to turn pink within 30 seconds and signifies nitrite produced by 105 or more organisms/ml. Urine that tests positive for nitrites should be cultured for bacteria. However, note that some organisms that cause UTIs do not convert nitrates to nitrites (e.g., *Staphylococcus* and *Streptococcus*).

Protein

The normally small amount of protein excreted by a healthy adult is usually not detectable by dipstick analysis until the patient excretes 150 to 300 mg/day. At this level the patient will show trace amounts. In healthy persons, urine contains no protein or only trace amounts of proteins, which consists of albumin and globulins from the plasma. Glomeruli usually prevent the passage of protein from the blood to the glomerular filtrate; therefore the persistent presence of protein in urine is a strong indication of renal disease. If more than a trace amount of proein is found, then a quantitative 24-hour evaluation is necessary. False positive results can occur with alkaline urine.

If the patient has trace levels of proteinuria, then the use of 20% sulfosalicylic acid testing for protein is appropriate. Add 8 drops of 20% sulfosalicylic acid to a sample of fresh, concentrated urine. Protein concentration is directly proportional to the degree of white turbidity produced. The absence of white turbidity indicates a false positive result by dipstick analysis.

A typical scale to indicate progressively increasing amounts of protein is 1+ (30 mg/dl), 2+ (100 mg/dl), 3+ (300 mg/dl), and 4+ (500 to 1000 mg/dl). Peripheral edema and ascites may be present in an adult who has 3+ or 4+ proteinuria and is typically excreting 3 g or more of protein per day. Proteinuria reported for a single urinalysis is not an absolute guide in a differential diagnosis because proteinuria may be glomerular or tubular.

Glucose

Glucose in the urine is indicative of an elevated serum glucose concentration greater than 200 mg/dl. If serum glucose levels are normal while urine glucose level is elevated, then proximal renal tubular damage should be suspected.

Ketones

Ketones are detected earlier in the urine than in the blood and may indicate starvation or diabetic ketoacidosis.

Blood

Reagent strips are calibrated to detect the red blood cells (RBCs) that are present. The strip detects heme at 0.05 to 0.3 mg of hemoglobin/dl (see later paragraph titled Red Blood Cells).

Urinalysis With Microscopic Examination

Color

The urine should be clear to yellow, depending on the concentration. The precipitation of calcium phosphate or urates can turn the urine milky, especially when stored in the refrigerator. Warming the urine to body temperature causes these precipitated salts to return to solution, removing the milky appearance. Methylene blue and indigo blue can make the urine blue. Vegetable dyes and paint from toys ingested by young children can turn their urine various colors. Brown urine is often observed in glomerulonephritis. Turbidity with a foul odor indicates infection. Color changes of the urine may result from various sources: hemoglobin from systemic red blood cell lysis; myoglobin from damaged muscle cells or rhabdomyolysis; vegetable pigments from food, such as red beets; pigments from drugs, such as rifampin and phenazopyridine; or porphyrins from porphyria.

Discoloration of the urine should be investigated with microscopic examination to determine if RBCs or any foreign substances are present. Pyuria results from white blood cell (WBC) debris and leukocytes in the urine, but cloudy urine can also result from other causes.

Sediment

Sediment for casts, blood cells, and bacteria can be detected by microscopic examination. Casts indicate hemorrhage or various conditions of the nephron. RBCs indicate acute inflammatory or vascular disorders of the glomerulus. More than 1 or 2 RBCs per high-power field (HPF) is abnormal and can indicate renal or systemic disease or trauma to the kidney. Sediment is labeled as active when an abnormal number of cells, tubular casts, crystals, or infectious organisms are found.

A healthy person's urinalysis usually contains no cells, although an occasional cell per HPF is seen. More than 1 tubular epithelial and transitional epithelial cell per HPF suggests damage to the tubules or bladder wall. More than 1 RBC or WBC per HPF is considered abnormal. The more cells per HPF, the more active may be the renal disease.

Microscopic examination of the urine resulting in 20 or more organisms per HPF indicates UTI. Fewer than 20 organisms per HPF merits further study such as culture and sensitivity (C & S).

Red Blood Cells

Hematuria is the presence of more than 3 RBCs/HPF. Distorted, irregularly shaped cells suggest a glomerular problem. The major causes of hematuria include acute and chronic prostatitis or urethritis, hemorrhagic cystitis, renal stones, or tumors of the kidney, renal pelvis, ureter, bladder, and urethra. Hematuria with proteinuria usually suggests a renal origin. Isolated hematuria is usually produced by sites outside the kidneys.

White Blood Cells

Pyuria (>5 WBCs/HPF) is highly sensitive for the presence of a UTI. However, it may occur with dehydration, renal stones, appendicitis, or other extrinsic ureteral irritation in the absence of demonstrable microbial infection.

Casts

Tubular casts are formed in the distal portion of the nephron. A hyaline cast is a wispy, translucent, cylindrical replica of the tubular lumen. Red cell casts are characteristic of glomerular origin. The presence of abnormal cells, protein, hemoglobin, myoglobin, or other debris with a cast helps identify the type of renal disease.

Urine Culture and Sensitivity

Culture is indicated in children if you are uncertain of a diagnosis of uncomplicated lower tract UTI based on clinical findings and urinalysis or if the patient has signs and symptoms of an upper UTI or complicated UTI.

Potassium Hydroxide (KOH) and Wet Mount/Preparation

Perform these procedures if you suspect vulvovaginitis as a cause of the urinary tract symptoms. See Chapter 21 for an explanation and a discussion of these procedures.

Vaginal Culture/Molecular Testing for Infectious Organisms

Use these testing procedures to diagnose or confirm vaginal infection (see Chapter 21).

Ultrasonography

Ultrasonography is a noninvasive technique than can provide information about the kidneys, ureters, bladder, and vascular structures. Renal ultrasound is a good first test to determine kidney size, contour, and the presence of calculi. Urinary bladder sonogram is used to identify tumors of the bladder, thickening of the bladder wall, posterior masses behind the bladder, or obstruction of the lower urinary tract showing residual urine.

Radiography

A flat plate of the abdomen can be used to identify structures of the kidney, ureters, and bladder. Urinary calculi are usually visible on radiographs.

Computed Tomography

Noncontrast helical (spiral) CT is the gold standard for evaluating kidney stones. It has 95% sensitivity and 98% specificity.

DIFFERENTIAL DIAGNOSIS

Uncomplicated Urinary Tract Infection (UTI)

Uncomplicated lower UTIs (bacterial cystitis) are common in women. Uncomplicated UTIs occur in individuals with normal urinary tract anatomy and function. Patients present with dysuria and may have urinary frequency, hematuria, back pain, mild nausea, nocturia, urgency, and voiding of small amounts. Fever is notably absent in adults but may be present in pediatric patients. Neonates may present with prolonged jaundice and failure to thrive.

The adult patient appears well on physical examination and may or may not have costovertebral angle (CVA) tenderness. Clinical diagnosis is supported by urine dipstick findings, which may include the presence of blood, leukocyte esterase, and nitrites. However, a negative dipstick result does not rule out UTI. Microscopic analysis may show the presence of RBCs and WBCs. No casts will be present. Urine culture and sensitivity will confirm the diagnosis. See Box 18-1 for evidence supporting the diagnosis of uncomplicated UTI.

Urethritis

Dysuria suggests urethritis, especially if accompanied by vaginal discharge. The history often includes a new sex partner, frequent sex, a partner with urethritis, or multiple sex partners. As with uncomplicated UTI, the patient appears well and on physical examination has no CVA tenderness or fever. On urinalysis using a dipstick, findings may include the presence of blood, leukocyte esterase, and nitrites, although the patient may have urethritis in the absence of these findings. Urine culture or molecular testing confirms the presence of the offending pathogens, usually *Chlamydia, N. gonorrhoeae, Trichomonas,* and herpes.

Box 18-1	**Evidence-Based Practice: Diagnosing Uncomplicated UTI**

In a systematic review, Bent et al. (2002) report four symptoms (dysuria, frequency, hematuria, and back pain) and one sign (costovertebral angle tenderness) that significantly increase the probability of uncomplicated UTI. In women who present with one or more of these symptoms, the probability of infection is about 50%. Specific combinations of symptoms, such as dysuria and frequency without vaginal discharge and irritation, raise the probability of UTI to more than 90%. If the dipstick result is positive, the probability of UTI is high, but if the dipstick result is negative, the probability of UTI is still high and a urine culture should be considered to rule out infection. The absence of dysuria, the absence of back pain, a history of vaginal discharge and irritation, and the presence of vaginal discharge on examination significantly decrease the probability of UTI.

Conclusion: History alone may effectively rule in the diagnosis of uncomplicated UTI. However, the history and physical examination and dipstick urinalysis cannot reliably rule out UTI in women who present with urinary tract symptoms.

Data from Bent S, Mallamothu BK, Simel DL et al: Does this woman have an acute uncomplicated urinary tract infection? *JAMA* 287(20):2701, 2002.

Vulvovaginitis

Vulvovaginitis is a common cause of dysuria. The patient often describes the dysuria as "external"—a burning sensation as the urine passes inflamed labia. The patient usually has a history of vaginal discharge, odor, and/or itching. On physical examination, discharge is usually present in the vagina or from the cervix. Wet mount, KOH, and vaginal culture or molecular testing for infectious organisms can confirm the diagnosis (see Chapter 21).

In older women, atrophic vaginitis may produce urinary tract symptoms. These women may be perimenopausal or post-menopausal. Women with atrophic vaginitis may complain of vaginal dryness or discomfort during sexual intercourse. On physical examination, the vaginal mucosa is thin, pale, and dry, with less rugation. Diagnosis is made on the basis of clinical findings.

Interstitial Cystitis

Interstitial cystitis produces diminished bladder capacity along with symptoms of frequent, painful urination. Hematuria may be present. The cause is unknown but may be related to collagen disease, may be an autoimmune disorder or an allergic manifestation, or may occur secondary to an unidentified infectious agent. The bladder wall becomes inflamed, with mucosal ulceration and scarring that produce contraction of the smooth muscle and cause the symptoms. Middle-age women are most often affected. Typically, the patient appears well and has no physical findings. Suprapubic tenderness may be present. Urinalysis is usually negative. This is a diagnosis of exclusion, and the patient is often frustrated because no cause has been previously found for her long-standing and persistent symptoms. The patient has no evidence of urological disease on radiographic and cystometric studies. Cystoscopic evidence of interstitial disease includes focal ulceration, edema, and perivascular infiltrates.

Pyelonephritis

The patient presents with fever and chills, appears toxic, and complains of back pain. Nausea and vomiting may be present. Some patients also complain of lower urinary tract symptoms, including frequency and dysuria. The patient feels and looks ill. On physical examination, CVA tenderness is usually present. The abdomen may also be tender. On microscopic examination, WBCs are usually present. White cell casts suggest pyelonephritis. Bacterial casts, although rare, are pathognomonic of pyelonephritis. Urine culture and sensitivity confirm diagnosis and identify the pathogen—usually *E. coli, Klebsiella, Proteus mirabilis,* or *Enterobacter.*

Urolithiasis

Urinary stones can occur anywhere in the urinary tract and may produce symptoms of acute pain, hematuria, and secondary infection. Many calculi are "silent" and may cause only hematuria, either microscopic or gross. Renal calculi may occur when a stone obstructs the urinary tract. Typical symptoms of renal colic include severe flank pain that radiates along the pathway of the ureter to the inner thigh. Chills, fever, and urinary frequency are common. The patient may have nausea, vomiting, and abdominal distention.

The clinical diagnosis is supported by urinalysis and imaging findings. The urine may be normal; however, gross or microscopic hematuria is common. Pyuria (WBCs) with or without bacteria may be present. Crystalline structures may be present. Noncontrast helical (spiral) CT is the gold standard for evaluating kidney stones.

Poststreptococcal Glomerulonephritis

This condition is an immune-mediated nephritis. It occurs most commonly in elementary school children. There is a history of recent streptococcal skin or pharyngeal infection within the past 1 to 3 weeks. Anorexia, vom-

iting, fever, abdominal pain, headache, and lethargy are reported. On physical examination, periorbital edema is usually present, as is hypertension. Orthopnea, dyspnea, cough, and rales may be present. Hematuria and proteinuria are present. A positive serum ASO titer confirms recent infection. A depressed serum concentration of C3 is found in the first few days of the disease.

Chemical Irritation

There is a history of the use of bubble baths, body lotions, soaps, and sprays. The patient experiences frequency, burning, and urgency with small volumes of voided urine. Children will frequently suppress voiding because of pain. Physical examination may reveal erythema of the labia and urethral outlet. Laboratory examination may reveal pyuria and bacteriuria as a result of local infection and denudation.

DIFFERENTIAL DIAGNOSIS OF *Common Causes of Urinary Problems in Females and Children*

CONDITION	HISTORY	PHYSICAL FINDINGS	DIAGNOSTIC STUDIES
Uncomplicated UTI	Dysuria, frequency, mild nausea, nocturia, urgency, voiding small amounts; neonates and young infants present with anorexia, irritability, fever	No fever; appears well; no CVA tenderness; may have suprapubic tenderness; Note: neonates and young infants may present with failure to thrive, bacteremia	Urine dipstick: + blood, + leukocyte esterase, + nitrites; microscopic analysis: RBCs, WBCs, no casts; urine C & S; in children, voiding cystourethrogram and renal ultrasound are recommended
Urethritis	Dysuria; vaginal discharge; history of new sex partner, frequent sex, partner with urethritis, multiple sex partners	Appears well; has no CVA tenderness or fever	Urine dipstick: may have + blood, + leukocyte esterase, + nitrites; urine culture; molecular testing vaginal specimen
Vulvovaginitis	History of vaginal itching, discharge, burning, dryness; postmenopausal	Inflamed or atrophic labia; vaginal or cervical discharge	Microscopic exam, vaginal cultures, molecular testing
Interstitial cystitis	Frequent painful urination; hematuria; most often middle-age women; often frustrated because no cause has been previously found for long-standing and persistent symptoms	Appears well and has no physical findings; suprapubic tenderness may be present	Urinalysis usually negative; x-ray and cystometric studies to rule out other urological disease; cystoscopy

Continued

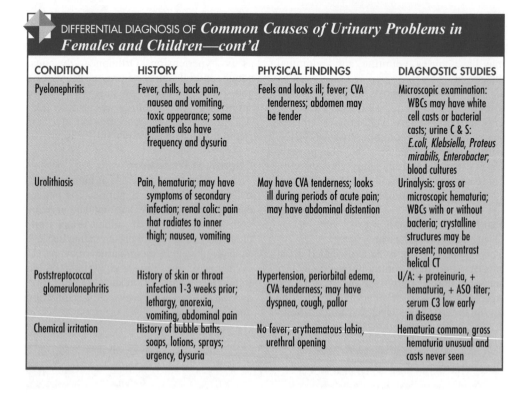

DIFFERENTIAL DIAGNOSIS OF *Common Causes of Urinary Problems in Females and Children—cont'd*

CONDITION	HISTORY	PHYSICAL FINDINGS	DIAGNOSTIC STUDIES
Pyelonephritis	Fever, chills, back pain, nausea and vomiting, toxic appearance; some patients also have frequency and dysuria	Feels and looks ill; fever; CVA tenderness; abdomen may be tender	Microscopic examination: WBCs may have white cell casts or bacterial casts; urine C & S: *E.coli, Klebsiella, Proteus mirabilis, Enterobacter,* blood cultures
Urolithiasis	Pain, hematuria; may have symptoms of secondary infection; renal colic: pain that radiates to inner thigh; nausea, vomiting	May have CVA tenderness; looks ill during periods of acute pain; may have abdominal distention	Urinalysis: gross or microscopic hematuria; WBCs with or without bacteria; crystalline structures may be present; noncontrast helical CT
Poststreptococcal glomerulonephritis	History of skin or throat infection 1-3 weeks prior; lethargy, anorexia, vomiting, abdominal pain	Hypertension, periorbital edema, CVA tenderness; may have dyspnea, cough, pallor	U/A: + proteinuria, + hematuria, + ASO titer; serum C3 low early in disease
Chemical irritation	History of bubble baths, soaps, lotions, sprays; urgency, dysuria	No fever; erythematous labia, urethral opening	Hematuria common, gross hematuria unusual and casts never seen

CHAPTER RESOURCES

Bartkowski DP: Recognizing UTIs in infants and children: early treatment prevents permanent damage, *Postgrad Med* 109:171, 2001.

Bent S, Mallamothu BK, Simel DL et al: Does this woman have an acute uncomplicated urinary tract infection? *JAMA* 287(20):2701, 2002.

Grossfeld GD, Wolf JS Jr, Litwan MS et al: Asymptomatic microscopic hematuria in adults: summary of the AUA best practice policy recommendations, *Am Fam Physician* 63:1145, 2001.

Lindbloom EJ: What is the best test to diagnose urinary tract stones? *J Fam Pract* 50:657, 2001.

Meyers K: Evaluation of hematuria in children, *Urol Clin North Am* 31(1):559, 2004.

Portis AJ, Sundaram CP: Diagnosis and initial management of kidney stones, *Am Fam Physician* 63:1329, 2001.

Roberts KB: The AAP practice parameter on urinary tract infections in febrile infants and young children. American Academy of Pediatrics, *Am Fam Physician* 62(8):1815, 2000.

Segura JW, Preminger GM, Assimos DG et al: Ureteral Stones Clinical Guidelines Panel summary report on the management of ureteral calculi. The American Urological Association, *J Urol* 158:1915, 1997.

The Institute for Clinical Systems Improvement (ICSI): *Uncomplicated urinary tract infection in women,* Bloomington, Minn, 2004, Institute for Clinical Systems Improvement (ICSI). Available at www.guideline.gov.

Genitourinary Problems in Males

Urinary tract problems in males represent a range of conditions from infections, inflammation, and urine outlet obstruction to congenital malformation, trauma, or neoplasm. Any part of the renal/urological/reproductive tract can be involved, and symptoms may often be localized to a single site. Symptoms may also be vague, reflect the involved area, or be referred from the actual site of involvement.

Dysuria in males is most commonly caused by urethritis, prostatitis, cystitis, and mechanical irritation of the urethra. Inflammation, although infrequent in young males, increases with age until elderly men are affected as frequently as elderly women.

Cystitis in men results from ascending infection of the urethra or prostate or occurs secondary to urethral instrumentation. The most common cause of recurrent cystitis in men is chronic bacterial prostatitis. *Escherichia coli* is the usual gram-negative pathogen. *Chlamydia trachomatis* is the major cause of prostatitis and nongonococcal urethritis in men under age 40 and is sexually transmitted. Recurrent urinary tract infections (UTIs) may involve resistant gram-negative *Klebsiella, Enterobacter, Pseudomonas,* or *Proteus mirabilis* or gram-positive *Enterococcus* and *Staphylococcus aureus*. Infection may involve the kidneys and cause pyelonephritis. Secondary infection can occur as the result of urinary stones.

The male patient with urinary problems may also present with symptoms involving urinary flow. Urine flow may be altered by compression of the urethra as it passes through an enlarged prostate, obstructing the flow of urine and producing hesitancy, slowing of the urinary stream, dribbling, and nocturia.

Benign prostatic hyperplasia (BPH) is common in men older than 50 and progresses with age until 80% of men over 80 are affected. Patients with BPH are more prone to UTIs and incontinence. Urinary stones may occur anywhere in the urinary tract and are common causes of obstructive symptoms, bleeding, and pain.

Trauma to the urinary tract may be caused by penetrating, straddle, blunt, or crushing injuries or by surgery or instrumentation. Hematuria, oliguria, and pain are the most common symptoms.

Neoplasms occur more often in males than in females. Kidney, prostate, and bladder neoplasms are more common in elderly men. Kidney and bladder neoplasms often produce painless hematuria. Prostate cancer may produce symptoms of outlet obstruction.

Kidney problems can range from asymptomatic blood chemical changes to life-threatening abnormal renal function that could manifest in fluid-electrolyte and acid-base imbalances. Patients with renal insufficiency may present with nonspecific complaints such as fatigue, anorexia, or weakness. A discussion of renal insufficiency and renal failure is beyond the scope of this chapter.

DIAGNOSTIC REASONING: FOCUSED HISTORY

Are Systemic or Acute Symptoms Present?

Key Questions

- Have you had fever, chills, nausea, or vomiting?
- Are you positive for HIV infection or receiving chemotherapy?

- Are you having acute pain?
- Have you been able to pass any urine?

Fever and Chills
The presence of fever and/or chills suggests a systemic inflammatory response and indicates that the patient may be acutely ill and should be aggressively treated. Specifically, suspect pyelonephritis or lithiasis of the upper urinary tract or prostatitis, orchitis, or epididymitis of the lower urinary tract.

Immunocompromised Patients
Immunocompromised patients are susceptible to overwhelming infections by both common and atypical organisms, and aggressive investigation is warranted.

Acute Pain
Acute pain in the abdomen or flank is characteristic of bladder, ureter, and kidney involvement. Acute pain in the scrotum or testicles may indicate infection or pathology of the scrotal contents or be referred pain from other sites in the urinary tract. Pain in the scrotum or testicles is characteristic of inflammation of the testicles, epididymitis, or torsion of a testicle (see Chapter 20).

Anuria
A sudden decrease in urinary output may result from compromised renal blood supply (prerenal); damaged interstitia, glomeruli, or tubules (intrarenal); or obstructed urine flow (postrenal). Patients with prerenal failure usually have a history of volume depletion or a reduction in arterial blood volume such as in low cardiac output states. Patients with intrarenal failure may present with history of renal damage from nephrotoxic agents. Postrenal failure is the least likely cause of anuria, but it should be ruled out first, because when failure results from obstructive causes, mechanical intervention may reestablish kidney function before permanent nephron damage occurs. Patients at greatest risk for acute renal failure are the elderly, diabetic patients, and those with a history of renal, heart, or liver disease.

Anuria may represent obstruction or renal failure.

Is There Hematuria?

Key Questions
- Have you noticed blood in your urine?
- Is there blood every time you urinate or just occasionally?
- Does the blood start with the beginning of urination, continue throughout urination, or occur only at the end of urination? Is there blood without urinating?
- Do you have pain with the blood?

Hematuria
Blood can enter the urinary tract at any site. The most common source of isolated hematuria is extrarenal. A lesion of the bladder or lower urinary tract is demonstrated in more than 60% of patients. The most common causes of gross hematuria from the kidney are nephropathy and polycystic kidney disease. No cause for hematuria can be found in 10% to 15% of patients.

Timing
Initial hematuria becomes clear during voiding and is indicative of anterior urethral lesions such as urethritis, stricture, or meatal stenosis. Terminal hematuria begins with clear urine and then becomes bloody and is suggestive of prostatic lesions or lesions in the prostatic urethra. Total hematuria is usually characteristic of lesions in the kidneys and ureters. Bladder lesions may produce bleeding independent of micturition. Recent trauma to the kidneys can also produce hematuria. Gross hematuria is often transient but may continue microscopically.

Pain
Hematuria with pain usually indicates the passage of a stone or sloughed renal papilla, often with concurrent infection. Painless gross hematuria is consistent with upper or lower tract tumor, systemic coagulopathy, or excessive anticoagulant effect. Less common causes include acute necrosis or sloughing of a papilla. In elderly men, painless hematuria may be a late presenting sign of renal cancer.

Can the Symptoms Be Localized to a Part of the Urinary Tract?

Key Questions

- Do you have trouble starting to urinate (e.g., slow/weakened urinary stream, dribbling of urine)?
- Do you have low back, flank, or abdominal pain?
- Do you have aching in the perineal area?
- Do you have suprapubic discomfort?
- Have you had involuntary urination?
- Do you have frequency, urgency, dysuria, or penile discharge?
- Do you have to urinate at night?
- Do you have an excessive volume of urine?

Hesitancy, Slow Urinary Stream, and Dribbling of Urine

In men older than 50, the presence of hesitancy, slow urinary stream, and dribbling of urine with a gradual onset over time indicates obstructive problems from benign prostatic hypertrophy. Have the patient complete the American Urological Association (AUA) Symptom Index (Table 19-1). Using the index, classify symptoms as mild (0 to 7), moderate (8 to 19), or severe (20 to 35).

Low Back, Flank, or Abdominal Pain

Patient reports of low back, flank, or abdominal pain are often indicative of ureteral and kidney involvement. Renal tract

---

Table 19-2	**The American Urological Association Symptom Index**

Patients rate their answers to each question on a scale of 0 to 5.

	AUA SYMPTOM SCORE (CIRCLE ONE NUMBER ON EACH LINE)[†]					
QUESTIONS	NOT AT ALL	LESS THAN 1 TIME IN 5	LESS THAN HALF THE TIME	ABOUT HALF THE TIME	MORE THAN HALF THE TIME	ALMOST ALWAYS
Over the past month, how often have you had a sensation of not emptying your bladder completely after you finished voiding?	0	1	2	3	4	5
Over the past month, how often have you had to urinate again less than 2 hours after you finished urinating?	0	1	2	3	4	5
Over the past month, how often have you found you stopped and started again several times when you urinated?	0	1	2	3	4	5
Over the past month, how often have you found it difficult to postpone urination?	0	1	2	3	4	5
Over the past month, how often have you had a weak urinary stream?	0	1	2	3	4	5
Over the past month, how often have you had to push or strain to begin urination?	0	1	2	3	4	5
Over the past month, how many times did you typically get up to urinate from the time you went to bed at night until the time you got up in the morning?	0	1	2	3	4	5

From Barry MJ, Fowler FJ Jr, O'Leary MP et al: The American Urological Association Symptom Index for benign prostatic hyperplasia. The Measurement Committee of the American Urological Association, *J Urol* 48(5):1549, 1992.
[†]AUA Symptom Score = sum of above circled numbers. Symptoms are classified as mild (0-7), moderate (8-19), or severe (20-35).

pain may present with a constant dull ache in the costovertebral angle (CVA) area. Dislodged kidney stones will produce an acute ureteral pain that is colicky and cyclic in nature. Gross blood in the urine and infection may accompany the ureteral pain. The pain can radiate to the abdomen, testes, and penis. However, renal disorders do not frequently cause pain. True renal pain can originate from the calyces or renal pelvis. Pain can result from stretching of the kidney capsule, interstitial edema, or inflammation of the capsule.

Aching in the Perineal Area

Prostate pain is often interpreted by the patient as a vague ache in the perineal area. The usual cause of perineal aching is infection; another cause may be prostatic stones with infection.

Suprapubic Discomfort and Urinary Incontinence

Discomfort in the suprapubic area is indicative of bladder involvement, whereas urinary incontinence is characteristic of bladder neck irritability caused by inflammation. Bladder pain is most often caused by infection; however, it can also be produced by obstruction and bladder distention as the result of tumor or stones.

Penile Discharge With Frequency, Urgency, and Dysuria

Penile discharge with frequency, urgency, and dysuria is characteristic of anterior urethral irritation in males and of exposure to a sexually transmitted infection (STI) (see Chapter 20).

Nocturia

Primary bladder disease from infection, stones, or tumors can produce nocturia. Prostate enlargement characteristically produces nocturia. Most adults do not need to void during the night, but some may get up once during the night depending on the amount and timing of fluid ingestion.

Patients who complain of daytime frequency without nocturia are usually free of organic disease.

Polyuria

Polyuria is defined as a volume greater than 3 L of urine/day and depends on fluid intake and the patient's state of hydration. Polyuria may be an early indication of renal disease progression because of the kidneys' inability to concentrate urine. Taking a history of fluid intake is important to identify possible causes of polyuria. Pseudopolyuria results from increased fluid ingestion and may present with certain personality disorders. With the current emphasis on water ingestion, however, a large fluid intake can also produce pseudopolyuria. Alcohol ingestion inhibits antidiuretic hormone; glycosuria promotes excess solute excretion. Diabetes insipidus may also be implicated. Nocturia can occur with the mobilization of fluid during sleep, secondary to congestive heart failure.

Are There Any Specific Risk Factors to Point Me in the Right Direction?

Key Questions

- Have you had this or similar problems before? If yes, when and how often have you had this problem?
- Do you have a family history of renal or kidney problems, prostatitis, or prostate cancer?
- How old are you? (What is the patient's age?)
- Have you been confined to bed (especially if elderly)?
- Are you sexually active? How many partners do you have?

History of Similar Problems

Patients with previous urinary problems are at risk for chronic relapsing conditions, such as unresolved infections, resistant strains of organisms, or reinfection. Recurrent infections, pyelonephritis, or complications warrant urological referral for workup and evaluation.

Family History of Urinary Problems

A family history of renal or kidney problems or prostatitis places the patient at increased risk for urinary problems. Familial disorders that may be implicated in kidney disease include diabetes mellitus, hypertension, collagen vascular disease, nephrolithiasis, and polycystic kidney disease.

Age
UTI in males increases with age. Slow development of prostatic obstruction is common in men older than 50 and is usually painless. Patients have difficulty starting the urine stream, and there is a decreased force of stream and dribbling after voiding. *Chlamydia* is the major cause of prostatitis, epididymitis, and nongonococcal urethritis in males under 40 years of age. Adolescents who are sexually active are at particular risk for STIs.

Confined to Bed
Elderly patients confined to bed are at an increased risk of infection. Likely mechanisms include urinary stasis and reflux.

Sexually Active
Sexually active males, especially those who engage in unprotected sex, are at risk for STIs, which can produce urethritis. The risk increases with multiple partners.

What Else Could This Be?

Key Questions
- Have you had recent instrumentation in the urethra or urinary tract?
- Have you had recent treatment for an STI?
- Have you been recently diagnosed with but not treated for an STI?
- What drugs have you taken (prescription, over the counter, or illicit)?
- What is your occupation? What are your hobbies (toxic exposure)?

Recent Instrumentation
Recent instrumentation in the urinary tract places the patient at risk for infections. Patients with indwelling catheters are also at risk for infection.

Recent Sexually Transmitted Infection
STIs can produce urethritis and urinary tract symptoms. Recent treatment for an STI

may indicate treatment failure, a coinfection that was not covered by the prescribed drug, or a reinfection.

Drug Review or History
The most prevalent nephrotoxic drugs include aminoglycosides, nonsteroidal anti-inflammatory drugs, iodinated radiocontrast media, and angiotensin-converting enzyme inhibitors. Less prevalent are antibiotics such as amphotericin B, chemotherapeutic agents, cocaine, H_2-receptor antagonists, phenytoin, sulfonamide diuretics, and volatile hydrocarbons.

Toxic Exposures
Occupational hazards that may cause kidney problems include exposure to volatile hydrocarbons, benzene, aniline, xylene, heavy metals, and ionizing radiation.

DIAGNOSTIC REASONING: FOCUSED PHYSICAL EXAMINATION
Note General Appearance
A patient who appears ill or who is in pain is likely to have an upper urinary tract problem such as pyelonephritis, urolithiasis, or acute prostatitis. Patients with lower urinary tract problems usually do not present with signs of systemic involvement, are free of fever, and generally appear well.

Obtain Vital Signs
Hypertension is seen in patients with nephritis.

Inspect Skin and Mucous Membranes
A pale skin color may suggest anemia caused by poor nutrition or chronic renal failure. Yellow-colored to brown-colored skin without scleral icterus may indicate severe chronic uremia. Other skin changes seen with renal problems may range from rash to purpura.

Hypertension and edema are two findings that usually indicate renal problems; however, a physical examination may not provide much data because few physical signs found on examination indicate the presence of kidney disease.

Palpate and Percuss for Flank Pain at the Costovertebral Angle

Pain that is reproducible is indicative of renal capsule distention and characterizes acute pyelonephritis or acute ureteral obstruction. Perinephric abscess may cause flank swelling and redness.

Palpate and Percuss the Abdomen

Abdominal distention suggests ascites or fluid collection in the bowel. Pain in the lower quadrant indicates lower ureter involvement. Perform deep palpation to identify kidneys or other abdominal masses. Normal kidneys are usually not easily palpated. A distended bladder rises above the symphysis pubis and is characteristic of residual urine from incomplete bladder emptying. Palpation of an enlarged bladder may cause pain. Chronic bladder distention is usually painless and cannot always be determined by manual palpation alone.

If the patient is hypertensive, auscultate at the subcostal anterior abdomen for bruit, which could indicate a renovascular cause of hypertension.

Inspect and Palpate the External Genitalia

Inspect the skin and hair for inflammation or lesions, parasites, or dermatitis. Note hair pattern distribution and level of development of structures for age-group. Palpate the shaft of the penis for strictures. Observe for phimosis if uncircumcised and retract the foreskin. Note inflammation or presence of smegma. Inspect glans, corona, and frenulum areas for lesions. Note personal hygiene, phimosis in uncircumcised males, and presence of urine, discharge, and fecal stains on undergarments. Check position of urethral meatus. Strip or milk the penis from the base toward the glans or head of the penis. Note any discharge for color, consistency, and amount.

Check scrotum skin surfaces and testicles for tenderness and masses; also check epididymis, spermatic cords, and inguinal canals. The left scrotal sac usually hangs lower than the right. Elevation of an affected testicle may relieve discomfort and is characteristic of epididymitis. A painful scrotal mass is usually associated with inflammation or testicular torsion.

Perform scrotal transillumination in a darkened room. Do not use a halogen light source because it may burn the patient. A solid mass prevents the passage of light and requires further examination. A hydrocele is a nontender firm mass that results from fluid accumulation. It will transilluminate but may make testicular palpation impossible. A spermatocele (a cystic swelling on the epididymis) is not as large as a hydrocele but does not transilluminate. Dilated veins in the scrotal sac, or varicocele, is the most common scrotal mass, usually occurring on the left side. A varicocele is often more prominent when the patient is standing and regresses with the patient in the prone position. It is classically described as a "bag of worms."

Observe Voiding

Observing the patient urinating may be useful to check for hesitancy in initiating the urine stream, force of stream, and dribbling at end of micturition. Observe the abdominal force used during urination. Patients will use abdominal muscles to increase the intraabdominal pressure to force urine from the bladder while holding their breath.

Perform Digital Rectal Prostate Examination

Digital rectal examination of the prostate is performed to identify irregularities of the prostate that are suggestive of cancer and to note any tenderness or inflammation. The size and consistency should be noted. The median sulcus and lateral margins should be palpated. Induration or firmness is characteristic of early prostate disease; a hard stony gland suggests advanced prostatic carcinoma. The gland may feel soft because of inflammation or infection. If hypertrophied, the prostate gland will extend into the rectal canal, and the median sulcus may be obliterated. **Do not massage the prostate if acute prostatitis is suspected because of the possibility of spreading the infection.**

Document the amount of prostate extension into the rectum using an acceptable clinical scale, such as the following:

- Grade I: protrudes less than 1 cm into the rectum
- Grade II: protrudes 1 to 2 cm into the rectum
- Grade III: protrudes 2 to 3 cm into the rectum
- Grade IV: protrudes more than 3 cm into the rectum

LABORATORY AND DIAGNOSTIC STUDIES

The history and the findings of the physical examination determine the extent of diagnostic investigation. The symptoms reported by the patient are taken into account when ordering diagnostic tests to corroborate or verify the diagnosis. General screening tests can be used to provide additional data for patients with urinary tract problems.

Specific tests for kidney function include urinalysis, screening blood chemistry tests such as urea nitrogen and serum creatinine, and hematological studies. Abnormal blood tests include elevated creatinine and blood urea nitrogen levels, hyperkalemia, and hypocalcemia.

Urine collected for urinalysis should be freshly voided and usually midstream. If not examined immediately, the specimen should be refrigerated because cells begin to disintegrate after 1 to 2 hours.

Urine Dipstick

Reagent strips can be used to screen urine in the clinical setting. See Chapter 18 for a complete discussion of each component. A positive leukocyte esterase or nitrite test result is indicative of urethritis. Urine that tests positive for leukocyte esterase should be cultured for bacteria. Proteinuria may indicate kidney involvement. Suspect proximal renal tubular damage if urine glucose is elevated while serum glucose levels are normal. Blood in the urine could be caused by acute or chronic prostatitis, urethritis, hemorrhagic cystitis, renal stones, or tumors of the kidney, renal pelvis, ureter, bladder, prostate, and urethra. Hematuria with proteinuria usually suggests a renal origin. Isolated hematuria is usually produced by sites outside the kidneys.

Urinalysis With Microscopic Examination

See Chapter 18 for a complete discussion of each component. Turbidity with a foul odor indicates infection. Color changes of the urine may result from various sources: hemoglobin from systemic red blood cell (RBC) lysis; myoglobin from damaged muscle cells or rhabdomyolysis; vegetable pigments from food, such as red beets; pigments from drugs, such as rifampin and phenazopyridine; and porphyrins from porphyria. RBCs indicate acute inflammatory or vascular disorders of the glomerulus. Casts indicate hemorrhage or conditions of the nephron. Red cell casts are characteristic of glomerular origin. The presence of abnormal cells, protein, hemoglobin, myoglobin, or other debris with a cast helps identify the type of renal disease. Significant proteinuria results from glomerulopathies, whereas tubular disorders cause little proteinuria. Therefore the sediment findings are helpful to correlate with the degree of proteinuria.

Segmented Urine Collection for Gram Stain and Culture and Sensitivity

Segmented urine collection is used to identify the site along the urinary tract where the colonization of organisms is occurring. The standard method for specimen collection and labeling is the following:

- Voided bladder specimen 1 (VB 1): 5 to 10 ml of first voided urine collected
- Voided bladder specimen 2 (VB 2): sterile midstream urine collected
- Expressed prostatic secretion (EPS): prostatic massage performed and prostatic secretion collected from meatal opening
- Voided bladder specimen 3 (VB 3): complete emptying of bladder; urine specimen collected

Another option is the premassage and postmassage urine test. The following two urine samples are collected:

- A midstream urine specimen before prostatic massage

■ A first-voided urine specimen immediately after prostatic massage

Label each of the specimens and perform culture and sensitivity (C & S) or Gram staining. Positive bacterial culture in VB 1 (premassage) suggests urethritis. Positive bacterial culture in VB 2 (premassage) suggests cystitis. Positive bacterial culture in EPS or VB 3 (postmassage) in the absence of positive bacterial culture in premassage specimens or a bacterial culture at least 10 times higher in postmassage samples than in premassage samples suggests bacterial prostatitis

Urine Flow Studies (Uroflowmetry)

Urine flow studies can be used as a screening tool to determine diminished force of urination and obstruction. Flow rate is defined as the volume of fluid expelled from the urethra per unit of time and is expressed in milliliters per second. The patient must have a full bladder because urine flow rate depends on voided volume. The patient urinates into an insert in the toilet, which measures the flow rate of the urine. The normal flow pattern exhibits a rapid increase to maximal flow rate, within one third of the ultimate voiding time. After achieving maximal rate, flow decreases more slowly; average flow rate should be approximately 50% of the maximal urine flow rate.

Gram Stain

Gram stain of urethral exudate or spun urine should be performed to determine inflammation (white blood cells [WBCs]) and the presence of either gram-negative or gram-positive bacteria. Gram-negative bacteria stain pink-red; gram-positive bacteria stain dark blue to purple. The nuclei of polymorphonuclear neutrophils (PMNs) (leukocytes) stain pink-red. A Gram stain with more than 4 PMNs/high-power field (HPF) is indicative of urethritis (defined by the presence of 5 to 10 PMNs/HPF). Practically, however, any number of WBCs is suggestive of urethritis. A symptomatic patient with risk factors but no positive laboratory results should be retested using the first voided urine of the day.

If the stain is positive for PMNs, then the smear is examined for gram-negative intracellular diplococci (GNICDCs). If GNICDCs are found, the smear is considered positive for gonococcal urethritis. A smear that is equivocal or atypical indicates a mixed gonococcal and nongonococcal urethritis. If there are no GNICDCs, then nongonococcal urethritis is indicated. The Gram stain has 95% specificity in gonococcal urethritis, with nearly 100% sensitivity in urethritis.

Culture and Sensitivity

Culture and sensitivity should be performed on specimens to identify the causative organism and its sensitivity to antibiotics. This is especially important in populations at increased risk for resistant organisms.

Molecular Testing for Infectious Organisms

Molecular testing using a sample taken from the urethra or first-voided urine provides rapid, sensitive, and specific results. Follow manufacturer's directions to collect and transport the sample.

Nucleic acid amplification tests (NAATs) are available to test for *Chlamydia trachomatis* and *Neisseria gonorrhoeae*. Single or dual organism tests are available.

Creatinine and Blood Urea Nitrogen

Serum creatinine and blood urea nitrogen levels are used to indicate kidney function.

Prostate-Specific Antigen

Tumor markers such as prostate-specific antigen (PSA) may be used to detect or monitor prostate cancer. PSA results should be correlated with the digital rectal examination (DRE). For normal-risk males, levels of 1 to 4 ng/ml are considered within reference range, whereas 4 to 10 ng/ml are elevated levels that fall into a gray zone and may require other tests such as transrectal ultrasound (TRUS) and prostate biopsy. PSA levels of 10 ng/ml or above are abnormal and indicate malignant activity of the prostate. The threshold level for African American males who are at risk may be lower than for other groups. The higher the PSA level, the more likely the presence of prostate cancer; however, men with prostate cancer can have a negative or borderline PSA level. In men taking finasteride, normal PSA is <2 ng/ml because finasteride halves the PSA level. A negative PSA and a negative DRE make the presence of cancer unlikely (Box 19-1).

Currently the use of PSA testing to screen men is under debate. Some authorities recommend screening males older than 50 and those at risk (i.e., patients with a family history or African American males). Others do not recommend routine screening based on lack of empirical evidence of the benefit. In either case, the patient should be told of the potential benefits, known harms, and treatment options available and should be assisted in making an individual decision about testing.

Radiography

If microscopic hematuria is present and the patient is under 50 years of age, obtain a flat plate of the abdomen to identify structures of the kidney, ureters, and bladder (KUB). Urinary calculi are usually visible on radiographs.

Ultrasound

Ultrasonography is noninvasive and provides information on the kidneys, ureters, bladder, vascular structures, prostate, and testicles. Renal ultrasound is a good first test to determine kidney size and contour, and the presence of calculi. A urinary bladder sonogram is used to identify tumors of the bladder, thickening of the bladder wall, posterior masses behind the bladder, and obstruction of the lower urinary tract evidenced by residual urine. A scrotal sonogram is used to evaluate chronic scrotal swelling; it can be

---

Box 19-1	**Evidence-Based Practice: PSA**

The use of PSA for diagnostic testing was approved in the United States by the FDA in 1992. However, PSA measurement for detecting cancer of the prostate is equivocal.
- With a cutoff of 4 ng/ml, overall sensitivity is 46%, specificity 91%, and positive predictive value 32%.
- False negative rate: More than 20% of patients with prostatic cancer have PSA levels <4 ng/ml.
- False positive rate: Of patients with benign prostatic hyperplasia (BPH), 30% to 50% have elevated PSA. Levels depend on prostate volumes, and each 1 g of BPH increases the PSA level by 0.2 ng/ml. PSA is elevated by transrectal biopsy, rigid cystoscopy, catheterization, and transurethral resection of the prostate; it is recommended that PSA is not checked for at least 6 weeks after these procedures. DRE can elevate PSA levels as well.

Some researchers have suggested lowering the cutoff levels that determine if a PSA measurement is normal or elevated:
- ≤2.5 ng/ml is low.
- 2.6 to 10 ng/ml is slightly to moderately elevated.
- 10 to 19.9 ng/ml is moderately elevated.
- ≥20 ng/ml is significantly elevated.

These cutoffs may also increase false positive test results.

New types of PSA tests have been developed that may be useful, particularly when the PSA result is borderline:
- **PSA density (PSAD).** PSA density considers the relationship of the PSA level to the size of the prostate. It is calculated by dividing the PSA number by the prostate volume (measured by transurethral ultrasonography [TRUS]).
- **Age-specific ranges.** These may be useful because older men have higher PSA levels than younger men, even in the absence of cancer. Generally, men younger than age 50 should have a PSA level below 2.4 ng/ml, whereas a PSA level up to 6.5 ng/ml would be considered normal for men in their 70s.
- **PSA velocity.** This measures how quickly the PSA level rises over time. Serial testing may be appropriate for managing borderline results. A sharp rise in the PSA level raises the suspicion of cancer.
- **Free versus bound PSA.** PSA circulates in the blood in two forms: free or bound to a protein molecule (complexed PSA). With benign prostate conditions, there is more free PSA, while cancer produces more of the bound form. Free PSA ratio indicates how much PSA circulates unbound and how much is bound. For PSA results in the borderline range, a low free PSA ratio increases the chance that prostate cancer is present and suggests the need for biopsy.

Data from National Cancer Institute (NCI): *Prostate cancer,* accessed on March 7, 2006, from http://www.cancer.gov/cancertopics/types/prostate.

used to identify abscess, infected testes, tumor, hydrocele, spermatocele, adherent scrotal hernia, and chronic epididymitis. However, because it does not assess perfusion, it is less helpful in the initial examination of an acute condition of the scrotum, where a Doppler blood flow is more appropriate. Transrectal prostate sonogram or ultrasound (TRUS) can be used to evaluate the prostate for tumors or nodules as well as to determine the volume of the prostate. It is also useful in diagnosing prostatitis, BPH, and cancer of the prostate.

Computed Tomography

Noncontrast helical (spiral) CT is the gold standard for evaluating kidney stones. It has 95% sensitivity and 98% specificity.

Doppler Flow Studies

Doppler blood flow studies are used to measure blood flow to the scrotal structures. Color Doppler provides a color image, depicting the direction of the flow and the velocity in shades of blue and red. It is useful in the differential diagnosis of testicular torsion and epididymitis. A Doppler of testicular torsion demonstrates reduced or absent blood flow, while epididymitis will show blood flow.

Biopsy

Biopsy of the prostate is necessary for definitive diagnosis of cancer. Guided biopsy is performed using transrectal ultrasound.

DIFFERENTIAL DIAGNOSIS

Cystitis/Urethritis

Males can have inflammation limited to the penile segment of the urethra. The history would include meatal burning and discharge. Classic symptoms are frequency, urgency, and dysuria. Nocturia with suprapubic or low back pain is common.

Screening can be done in most settings with urine dip strips. A positive leukocyte esterase and nitrate test indicates infection. Urine culture and sensitivity confirms diagnosis and identifies the causative organism(s). Urinalysis with microscopic examination can determine if 20 or more organisms/HPF

are present, which is indicative of UTI. Less than 20 organisms/HPF merits further study such as culture and sensitivity. Colonization has taken place if 103 or more organisms/ml are present in the culture.

Pyelonephritis

The patient with pyelonephritis has fever and chills, appears toxic, and complains of back pain. Nausea and vomiting may be present. Some patients also complain of lower urinary tract symptoms, including frequency and dysuria. The patient feels and looks ill. On physical examination, CVA tenderness is usually present. The abdomen may also be tender. On microscopic examination, WBCs are usually present. White cell casts suggest pyelonephritis. Bacterial casts, although rare, are pathognomonic of pyelonephritis. Urine culture and sensitivity confirm the diagnosis and identify the pathogen, which is usually *E. coli, Klebsiella, Proteus mirabilis,* or *Enterobacter.*

Urolithiasis

Urinary stones can occur anywhere in the urinary tract and may produce symptoms of pain, hematuria, and secondary infection. Many calculi are "silent" and may cause only hematuria, either microscopic or gross. Renal calculi may occur when a stone obstructs the urinary tract. Typical symptoms of renal colic include severe flank pain that radiates along the pathway of the ureter to the scrotum or inner thigh. Chills, fever, and urinary frequency are common. The patient may have nausea, vomiting, and abdominal distention. There may be a history of hematuria. Painful hematuria is characteristic of a stone, and the pain is described as colicky. Evaluate if the hematuria occurs at the time of urine initiation, at termination of micturition, or throughout micturition. This may be helpful in localizing the stone.

The clinical diagnosis is supported by urinalysis and imaging findings. The urine may be normal; gross or microscopic hematuria is common. Pyuria (WBCs) with or without bacteria may be present. Crystalline structures may be present. Noncontrast helical (spiral) CT is the gold standard for evaluating kidney stones.

Acute Bacterial Prostatitis

The patient with acute prostatitis is obviously ill and presents with chills, high fever, urinary frequency and urgency, perineal pain, and low back pain. The patient may exhibit varying degrees of obstructive symptoms, dysuria or burning, nocturia, hematuria, arthralgia, and myalgia. On examination, the prostate gland is tender, swollen, indurated, and warm. Do not massage the gland because bacteremia can result from the expression of microorganisms. Urine or prostate secretion culture can confirm the diagnosis. The most common causative organism is *E. coli*. Other common organisms include *Klebsiella* spp, *Enterobacter* spp, and *Proteus* spp. See Box 19-2 for the classification of prostatitis.

Chronic Bacterial Prostatitis

Chronic prostatitis is a common cause of recurrent cystitis in men. The patient may present with recurrent urinary tract infections caused by the same pathogen. Chronic bacterial prostatitis is caused by the same pathogens seen in acute prostatitis. Patients may be asymptomatic. Common symptoms, if evident, include low back pain and perineal discomfort, urinary frequency, and painful urination. Traditionally, symptoms are present for at least 3 months for a diagnosis of chronic prostatitis. Infection can involve the scrotal contents, producing epididymitis. Palpation of the prostate may reveal no specific findings. It may be moderately tender and irregularly indurated or boggy. Copious secretion may be present. Diagnosis is made on the basis of clinical symptoms and by culture of prostatic secretion or positive bacteria culture from postmassage urine. WBCs will be present in expressed prostatic secretions (EPSs) and voided bladder sample 3 (VB 3)

Chronic Prostatitis, Chronic Pelvic Pain Syndrome (CP-CPPS)

The diagnostic criterion for CP-CPPS is pelvic pain that has been present for at least 3 of the preceding 6 months, with no bacterial cause. The pain may be accompanied by additional symptoms such as dysuria, urgency, frequency, and backache. Patients may or may not have had obstructive voiding symptoms. Inflammatory CP-CPPS is characterized by the absence of bacteria and the presence of WBCs in the semen, expressed prostatic secretion (EPS), or voided bladder urine specimen 3 (VB 3). This category was previously called nonbacterial prostatitis. Noninflammatory CP-CPPS is characterized by the absence of both bacteria and WBCs in the semen, EPS, or VB 3. This condition was formerly called prostadynia. The prostate may feel normal on clinical examination.

Asymptomatic Inflammatory Prostatitis

This condition is diagnosed in patients during the evaluation of another genitourinary (GU) problem such as benign prostatic hypertrophy. These patients do not experience genitourinary pain. WBCs are found in the expressed prostatic secretions.

Box 19-2	**NIH Classification of Prostatitis**
I	Acute bacterial prostatitis (acute symptoms)
II	Chronic bacterial prostatitis (symptoms present for 3 months)
III	Chronic prostatitis chronic pelvic pain syndrome (CP-CPPS) (no bacterial cause)
IIIA	Inflammatory chronic pelvic pain syndrome (WBCs found in semen, expressed prostatic secretions, or final voided specimen)
IIIB	Noninflammatory chronic pelvic pain (no WBCs in semen, expressed prostatic secretions, or final voided specimen)
IV	Asymptomatic inflammatory prostatitis (no subjective symptoms; incidental detection of WBCs in expressed prostatic secretions or prostate tissue)

Modified from National Institute of Diabetes and Digestive and Kidney Diseases: *Chronic prostatitis workshop*, Bethesda, Md, December 7-8, 1995, National Institutes of Health. Available at http://kidney.niddk.nih.gov/kudiseases/pubs/chronicprostatitis/index.htm.

Epididymitis/Orchitis

The patient with epididymitis/orchitis is usually a sexually active young male, and pain is the likely presenting symptom. The patient may be febrile. The history usually indicates a slow onset of discomfort over hours or days compared with testicular torsion, which has a rapid onset of symptoms. Elevation of the affected testicle may reduce the discomfort. Swelling of the scrotum and testicle may be present. Palpable swelling of the epididymis is usually present. Doppler flow studies with color can locate hot spots and identify intact blood flow. Urethral discharge or an intraurethal swab specimen should be Gram stained for a diagnosis of urethritis. A nucleic acid amplification test (either on the intraurethral swab or with the first-void urine) should be used to test for *N. gonorrhoeae* and *C. trachomatis*.

Testicular Torsion

The patient with testicular torsion is usually a pubescent male, with previous episodes of testicular pain. The history indicates a rapid onset of acute pain. Nausea and vomiting may have occurred or be present. Doppler blood flow studies may support the diagnosis by identifying lack of blood flow to the affected testicle. **This is an emergent condition, and intervention must take place within the first 4 to 6 hours to salvage the testicle from infarction.**

Benign Prostatic Hyperplasia

Prostatic hypertrophy is common in men over age 50. Presenting symptoms include hesitancy, slow urine stream, and dribbling. Digital rectal examination reveals an enlarged prostate with a reduced or obliterated median sulcus. Induration or firmness is characteristic of early prostate disease, and a hard stony gland suggests advanced prostatic carcinoma. The gland may feel soft because of inflammation or infection. The American Urological Association Symptom Index (Table 19-1) is useful in determining treatment options based on severity of symptoms, ranging from mild to severe. Digital rectal examinations combined with PSA tests are done annually by many clinicians for men older than 50 and for men at risk, including African American males starting at age 40, to differentiate between BPH and prostate cancer.

Prostate Cancer

Patients with prostate cancer often present with the same obstructive symptoms as BPH but may also be asymptomatic. Males presenting with complaints of lower abdominal pain probably represent extension of the cancer with metastasis. On examination, the prostate is stony hard and protrudes into the colon. PSA levels may be elevated, and TRUS indicates enlargement or nodules. PSA levels between 4 and 10 ng/ml may necessitate a biopsy to determine or rule out prostate cancer (see Box 19-1).

Bladder or Kidney Tumor

Silent hematuria in elderly patients is often a late presenting indication of cancer. It is more common in men than women. Patients often have a history of smoking or alcohol abuse.

DIFFERENTIAL DIAGNOSIS OF *Common Causes of Genitourinary Problems in Males*

CONDITION	HISTORY	PHYSICAL FINDINGS	DIAGNOSTIC STUDIES
Cystitis/urethritis	Frequency, urgency, dysuria; nocturia with low back pain	Discharge may be present; may have suprapubic tenderness	Urine dipstick: positive leukocyte esterase; hematuria; urinalysis with microscopic examination; segmented urine collection; Gram stain; C & S

Continued

DIFFERENTIAL DIAGNOSIS OF *Common Causes of Genitourinary Problems in Males—cont'd*

CONDITION	HISTORY	PHYSICAL FINDINGS	DIAGNOSTIC STUDIES
Pyelonephritis	Fever, chills, back pain, nausea and vomiting, toxic appearance; some patients also have frequency and dysuria	Feels and looks ill; temperature >101° F; CVA tenderness; abdomen may be tender	Microscopic examination: WBCs may have white cell casts or bacterial casts; urine C & S; blood cultures
Urolithiasis	Pain, hematuria; may have symptoms of secondary infection; renal colic: pain that radiates to inner thigh; nausea, vomiting	May have CVA tenderness; looks ill during periods of acute pain; may have abdominal distention	Urinalysis: gross or microscopic hematuria; WBCs with or without bacteria; crystalline structures may be present; radiograph or ultrasound
Acute bacterial prostatitis	Chills, high fever, urinary frequency; urgency; perineal pain and low back pain; varying degrees of obstructive symptoms, dysuria or burning, nocturia, hematuria, arthralgia, and myalgia	Temperature >101° F; prostate gland tender, swollen, indurated, warm; do not massage as can cause bacteremia	Urinalysis; urine culture; prostate secretion culture
Chronic bacterial prostatitis	Common cause of recurrent cystitis in men; same pathogen as in prostate secretion; may be asymptomatic; commonly have low back pain and perineal pain, urinary frequency, and painful urination	Infection can involve scrotal contents, producing epididymitis; palpation of prostate reveals no specific findings; may be moderately tender and irregularly indurated or boggy; may have copious secretion	Culture prostatic secretion; culture postmassage urine; WBCs present in EPS and VB 3
Chronic prostatitis, chronic pelvic pain syndrome (CP-CPPS); can be inflammatory or noninflammatory	Pelvic pain present for at least 3 of preceding 6 months, with no bacterial cause; may be accompanied by additional symptoms such as dysuria, urgency, frequency, and backache; may or may not have had obstructive voiding symptoms	Normal prostate examination	Inflammatory: absence of bacteria and presence of WBCs in semen, EPS, or VB 3 Noninflammatory: absence of both bacteria and WBCs in semen, EPS, or VB 3
Asymptomatic inflammatory prostatitis	Symptoms of another genitourinary problem; no pain	Specific for another genitourinary disorder	WBCs found in expressed prostatic secretions
Epididymitis/orchitis	Abrupt onset over several hours; febrile; pain in scrotum and/or testicles	Tender, swollen epididymitis and/or testicles; elevation of affected testicle may lessen discomfort; may have fever	Doppler flow studies with color
Testicular torsion	Sudden onset of testicular pain that radiates to groin; may also have lower abdominal pain	Exquisitely tender testicle; testicle may ride high because of shortened spermatic cord; cremasteric reflex absent	Scrotal ultrasonography; this is a surgical emergency

Continued

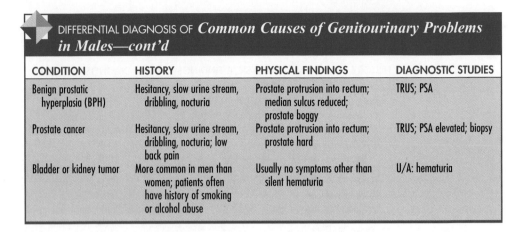

DIFFERENTIAL DIAGNOSIS OF *Common Causes of Genitourinary Problems in Males—cont'd*

CONDITION	HISTORY	PHYSICAL FINDINGS	DIAGNOSTIC STUDIES
Benign prostatic hyperplasia (BPH)	Hesitancy, slow urine stream, dribbling, nocturia	Prostate protrusion into rectum; median sulcus reduced; prostate boggy	TRUS; PSA
Prostate cancer	Hesitancy, slow urine stream, dribbling, nocturia; low back pain	Prostate protrusion into rectum; prostate hard	TRUS; PSA elevated; biopsy
Bladder or kidney tumor	More common in men than women; patients often have history of smoking or alcohol abuse	Usually no symptoms other than silent hematuria	U/A: hematuria

CHAPTER RESOURCES

Aldmen W, Joffe A: The adolescent male genital examination: what's normal and what's not, *Pediatr Rev* 20:125, 1999.

Diaz-Parker C, Bratslavsky G: Male genitourinary disease: urethritis, epididymitis, and prostatitis, *Clin Rev* 15(3):40, 2005.

Epperly TD, Moore KE: Health issues in men, part I: common genitourinary disorders, *Am Fam Physician* 61:3657, 2000.

Fracchia MS, Pareek G, Armenakas N: Scrotal pathology in children: benign or serious? *Consultant* July:1114, 2004.

Lan G: Scrotal swelling in children, *Pediatr Rev* 21:311, 2000.

Mulle BA: Prostatitis: what NPs need to know about diagnosis and treatment, *Am J Nurse Practitioners* 9(11/12):33, 2005.

Ogunfidmitmi F: Testicular disorders: what you should know, *Clinical Advisor* September 31, 2005.

Stevemer JJ, Easley SK: Treatment of prostatitis, *Am Fam Physician* 61(10):3015, 2000.

Penile Discharge

Penile discharge results from an infectious or inflammatory process secondary to exposure or contact with secretions containing causative organisms that enter and ascend the urethra. Males infected with *Chlamydia trachomatis* may be asymptomatic 25% of the time, and symptoms may be absent in a few men with gonorrhea infections. Coinfections with both *Neisseria gonorrhoeae* and *Chlamydia* organisms may be present in up to 25% of heterosexual males.

Urethritis in males, usually related to a sexually transmitted infection (STI) that is acquired during unprotected sexual contact, is classified as either gonococcal urethritis or nongonococcal urethritis (NGU). It is not possible to accurately determine the causative organism based on symptoms or physical examination alone. Although patients may be tentatively classified clinically, laboratory tests are used to direct diagnosis and treatment. The most frequently identified organism (40%) in nongonococcal infection is *Chlamydia trachomatis*. Other organisms identified in NGU include *Ureaplasma urealyticum* and, less frequently, *Trichomonas*.

DIAGNOSTIC REASONING: FOCUSED HISTORY

Is This Likely a Sexually Transmitted Infection?

Key Questions
- When did you last have sex? Is this a sexually active adolescent?
- How many sexual partners do you have?
- Do you have any new partners?
- When is the last time you had sex that was risky, such as unprotected sex, a same-sex partner, or oral or anal sex?
- How many days from exposure to onset of symptoms?

Sexual History
A history of multiple sexual partners signifies a risk for exposure to sexually transmitted infections (STIs). The incidence of *Ureaplasma urealyticum* increases with the number of sexual partners. A new partner also is a risk factor, as is a sexual partner who has other sexual partners. Sexually active adolescents, about 40% of persons between 14 and 18 years, are at risk for STIs because of their lack of barrier protection use, impetuous sexual activities, and use of alcohol or drugs. STIs are a serious health problem, occurring in about 25% of sexually active adolescents.

Risky Sexual Preferences and Practices
Unprotected sex increases the chances of STIs. A same-sex partner provides information about risk as does unprotected sex. Oral and anal sexual practices increase the possibility of STI at these sites.

Number of Days Between Exposure and Symptom Onset
For patients with a single exposure, a shorter incubation period is characteristic for *N. gonorrhoeae* (2 to 6 days) and a longer period (2 to 3 weeks) for *C. trachomatis*. For patients with multiple or unknown exposures, the time interval may not be useful.

Are There Any Risk Factors That Point Me in the Right Direction?

Key Question
- Have you used street or illicit drugs?

History of Drug or Substance Abuse

Substance or drug abuse is a risk factor for unprotected and indiscriminate sexual relations. Substance or drug abuse may produce a scant, whitish penile discharge.

What Do the Characteristics of the Discharge Tell Me?

Key Questions

- What color is the discharge?
- How much discharge are you having?
- What is the consistency of the discharge?

Color, Consistency, and Amount of Discharge

The presence of copious amounts of spontaneous yellow-greenish drainage is indicative of a gonococcal infection. A scant mucoid discharge is characteristic of a nongonococcal infection.

Is This a Local Infection or Process?

Key Questions

- Is the end of your penis red and inflamed?
- Tell me how you clean yourself.

Red, Inflamed Glans Penis

A beefy-red, inflamed glans penis is indicative of a yeast infection or a fixed drug reaction often caused by tetracycline. Lubricated condoms or spermicidical gel can cause contact dermatitis.

Hygienic Practices

Poor hygiene or aggressive hygiene with inappropriate or harsh cleansers can cause local irritation and result in inflammation.

Is This Complicated Urethritis?

Key Questions

- Do you have frequency, urgency, or nocturia?
- Do you have rectal, testicular, or low back pain?
- Do you have pain in any joints or muscles? Do you have any skin sores or lesions?

Symptoms That May Indicate Complicated Urethritis

Symptoms of urinary frequency, urgency, and nocturia may indicate complications of a urethral infection caused by spreading of the infection to other urinary tract structures such as the prostate (see Chapter 19). Further involvement may include symptoms of perirectal, testicular, or low back pain, indicating involvement of the vas deferens and the epididymis, which can lead to acute epididymitis and/or the involvement of the testicle and the development of orchitis.

Symptoms That May Indicate Reiter Syndrome

Reiter syndrome is a complication of NGU that follows urogenital infection and classically includes arthritis, conjunctivitis, oral mucosal ulcers, and dermatitis. More common is the joint and tendon involvement after *C. trachomatis* infection. This complication has also been reported in HIV-positive patients. It is less common in non-Caucasian populations, and the incubation period is usually 1 to 4 weeks after the onset of urethritis.

Disseminated Systemic Urethral Infection

A disseminated gonococcal infection can produce papules or petechiae that progress to pustules on the skin surfaces of the hands, arms, and legs.

Is This an Upper Urinary Tract Problem?

Key Questions

- Have you had a fever or chills?
- Have you noticed any blood in your urine?
- Are you having any acute pain? Where is the pain?

Fever

The presence of fever indicates an ascending infection of the upper urinary tract (e.g., pyelonephritis) or a descending infection of the lower urinary tract (e.g., prostatitis, epididymitis). A fever with a temperature of greater than 101° F (39° C) should be cause for concern and aggressive treatment.

Hematuria

Blood in the urine signifies renal involvement—specifically, pyelonephritis or lithiasis. Painless hematuria in the elderly is characteristic of bladder tumor or is a late symptom of carcinoma of the kidney.

Acute Pain

Abdominal pain, flank pain, and costovertebral angle pain are characteristic of bladder, ureter, and kidney involvement. Urinary tract pain is usually perceived locally in the area where sensory fibers of nerves are located. However, pain can be referred to a site distant from the area that is affected because sensory nerves of the lower body are concentrated in the same segments of the spinal cord. Most pain in the urinary tract is referred pain and may not actually be perceived by the patient in the site where the problem actually occurs. A dull ache may be felt at the costovertebral angle or flank. Pain may be elicited by applying tension to the renal capsule, pelvis, or ureter. Ureter pain may be perceived in the bladder, penis, scrotum, or perineum. Testicular pain may be a result of renal calculi. Pain may vary in intensity from a dull ache to a sharp, stabbing, colicky pain that is unbearable.

What Else Could This Be?

Key Questions

- Do you have scrotal pain and/or fever with the discharge?
- Have you had recent instrumentation in the urethra (e.g., catheterization)?
- Have you been treated recently for an STI?
- Are you or your partner an immigrant, or have you recently engaged in foreign travel?

Scrotal Pain or Fever

Epididymitis usually presents with scrotal pain that developed over a period of several hours. The patient is also often febrile.

Recent Treatment or Instrumentation

Recent treatment or instrumentation of the urethra produces a risk for infection. Elderly males are especially at risk because they often undergo urinary tract treatment or instrumentation secondary to benign prostatic hypertrophy.

Recent Treatment for an STI

Recent treatment for an STI may indicate treatment failure, a coinfection that was not covered by the prescribed drug, or recent exposure. The appropriate laboratory test may not have been done or was not available, or treatment may have been empirically based on presenting symptoms. Infection with more than one organism or a coinfection may take place. Urethritis can also develop from a nongonococcal organism that has a longer incubation period and was not sensitive to the drug prescribed. The urethritis episode may also represent a recent exposure after treatment. Another possibility could be lack of patient compliance with treatment. The patient does not take the medication as directed or stops taking the medication when the symptoms disappear but before the causative organism is eliminated from the urethra.

Immigrant Patient or Partner or Recent Foreign Travel

Immigrants, partners of foreigners, or patients with a history of foreign travel may have exposure to other STIs that are not seen as frequently in the United States but have a higher incidence and prevalence in foreign countries. Resistant strains of common organisms are also prevalent in foreign countries. Referral or infectious disease consultation may be necessary from urologists, infectious disease departments, or public health departments to identify and treat patients with unusual STIs.

DIAGNOSTIC REASONING: FOCUSED PHYSICAL EXAMINATION

Note General Appearance

If the patient appears systematically ill, a more aggressive and immediate approach should be taken and an expanded examination becomes appropriate. An ascending infection is usually limited to the anterior portion of the male urethra and is most likely to cause local signs and symptoms in the male patient. The patient who appears to be in acute pain from sites other than the urethra warrants more than a focused physical examination.

Examine skin surfaces, exposed orifices, and eyes as well as mucous membranes and bordering areas around sites that may have been exposed during sexual activity.

Note eyes for discharge or infection. Check around nares and lips for signs of infection or lesions. Inspect the chest, back, palms, and bottoms of the feet for rashes or lesions. Secondary syphilis produces typical rashes and lesions in these areas, as does Reiter syndrome. Spontaneous greenish-yellow discharge from the eyes is indicative of gonococcal infections.

Inspect the skin of the abdomen, inguinal areas, and thighs for lesions or rashes. Disseminated gonococcal infections may produce papules, petechiae, and pustules on the hands, arms, and feet. *Chlamydia* may produce hyperkeratotic lesions on skin surfaces and a rash on the penis in the uncircumcised male.

Palpate Lymph Nodes
Palpate the cervical, axillary, inguinal, and femoral lymph nodes for adenopathy. Although a nonspecific indicator of infection, lymph nodes may enlarge in response to exposure from several organisms. Virus exposure may cause lymph node enlargement, or there may be extension of bacterial organisms into adjacent lymph chains, indicating regional infections. It is important to ascertain how long the nodes have been enlarged and what symptoms have appeared during the course of enlargement. Assess the state of the nodes, such as any redness, swelling, heat, or pain, or if they are firm, mobile, or boggy. Sexually active males may have some inguinal lymph node enlargement, and the patient may or may not be aware of the enlargement. Lymph node enlargement should be documented and described.

Examine Body Hair
Examine hair on the head and in the pubic area and inspect underlying skin areas. Hair shafts can be infected with lice and nits. Hair follicles can be irritated from scratching and from secondary infection by other organisms.

Examine the Penis and Urethral Meatus
Inspect penile skin surfaces for lesions, especially the underside of the head of the penis around the area of the frenulum, where viral lesions may be found. Palpate the shaft of the penis for tenderness or for strictures of the urethra. Retract the foreskin if present and inspect the glans penis, corona, and frenulum for lesions. Inspect the meatus for redness, discharge, patency, or growths. If there is discharge, note if it is spontaneous or produced by milking or stripping the penis. Document a tender urethra and describe the character of any discharge. Note whether the discharge is profuse and yellow-green, which indicates gonococcal infection, or scant and mucoid like, which is characteristic of *C. trachomatis* and nongonococcal infection.

Examine the Scrotum and Testicles
Inspect and palpate the scrotum for lesions. Palpate the testicles and epididymis for tenderness and any signs of inflammation. Elevating a tender testicle may alleviate pain and reduce discomfort in epididymitis. The testicle may not be able to be defined when there is an acute infection present because of examiner-produced pain with palpation. The borders of the testicle may also be obliterated from swelling and edema.

Inspect and Examine Other Sites for Lesions and Discharge
Inspect other sites such as the mouth and pharynx, using a tongue depressor to visualize buccal skinfolds for any lesions. The pharyngeal area may be asymptomatic. Depending on the patient's sexual practices and preferences, other sites exposed to sexual contact, such as the rectum, need to be examined. Rectal bleeding, pus, and mucus may indicate proctitis and require further anoscopic examination and special cultural and laboratory consideration (see Chapter 16). Examine any joints or tendons that are inflamed or tender or have limited range of motion.

LABORATORY AND DIAGNOSTIC STUDIES

To improve the probability of identifying the causative organism, the patient should be examined and specimens obtained at least 1 hour after the last voiding, ideally up to 4 hours after voiding. Manufacturer directions should be followed for all materials used to collect specimens, and policies and procedures should be followed to obtain valid and reliable results from laboratory and diagnostic tests.

Urine Dipstick

Urine dipstick is used as a screening test for urethritis. The leukocyte esterase strip is calibrated to turn purple in 60 seconds, indicating 5 or more white blood cells (WBCs) in the urine. A positive result is indicative of urethritis (75% to 90% sensitivity, 95% specificity). The nitrite strip is calibrated to turn pink within 30 seconds and signifies nitrites produced by 105 or more organisms per milliliter. Urine that tests positive for leukocyte esterase and nitrites should be cultured for bacteria. However, note that some organisms that cause UTIs do not convert nitrate to nitrites (e.g., *Staphylococcus* and *Streptococcus*).

Urinalysis With Microscopic Examination

Look for proteinuria and glycosuria, which suggest kidney involvement. The presence of casts, red blood cells (RBCs), and bacteria is also important. Casts indicate hemorrhage or pathological conditions of the nephrons. RBCs indicate acute inflammatory or vascular disorders of the glomerulus. More than 1 or 2 RBCs/high-power field (HPF) is abnormal and can indicate renal or systemic disease or kidney trauma. Microscopic examination of the urine resulting in 20 or more organisms/HPF indicates urinary tract infection. Fewer than 20 organisms/HPF merits further study such as culture and sensitivity.

Segmented Urine Collection for Culture and Sensitivity

Obtaining segmented urine specimens is a procedure used to identify the site along the urinary tract where the colonization of organisms is occurring and is useful in diagnosing prostatitis (see Chapter 19).

Gram Stain of Specimens

The Gram stain has 95% specificity in gonococcal urethritis. Sensitivity in urethritis is nearly 100%. Gram stain of urethral discharge should be performed to determine inflammation (WBCs) and the presence of either gram-negative or gram-positive bacteria.

If the stain is positive for polymorphonuclear neutrophils (PMNs), then the smear is examined for gram-negative intracellular diplococci (GNICDCs). If diplococci are found, the smear is considered positive for gonococcal urethritis. A smear that is equivocal or atypical indicates a mixed gonococcal and NGU. If there are no GNICDCs, then an NGU is indicated.

Culture and Sensitivity

Culture and sensitivity should be performed on specimens to confirm the identity of the causative organism and its sensitivity to antibiotics. This is especially important in populations with resistant organisms. Cultures are necessary in cases of suspected rectal or pharyngeal infection, as well as a typical urethral swab.

Molecular Testing for Infectious Organisms

Molecular testing using a first-void sample or a sample taken from the urethra or rectum provides rapid, sensitive, and specific results. A number of products are available. Follow manufacturer directions to collect and transport the sample. Nucleic acid amplification tests (NAATs) are available to test for *Chlamydia trachomatis* and *N. gonorrhoeae*. Single or dual organism tests are available.

Doppler Blood Flow

Doppler blood flow studies can be performed to support the diagnosis of testicular torsion and epididymitis. Testicular torsion results in a lack of blood flow to the testicle, whereas in epididymitis the blood flow is intact. Color Doppler flow studies also provide information concerning blood flow to the testicles and identify hot areas of infection.

Complete Blood Cell Count

Complete blood cell count with differential can be performed to indicate a systemic response to infection.

Serology for Syphilis

Serological tests are used for screening and diagnosing syphilis and are recommended if other STIs are found or suspected. The screening tests are nontreponemal and include VDRL (Venereal Disease Research Laboratory), RPR (rapid plasma reagin), and EIA (enzyme immunoassay) tests. Diagnostic tests are *Treponema pallidum* specific and include FTA-ABS (fluorescent treponemal antibody absorption test) and TPPA (*Treponema pallidum* particle agglutination assay).

Human Leukocyte Antigen

The human leukocyte antigen (HLA) test is done to determine antigens that are present for specific diseases. Histocompatibility locus A (HLA-B27) tissue haplotype is associated with sexually acquired reactive arthritis seen in Reiter syndrome. This test is not specific but is used to confirm the diagnosis.

DIFFERENTIAL DIAGNOSIS

Urethritis

Urethritis presents with itching, burning, or pain around the urethral opening. Symptoms vary in severity. Discharge may range from copious amounts of greenish-yellow discharge to scant mucoidlike discharge that may only be visible before the first voiding of the day. Patients commonly present with complaints of urinary frequency, urgency, and/or burning with urination as well as penile discharge. Patients may also report a known sexual partner or that the public health department has contacted them indicating that they need to be checked for an STI. If you are unable to make a diagnosis based on history and physical findings, diagnostic testing is necessary for specific organism identification.

N. gonorrhoeae and NGU caused by *C. trachomatis* are the two most common infectious causes of urethritis. A coinfection with both organisms is common in up to 25% of the cases.

Gonococcal Urethritis

Gonococcal STIs are usually the easiest to diagnose because the patient often presents with complaints of a yellow-green discharge and burning on urination. Unprotected sexual relations increase the risk for contracting this STI. Gonococcal infection often becomes symptomatic in 2 to 6 days after exposure and produces the classic yellow-green profuse spontaneous drainage. On examination, the penis will be normal in appearance except for the copious discharge. Diagnosis is established by molecular testing and is confirmed by Gram stain and urethral culture.

Nongonococcal Urethritis

NGU can produce penile discharge, although on examination discharge may not be present. NGU typically develops over a longer incubation period of 8 to 21 days, and 75% of patients present with a clear or mucoid discharge.

Chlamydia is the most common nongonococcal causative organism. The resulting urethritis is characterized by a scant mucoid discharge visible before the first urination of the day. The patient may complain of irritation around the meatus of the urethra or have vague symptoms. On examination, stripping the penis may produce scant mucoid discharge. Molecular testing is used to diagnose *Chlamydia,* and Gram stains are used to rule out and establish nongonococcal disease, of which chlamydial infection is the most frequent. Urine screening tests can be used to identify DNA chlamydial particles.

Complicated Urethritis

The examiner should recognize common complications of urethritis. Periurethritis may progress to urethral stricture in untreated cases, causing banding of the penile urethra in the shaft of the penis. Prostatitis can develop and progress to a systemic inflammatory response, causing chills and fever. Extension of inflammation to other structures of the urinary tract may result in acute infection of the epididymis and testicles. Orchitis, a testicular inflammation, presents with a swollen and tender testicle. Disseminated systemic urethral infection produces small tender papules or petechiae on the skin surfaces of the hands, arms, and legs. They may further develop into pustules and become hemorrhagic or necrotic. Joints can become involved with tenosynovitis and arthritis with synovial effusion in Reiter syndrome. Monarticular joint or tendon involvement should be further investigated.

Prostatitis

Patients with acute bacterial prostatitis are likely to look and feel sick and be febrile. They usually complain of dysuria, burning, frequency, and nocturia (see Chapter 19). Prostatic massage is contraindicated in acute bacterial prostatitis.

Patients with chronic prostatitis do not present as acutely ill but have a history of prostate problems. A causative organism may not be identified (see Chapter 19).

Epididymitis and Orchitis

The patient with epididymitis/orchitis is usually a sexually active young male, and pain is the likely presenting symptom. The patient may also have a urethral discharge. The patient may be febrile. The history usually indicates a slower onset of discomfort

over hours or days compared to torsion testicle, which has a rapid onset of symptoms. Elevation of the affected testicle may reduce the discomfort. Swelling of the scrotum and testicle may be present. Doppler flow studies with color can locate hot spots and identify intact blood flow (see Chapter 19).

Reiter Syndrome

As a complication of a urethral infection, Reiter syndrome commonly includes joint or tendon involvement, but conjunctivitis and skin lesions may also be present. History includes a urethral infection within 1 to 3 weeks. HLA-B27 antigen typing may support confirmation of the diagnosis.

Balanitis

Balanitis is inflammation of the glans penis. Balanitis involving the foreskin or prepuce is called balanoposthitis. Uncircumcised men with poor personal hygiene are most affected by balanitis. Lack of aeration and irritation because of smegma and discharge surrounding the glans penis cause inflammation and edema. The most common complication of balanitis is phimosis, or inability to retract the foreskin from the glans penis.

DIFFERENTIAL DIAGNOSIS OF *Common Causes of Penile Discharge*

CONDITION	HISTORY	PHYSICAL FINDINGS	DIAGNOSTIC STUDIES
Balanitis	Not circumcised; poor hygiene practices	Localized erythema and edema; presence of smegma	None; history and physical examination
Urethritis			
Gonococcal urethritis	Unprotected sexual activity; abrupt onset of symptoms 3-5 days after exposure; yellow-green discharge; classic symptoms reported by males: frequency, urgency, dysuria; dysuria may be worse at beginning of urine flow	Yellow-green discharge; spontaneous or copious amounts with stripping of penis	Collect specimens at least 1 hr, preferably 4 hr, after last voiding; Gram stain, culture; molecular testing for gonococcus

Continued

DIFFERENTIAL DIAGNOSIS OF *Common Causes of Penile Discharge—cont'd*

CONDITION	HISTORY	PHYSICAL FINDINGS	DIAGNOSTIC STUDIES
Nongonococcal urethritis	Unprotected sexual activity; longer incubation period (8-21 days); meatal itching or irritation; scant mucoidlike discharge, if present, before first voiding of day; symptoms vary and range in severity for urgency, frequency, and dysuria	Thin mucoid discharge may be absent or minimal with penile milking or stripping	Gram stain; culture; molecular testing for *Chlamydia*
Complicated Urethritis			
Acute bacterial prostatitis	Chills, fever; 30-50 yr of age; onset of symptoms over days; pain in rectal, perianal area, low back, and abdomen	May have fever; painful prostate; do not massage	Segmental urine specimens; culture and sensitivity
Epididymitis/orchitis	Abrupt onset over several hours; febrile, pain in scrotum and/or testicles	Tender, swollen epididymis and/or testicles; elevation of affected testicle may lessen discomfort; may have fever	Doppler flow studies with color
Reiter syndrome	Joint and tendon involvement; urethritis	Joint and tendon involvement, decreased range of motion; skin and mucous lesions; conjunctivitis	Blood, synovial fluid, HLA-B27 antigen; radiographs
Balanitis	Not circumcised; poor hygiene practices	Localized erythema and edema, presence of smegma	None; history and physical examination

CHAPTER RESOURCES

Blake D: The future is here: noninvasive diagnosis of STDs, *Contemp Pediatr* 2:71, 2001.

Bremnor JD, Sadovsky R: MD evaluation of dysuria in adults, *Am Fam Physician* 65(8):1589, 2002.

Diaz-Parker C, Bratslavsky G: Male genitourinary disease: urethritis, epididymitis, and prostatitis, *Clin Rev* 15(3):40, 2005.

Luzzi GA, O'Brien TS: Acute epididymitis, *BJU Int* 87(8):747, 2001.

Parker CT, Thomas D: Reiter's syndrome and reactive arthritis, *J Am Osteopath Assoc* 100:101, 2000.

Richens J: Main presentations of sexually transmitted infections in men, *BMJ* 328:1251, 2004.

Simpson T, Oh MK: Urethritis and cervicitis in adolescents, *Adolesc Med Clin* 15(2):253, 2004.

Wren T: Penile and testicular disorders, *Nurs Clin North Am* 39:319, 2004.

VIII

Common Gynecological Problems

21

Vaginal Discharge and Itching

Vaginitis is an inflammation of the vagina that can cause a vaginal discharge. Vaginal infections are common in postpubertal women. *Trichomonas vaginalis, Candida,* and bacterial vaginosis (BV) (the epithelium is not inflamed with this syndrome) account for 95% of all vaginal infections in U.S. women. Often patients have more than one infection at a given time.

In women of childbearing age, the three most common vaginal discharges are associated with BV, *Candida,* and *Trichomonas.* Some studies suggest that pregnant women with BV have premature rupture of membranes and early delivery. The most common cervical infections are *Chlamydia trachomatis, Neisseria gonorrhoeae,* and herpes simplex. Postmenopausal women often have discharge related to atrophic vaginitis, caused by the deficiency of estrogen in the vaginal tissues.

Vulvar itching, burning, and a foul odor often accompany vaginal discharge. Pubic lice, scabies, pinworms, and genital warts (condylomata acuminata) can all cause itching. Common foreign bodies found in the vagina of adults are lost or forgotten tampons, which can produce a foul-smelling discharge.

Chemical vaginitis in a young girl is usually caused by sensitivity to "bubble bath," whereas in the adolescent or woman it occurs because of the use of scented douches, lubricants, or hygiene sprays. Vulvovaginitis is one of the most common gynecological disorders in girls as a result of their hypoestrogenic state and their perineal hygiene, which is often poor. The vaginal mucosa is thin and less resistant to infectious organisms. The postmenopausal woman can experience these same symptoms with estrogen deficiency.

In childhood and adolescence, complaints of vulvar itching, soreness, or vaginal discharge are common. The lack of estrogen stimulation, neutral pH of the vaginal secretions, lack of protective thick labia and pubic hair of women, and daily living habits (e.g., wiping, clothing, play equipment and environment, baths, foreign bodies, and pinworms) lead to this complaint.

DIAGNOSTIC REASONING: FOCUSED HISTORY

What Kind of Vaginitis Might This Be?

Key Questions

- What is the amount, color, and consistency of your discharge?
- Do you have itching, swelling, or redness?
- Is there an odor?

Characteristics of Discharge

Copious amounts of greenish, offensive-smelling discharge are most consistent with *T. vaginalis.* Mucopurulent or purulent discharges are associated with gonorrhea and *Chlamydia.* A moderate amount of white, curd-like discharge is consistent with *Candida* vulvovaginitis. BV typically produces a discharge that is thin and either white, green, gray, or brownish. Although characteristic symptoms associated with each type of vaginal discharge can be helpful in arriving at a diagnosis, they are not diagnostic in and of themselves. Microscopic examination of the vaginal discharge is more sensitive than the clinical picture in confirming the diagnosis (Figure 21-1).

Itching, Swelling, and Redness

Vaginitis causes inflammation of the tissues, resulting in erythema and edema.

281

FIGURE 21-1 Microscopic differential diagnosis of vaginal infections. **A,** Clue cells (epithelial cells with clumps of bacteria) are evident in bacterial vaginosis. **B,** Budding, branching hyphae characterize candidiasis. **C,** Motile trichomonads are seen with trichomoniasis. (From Zitelli BJ, Davis HW: *Atlas of pediatric physical diagnosis,* ed 3, St Louis, 1997, Mosby-Wolfe.)

Because of the inflammatory process, the amount of discharge will produce a concomitant amount of swelling and redness of the vulva and vagina. Itching is consistently present with candidiasis. Scratching can lead to excoriations and satellite lesions. BV does not involve the inflammatory process and results in discharge with little vulvovaginal erythema and edema.

Odor

A fishy odor caused by the release of amines from organic acids is prominent with BV. It is accentuated by the addition of potassium hydroxide (KOH) to the wet mount slide and is considered a positive "whiff" test. Odor commonly accompanies trichomonal infections. Retained tampons or other foreign bodies can also cause a foul odor.

Is This Likely a Sexually Transmitted Infection?

Key Questions

- Are you sexually active? Do you have multiple partners? Do you have a new partner?
- Have you had sex against your will? If a child: You might ask, "Has anyone touched your private parts?"
- What form of protection do you use? How often do you use protection?

- Have you or your partner(s) ever been tested or treated for a sexually transmitted infection (STI)?
- Do you have any rashes, blisters, sores, lumps, or bumps in the genital area?

Sexual History

Early-age onset of sexual activity, multiple partners, and nonuse of barrier contraceptives, particularly condoms, increase the risk of vaginal infection. STIs are common in women of childbearing age (12 to 50 years) who have acquired a new partner. The patient who frequently changes sexual partners or participates in risky sexual practices (e.g., rectal intercourse without a condom) is at high risk for STIs.

Do not ignore the possibility of an STI in older women or children. An older woman may be sexually active after a divorce or widowhood. Also, 50% of all children with an STI have been found to be sexually abused. *T. vaginalis* is rare in children but can be transmitted to the neonate from an infected mother.

Recent Treatment for a Sexually Transmitted Infection

Recent treatment for an STI may indicate treatment failure, a coinfection that was not covered by the prescribed drug, or recent exposure.

Lesions

Vesicles usually indicate herpes infection. Patients typically notice them on the external labia and complain that they itch or burn. Condylomata lata, condylomata acuminata, and molluscum contagiosum are all papular lesions found on the labia, perineum, and anal regions. Molluscum contagiosum, when occurring in the genital area, may extend to include the inner thighs. Typically, condylomata acuminata (genital warts) are rough, verrucous lesions that are usually located inferiorly from fossa navicularis to the fourchette and the perineal area. A painless ulcer suggests syphilis and classically appears as a solitary lesion. However, there can be more than one chancre, especially if the patient is immunocompromised.

Can This Be Vaginitis That Is Not Related to an STI?

Key Questions

- Have you ever been told that you have diabetes or Cushing's syndrome or that you are positive for HIV infection?
- Have you been ill recently?
- Are you taking antibiotics, hormones, or oral contraceptive pills?
- Have you received chemotherapy?
- Does the itching seem to be worse at night?
- Describe some of your recent activities.
- Is the patient premenarche?

Immunocompromised States

Refractory fungal vulvovaginitis may indicate undiagnosed diabetes or an immunocompromised state.

Recent Illness

Chickenpox, scarlet fever, and measles can cause vaginitis.

Medications or Chemotherapy

Birth control pills, corticosteroids, antibiotics, and chemotherapy are associated with candidal vulvovaginitis. Oral contraceptives may alter the vaginal pH, and antibiotics may alter the normal vaginal flora; both predispose to fungal infection. Corticosteroids and chemotherapy can produce an immunocompromised state and provide the opportunity for fungal infection.

Night Itching

Pinworms are intestinal parasites that inhabit the rectum or colon and emerge to lay eggs in the skinfolds of the anus. Perianal pruritus, especially at night, along with pain or itching of genitals is common (Figure 21-2).

Activities

Riding a bicycle, using pools or hot tubs, or wearing tight-fitting pants or pantyhose can lead to heat and moisture in the genital area, causing mechanical irritation and infection such as candidiasis or BV.

Premenarche

Girls who have not yet reached menarche are prone to vulvovaginal infections because of a nonestrogenized vagina and the lack of labial development and hair growth.

Is This Condition Acute, Recurring, or Chronic?

Key Questions

- How long have you had these symptoms? Are they getting better or worse?
- Have you ever had these symptoms before?
- How many episodes have you had in the past year?
- Are the episodes related to any particular activity or time?

Chronology of Symptoms

The occurrence of a vaginal discharge after having a new sex partner suggests an acute condition, such as a sexually transmitted infection. Symptoms associated with use of condoms or spermicidal jelly suggest sensitivity to the product. If the discharge occurs monthly, becoming worse after menses, suspect a chronic condition such as vulvovaginitis candidiasis. Recurrent episodes related to bathing activities point to chemical irritation.

A

B

FIGURE 21-2 Pinworms (*Enterobius vermicularis*). On this wet mount a mature worm is shown surrounded by eggs **(A)**, which are shown more clearly at higher power **(B)**. (From Zitelli BJ, Davis HW: *Atlas of pediatric physical diagnosis*, ed 3, St Louis, 1997, Mosby-Wolfe.)

If This Is Acute, Could It Be Related to a Previous Infection?

Key Questions

■ Have you been tested and treated for this condition recently?
■ What medication was prescribed? When was it prescribed?
■ Did you take all of the medication?
■ What other prescriptions were you taking at that time?

Adequate Diagnosis

Diagnoses made clinically on the basis of the color or appearance of a discharge may be incorrect, or a concomitant vaginal infection may have been missed. However, self-diagnosis and treatment are common, especially with the over-the-counter medicines for "yeast infection."

Adequate Therapy

Most medications that are prescribed are not taken exactly as directed. Women may stop using their vaginal medications when menses begins and resume after it ends. This practice can lead to treatment failure. They may also discontinue the therapeutic agent early, as soon as relief from symptoms takes place or a drug side effect is experienced (e.g., the metallic taste of metronidazole). Drug interactions may account for inadequate therapy, or there may be the need to alter dietary regimen (e.g., abstinence from alcoholic beverages).

If This Is Chronic, What Should I Suspect?

Key Questions

■ Do any family members or sexual partners have vaginal or urinary tract infections? Do they have any itching, rashes, sores, lumps, or bumps?
■ Do you have a new or untreated partner?
■ What are your sexual practices (e.g., vaginal, oral, and/or anal sex)?
■ How many yeast infections have you had this year?

Transmission

Caregivers, parents, and siblings can spread infections such as candidiasis, molluscum contagiosum, herpes, lice, and pinworms to children through poor hygiene practices. Autoinoculation is also possible, especially for herpes, genital warts, and molluscum contagiosum.

New or Untreated Partner

The most common cause of reinfection is intercourse with a new or untreated partner.

Sexual Practices

Possible infection reservoirs are oral and anal cavities, which may need to be cultured for herpes or gonorrhea. Additionally, materials used during intercourse may need to be disinfected (e.g., diaphragm). Less common modes of transmission include shared intimate clothing.

Chronic Vulvovaginitis

If the patient has had more than three separate episodes of candidal vulvovaginitis in 1 year, consider diabetes or the immunocompromised state of HIV/AIDS as the underlying cause. Yeast grows best in areas that are dark, moist, warm, and high in glucose—areas where the normal flora has been compromised. The use of oral contraceptive pills or hormone replacement therapy, antibiotic (e.g., tetracycline for acne) or steroid therapy, diets high in carbohydrates or artificial sweeteners, and clothing that holds moisture against the vulva (e.g., pantyhose, tight jeans) are excellent potentiators for infection.

What Are Other Possible Causes for This Vaginitis?

Key Questions

- What are your personal hygiene practices?
- Do you douche?
- Have you changed brands of contraceptive products?
- Could you have forgotten to remove your diaphragm or tampon?

Hygiene Practices

Feminine hygiene practices may contribute to vaginitis by causing a local allergic reaction, altered vaginal flora, or contamination of the vagina from the rectum. Perfumes in douches, sprays, lubricants, and bubble baths are frequent offenders in allergic vaginitis.

Once a child is out of diapers, toileting is less closely assisted, and wiping techniques may be poor, leading to contamination of the vagina with bowel flora.

Douching

Frequent douching may change the balance of normal vaginal flora by altering the pH. This allows recolonization of the vagina with enteric bacteria, leading to pruritus and discharge. Douching can cause an allergic reaction. Colored or perfumed toilet paper can irritate the perineum, causing redness and itching. Wiping with tissue after urination or defecation in the direction from the anus toward the vagina can inoculate the vagina with rectal microbes.

Contraceptive Products

Contraceptive products (e.g., spermicidal jellies, suppositories, foam, or condoms) may cause an allergic inflammation of the sensitive mucosa and produce itching, erythema, tenderness, and an increase in usual vaginal secretions.

Foreign Body

A foul-smelling vaginal discharge can be caused by a lost tampon or condom or a forgotten diaphragm. A child who puts a foreign object into her vagina may have pruritus, burning, or a foul, purulent vaginal discharge. Foreign bodies in the vagina are associated with vaginal bleeding or spotting. If the object is left for some time, it can imbed and perforate the vaginal wall.

Are There Any Associated Symptoms That Point to a Cause?

Key Questions

- Do you have burning or pain with urination? Do you have urinary frequency or hesitation, or nocturia?
- Do you have painful intercourse?
- Do you have abdominal or pelvic pain?
- If an infant: Does the infant have an eye infection?
- If an infant: Does the infant have a cough?

Urinary Tract Symptoms

Atrophic vaginitis is often accompanied by dysuria, dyspareunia, and vaginal dryness. Estrogen deficiency affects the woman's entire lower genital tract and may produce symptoms that can be confused with a urinary tract infection. Low estrogen levels may exacerbate stress and urge incontinence. *Trichomonas* and *Chlamydia* may produce a coexisting urethritis that causes frequency and dysuria.

Dyspareunia and Pain
Vaginal atrophy, genital warts, or vaginal infections can cause introital dyspareunia. A more likely reason for deep vaginal dyspareunia is endometriosis, pelvic inflammatory disease (PID), or fibroids. Sexually transmitted infections like gonorrhea and *Chlamydia* can cause cervicitis, which, if left untreated, can progress to PID and produce abdominal and/or pelvic pain (see Chapter 13).

Eye Infection
Eye infections in the newborn may be associated with gonorrhea and *Chlamydia* (see Chapter 6).

Cough
Pneumonia in the newborn may be an indication of chlamydiosis (see Chapter 12).

DIAGNOSTIC REASONING: FOCUSED PHYSICAL EXAMINATION

Note Vital Signs
The presence of a fever may alert you to a serious infection such as PID. Fever is uncommon with vaginitis.

Perform an Oral Examination
Oral thrush may accompany vulvar candidiasis, particularly in children. Look for white patches that bleed when you try to scrape them off.

Perform an External Genitalia Examination
Palpate for inguinal lymphadenopathy and tenderness, which can be present with vaginal infections. Inspect the vulva and labia, looking for erythema, excoriations, and induration. The skin is often bright red and swollen with small fissures or excoriations from candidiasis. Also, thick white curds of discharge are often noted in the labial folds. BV often produces a profuse, thin, whitish discharge that will leak out of the vagina onto the perineum. Palpate Bartholin's and Skene's glands and milk the urethra for discharge. Palpable Bartholin's glands often coexist with STIs. If purulent discharge is seen, consider the diagnoses of gonorrhea or *Chlamydia* and obtain specimens for diagnostic tests.

Condolymata lata, condolymata acuminata, and molluscum contagiosum are all papular lesions found on the labia, perineum, and anal regions. Molluscum contagiosum, when occurring in the genital area, may extend to include the inner thighs. Herpes lesions are usually ulcerative in nature when seen clinically and need to be differentiated from other similar lesions (e.g., syphilitic chancre can be more than one lesion and tender if secondarily infected). Herpetic lesions are found in clusters and can extend from the labia into the vagina. Typically, condylomata acuminata (genital warts) are rough, verrucous lesions that are located inferiorly from the fossa navicularis to the fourchette and the perineal area.

In the overweight patient, vulvovaginitis candidiasis is frequently accompanied by intertriginous candidiasis (e.g., under the breasts and the abdominal apron).

Perform an Internal Vaginal Examination
Note the condition of the vaginal walls. A plastic speculum makes vaginal wall inspection easy and helps in the identification of a foreign body for removal. In children, the knee-chest position is very useful for inspecting the vagina. In children, an otoscope or a nasal speculum may be used; rarely is a hysteroscope (under anesthesia) needed. Pale or mottled red splotches of the vaginal mucosa are associated with atrophic vaginitis, and the sticky discharge is yellow or brown. In severe cases of atrophic vaginitis, the pale, thin mucosa may have adhered to the opposing vaginal wall, and the speculum examination often causes an oozing bloody discharge.

The appearance of the cervix should be noted. A friable or "strawberry" appearance of cervical petechiae with a frothy, foul-smelling discharge is descriptive of a *Trichomonas* infection. A mucopurulent discharge from the cervical os is an indication to obtain an endocervical sample for gonorrhea and *Chlamydia* testing. This discharge is yellowish green when collected on an endocervical swab. The character of the discharge does not consistently identify common infectious causes of vaginitis. Treat vaginal infections before the Papanicolaou test is obtained because BV and trichomoniasis may cause inflammatory atypia results.

The wet mount is a valuable diagnostic tool, and a sample of vaginal discharge is best obtained from the lateral vaginal fornices. Three positive characteristics for any one etiology can correctly identify the causative agent (e.g., increased pH; the presence of "clue cells," which are epithelial cells full of bacteria that obscure the cell border; and a thin gray discharge seen in BV) (see Differential Diagnosis).

DNA probes and nucleic acid amplification tests (NAATs) are available to test for *Chlamydia trachomatis* and *N. gonorrhoeae*. A combination organism DNA probe is available for *Trichomonas vaginalis, Gardnerella vaginalis,* and *Candida* species. Cultures for BV, fungal infections, and *T. vaginalis* are not routinely recommended and are usually reserved for determining resistant organisms.

Perform a Bimanual Examination

Assess the condition of the uterus, fallopian tubes, and ovaries by checking for uterine and cervical motion tenderness (CMT), ovarian size, and presence of masses. CMT or pain on palpation of the uterus and adnexa confirms the spread of vaginitis or cervicitis to the upper genital tract and results in PID. **This warrants immediate evaluation, treatment, or referral to prevent tubal scarring, ectopic pregnancy, and infertility.**

Perform a Vaginal-Rectal Examination

Vaginal-rectal examination is an important technique in assessing the posterior uterus and condition of the cul-de-sac as well as the rectum. Make sure that the internal examination glove is changed before rectal insertion to prevent contamination of the rectum with vaginal discharge organisms. A rectal examination is used to palpate a foreign body and to check for normal pelvic anatomy in the child.

LABORATORY AND DIAGNOSTIC STUDIES
Potassium Hydroxide (KOH) and Wet Mount/Preparation

Obtain a discharge sample from the lateral fornices of the vagina, using a cotton-tipped applicator. There are several acceptable techniques for preparing a KOH and wet mount. One technique is to prepare two slides with a smear of vaginal discharge. To one slide, add a drop of 10% KOH and put a coverslip in place. To the other slide, add a drop of normal saline and put a coverslip in place. The whiff test is positive when the addition of the 10% KOH produces a fishy odor, which is caused by the release of amines. The whiff test has a positive predictive value of 76% for BV. Look under the microscope at the KOH slide for the presence of branching and budding hyphae that are characteristic of yeast infection. Examine the saline wet mount microscopically for motile trichomonads that signal the presence of *Trichomonas*. Clue cells are characteristic of BV (see Figure 21-1).

Test for pH

Most litmus paper reads the pH range from 3.0 to 9.0. This is a simple inexpensive test to aid in determining the cause of the vaginal discharge. Normal vaginal secretions are less than pH 4.5. A pH greater than 4.5 is consistent with BV, trichomoniasis, or atrophic vaginitis.

Fungal Culture or Sabouraud's Agar Culture

Fungal culture may be needed in the diagnosis of non–*Candida albicans* (e.g., *C. glabrata, C. tropicalis, C. krusei*) that are refractory to medication regimens.

Herpes Viral Culture

Viral culture is the most specific method of diagnosing herpes. Results may take from 1 to 7 days, with maximum sensitivity achieved at 5 to 7 days. The herpes culture will probably not be able to identify the causative agent if the specimen is taken from a lesion that is 5 or more days old. It is important to document positive genital herpes infections in the pregnant woman and in skin lesions of the newborn. Collect cells or fluid from a fresh sore with a cotton swab and place them in the culture container.

Herpesvirus Antigen Detection Test

This test detects antigens on the surface of cells infected with the herpes virus. Cells from a fresh sore are scraped off and then smeared onto a microscope slide. This test may be done in addition to or in place of a viral culture.

Tzanck Smear

Tzanck smear characteristic findings are multinucleated giant cells that are likely to be found if the specimen is from an intact herpes lesion. Prepare the Tzanck smear by removing the roof of the vesicle and scraping the skin with a scalpel blade. Make sure that the base and the margins of the vesicle are scraped; do not use the vesicular fluid for this specimen. The cellular material is spread onto a glass slide, fixed with absolute alcohol for 1 minute, and then stained with Wright's stain. Alternative staining methods are available, and guidelines can be obtained from local laboratories.

Modified Diamond's Culture

Diamond's culture is used to identify *Trichomonas*. However, it is seldom needed to make the diagnosis.

Thayer-Martin Culture

Thayer-Martin medium is a bacterial culture that identifies gonococcal infections. A culture is taken from the endocervical canal of the uterine cervix. First remove excess mucus from a portion of the cervix, using a cotton ball held in ring forceps or a large cotton-tipped procto-swab. Insert a sterile cotton-tipped applicator (Q-tip) into the endocervical canal and allow it to absorb the mucus for 10 to 30 seconds before inoculating the medium. Inoculate the medium bottle or plate in a zigzag manner while simultaneously rolling the small cotton-tipped applicator. When opening the Thayer-Martin culture bottle, avoid holding the bottle totally upright, which will allow for the loss of the carbon dioxide from the specimen collection bottle.

Molecular Testing for Infectious Organisms

Molecular testing using a sample taken from the vagina provides rapid, sensitive, and specific results. A number of products are available. Follow manufacturer directions to collect and transport the sample.

DNA probes and nucleic acid amplification tests (NAATs) are available to test for *Chlamydia trachomatis* and *N. gonorrhoeae*. Single or dual organism tests are available. For gonorrhea testing, the sample should be taken from the endocervical canal because *N. gonorrhoeae* has a predilection for the columnar and transitional cells.

A multiorganism DNA probe is available to test for *Trichomonas vaginalis, Gardnerella vaginalis,* and *Candida* species.

Serology for Syphilis

Serological tests are used for screening and diagnosing syphilis and are recommended if other STIs are found or suspected. The screening tests are nontreponemal and include VDRL (Venereal Disease Research Laboratory), RPR (rapid plasma reagin), and enzyme immunoassay (EIA) tests. Diagnostic tests are *Treponema pallidum* specific and include FTA-ABS (fluorescent treponemal antibody absorption test) and TPPA (*Treponema pallidum* particle agglutination assay).

Urinalysis (U/A)

Obtain a U/A if the patient has dysuria. However, external pain on urination may originate from urine on inflamed vulvar tissue, eliminating the need for urinalysis.

Microscopy and Skin Scraping

Viewing a skin scraping under the microscope is used to assist with the differential diagnosis of scabies and pubic lice (see Chapter 8).

Scotch Tape Test

Use this test when you suspect pinworms (*Enterobius vermicularis*), which occur most commonly in children. Instruct the adult to apply adhesive cellophane tape to the child's perianal region early in the morning when the child awakens. The tape is then recovered and brought in. Place it on a glass slide and examine under a microscope for the presence of eggs. Parents may also be able to see the worms by shining a flashlight on the external anus of the child at night. The female worm is about 10 mm long (see Figure 21-2).

Acetic Acid Test (Acetowhite)
The acetic acid test is best used to detect subclinical lesions caused by human papillomavirus (HPV) when a genital wart has been identified on the patient, when there has been sexual contact, or when the Pap test indicates dysplasia. The application of 5% acetic acid (vinegar) to the cervix, labia, or perianal area causes the lesion to turn white (acetowhite). Saturate a gauze pad with vinegar and place on the lesion for 5 to 10 minutes. After this soaking, the white wart will have a sharp circumscribed macular or papular border. The surface will appear verrucous. False positive results can occur with candidiasis, psoriasis, lichen planus, and sebaceous glands.

Follicle-Stimulating Hormone
Follicle-stimulating hormone (FSH) levels that are greater than 30 milliunits/ml are diagnostic of perimenopause, and levels of 40 milliunits/ml or higher represent menopause. This test is particularly helpful in establishing the hypoestrogenic status of a young woman who is experiencing premature menopause and atrophic vaginitis (Box 21-1).

DIFFERENTIAL DIAGNOSIS
Discharges
Physiological Discharge
Normal vaginal discharge is produced by the cervical and vulvar glands. It is mucoid, clear, or white in color and has no foul odor. The amount varies from scant to profuse, depending on the amount of estrogen stimulation to the tissues. On occasion physiological discharge can lead to slight vulvar irritation and mild itching secondary to wetness. The vaginal pH is less than 4.5. Wet mount reveals up to 3 to 5 white blood cells (WBCs)/high-power field (HPF) and the presence of epithelial cells and lactobacilli.

Bacterial Vaginosis
BV is the most common cause of vaginal discharge and is considered a disturbance in normal vaginal flora. It is often found after intercourse with a new partner or in conjunction with other STIs. Fifty percent of women are asymptomatic; hence treatment may not

---

Box 21-1	**Evidence-Based Clinical Diagnosis of Vaginitis**

Vaginal candidiasis, bacterial vaginosis, and trichomoniasis are the three most common causes of vaginitis.

In a systematic review of the literature, Anderson et al. (2004) report that symptoms alone are not able to adequately distinguish between the causes of vaginitis and that physical findings are limited in their diagnostic power. Laboratory examination and microscopy of vaginal discharge are the most useful ways of diagnosing the three conditions.

However, the following symptoms and signs can suggest a particular diagnosis:

- Candidiasis is associated with itching, a cheesy discharge, redness, and self-diagnosis. A watery discharge makes candidiasis unlikely. Inflammatory signs are relatively specific for vaginal candidiasis but are not always present. Odor on physical examination is absent.
- Bacterial vaginosis is associated with increased discharge and a patient complaint of odor. An absent or mild discharge makes bacterial vaginosis unlikely. Odor is noted on physical examination.

Most diagnoses are made by microscopy and the whiff test. Anderson et al. (2004) also report the following findings:

- Most studies (but not all) support that candidiasis is associated with a normal pH.
- While the microscopic identification of yeast or trichomonads is diagnostic, negative findings do not rule out the condition.
- The presence of clue cells makes candidiasis less likely.
- A lack of lactobacilli and the presence of bacilli with corkscrew motility are highly associated with bacterial vaginosis.

The authors conclude that the likelihood ratios found in the review were not particularly robust, that the current research on vaginitis has a number of weaknesses, and that the existing diagnostic approach fails to diagnose approximately 30% of women with vaginal symptoms.

Data from Anderson MR, Klink K, Cohrssen A: Evaluation of vaginal complaints, *JAMA* 291(11):1368, 2004.

be necessary except for pregnant patients (increased preterm labor) or patients undergoing vaginal surgical procedures (increased infection). Consistent symptomatology includes a thin homogeneous white, gray, green, or brownish discharge that has a foul odor; there can be pelvic tenderness or pain but no CMT. The vaginal pH is greater than 4.5. Wet mount shows clue cells and a few lactobacilli; the "whiff" test is positive (see Figure 21-1).

Candida Vulvovaginitis

Ninety percent of women with *Candida* vulvovaginitis present with vulvar pruritus. In children, it may be accompanied by oral thrush. The discharge is often thick, white, and "curdy"; the labia are erythematous and edematous. Vaginal pH is 4.0 to 4.7. A KOH wet mount shows pseudohyphae and spores (see Figure 21-1).

Trichomoniasis

Trichomoniasis is asymptomatic in about half of the women affected and 90% of the men. It is usually transmitted via sexual contact but can also be spread by fomites. Women with chronic infections will have copious amounts of discharge and little or no inflammation of the vaginal tissues. When there is an acute infection, they will complain of vulvar itching, swelling, and redness. The pH is greater than 5; the discharge is white, grayish-green, or yellow and sometimes frothy; infrequently there will be a "strawberry cervix" (cervical petechiae). If the woman has douched within the past 24 hours, the sensitivity of tests will be greatly decreased. Wet mount shows "gyrating" motile protozoa and often greater than 10 WBCs/HPF (see Figure 21-1).

Atrophic Vaginitis

In atrophic vaginitis, there is a dry (shiny), pale, thin vaginal wall caused by an insufficient amount of endogenous estrogen. During menopause, the vaginal mucosa and vulva, which lack glycogen, become fragile and are susceptible to injury and infection. Patients may experience burning, dryness, irritation, or dyspareunia. This also occurs in post-partum women, those who are breastfeeding, and prepubertal girls. The pH is alkaline and ranges from 6.5 to 7.0. Wet mount shows a few WBCs and is negative for pathogens.

Allergic Vaginitis

The causes for allergic vaginitis are different for the child and the adult. In the child, the most common offending agents are bubble baths and perfumed soaps. Adult vulvovaginitis involves any harsh or caustic substance that has direct contact with the area. Often a new brand of vaginal lubricant, douche, spermicide, or condom will cause the inflammation and edema. Vinegar douches stronger than 1 to 2 tablespoons per quart of water may also irritate tissues. The wet mount is positive for WBCs and negative for pseudohyphae.

Foreign Body

The presenting symptom in foreign body retention is a very malodorous, whitish discharge. In children, the foreign body is as variable as those objects found in the ears and nose. However, children younger than 12 months do not have the coordination to insert anything into their vagina, so suspect child abuse in such cases and inspect for bruising or excoriations. Wet mount reveals many WBCs.

Chlamydia

Chlamydia is the most prevalent STI in the United States. About 30% of infected women are asymptomatic. Gonorrhea and *Chlamydia* coexist in up to 60% of patients. Women with *Chlamydia* have an increasing amount of vaginal discharge and bleeding after intercourse. Those patients at greatest risk for infection are young (younger than 25 years) and sexually active (three or more partners) and are not using barrier methods of contraception. Wet mount shows greater than 10 WBCs/HPF and few microscopic bacteria. Except for perinatal syndromes, nonsexual transmission has not been reported; therefore suspect child abuse.

Gonorrhea

Gonorrhea is one of the most common reportable diseases. Women are asymptomatic

50% to 80% of the time. However, the patient may have a purulent discharge that originates from the endocervical columnar and transitional cells. Patients often experience inflammation of Skene's glands, Bartholin's glands, or the urethra, which causes pain and dysuria. Culture or DNA probe confirms the diagnosis. A finding of gonorrhea in children is considered specific evidence of sexual abuse.

Pelvic Inflammatory Disease

PID is most commonly caused by *Chlamydia trachomatis* and *N. gonorrhoeae* (see Chapter 13) and can produce bleeding, abdominal pain, fever, and vaginal discharge. Women with PID have an increasing amount of vaginal discharge and bleeding after intercourse. Infection begins intravaginally in most cases and then spreads upward, causing salpingitis. In the early stages, women may be asymptomatic. Patients may have a purulent discharge that originates from the endocervical columnar and transitional cells. With gonorrhea, patients often experience inflammation of Skene's glands, Bartholin's glands, or the urethra, which causes pain and dysuria. On examination, abdominal tenderness, CMT, and adnexal tenderness is present. As with peritonitis, patients may also have guarding and rebound tenderness. WBCs and erythrocyte sedimentation rate are usually elevated. Cultures and Gram staining can assist with diagnosis.

Itching and Lesions
Syphilis

The chancre of primary syphilis is an ulcerative lesion that most often develops at the site of initial inoculation. The syphilitic chancre begins as a papule and progresses to a painless to tender, hard, indurated ulcer. The infection causes inguinal lymphadenopathy. Even without treatment, the lesion will heal in 3 to 6 weeks. Many chancres go unnoticed until the appearance of condylomata lata, the warty papule of secondary syphilis, or a maculopapular rash on the palms of the hands and soles of the feet. Diagnosis is confirmed with serological testing for syphilis.

Genital Warts

Genital warts (condylomata acuminata) are caused by the human papillomavirus and may be precursors to genital cancers. The warts may involve the vagina, cervix, perineum, or perianal areas. Condylomata can be flat or raised verrucous lesions. The patient usually notices a bump on the genital region, accompanied by itching and leukorrhea. A wet mount should be performed to rule out any coexisting vaginal infections. An acetic acid test is helpful in identifying flat warts. Referral to a dermatologist or gynecologist is indicated for treatment of warts of the urethra or anus.

Herpes

Herpetic lesions can be difficult to distinguish from ulcerative lesions. The most typical presentation is that of grouped vesicles that rupture and leave an erosion. A prodrome of tingling or itching occurs before the outbreak of the vesicles. On the vulva, the erosions are covered with a whitish, exudative layer. Herpetic outbreaks can involve the cervix, vagina, vulva, anus, or extragenital organs, like the pharynx. Culture, antigen test, or Tzanck smear confirms the diagnosis.

If the mother has an active primary herpes simplex virus infection at the time of birth, the infant has a 50% risk of becoming infected. Recurrent maternal infections impart less than a 5% risk of transmission. Clinical signs of the infant's infection become apparent in the first week of life and pose the possibility of death.

Molluscum Contagiosum

Molluscum are small (2 to 5 mm in diameter), umbilicated, flesh-tone papules. These characteristic lesions are the hallmark of the diagnosis. Scratching can spread them. Molluscum is an STI of adults and is a likely finding in HIV-infected patients. When children are found with genital molluscum, suspect child abuse.

DIFFERENTIAL DIAGNOSIS OF *Common Causes of Vaginal Discharge and Itching*

CONDITION	HISTORY	PHYSICAL FINDINGS	DIAGNOSTIC STUDIES
Discharges			
Physiological discharge	Increase in discharge; no foul odor, itching, or edema	Clear or mucoid; pH <4.5	Up to 3-5 WBCs/HPF; epithelial cells, lactobacilli
Bacterial vaginosis	Foul-smelling discharge	Homogeneous thin white or gray discharge; pH >4.5	Presence of KOH "whiff" test; presence of clue cells; few lactobacilli (see Figure 21-1)
Candida vulvovaginitis	Pruritic discharge	White, curdy discharge; pH 4.0-5.0	KOH prep: mycelia, budding, branching yeast, pseudohyphae (see Figure 21-1)
Trichomoniasis	Watery discharge; foul odor	Profuse, frothy, greenish discharge; red friable cervix; pH 5.0-6.0	Round or pear-shaped protozoa; motile "gyrating" flagella (see Figure 21-1)
Atrophic vaginitis	Dyspareunia; vaginal dryness	Pale, thin vaginal mucosa; pH >4.5	Folded, clumped epithelial cells
Allergic vaginitis	New bubble bath, soap, douche, for example	Foul smell, erythema; "lost tampon"; pH <4.5	WBCs
Foreign body	Red and swollen vulva; vaginal discharge; history of use of tampon, condom, or diaphragm	Bloody, foul-smelling discharge	WBCs
Chlamydia	Partner with nongonococcal urethritis; asymptomatic	May or may not have purulent discharge	Molecular testing; >10 WBCs/HPF
Gonorrhea	Partner with STI; often asymptomatic	Purulent discharge; inflammation of Skene's/Bartholin's glands	Gram stain; culture
Pelvic inflammatory disease (PID)	Bleeding, abdominal pain, fever, and vaginal discharge; increasing amount of vaginal discharge and bleeding after intercourse	CMT and adnexal tenderness; may also have guarding and rebound tenderness	WBC; culture; molecular testing; Gram staining
Itching and Lesions			
Syphilis	History of painless ulcerative lesion; rash on palms and soles of feet; warty growth on vagina or anus	Chancre: usually 1 but can be more, painless ulceration; condylomata lata: flat, whitish papule or plaque; maculopapular rash: palm, soles, body	Serology for syphilis
Genital warts	Mild-to-moderate itching, foul vaginal discharge; child: history of sexual abuse; adult: new or multiple partners; history of warts	Moist, pale-pink, verrucous projections on base; located on vulva, vagina, cervix, or perianal area	Acetic acid test: white

Continued

DIFFERENTIAL DIAGNOSIS OF *Common Causes of Vaginal Discharge and Itching—cont'd*

CONDITION	HISTORY	PHYSICAL FINDINGS	DIAGNOSTIC STUDIES
Herpes	History of prodromal syndrome, paresthesias, burning, itching; may have mucoid vaginal discharge	Grouped vesicles on red base, erode to an ulcer; if on mucous membrane, exudates form; if on skin, crusts form; redness, edema, tender inguinal lymph nodes	Viral culture; Tzanck smear
Molluscum contagiosum	History of contact with infected person; if inflamed: itching	Flesh-colored, dome-shaped papules, some with umbilication; usually 2-5 mm in diameter	None

CHAPTER RESOURCES

Anderson MR, Klink K, Cohrssen A: Evaluation of vaginal complaints, *JAMA* 291(11):1368, 2004.

Bachmann GA, Nevadunsky NS: Diagnosis and treatment of atrophic vaginitis, *Am Fam Physician* 61:3090, 2000.

Burstein G, Murray P: Diagnosis and management of sexually transmitted diseases among adolescents, *Pediatr Rev* 24(4):19, 2003.

Coco AS, Vandenbosche M: Infectious vaginitis: an accurate diagnosis is essential and attainable, *Postgrad Med* 107(4):63, 2000.

Egan ME, Lipsky MS: Diagnosis of vaginitis, *Am Fam Physician* 62(5):3090-3096, 2000.

Nyirjesy P: Chronic vulvovaginal candidiasis, *Am Fam Physician* 63(4):697-702, 2001.

Parks D, Yetman R: Diagnosis and management of pelvic inflammatory disease in adolescents, *J Pediatr Health Care* 17(3):145, 2003.

Teran S, Walsh C, Irwin KL: *Chlamydia trachomatis* infection in women: bad news, good news, and next steps in prevention, *J Am Med Womens Assoc* 56(3):100-104, 2001.

Vaginal Bleeding

The average menstrual cycle is 28 days. It is considered abnormal if the cycle occurs more often than every 21 days (polymenorrhea) or less often than every 35 days (oligomenorrhea). Bleeding at irregular intervals is known as metrorrhagia. Intermenstrual bleeding is bleeding between cycles. The average duration of menses is 4 days; a duration of longer than 7 days or blood loss heavier than 80 ml is considered excessive and is classified as menorrhagia. Hypomenorrhea occurs when the frequency of periods remains normal but the menstrual flow decreases in amount. Systemic disorders that cause an imbalance in the hypothalamic-pituitary-ovarian (HPO) axis may lead to menses that are too heavy (menorrhagia/hypermenorrhea), too often (polymenorrhea), or too heavy and irregular (menometrorrhagia).

Other systemic reasons for vaginal bleeding include blood dyscrasias, liver and kidney diseases, and medications (e.g., hormones, anticoagulants, and nonsteroidal anti-inflammatory drugs [NSAIDs]). Organic causes for aberrant menstrual cycles are multiple and include problems such as vaginitis, ectopic pregnancy, fibroids, and polyps. Vaginal bleeding in perimenopausal and postmenopausal women may indicate gynecological cancer. When organic and systemic reasons for abnormal vaginal bleeding are not found, the diagnosis of dysfunctional uterine bleeding (DUB) is warranted.

DIAGNOSTIC REASONING: FOCUSED HISTORY

Is This Related to Age? Where Is the Woman in Her Reproductive Life Cycle?

Key Question
- How old are you?

Age Today

Knowing the woman's present age is the first step in determining the most common causes of vaginal bleeding. The majority of adolescents with abnormal bleeding are experiencing anovulatory cycles. This is caused by estrogen stimulating the uterine lining with no opposing progesterone. This condition leads to a thicker, more vascular, and less stable endometrium, predisposing the adolescent to dyssynchronous bleeding. A young woman's bleeding is most frequently caused by pregnancy, contraceptive methods, or infection. The woman older than age 40 is more likely to have problems related to polyps, fibroids, or ovarian dysfunction. If the patient is more than 50 years of age, the origin of bleeding irregularities is often hormone therapy (HT) or endometrial hyperplasia, which has the potential for endometrial cancer.

Is This Prepubertal Bleeding?

Key Questions
- How old is the child?
- Is there a family history of early sexual development?
- Is there a family history of bleeding problems or blood dyscrasias?
- Did the child ingest any birth control pills or estrogens?
- Are there any accompanying symptoms?

Pediatric Vaginal Bleeding

In the United States, the average age of menarche is 12 years old. Vaginal bleeding before age 9 is abnormal and may indicate foreign body or injury. The presence of secondary sexual characteristics indicates sexual precocity. Newborn girls may experience breast bud enlargement, galactorrhea, and a small amount of vaginal bleeding from maternal exogenous hormones. These symptoms resolve without intervention within a few weeks.

Although uncommon, malignant genital tract tumors in girls can cause vaginal bleeding. Vaginal adenosis and adenocarcinoma are the most common tumor types.

Bleeding Problems

A family history of bleeding problems or a positive review of systems and physical examination indicating the presence of petechiae or bruises may suggest a bleeding tendency. Platelet counts or clotting studies are indicated.

Accompanying Symptoms

Vulvovaginitis is the most common pediatric gynecological problem. A vaginal discharge, vaginal itching, vulvar erythema, and lesions often accompany vulvovaginal bleeding. A foul-smelling discharge is noted with bacterial vaginosis, trichomoniasis, and a foreign body. Wet mounts and cultures should be taken for all vaginal discharges of a child, including cultures for gonorrhea and *Chlamydia*. If a sexually transmitted infection (STI) and sexual abuse are suspected, syphilis and human immunodeficiency virus (HIV) testing should be done. Throat and rectal cultures for gonorrhea and *Chlamydia* should also be obtained.

Trauma to the perineum is more common in children because there is less subcutaneous fat of the vulva. Large lacerations and hematomas warrant referral for examination and repair under anesthesia.

Prolapse of the urethra may cause bleeding. It is accompanied by pain at the meatus and pain with urination.

What Is the Character of the Bleeding?

Key Questions

- When did it begin?
- How long have you been bleeding?
- What is the flow like?
- How many pads do you use?
- Are there any accompanying problems?

Symptom Analysis

Determine the amount of flow and its duration to establish if there is menorrhagia, metrorrhagia, or menometrorrhagia. Menorrhagia is considered to be 80 ml of menses, which is estimated as saturating a sanitary pad hourly, over several hours. Metrorrhagia is defined as bleeding at irregular intervals or intermenstrual bleeding. When the menstruation has an unpredictable schedule and lasts for a prolonged time, it is termed menometrorrhagia.

Associated Complaints

Patients may experience postcoital bleeding with cervical infections, cervical polyps, or cervical cancer. Accompanying dyspareunia may indicate endometriosis. Dysmenorrhea can be caused by an intrauterine device (IUD) or adenomyosis. Pelvic pressure or pain is suspicious for persistent corpus luteum cyst. Uterine prolapse causes pelvic pressure, which is subjectively described as "something falling out of the vagina." Fever is associated with a pelvic infection. Menorrhagia, accompanied by fatigue, weight gain, hair loss, cold intolerance, decreased libido, and constipation, is a symptom of hypothyroidism. Bleeding disorders may become apparent for the first time in the teenager, with severe menorrhagia accompanied by bruising, petechiae, and gingival bleeding.

Is This Problem Acute or Chronic? How Does It Compare With Usual Menses?

Key Questions

- Has this kind of vaginal bleeding occurred before?
- Were your periods regular before this episode?
- How long did they last?
- What was the amount and pattern of bleeding?

Irregular Menses

In anovulatory cycles, the endometrium proliferates under the influence of high estrogen levels until it can no longer be supported—then bleeding occurs. This results in a menstrual pattern that is longer than 28 days with a very heavy flow that lasts 7 to 14 days. If the patient's estrogen levels are fluctuating, she may have two periods a month. Both of these patterns are consistent with DUB. However, organic problems with any component of the reproductive tract must be ruled out.

Acute Bleeding

One episode of acute bleeding in a woman with normally regular menstrual cycles suggests uterine fibroids or a complication of pregnancy such as threatened abortion. In a postmenopausal women with an intact uterus, an episode of vaginal bleeding is indicative of endometrial hyperplasia and is suspicious for endometrial cancer.

Chronic Bleeding

Chronic, irregular menstrual cycles coupled with obesity are likely to be caused by polycystic ovary syndrome (PCOS), also known as Stein-Leventhal syndrome. Chronic midcycle spotting can occur secondary to the normal midcycle drop in estrogen levels and usually is not bothersome to the patient because the amount of vaginal bleeding is very scant and the duration is short.

Could This Be Related to Pregnancy?

Key Questions

- Do you have any symptoms of pregnancy (e.g., missed period, breast tenderness, nausea and vomiting)?
- When was your last normal menstrual period?
- What are you using for birth control?
- Have you recently delivered a baby?

Pregnancy

A small amount of bleeding can occur at the time of implantation. The blastocyst burrows into the endometrium and invades the maternal blood supply; the formation and implantation of the placenta follow this. If bleeding occurs from implantation, it happens about 1 week before the expected menstrual cycle. Regard women of childbearing age as pregnant until pregnancy is ruled out. It is estimated that up to 50% of all fertilized eggs die and are aborted spontaneously, usually before the woman knows she is pregnant. About 20% of pregnant women have some vaginal bleeding during the first trimester.

Recent Delivery

If the patient has recently delivered an infant, the abnormal vaginal bleeding could likely be from retained placenta, infection of the uterus (endometritis), or a laceration.

If the Patient Is Pregnant, Is This a Complication?

Key Questions

- How old are you?
- How many weeks pregnant are you?
- Do you have any chronic health problems?
- Are you experiencing any pain or cramping?
- Have you passed any tissue?
- Are you having any other symptoms?
- Have you ever had any STIs?
- Have you ever had an infection of your tubes (pelvic inflammatory disease [PID])?
- Have you ever been pregnant? What were the number of times and outcomes of your pregnancies?

Age

The risk for spontaneous abortion is higher in women older than 35. Most ectopic pregnancies occur in women ages 25 to 34 years. However, women older than age 35 have a higher rate of death from ectopic pregnancy.

Weeks of Gestation

Among known pregnancies, the rate of spontaneous abortion is approximately 10% and usually occurs between the seventh and twelfth weeks of pregnancy. An estimated 10% to 15% of clinically recognized pregnancies result in first trimester loss. The patient experiencing an ectopic pregnancy typically presents at about 6 to 8 weeks of gestation.

Chronic Health Conditions

The risk for spontaneous abortion is higher in women with systemic diseases such as diabetes or thyroid problems.

Pain

Low back pain or abdominal pain that is dull, sharp, or cramping may indicate spontaneous abortion or ectopic pregnancy If there is any pain associated with ectopic pregnancy, it will usually be described as "crampy," pelvic pressure, or "soreness" in the lower abdomen. In ectopic pregnancy, the pain may lateralize to one side. Severe, sharp, and sudden pain in the lower abdominal area may indicate rupture of the ectopic pregnancy.

Passing Tissue

The passage of tissue of clotlike material from the vagina suggests spontaneous abortion. Ectopic pregnancies can be accompanied by sloughing material.

Other Symptoms

Pain referred to the shoulder is suggestive of ectopic pregnancy rupture with peritoneal free fluid and significant hemorrhage. Other symptoms of rupture include feeling dizzy or faint or actually fainting. **Ruptured ectopic pregnancy is a surgical emergency.**

Sexually Transmitted Infections

STIs may have been unnoticed or untreated or have been inadequately treated and caused scarring of the fallopian tubes, which would place the patient at greater risk for ectopic pregnancy. Ectopic pregnancy occurs in about 1 of every 200 pregnancies (Box 22-1). However, if the woman has had PID, the rate is as high as 1 of every 40 pregnancies.

Previous Pregnancies

The risk for spontaneous abortion is higher in women older than age 35 and in women with a history of three or more prior spontaneous abortions.

Could This Be Caused by the Patient's Birth Control Method?

Key Questions

- Do you use a method of birth control?
- Which kind(s) of birth control do you use?
- How do you use it?

Birth Control

Menorrhagia from IUD contraception is accompanied by increased cramping and pain. If spotting or cramping is not of a usual pattern, ectopic pregnancy or infection must be considered. Displacement or perforation of the uterus by the IUD can be verified by pelvic ultrasound. Women who have recently discontinued the use of oral contraceptive (OC) pills after several years of use may experience heavier menstrual bleeding than when they were on OC pills. Breakthrough bleeding caused by OC pills may occur in the first 2 weeks of the cycle because of low estrogen level or in the last 2 weeks because of low progesterone level. Long-acting progestin contraceptives (Norplant [medroxyprogesterone acetate]) may cause irregular heavy menses because there is a lack of estrogen to stabilize the endometrium. Changes in bleeding patterns for progestin users necessitate ruling out pregnancy.

Is the Patient Experiencing Anovulatory Cycles?

Key Questions

- Have you experienced irregular menstrual cycles?
- Are you having symptoms of menopause (e.g., vaginal dryness, hot flashes, night sweats)?
- At what age did your mother or grandmother go through menopause?

Irregular Menstrual Cycles

Anovulatory cycles are the most common cause of irregular bleeding patterns among

---

Box 22-1	**Risk Factors for Ectopic Pregnancy**

History of PID
Previous ectopic pregnancy
History of tubal surgery
Infertility
In utero diethylstilbestrol exposure
Present use of IUD
Smoking

females beginning (adolescent) or ending (perimenopausal) their menstrual cycles. It is estimated that 80% of young adolescents will be anovulatory during the first year of their menstruation. Regular ovulatory cycles are usually established by the second year of menses but may take up to 5 years.

Menopause Symptoms

The hot flash is the most commonly experienced symptom of menopause. It is a sensation of increased upper body warmth that begins in the chest area and progresses upward to the neck and face. Sweating, which can be so profuse as to leave clothing wet, follows the hot flash. Hot flashes often lead to disturbed sleep patterns, insomnia, and fatigue. Vaginal atrophy is experienced by the patient as vaginal dryness, dyspareunia, and atrophic vaginitis (see Chapter 21). Atrophic changes can affect the urinary system, causing urinary frequency, urgency, and exacerbation of stress incontinence.

Menopausal Syndrome

The frequency of monthly ovulation begins to become irregular at about 40 years of age, and this leads to intermittent symptoms of menopause. The time frame from onset of symptoms to complete cessation of menstruation is termed the perimenopause or climacteric phase. The perimenopause can last up to 10 years. If menopause is completed before age 40, it is considered premature ovarian failure. The age of menopause is genetically determined and will be similar to those of the woman's mother and grandmother. Menopause is unrelated to age of menarche, pregnancies, or contraceptive methods used.

Is the Patient Experiencing Postmenopausal Bleeding?

Key Questions

- How old were you when you stopped menstruating?
- Do you still have a uterus?
- Did you have a hysterectomy? Why did you have surgery? Were your ovaries removed?
- Are you using hormones?

Age at Menopause

The average age for a woman in the United States to go through menopause is 51 years. Menopause is defined as 1 year without menstrual cycles. However, a diagnosis can be accurately made earlier by measuring the rising follicle-stimulating hormone (FSH) and the falling estradiol levels. Postmenopausal bleeding is any bleeding that occurs after the establishment of menopause. Vaginal bleeding after menopause warrants investigation to rule out endometrial cancer. Box 22-2 lists risk factors for endometrial cancer.

Intact Uterus

In postmenopausal women with an intact uterus, unexplained vaginal bleeding suggests endometrial hyperplasia with a suspicion for endometrial cancer.

Hysterectomy

Any vaginal bleeding after a hysterectomy justifies suspicion of cancer, but the bleeding will most likely be a symptom of atrophic vaginitis. If the ovaries were left in place at the time of the hysterectomy, the woman may not experience menopausal syndrome until about 8 to 10 years after the surgery. The ovaries become atrophic and nonfunctional over time, probably secondary to altered blood flow resulting from the surgery. The bleeding of atrophic vaginitis occurs from the slightest trauma; even wiping the perineum with tissue after urination can cause spotting.

Hormone Therapy

Hormone therapy for menopausal symptoms may cause vaginal bleeding in women

Box 22-2	**Risk Factors for Endometrial Cancer**

Postmenopausal with intact uterus and abnormal vaginal bleeding
Family history of endometrial cancer
Hypertension, diabetes mellitus, liver disease
Obesity
Chronic anovulatory cycles
Unopposed estrogen therapy with intact uterus
Tamoxifen therapy

with an intact uterus. Regimens for women with an intact uterus include the cycling of estrogen and progestin and continuous daily doses of both hormones. The cycled hormones produce a regular scheduled bleeding. However, the continuous daily combination therapy will often cause amenorrhea after 3 to 6 months of use. After a pattern of amenorrhea has been established, new bleeding should be investigated.

Unopposed estrogen therapy in a woman with an intact uterus predisposes her to endometrial cancer from a thick, built-up endometrium. Endometrial hyperplasia accounts for about 20% of postmenopausal women who complain of abnormal vaginal bleeding. Endometrial hyperplasia can be diagnosed with endometrial biopsy, ultrasonography, or dilation and curettage (D&C).

Vaginal bleeding can also be caused by a cancerous cervical lesion (diagnosed with colposcopy and biopsy), cervical polyps, or endometrial polyps. Ovarian tumors can excrete estrogens and progestins, causing vaginal bleeding. Fallopian tube cancer more commonly presents with scant vaginal bleeding or watery vaginal discharge with a pelvic mass.

Could This Be From Infection or Inflammation?

Key Questions

- Have you noticed any sores, rashes, or lumps in the vaginal area?
- Do you have a vaginal discharge or vulvar itching or burning?
- What were the results of your last Papanicolaou test?

Lesions and Lumps

Genital warts (condylomata acuminata) can cause bleeding secondary to trauma that has been induced. Typically, genital warts are located inferiorly from the fossa navicularis to the fourchette and perineal area and internally on the walls of the vagina and cervix. A painless ulcer suggests syphilis and classically appears as a solitary lesion; however, there can be more than one chancre, especially if the patient is immunocompro-

mised. Lesions secondarily infected by bacteria may bleed. Inguinal lymphadenopathy can signal a sexually transmitted infection of the genitourinary tract.

Vaginal Discharge

Acute or chronic endometritis and PID may cause heavy menstrual bleeding. An endometrial infection disturbs the clotting properties, resulting in painful, heavy bleeding. *Chlamydia* and gonorrhea are the most frequent causes of PID.

Last Pap Test

The last Pap test result may provide clues to a chronic vaginal infection showing a predominance of coccobacilli or atrophy with inflammation; a progressive, low-grade, squamous, intraepithelial lesion; or a cancerous condition. However, the accuracy of a normal Pap test is unreliable if a cervical lesion or abnormal cervical vascular patterns are noted on physical examination.

What Other Causes of Bleeding Should I Consider?

Key Questions

- Could this bleeding be from the urethra or rectum?
- Are you taking tamoxifen?
- What other medications are you taking?
- Do you have a history of anemia, or do you bleed easily with dental work?
- Did your mother take diethylstilbestrol (DES) when she was pregnant with you?

Urinary or Rectal Bleeding

Bleeding from the urethra or rectum can be misinterpreted as vaginal bleeding. A prolapsed cystocele or rectocele might be subject to drying, abrasion, and bleeding. These causes can be documented through physical examination, urinalysis, fecal testing for occult blood, and colonoscopy.

Tamoxifen

Tamoxifen, used for primary or secondary prevention of breast cancer, can cause endometrial hyperplasia and produce vaginal bleeding. Endometrial biopsy is required.

Medications

Antibiotics, phenobarbital, rifampin, phenytoin, carbamazepine, and other drugs that induce hepatic microsomal enzymes may produce lower estrogen levels and cause bleeding irregularities. Drugs containing aspirin can increase menstrual flow.

Blood Dyscrasias

Some females with a coagulation defect have excessive menstrual bleeding as the first symptom of a blood disorder; also most platelet abnormalities will cause vaginal bleeding. If the patient has severe anemia (hemoglobin <10 g/dl) resulting from the vaginal bleeding, it is highly probable that a coagulopathy is present. If this occurs in the perimenarcheal or second or third decade of life, suspect von Willebrand's disease—a congenital bleeding disorder caused by deficiency in factor VIII.

DES Exposure in Utero

In utero exposure to diethylstilbestrol (DES) has been associated with adenocarcinoma of the vagina in daughters of women who took the drug during pregnancy.

DIAGNOSTIC REASONING: FOCUSED PHYSICAL EXAMINATION

Perform a General Assessment

Determine whether the patient's general state of health includes problems of nutrition (e.g., obesity or muscle wasting), hirsutism, hypothyroidism, or hyperthyroidism, all of which may cause an endocrinopathy with consequent vaginal bleeding.

Assess Vital Signs

In patients who are tachycardic and tachypneic, suspect a ruptured ectopic pregnancy. The patient will show signs of hemorrhage and shock.

Determine Patient Weight and Calculate Body Mass Index

A body mass index (BMI) of greater than 27% corresponds to being more than 20% overweight. (See nomogram in Appendix C for calculation of BMI.) Obesity causes anovulatory cycles because the adipose cell stroma converts androstenedione to estrogen (estrone) as the body fat increases. Obesity also increases sex hormone binding globulin, thereby increasing free steroid levels. Both processes can cause an imbalance in the HPO axis and increase the probability of an anovulatory cycle and heavy vaginal bleeding. Amenorrhea in anorexia nervosa may precede weight loss by many months.

Perform a Lymph Node Examination

Lymph node examination should be performed to assess for leukemia or metastatic gynecological cancer. Inguinal lymph nodes can be enlarged from an STI or a vulvar infection (e.g., bartholinitis).

Perform a Thyroid Examination

Observe and palpate the thyroid gland. Hypertrophy (enlargement) may be found in hypofunctioning glands. Hypothyroidism is known to be present in 22% of women with severe menorrhagia.

Perform a Breast Examination

The finding of spontaneous, bilateral, clear, or nonbloody nipple discharge on breast examination could be indicative of hyperprolactinemia, which may cause amenorrhea or irregular vaginal bleeding.

Perform a Pelvic Examination

If practitioners and patients believe bleeding to be uterine in origin, the external and internal pelvic examination can verify that etiology. Perform an examination of the external genitalia, noting whether the bleeding is coming from external hemorrhoids or a painless labial lesion such as a squamous cell cancer or condylomata acuminata. Note bruising, lacerations on the vaginal walls, or other signs of sexual abuse. Observe the introitus for signs of a prolapsed uterus or cystocele or rectocele that might be subject to drying, abrasion, or bleeding. These signs are usually accompanied by pelvic pressure or urinary or bowel symptoms.

Observe the external genitalia for signs of estrogen deficiency: sparse hair distribution, graying or white hair color, clitoral atrophy, and thin, small labia minora. These signs strongly suggest atrophic vaginitis as the cause for bleeding.

Next perform a vaginal examination to determine if the bleeding may be caused by a vaginal infection. Note the color and condition of the vaginal walls. Pale, nonrugated vaginal walls are a sign of an atrophic vagina, which is easily abraded to cause bleeding. Pale vaginal mucosa with splotchy red patches is also a sign of vaginal atrophy. Bleeding from atrophic vaginitis most commonly follows intercourse or douching. It often is a whitish-brown discharge with no particular foul odor. The patient may also have pruritus and a burning sensation of the vagina, labia, and urinary tract because of a lack of estrogen.

Note the amount, color, consistency, and odor of the vaginal discharge. Take samples for wet mount examination from the pooled discharge in the lateral fornices. Note cervical friability and discharge from the cervical os. Take samples of the discharge and assess as noted in Chapter 21. Cervical polyps are red, glossy, nontender masses protruding from the cervical os. They are usually benign and can be removed by twisting them off with ring forceps. The specimen should be sent for pathological evaluation.

If a threatened or spontaneous abortion is suspected, check the internal cervical os to determine if it is closed or open.

Ectopic pregnancy will cause adnexal or cervical motion tenderness. However, uterine enlargement is not often appreciated. Uterine size and contour can be grossly assessed via bimanual examination. On pelvic examination, the uterus is enlarged but smaller than anticipated from dates provided. The cervix is tender to motion, and a tender adnexal mass may be palpable. Diagnosis is confirmed by positive human chorionic gonadotropin (hCG) test results and ultrasound. Serial quantitative serum hCG levels may be useful. **A ruptured ectopic pregnancy is a surgical emergency.**

Uterine leiomyomas (myomas, fibroids) typically feel firm and may make the uterus asymmetrical. These tumors can progress to a size that mimics an advanced pregnant uterus. The uterine size is measured in weeks, just as the pregnant uterus is measured. When the uterus reaches 12- to 14-week size, referral to a gynecologist for surgery (myomectomy or hysterectomy) is appropriate. The patient may experience urinary or bowel problems (e.g., urinary frequency and constipation) because the fibroid is distorting or obstructing those systems. Carcinogenic tumors of the uterus are classically firm, hard, and rapidly growing, becoming fixed masses. Ultrasound is a valuable tool in documenting the size and growth patterns of tumors.

The average-size adult uterus measures 8 cm long, 5 cm wide, and 2.5 cm deep for the nulliparous woman. Add 1 cm to each dimension for the average size of the multiparous uterus (9 × 6 × 3.5 cm). The uterus with adenomyosis is increased in size to 2 to 3 times that of normal, may be globular, and has a uniform consistency. Adenomyosis is accompanied by worsening menorrhagia and dysmenorrhea.

The rectovaginal examination can detect lesions or nodularity of the cul-de-sac, which is present with endometriosis or the presence of a primary rectal tumor.

Pediatric Examination: Perform a Breast and Genital Examination

Assess for signs of sexual precocity by determining the presence and stage of secondary sexual characteristics of the breasts and pubic hair. Assess development using Tanner staging (see Chapter 23, Figure 23-3). Inspect the vulva, noting the hygiene status—presence of smegma in the labial folds, urine, fecal material, or erythema and lesions. Examine the urinary meatus. A prolapsed urinary meatus is noted by the presence of a dark red tissue surrounding the urinary opening. This tissue is usually tender. Use an appropriate pediatric size speculum, long otoscope, or nasal speculum. It may be necessary to refer the patient for a vaginoscopy or cystoscopy under anesthesia for a complete assessment of the vagina and uterus.

Consider the possibility of infection or sexual abuse. See Chapter 21 for assessment of vaginal discharges.

LABORATORY AND DIAGNOSTIC STUDIES

Qualitative Urine/Serum hCG Tests

Qualitative urine/serum hCG tests are monoclonal antibody tests using radioimmunoassay (RIA) to determine or exclude pregnancy. The serum hCG test is more sensitive than the urine hCG test. The serum test can be performed in about 2 hours, and hCG can be detected as early as 6 days after conception. The result is reported as either negative or positive. Because the β-subunits are measured, it is highly specific and does not cross-react with luteinizing hormone.

Depending on the specific test used, urine testing can detect pregnancy from before to several days after a missed period. The results are obtained in minutes. A positive test (usually a color change) indicates pregnancy.

Quantitative Serum Human Chorionic Gonadotropin Test

A quantitative human chorionic gonadotropin (β-hCG) test is the first step in determining a complication of pregnancy. The test is a fluorometric enzyme immunoassay that is highly specific for the β-receptors of hCG, with almost no cross-reactivity with other hormones. Results are provided as values. The reference ranges for determining an abnormal pregnancy are as follows:

Not significant: 0 to 5.0 mIU/ml
Borderline significance: 5.0 to 25 mIU/ml
Evaluate with serial determinations: more than 25 mIU/ml

A rapid β-hCG test (with a sensitivity of at least 5 milliunits/ml) that measures less than 5 milliunits/ml is highly predictive in excluding ectopic pregnancy. The β-hCG levels have a doubling time of 58 hours with pregnancy. Ectopic pregnancy causes an increase in hCG levels at the same rate as a normal pregnancy but only up to a certain point. In ectopic pregnancy, that point is usually less than 4 to 6 weeks, at which time the hCG levels plateau or begin to fall. Therefore serial determinations are more useful than a single determination.

The β-hCG test and ultrasound are used together to determine the possibility of ectopic pregnancy. If the discriminatory threshold of β-hCG is 1500 milliunits/ml and a vaginal ultrasound determines the absence of a gestational sac (gestational age, 35 days) or a value of 6500 milliunits/ml and negative transabdominal ultrasound (gestational age, 42 days), the presumptive diagnosis of ectopic pregnancy can be made. A drop in serial hCG levels and an ultrasound that does not identify an intrauterine gestational sac support the diagnosis of spontaneous abortion.

Hematocrit and Hemoglobin Levels

Hematocrit and hemoglobin levels are used to determine anemia caused by blood loss from long-standing menorrhagia. Hematocrit and hemoglobin levels are not useful in evaluating acute blood loss from a single episode of heavy bleeding caused by a spontaneous abortion or ectopic pregnancy.

Complete Blood Cell Count With Indices and Differential

Complete blood cell count with indices will provide information about the degree and cause of anemia. Typically, the hematocrit and hemoglobin levels reflect the degree of anemia, with erythrocyte indices suggesting the cause. Microcytic hypochromic anemia is reflective of chronic blood loss, whereas normocytic normochromic anemia suggests acute hemorrhage. Microcytic hypochromic anemia is indicated by a mean corpuscular volume (MCV) of less than 80 μ^3 and a mean corpuscular hemoglobin (MCH) level of less than 27 pg. The MCV and MCH values are within reference range in normocytic normochromic anemia.

An increased white blood cell (WBC) count with a shift to the left (an increase in the number of bands that are immature neutrophils) points to infection as a cause of the vaginal bleeding. Additionally, the CBC can rule out leukemia and thrombocytopenia, both of which can produce abnormal vaginal bleeding.

Prothrombin Time/Partial Thromboplastin Time/Bleeding Time (PT/PTT/BT)

If the history and/or the physical examination is suggestive of a bleeding problem, prothrombin time (PT), partial thromboplastin time (PTT), and bleeding time (BT) can differentiate between blood dyscrasias, hepatic or renal diseases, or iatrogenic causes (e.g., anticoagulants, nonsteroidal anti-inflammatory drugs).

Serum Progesterone Levels

A serum progesterone level of greater than 25 ng/ml is predictive of an intrauterine pregnancy; however, a level less than 15 ng/ml suggests an ectopic pregnancy.

Serum Follicle-Stimulating Hormone Levels

Ovarian failure, which causes a low estradiol secretion, will raise the FSH level greater than 40 mIU/ml. If both the follicle-stimulating hormone (FSH) and luteinizing hormone (LH) levels are greater than 50 mIU/ml, primary ovarian failure is established. If the patient is older than 30 years, menopause is diagnosed; if she is younger than 30 years, a chromosomal karyotype should be obtained. An FSH measurement of less than 40 milliunits/ml denotes a hypothalamic-pituitary dysfunction and secondary ovarian failure.

Serum Luteinizing Hormone Levels

A serum LH level of greater than 35 mIU/ml is frequently seen in patients with PCOS. An LH/FSH ratio higher than 2:1 is suggestive of PCOS, whereas a ratio greater than 3:1 is considered diagnostic of PCOS.

Serum Estradiol Levels

Serum estradiol levels less than 15 pg/ml are found with menopause.

Fecal Occult Blood Test (FOBT) or Fecal Immunochemical Test (FIT)

A negative FOBT or FIT rules out the cause of bleeding being located in the colon or rectum (see Chapter 16).

Vaginal/Lower Abdominal Ultrasound

Ultrasonography is used to determine endometrial thickness. A thickness greater than 3 mm indicates hyperplasia. In postmenopausal women, 5 mm is the cutoff for a normal unilateral stripe. It is also helpful in identifying cystic enlargement of the uterus, the presence of leiomyomas, and the presence or absence of the products of conception. Ultrasonography is used to determine complications of pregnancy such as ectopic pregnancy, placenta previa, or threatened abortion. When the intrauterine sac is identified within the uterus by ultrasound, an ectopic pregnancy is rarely the diagnosis, even though it is possible to have simultaneous intrauterine and ectopic pregnancies.

Endometrial Biopsy

Endometrial biopsy (EMB) is used to detect cancer in any perimenopausal or postmenopausal woman who is experiencing abnormal vaginal bleeding. It is used to exclude endometrial cancer in women taking tamoxifen who experience vaginal bleeding. EMB can be performed on women who are in their thirties if they are at increased risk for endometrial cancer (see Box 22-2). The sensitivity of this biopsy for endometrial carcinoma is 95% to 97%. If the test results are abnormal or inadequate in terms of amount of tissue, the next diagnostic test would be dilation and curettage (D&C). If the test is normal and abnormal bleeding continues, further workup is indicated to exclude neoplasia.

Dilation and Curettage

D&C is useful in determining the cause of abnormal uterine bleeding and for the removal of retained products of conception. The curetting of the entire uterus provides specimens to send to pathology to rule out carcinogenic causes for the uterine bleeding.

Hysteroscopy

Hysteroscopy allows for visualization of the uterine cavity. Endometrial biopsies, endometrial polyps, and submucosal leiomyomas can be obtained and/or removed by hysteroscopy.

DIFFERENTIAL DIAGNOSIS
Organic Causes of Vaginal Bleeding
Pregnancy
A small amount of bleeding can occur at the time of implantation. The blastocyst burrows into the endometrium and invades the maternal blood supply; the formation and implantation of the placenta follow this. If bleeding occurs from implantation, it happens about 1 week before the expected menstrual cycle. Regard women of childbearing age as pregnant until pregnancy is ruled out.

Spontaneous Abortion
A spontaneous abortion (or miscarriage) is the natural termination of a pregnancy before fetal viability (before 20 weeks). Approximately 15% of diagnosed pregnancies abort spontaneously. It is a complete spontaneous abortion if the fetus and the placenta are completely expelled and incomplete if partial tissue remains within the uterus. Most often the woman will present with persistent uterine cramping and bleeding that is increasing in severity and amount. She may have experienced passage of tissue. The typical patient experiencing a spontaneous abortion presents to the clinic at about 10 to 12 weeks of gestation. The pregnancy test may remain positive for weeks after fetal death. Serial serum hCG levels and ultrasound are useful in establishing the diagnosis.

Threatened Abortion
Threatened abortion produces menstruation-like cramping and bleeding but the cervical os remains closed. The pain is often midline or suprapubic. Perform a sterile speculum examination to inspect the external cervical os. **Only if the facility is prepared to deal with the possibility of surgical intervention** should a cotton-tipped applicator or ring forceps be passed through the os to verify its closed status. In addition to the bleeding and cramping, if the cervical os is open or if tissue is in the cervical canal, the woman is diagnosed with an inevitable abortion.

Placenta Previa
Placenta previa occurs in the third trimester of pregnancy and presents with bright red painless bleeding. The placenta is implanted in the lower segment of the uterus. When the cervix begins to dilate, the placenta is pulled away from the endometrial wall, and bleeding can occur. Any significant bleeding that leads to hemorrhage can endanger the mother and may interfere with uteroplacental sufficiency. Fetal activity is present. The uterus is nontender with a normal resting tone. Diagnosis is made by sonogram. Pelvic examination should not be performed to avoid dislodging any clot that may have formed at the cervix.

Placenta Abruptio
Placenta abruptio can occur any time after 20 weeks of gestation. As the placenta detaches from the uterine wall, the patient experiences dark red, painful bleeding. The amount of bleeding varies from scant to profuse. On physical examination, vaginal bleeding is apparent, and the uterus may be tender and demonstrate increased tone. Signs of fetal distress may be apparent. **Vaginal examination is not performed until placenta previa is ruled out as a diagnosis through the use of ultrasound.**

Ectopic Pregnancy
Ectopic pregnancy occurs in about 1 of 200 pregnancies. Ectopic pregnancy is the second most common cause of maternal death in the United States. Maintain high suspicion for this life-threatening condition. A ruptured ectopic pregnancy is a surgical emergency (see Chapter 13). Ectopic pregnancy symptoms can be the same as normal pregnancy symptoms; therefore any pregnancy accompanied by bleeding or pain must be considered high risk for ectopic pregnancy and must be evaluated to rule out the condition. Persistent one-sided pain or pain that radiates toward the midline of the abdomen is indicative of ectopic pregnancy. The patient experiencing an ectopic pregnancy typically presents at about 6 to 8 weeks of gestation. The menstrual pattern for these patients begins with a time of amenorrhea, followed by abnormal bleeding. They may have some symptoms of pregnancy (e.g., breast tenderness, nausea, and vomiting), have passed some tissue (decidual cast), or have experienced fainting

or dizziness. Ninety percent of ectopic pregnancies are implanted in the fallopian tube. About half of these women will have an adnexal mass.

Leiomyomas (Myomas or Fibroids)

Fibroids are found in about 1 of 4 women over age 35. They are more frequently found in African American women than in Caucasian women, and they usually decrease in size after menopause. Depending on location, they are associated with infertility in 2% to 10% of patients. These benign tumors are estrogen dependent and may grow during HT. The most frequent symptom of leiomyomas is bleeding, which ranges from slightly heavier menstrual flow to continuous bleeding. Fibroids may occur as single or multiple tumors within the uterine layers, or they can be pedunculated. Pain is not a common complaint of women with fibroids unless there has been strangulation of a pedunculated fibroid, degeneration of a large fibroid, or compression of other organ systems.

Adenomyosis

Adenomyosis is a condition in which there are endometrial glands and stroma within the myometrium of the uterus. It is a condition, more common in multiparous women, that occurs in the later reproductive years. The uterus is 2 to 3 times its normal size, and there is often dysmenorrhea and infertility. Adenomyosis often coexists with uterine fibroids. Ultrasound may not identify this diffuse intramural lesion. Adenomyosis is found in 20% of hysterectomy specimens.

Uterine/Endometrial Cancer

Endometrial cancer is presently the most common female genital cancer in the United States. The average age at diagnosis is 61 years, but it occurs throughout the reproductive and postmenopausal years. Uterine cancer risk factors are anovulatory states (e.g., obesity), endometrial hyperplasia (e.g., unopposed estrogen), and family history (see Box 22-2). Classic symptoms include pain-

less vaginal bleeding and a rapidly enlarging uterus. Late symptoms, such as weight loss and weakness, are those of systemic disease.

Systemic Causes of Vaginal Bleeding

Anovulatory Cycles

Perimenopause

The perimenopausal years occur from ages 40 to 50 and last about 7 to 10 years. The perimenopausal woman experiences irregularities in her menstrual flow. Often she has spotting, followed by 1 or 2 days of heavy bleeding, or has her regular menstrual flow and a few days of spotting at the end of the cycle. These types of irregular patterns are characteristic of a degenerating corpus luteum function. A woman who has had 1 year of irregular periods and who has missed the past three cycles can be clinically diagnosed as being in perimenopause (a synonymous term is climacteric). The perimenopause progresses to menopause when the FSH level is elevated above 40 milliunits/ml or there has been an absence of periods for 1 full year. An FSH level of 30 milliunits/ml is typical of perimenopause.

Perimenarche

With perimenarche, the patient has a history of beginning her menstrual cycles and then experiencing months of amenorrhea, followed by resumption of regular cycles. The menstrual flow may be heavier, more frequent, or longer in duration. The young adolescent has appropriate secondary sexual characteristics and sexual maturity ratings. These symptoms are characteristic of anovulatory cycles.

Newborn

A bloody vaginal discharge may occur normally in the female newborn because of maternal estrogen hormone withdrawal during the first few weeks of life.

Endocrinopathies

Polycystic Ovary Syndrome

In PCOS, the patient typically is obese and hirsute and has oligomenorrhea and large cystic ovaries. However, women with chronic anovulatory cycles and hyperandro-genemia meet the criteria for PCOS even if they are slim and without hirsutism. The LH/FSH ratio is greater than 3:1.

Thyroid Dysfunction
Both hypothyroidism and hyperthyroidism are associated with abnormal menstrual bleeding. Menorrhagia can occur with hypothyroidism, whereas oligomenorrhea or scant menses may occur with hyperthyroidism.

With hypothyroidism, the patient may also experience delayed growth, weight gain, fatigue, constipation, and cold intolerance. On physical examination, you may note dry skin, coarse hair, and galactorrhea. The TSH level will be high.

With hyperthyroidism, the patient may experience weight loss, nervousness, heat intolerance, and palpitations. On physical examination, the skin may be moist and sweaty, the hair thin, and the pulse rate rapid. The thyroid gland may be enlarged or nodular. The TSH level will be low, with high triiodo-thyronine (T_3) and thyroxine (T_4) levels.

Hyperprolactinemia
Prolactin inhibits gonadotropin release and causes anovulatory cycles that may be associated with irregular and sometimes heavy bleeding or with amenorrhea (see Chapter 23). Galactorrhea often accompanies hyperprolactinemia. Nipple discharge will be negative for red blood cells. Prolactin levels will be elevated. Thyroid function tests can rule out hypothyroidism. Magnetic resonance imaging or computed tomography scan along with a cone view of the sella turcica assists in the diagnosis of pituitary tumor.

Vaginal Infection
Atrophic Vaginitis
In atrophic vaginitis, there is a dry (shiny), pale, thin vaginal wall caused by an insufficient amount of endogenous estrogen. During menopause, the vaginal mucosa and vulva, which lack glycogen, become fragile and are susceptible to injury and infection. The patient may experience burning, dryness, irritation, dyspareunia, or atrophic vaginitis.

This also occurs in the postpartum woman, the woman who is breastfeeding, or the prepubertal girl. The pH is alkaline and ranges from 6.5 to 7.0. Wet mount reveals a few WBCs and is negative for pathogens.

Endometritis
Endometritis is an infection of the endometrium, in which *Chlamydia* is the cause about 25% of the time. Group A or B *Streptococcus* produces puerperal sepsis and may lead to peritonitis, abscess, thrombophlebitis, disseminated intravascular coagulation, septic shock, and infertility. The woman has a slight vaginal discharge (lochia) that is bloody or purulent. The bleeding is accompanied by fever (temperature 39° C to 39.8° C; 102° to 103° F) and uterine tenderness often within the first 24 hours after delivery. Endometritis should be suspected in a woman with these symptoms, especially if she has undergone an emergency cesarean section or an intrauterine manipulative procedure. Other contributing factors for endometritis are premature rupture of membranes and prolonged labor.

Pelvic Inflammatory Disease
PID is most commonly caused by *Chlamydia trachomatis* and *Neisseria gonorrhoeae* (see Chapter 13) and can produce bleeding, abdominal pain, fever, and vaginal discharge. Women with PID have an increasing amount of vaginal discharge and bleeding after intercourse. Infection begins intravaginally in most cases and then spreads upward, causing salpingitis. In the early stages, women may be asymptomatic. Patients may have a purulent discharge that originates from the endocervical columnar and transitional cells. With gonorrhea, patients often experience inflammation of Skene's glands, Bartholin's glands, or the urethra, which causes pain and dysuria. On examination, abdominal tenderness, CMT, and adnexal tenderness are present. As with peritonitis, patients may also have guarding and rebound tenderness. WBCs and erythrocyte sedimentation rate are usually elevated. Cultures and Gram staining can assist with the diagnosis (see Chapter 21).

Genital Warts

Genital warts (condylomata acuminata) are caused by the human papillomavirus and may be precursors to genital cancer. The warts may involve the vagina, cervix, perineum, or perianal areas. Condylomata can be flat or raised verrucous lesions. The patient usually notices a bump on the genital region accompanied by itching and leukorrhea. A wet mount should be performed to rule out any coexisting vaginal infections. An acetic acid test is helpful in identifying flat warts. Refer to a dermatologist or gynecologist for treatment of warts of the urethra or anus.

Foreign Body

In foreign body retention, the presenting symptom is a very malodorous, whitish discharge. In children, the foreign body is as variable as those objects found in the ears and nose. Children younger than 12 months do not have the coordination to insert anything into their vagina; suspect child abuse in those cases and inspect for bruising or excoriations. Wet mount reveals many WBCs.

Blood Dyscrasias

von Willebrand's Disease

von Willebrand's disease is a congenital autosomal dominant bleeding disorder. Altered factor VIII activity and deficient platelet function characterize it. The patient has a prolonged bleeding time. Hypermenorrhea may occur at menarche or may begin in women 20 to 30 years of age.

Leukemia

Hypermenorrhea may be one of the chief complaints of the woman presenting with leukemia. Other symptoms may include fatigue, bruising, and lymph node enlargement. The CBC and bleeding times will direct the workup for this diagnosis.

Other

Medications

Drugs such as rifampin, phenytoin, carbamazepine, and phenobarbital reduce the efficacy of oral contraceptives. If the woman is on a low-estrogen dose oral birth control pill, these medications are likely to be the cause of irregular vaginal bleeding. Changing the oral contraceptive to one of higher estrogenic potency will alleviate the bleeding. Tamoxifen, which acts as an anti-estrogen on breast tissue, has estrogenic effects on the endometrium and can cause endometrial hyperplasia and/or endometrial cancer. The symptom is vaginal bleeding.

DIFFERENTIAL DIAGNOSIS OF *Common Causes of Vaginal Bleeding*

CONDITION	HISTORY	PHYSICAL FINDINGS	DIAGNOSTIC STUDIES
Organic Causes of Vaginal Bleeding			
Pregnancy	Implantation bleeding; breast tenderness, nausea and vomiting	Internal cervical os closed; minimal spotting; globular, enlarged uterus; soft, bluish color cervix	Pregnancy test; β-hCG positive
Spontaneous abortion	Vaginal bleeding following time of amenorrhea; cramping, passage of tissue; history of miscarriages	Internal cervical os open; blood from cervical os	Serial β-hCG declining levels; ultrasound negative
Threatened abortion	Vaginal bleeding following time of amenorrhea; mild cramping	Fetal activity present; internal cervical os may be open	β-hCG positive; ultrasound positive
Placenta previa	Late pregnancy: bright red, painless bleeding	Fetal activity present; uterus is nontender, normal resting tone	Ultrasound

Continued

DIFFERENTIAL DIAGNOSIS OF *Common Causes of Vaginal Bleeding—cont'd*

CONDITION	HISTORY	PHYSICAL FINDINGS	DIAGNOSTIC STUDIES
Placenta abruptio	Dark red, painful bleeding; any time after 20 wk of gestation	Vaginal bleeding; uterus tender with tone; signs of fetal distress	Rule out placenta previa with ultrasound
Ectopic pregnancy	Painless vaginal bleeding; multiparity, older gravida, multiple gestation; history of PID, infertility, STIs	Internal cervical os closed; bloody discharge present	β-hCG positive; ultrasound; laparoscopy
Leiomyomas	Heavier menstrual bleeding; menorrhagia	Enlarged uterine size; firm, spherical masses; nontender	Pelvic examination; ultrasound
Adenomyosis	Worsening menorrhagia; dysmenorrhea	Pelvic enlargement (2-3 times normal size)	Pelvic examination; ultrasound not always helpful
Uterine/endometrial cancer	Rapidly enlarging uterus; painless menorrhagia; pelvic pressure; weight loss, weakness	Enlargement of uterus, often symmetrical; fixed with advanced disease	Endometrial biopsy; D&C; ultrasound; CT or MRI
Systemic Causes of Vaginal Bleeding ***Anovulatory Cycles***			
Perimenopause	Irregular menses, amenorrhea couples with heavier and longer menstrual cycles; hot flashes, night sweats, insomnia, mood changes	Pale, dry vaginal mucosa, few rugae	FSH and LH high; estradiol low
Perimenarche	History of beginning menses within last 1-2 yr; has period of amenorrhea followed by irregular menstrual cycles that are of heavy, frequent, or long duration	Physical examination normal; secondary sexual characteristic present	History and examination
Newborn	Less than 2 month old	Small amount of vaginal spotting	History and examination
Endocrinopathies			
Polycystic ovary syndrome	Infertility; irregular menstrual cycles	Hirsute; obese; enlarged ovaries	Pelvic examination; ultrasound; enlarged ovaries with multiple fluid-filled cysts
Thyroid dysfunction	Hypothyroid: menorrhagia, delayed growth, weight gain, fatigue, constipation, cold intolerance	Hypothyroid: dry skin, fine hair, galactorrhea	TSH high
Hyperprolactinemia	Menometrorrhagia, oligomenorrhea	Bilateral, multiduct, clear-to-white nipple discharge	Serum prolactin level; MRI if indicated
Vaginal Infection			
Atrophic vaginitis	Dyspareunia; vaginal dryness	Pale, thin vaginal mucosa; brown or bloody discharge; pH >4.5	Folded, clumped epithelial cells
Endometritis	History of emergency cesarean section, PROM, prolonged labor, intrauterine manipulative procedures	Tenderness of uterus on bimanual examination; temperature 102-103° F; discharge or lochia may be purulent	WBC >10,000/mm³

DIFFERENTIAL DIAGNOSIS OF *Common Causes of Vaginal Bleeding—cont'd*

CONDITION	HISTORY	PHYSICAL FINDINGS	DIAGNOSTIC STUDIES
Pelvic inflammatory disease	History of PID; chronic vaginitis; STIs	Bilateral abdominal pain following menses; pelvic mass; cervical motion tenderness; vaginal discharge; temperature >100.4° F	WBC, ESR; Gram staining, cultures, molecular testing
Genital warts	Mild-to-moderate itching; foul vaginal discharge; child: history of sexual abuse; adult: new or multiple partners; history of warts	Moist, pale pink, verrucous projections on base; located on vulva, vagina, cervix or perianal area; bleeding with trauma	Acetic acid test: white
Foreign body	Red and swollen vulva; vaginal discharge; history of use of tampon, condom, or diaphragm	Foreign body present (tampon, condom); bloody, foul-smelling discharge	Wet mount: many WBCs, no pathogens; history and examination
Blood Dyscrasias			
von Willebrand's disease	Menorrhagia, adolescent	Bruising; petechiae; gingival bleeding	Bleeding time, factor VIII deficiency, decreased platelets
Leukemia	Menorrhagia; fatigue usually less than 3 months duration	Fever, bruising, pallor; lymph node enlargement; hepatic or splenic enlargement	WBCs: 1000- 400,000/mm³ leukocytosis with immature blasts or cells; anemia, thrombocytopenia, decreased factor V or VIII
Other			
Medications	Taking rifampin, phenytoin, carbamazepine, or phenobarbital while on low-estrogen dose oral contraceptives; tamoxifen	Normal gynecological exam	Bleeding stops with higher estrogen dose oral contraceptive; endometrial biopsy

CHAPTER RESOURCES

Albers JR, Hull SK: Abnormal uterine bleeding, *Am Fam Physician* 69(8):1916, 2004.

Alexander JD, Schneider FD: Vaginal bleeding associated with pregnancy, *Prim Care* 27:137, 2000.

Kilbourn CL, Richards CS: Abnormal uterine bleeding: diagnostic considerations, management options, *Postgrad Med* 109(1):137, 2001.

Mahoney S, Parker C, Potlog-Nahari C et al: Abnormal uterine bleeding: a primary care primer, *Consultant* 46(2):225, 2006.

Munday PE: Pelvic inflammatory disease: an evidence-based approach to diagnosis, *J Infect* 40:31, 2000.

Rimsza M: Dysfunctional uterine bleeding, *Pediatr Rev* 23:227, 2003.

Scott LD, Hasik KJ: The similarities and differences of endometritis and pelvic inflammatory disease, *J Obstet Gynecol Neonatal Nurs* 30:332, 2001.

Amenorrhea

A menorrhea is a lack of menstruation that may be the result of primary or secondary causes. Primary amenorrhea can be defined as the absence of menarche by 16 years of age with normal pubertal growth and development, the absence of menarche by 14 years of age with lack of normal pubertal growth and development, or the absence of menarche 2 years after sexual maturation is complete. Primary amenorrhea is a rare condition, with constitutional puberty delay the most common cause. One third of primary amenorrhea cases are genetic in nature, such as Turner's syndrome or abnormality of the X chromosome.

Secondary amenorrhea is defined as the absence of menstruation for at least three cycles or 6 months in females who have already established menstruation. The most common causes of secondary amenorrhea are the physiological events of pregnancy, lactation, and menopause. Traditionally, the primary care provider would begin investigation of etiological reasons for amenorrhea and use that knowledge to determine the type of amenorrhea. In turn, the suspected cause would guide diagnostic tests, treatment, and referrals. This method of classification looks first at the lower genital tract and then for a dysfunction of any component of the hypothalamic-pituitary-ovarian (HPO) axis.

The normal menstrual cycle begins with the pulsatile delivery of gonadotropin-releasing hormone (GnRH) by the medial-basal hypothalamus. In response, the posterior pituitary releases luteinizing hormone (LH) and follicle-stimulating hormone (FSH). These influence the growth and development of a follicle and its release of estradiol, which causes the uterine endometrium to proliferate,

and initiates the LH surge, which is followed by ovulation and menstruation (Figure 23-1 and Table 23-1).

The hypothalamus is also affected by the central nervous system and the thyroid gland, which can determine the amount of GnRH received by the pituitary. Alterations in the pattern of GnRH pulsatile release will decrease circulating LH and FSH levels; the consequence will be an anovulatory menstrual cycle and amenorrhea.

About 66% of all amenorrheic women are hypoestrogenic because of either hypothalamic-pituitary hypofunction or end-organ failure. Determining whether the patient is hypoestrogenic can expedite finding the reason for her amenorrhea and setting the sequencing of laboratory tests. The progesterone challenge test (PCT) will cause withdrawal bleeding if there is estrogen production and an adequate outflow tract. The functional status of the pituitary-ovarian unit is assessed by measuring the gonadotropins.

DIAGNOSTIC REASONING: FOCUSED HISTORY

Is There a Pregnancy?

Key Questions
- Are you sexually active?
- Are you using any birth control methods?
- Are you trying to become pregnant?

Pregnancy
For any female with a uterus, it is important to rule out pregnancy as the first step in determining the cause of amenorrhea. It is rare, but a young girl can become pregnant before the onset of menses. Pregnancy should

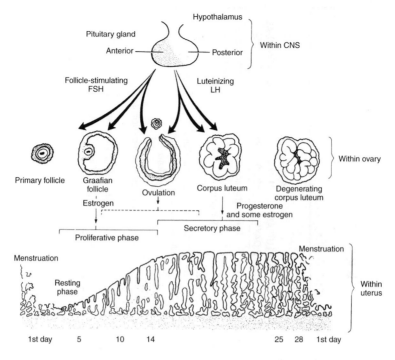

FIGURE 23-1 Interrelationships among cerebral hypothalmic, pituitary, ovarian, and uterine functions throughout the menstrual cycle. (Modified from Lowdermilk DL, Perry SE, Bobak IM: *Maternity and women's health care*, ed 6, St Louis, 1997, Mosby.)

be ruled out before the administration of androgenic challenge tests. If the woman is pregnant and there is accompanying bleeding, determination of whether the pregnancy is uterine or ectopic is the next priority (see Chapter 22). Be cognizant of domestic violence and sexual abuse, with consequent unintended pregnancy. Ask direct questions in private about being hit, pushed, or slapped or about having nonconsensual sex.

Contraceptive Use

The type and use patterns of contraceptives are important in the search for the cause of amenorrhea. Contraceptive failures may account for an unintended pregnancy. Amenorrhea can occur after discontinuation of oral contraceptives. Measurement of serum gonadotropins is affected by long-acting contraceptives such as Depo-Provera (medroxyprogesterone acetate [DMPA]), implants, or intrauterine devices (IUDs) containing progestagens; these must be discontinued before testing.

Seeking Pregnancy

Knowing that the patient is seeking pregnancy or, if the patient is pregnant, whether it is intended or unintended will allow the interview to be structured appropriately. It will also aid in proper counseling and referral. Amenorrheic patients seeking pregnancy who do not bleed after androgen challenge tests are most successfully treated by an infertility specialist. Young maternal age and early referral to a specialist increase a woman's conception rate.

Is This Primary or Secondary Amenorrhea?

Key Questions

- Have you ever had a menstrual cycle?
- Have you started pubertal development? Can you show me how your breast and pubic hair (PH) look compared with these pictures? (Use Tanner Sexual Maturity Rating [SMR] scales [Figures 23-2 and 23-3].)

Table 23-2 Correlation of Ovarian and Endometrial Cycles (Ideal 28-Day Cycle)

	MENSTRUAL (1-3 TO 5 DAYS)	EARLY FOLLICULAR (4 TO 6-8 DAYS)	ADVANCED FOLLICULAR (9 TO 12-16 DAYS)	OVULATION (12-16 DAYS)	EARLY LUTEAL (15-19 DAYS)	ADVANCED LUTEAL (20-25 DAYS)	PREMENSTRUAL (26-32 DAYS)
Ovary	Involution of corpus luteum	Growth and maturation of graafian follicle		Ovulation	Active corpus luteum		Involution of corpus luteum
Estrogen	Diminution	Progressive increase		High concentration	Secondary rise		Decreasing
Progesterone	Absent	Absent	Absent	Appearing	Rising	Rising	Decreasing
Endometrium	Menstrual desquamation and involution	Reorganization and proliferation	Further growth and watery secretion		Active secretion and glandular dilation	Accumulation of secretion and edema	Regressive
Pituitary secretion							
Follicle-stimulating hormone (FSH)	Fairly constant until just before ovulation			Moderate increase just before	Rapid decrease in previous levels		
Luteinizing hormone (LH)	Fairly constant until just before ovulation			Marked increase just before	Rapid decrease in previous levels		

From Thompson JM et al: *Mosby's clinical nursing,* ed 4, St Louis, 1997, Mosby.

- At what age did you start your periods?
- When was your last normal menstrual period?
- What is the nature of your periods (e.g., frequency, duration, amount of flow)?

Onset of Menstruation

The age range for menarche in the United States is 9 to 17 years. If the woman has had established menses at intervals of every 21 to 38 days, then the classification of secondary amenorrhea would apply. Established menses indicate that there is no outlet flow problem and that the HPO axis and endometrium are functioning.

Pubertal Development

Female pubertal development begins with a growth spurt 1 year before the development of breast buds (thelarche) at around age 11 years. Then there is continued growth for 1 year until the peak height velocity is achieved. Pubic hair appears (pubarche), followed by axillary hair and the beginning of menarche. The average age of menarche for U.S. girls is 12 years 4 months. The length of time from thelarche to menarche is 2 to 3 years.

A thorough review of pediatric growth charts is helpful in determining the young girl's norm of growth and development and the centimeters attained by her latest growth spurt. Most adolescent girls have a mean height gain of 29 cm (64.8 inches) and the growth spurt lasts approximately 4 years. Asking adolescents to self-identify their Tanner SMR scales for breast and pubic maturity provides very accurate staging (Figures 23-2 and 23-3). Additionally, it gives the opportunity for insight into their feelings about their body and self-esteem.

Age of Menarche

The lack of menstrual periods and secondary sex characteristics by age 14 or the lack of menses by age 16 in the presence of secondary sex characteristics is considered primary amenorrhea. Fifty-six percent of all adolescents start menses when PH development is at PH stage 4 and 19% at PH stage 3 (see Figure 23-3). If the adolescent is PH stage 4 but has not had a menses, then primary amenorrhea should be diagnosed. However, if the adolescent does not meet the age and maturation criteria, then suspect she is experiencing delayed puberty or is a so-called "late bloomer." She is likely to have a family history in her mother and sisters of delayed menarche. Almost 80% of amenorrheic adolescents with intact female genitalia and developed breasts have an inappropriate LH feedback, anovulatory cycles, or high levels of androgenic hormones. They will bleed after a PCT and should be monitored for continued menses to avoid endometrial hyperplasia.

Menstrual History

Absence of a menstrual period for the past 6 months or a cycle interval exceeding 35 days (a time frame that is equal to 3 missed cycles) is considered secondary amenorrhea. Sudden cessation of menstruation is more likely to indicate pregnancy or stress as a cause, whereas a gradual cessation suggests polycystic ovarian syndrome (PCOS) or premature ovarian failure.

Are There Any Constitutional Delays Causing the Amenorrhea?

Key Questions

- Has there been a change in weight, percentage of body fat, or athletic training intensity?
- Are you under unusual stress at school, home, or work?
- Do you or anyone in your family have any congenital disorders or chronic diseases?

Change in Weight, Percentage Body Fat, and Athletic Training Intensity

Underweight persons typically have a low body fat–to–lean muscle ratio. Body fat can be assessed by measuring the body mass index (BMI). The severe stress of anorexia nervosa can produce prolonged amenorrhea. Exercise from various sports—jogging, middle and long distance running, ballet dancing, gymnastics, and track and field events—can lower body fat sufficiently to cause menstrual

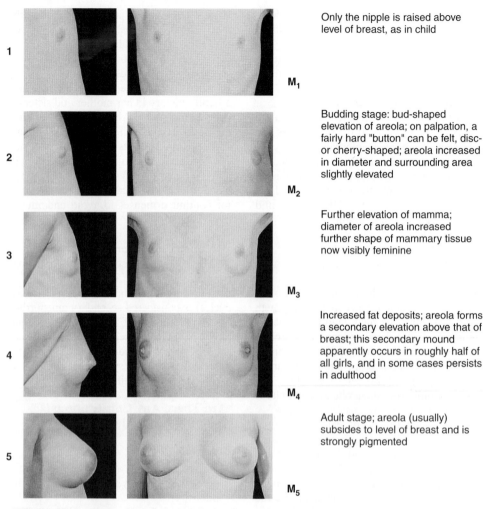

1   M₁   Only the nipple is raised above level of breast, as in child

2   M₂   Budding stage: bud-shaped elevation of areola; on palpation, a fairly hard "button" can be felt, disc- or cherry-shaped; areola increased in diameter and surrounding area slightly elevated

3   M₃   Further elevation of mamma; diameter of areola increased further shape of mammary tissue now visibly feminine

4   M₄   Increased fat deposits; areola forms a secondary elevation above that of breast; this secondary mound apparently occurs in roughly half of all girls, and in some cases persists in adulthood

5   M₅   Adult stage; areola (usually) subsides to level of breast and is strongly pigmented

FIGURE 23-2 Five stages of breast development in females. (Photographs from Van Wieringen JC: *Growth diagrams 1965 Netherlands Second National Survey on 0- to 24-year-olds*, Groningen, The Netherlands, 1971, Wolters-Noordhoff; reprinted by permission of Kluwer Academic Publishers.)

aberrations. Long distance runners and ballerinas are more apt to be amenorrheic than are swimmers; however, even moderate exercise can cause one or two missed periods a year. The mechanism of action on the HPO axis is unknown but is expressed by delayed puberty, shortened luteal phase, anovulation, and amenorrhea. Obesity may be the cause of amenorrhea or be a sign of PCOS. PCOS will cause ovarian dysfunction— elevated androgens, hirsutism, low sex steroid binding globulin (SSBG), and an elevated LH/FSH ratio.

Emotional State

The stress of athletic competition, family situations, school performance, peer relations, and work can disrupt normal cyclic menses. The HPO axis of a teenager is more sensitive to physical and psychological stress than that of an adult female.

Congenital or Chronic Diseases

Turner's syndrome stigmata (see Perform a Head and Neck Examination) or similar physical findings suggest the probability of an abnormality of one or all components

1   No growth of pubic hair

2   Initial, sparse, straight, downy, and slightly pigmented pubic hair, especially along labia

3   Pubic hair is darker, coarser, and curly, and spread sparsely over entire pubis in typical female triangle

4   Pubic hair is denser, curly, and in an adult distribution, but less abundant and restricted to pubic area

5   Pubic hair is adult in quantity, type, and pattern, with lateral spreading to inner aspect of thighs

6   Further extension laterally, upward, or over the upper thighs (this stage may not occur in all women)

FIGURE 23-3 Tanner sexual maturity development in females. (Photographs from Van Wieringen JC: *Growth diagrams 1965 Netherlands Second National Survey on 0- to 24-year-olds,* Groningen, The Netherlands, 1971, Wolters-Noordhoff; reprinted by permission of Kluwer Academic Publishers.)

(central nervous system, structural anomalies, or HPO axis) necessary for menstruation. Most structural anomalies that would prevent outflow of the menstrual blood are detectable on physical examination. Chronic diseases such as anorexia nervosa, diabetes mellitus, Crohn's disease, systemic lupus erythematosus, glomerulonephritis, cystic fibrosis, pituitary adenoma, adrenal diseases, and thyroid dysfunction can cause amenorrhea.

Could This Be Thyroid Dysfunction?

Key Questions

- Have you noticed changes in the texture of your hair or skin?

- Are you bothered by hot or cold temperatures?
- Have you had any changes in your energy level?
- Have you had any changes in your bowel function?

Hair and Skin Changes and Temperature Intolerance

Hypothyroidism and hyperthyroidism are expressed by changes in hair and skin texture. Hyperthyroidism often makes women intolerant of the heat, and this is sometimes confused with menopausal syndrome symptoms. Cold intolerance is frequently exhibited by persons with low-functioning thyroids.

Energy and Bowel Changes

Increased functioning of the thyroid causes restlessness and diarrhea, whereas decreased functioning results in constipation and fatigue. Even mild thyroid dysfunction can cause menstrual irregularities; therefore a thyroid function test is needed to assess the thyroid status.

Could This Be Caused by Hyperprolactinemia?

Key Questions

- Are you able to express a discharge or liquid from your nipples?
- Is there increased stimulation to your nipples?
- Have you had any surgery or disease of the breasts or chest wall?

Galactorrhea

Women may notice breast nipple discharge that is not associated with breastfeeding or medications. Offensive medications are listed in Box 23-1 and include primarily the dopamine antagonist agents and estrogens.

Nipple Stimulation and Chest Wall Stimulation

Nipple stimulation from clothing irritation during jogging or nipple manipulation during sexual activity may cause galactorrhea. Surgical interventions such as lymph node dissection or disease processes such as herpes zoster may also lead to galactorrhea, triggered by peripheral neural stimulation.

Could the Hyperprolactinemia Be Caused by Medications?

Key Questions

- What prescription medicines are you taking?
- Have you used any street drugs? What kind of drugs have you used?

Medication History

Medications such as phenothiazines or contraceptives may cause amenorrhea. These drugs increase prolactin levels, induce an estrogenic effect, or are toxic to the ovaries (see Box 23-1). Illicit drugs such as heroin and methadone also lead to menstrual abnormalities.

Is a Pituitary Tumor Causing the Amenorrhea?

Key Questions

- Have you experienced any visual changes?
- Are you having an increased number of headaches?

Visual Changes and Headaches

A pituitary tumor may be responsible for the hyperprolactin state. Enlarging pituitary tumors cause headache. As the tumor grows

---

Box 23-1	**Drugs That May Cause Amenorrhea**

Prolactin Increase
Antipsychotics: Phenothiazines, haloperidol, pimozide, clozapine
Antidepressants: Tricyclic antidepressants, monoamine oxidase inhibitors
Antihypertensives: Calcium channel blockers, methyldopa, reserpine
Estrogenic Effect
Digitalis, marijuana, flavonoids, oral contraceptives
Ovarian Toxicity
Busulfan, chlorambucil, cisplatin, cyclophosphamide, fluorouracil

Modified from Kiningham RB, Apgar BS, Schwenk TL: Evaluation of amenorrhea, *Am Fam Physician* 53(4):1186, 1996.

out of the sella turcica, it compresses the optic chiasm and nerves. The common visual defect is bitemporal hemianopia, although other defects may occur. Changes in visual fields are often self-diagnosed when the patient recognizes vision problems while reading or driving an automobile. Clinical changes in vision warrant a referral to an ophthalmologist and computed tomography (CT) or magnetic resonance imaging (MRI) work-up for a tumor of the sella turcica. A high prolactin level will indicate a pituitary adenoma that presents with or without galactorrhea.

Is This a Problem of the HPO Axis?

Key Questions

- Have you experienced any problems with infertility?
- Do you have excess hair on your face or chest?
- Are you having any menopausal symptoms (e.g., hot flashes, vaginal dryness)?
- Did you hemorrhage during childbirth?

Infertility

Many cases of infertility are caused by failure of ovulation. PCOS affects women between the ages of 15 and 30 years. Basal body temperature charts and endometrial biopsies can reveal anovulatory cycles. Vaginal ultrasound will show enlarged ovaries with multiple small, fluid-filled cysts. Infertility can be caused by low or high estrogen levels. Measurement of gonadotropins, vaginal maturation index, and progesterone levels will provide insight into the functioning of the HPO axis.

Androgen Excess

About 50% of women diagnosed with PCOS are hirsute and obese and have difficulty conceiving. Few other signs of masculinization are present. LH is elevated with PCOS. Truncal obesity, acne, and male pattern baldness can signify androgen excess.

Estrogen Deficiency

Hot flashes or flushes, changes in mood, and difficulty sleeping are common menopausal symptoms that women with low estra-diol levels may experience. A dry vagina is often accompanied by dyspareunia and sometimes dysuria. The dysuria may be secondary to the hypoestrogenic state of the urethra and not be the result of a urinary tract infection. Prolonged hypoestrogenic status leads to osteopenia, regardless of age.

Hemorrhage at Childbirth

Amenorrhea can occur subsequent to a pregnancy and delivery if, at the time of delivery, there was severe hemorrhage. Obstetric hemorrhage causes pituitary ischemia and infarction and results in pituitary insufficiency. This pathological process is known as Sheehan's syndrome. In this instance, refer the patient to an endocrinologist.

Is This a Problem of the Uterus?

Key Question

- Have you had a miscarriage or abortion, uterine infection, or any surgery or procedure involving your uterus?

Gynecological Problem

Endometritis, incomplete abortion, or aggressive curettage of the uterus can lead to denuding of the endometrial layer, scarring, and Asherman's syndrome. The patient with Asherman's syndrome will not bleed after the PCT, nor will she bleed after the uterus is primed with estrogen and challenged with medroxyprogesterone acetate. The diagnosis can be made by performing weekly serum progesterone tests to determine if any value is within the ovulatory range (>3 ng/ml) yet there are no periods. The diagnosis can also be made by the gynecologist via hysteroscopy, hysterosalpingography, or measuring endometrial thickness by ultrasonography.

What Symptoms Support a Structural Outflow Problem?

Key Questions

- Do you have cyclic abdominal bloating or cramping?
- Have you been amenorrheic since you had a cervical procedure?

Presence of Premenstrual Symptoms or Dysmenorrhea

Cyclic symptomatology of dysmenorrhea in the absence of menses may be caused by an incomplete outflow tract. Physical examination will validate a vaginal opening, imperforate hymen, intact uterus, or congenital imperforate cervical os. If there is no indication of a uterus by examination or lower abdominal ultrasound, a karyotype is needed to determine the congenital disorder. A referral to an endocrinologist or gynecological surgeon may be indicated for removal of any abdominal male gonads, which would be a risk for cancerous degeneration.

Amenorrhea Since Cervical Procedure

Stenosis of the cervical os can occur after gynecological office surgeries such as cervical biopsies and cryotherapy. However, it is more common after cone biopsies of the cervix, such as the loop electrosurgical excision procedure (LEEP), or carbon dioxide laser treatment.

DIAGNOSTIC REASONING: FOCUSED PHYSICAL EXAMINATION

Note General Appearance

The body morphology of the patient can provide clues to the cause of amenorrhea; often diseases can be diagnosed secondary to short stature, underweight, or overweight. A height less than 5 feet (short stature) in a girl who is 14 years old or older may indicate a congenital chromosomal problem. Assess the woman's general state of health to determine if there are signs of systemic, chronic, or congenital disease.

Assess Nutritional Status and Plot Measurements on Growth Chart in Adolescents

Assess nutritional status, looking for signs of undernutrition or overnutrition. Measure the height, weight, and arm span of the adolescent. Plot on a growth chart if delayed puberty is a consideration. Anorexia nervosa is often found while evaluating an adolescent who has short stature and is underweight.

Assess Sexual Maturity

Use the Tanner SMR scales to assess and rate the stage of breast and PH development. An SMR may be calculated by averaging the girl's stage of PH and breast development. The stage of breast and PH development in the adolescent girl is related to her chronological age, age at menarche, and evidence of growth spurt. The breasts often develop at different rates, so some asymmetry is common. Menarche generally occurs at SMR 4 or breast stage 3 to 4. Plot these physiological events on the growth curve.

Screen for Eating Disorders

If you suspect anorexia nervosa or bulimia, administer a screening instrument to help determine the diagnosis. Refer to the *DSM-IV* for diagnostic criteria. About half of the females with eating disorders will have short stature.

Calculate the Body Mass Index

Seventeen percent body fat is needed for most females to be menarchal, and about 22% body fat is necessary for ovulation. Calculate the BMI (Box 23-2; also see Appendix C). A BMI of 19 kg/m^2 compares with 17% body fat, which may cause amenorrhea. A weight loss of 10% to 15% of the woman's body weight corresponds to a loss of approximately one third of her body fat and consequently a BMI of less than 22% and anovulatory cycles.

Obesity causes amenorrhea secondary to ovarian dysfunction. A BMI of greater than 27% corresponds to being more than 20% overweight. Adipose cell stroma convert androstenedione to estrogen (estrone) as the body fat increases. Obesity also increases sex hormone binding globulin, thereby increasing free steroid levels. Both processes may cause an imbalance in the HPO axis and lead to amenorrhea.

Examine the Skin and Hair

Observe for signs of thyroid dysfunction or adrenal excess. Features of hypothyroidism include dry, coarse, flaky skin; coarse hair that tends to break; and thick, brittle nails. Hyperthyroidism is characterized by fine,

Box 23-2	**Body Mass Index (BMI)**

BMI is helpful in assessing the nutritional status and total body fat of the patient. You can use the BMI chart, Appendix C, to determine the BMI. You can also calculate the BMI by using the following formula:
Multiply the patient's weight in pounds by 704. Take that number (product) and divide by the height in inches. Once again, divide by the height in inches.
Example: Weight = 75 pounds; height = 4 feet 2 inches or 50 inches
$$75 \times 704 = 52,800$$
$$52,800 \div 50 = 1056$$
$$1056 \div 50 = 21.12$$
$$BMI = 21$$

warm skin that is hyperpigmented at pressure points. Nails will often separate from the nail plate (onycholysis), and hair will be fine, thin, and limp. Cushingoid features include truncal obesity, striae, and moon face. Observe for other signs of androgen excess, which include hirsutism, acne, and male pattern baldness.

Perform a Head and Neck Examination

During the head and neck examination, note any visual changes, including visual field defects, that might indicate a pituitary tumor. Anosmia might denote a congenital absence of luteinizing hormone–releasing hormone (LHRH), producing no secretion of LH or FSH from the pituitary. Without LH or FSH production, there is no ovulation; anovulatory cycles are amenorrheic. Also look for Turner's syndrome stigmata—webbed neck and low-set ears (other signs are shieldlike chest and short fourth metacarpal).

Palpate the Thyroid Gland and Lymph Nodes

Palpate the thyroid gland for diffuse enlargement, asymmetry, and nodules. Auscultate for thyroid bruits and count the pulse rate. Assess for supraclavicular and infraclavicular lymphadenopathy or carcinogenic masses of the sternal notch and abdomen, which might arise from a tumor of germ cell, adrenal, or pituitary origin.

Perform Clinical Breast Examination

Physical examination verifies sexual maturation level. The growth spurt occurs before breast development (thelarche), which is followed by the appearance of axillary hair. Perform a breast examination and assess breast maturity level using Tanner staging. More than 95% of adolescents are menarchal 1 year after they reach a breast maturity rating of 4. Check for galactorrhea (see Chapter 24).

Perform a Pelvic Examination

Observe for maturation of the female genitalia and secondary sex characteristics. Assign a Tanner stage for PH development. A congenital problem might manifest as vaginal or uterine agenesis and is identified by the absence of a vagina, cervix, or uterus. There may be a small invagination of the perineum below the urinary meatus. It can be explored using a cotton-tipped applicator and otoscope with a large ear speculum or nasal speculum to determine the dimensions of the vault and presence of a cervix. A clitoris larger than 1 cm is suggestive of androgen excess.

Assess for other outlet problems, including an imperforate hymen (painful, bluish bulging of the perineum), stenotic cervix (bulging os or inability to pass a cotton-tipped applicator through the os), or a transverse vaginal septum. The development of hematocolpos, hematometra, or hematoperitoneum from menses behind an obstructed outflow tract needs immediate intervention to prevent inflammatory changes and endometriosis. Needle aspiration is NOT recommended because it might potentiate infection. Refer to a reconstructive gynecological surgeon for MRI and, often, extensive surgery.

If the introitus is small, use a pediatric Pedersen, Huffman-Graves, or Graves' speculum (which measures approximately ½ inch wide and 3¾ inches long) or a Huffman vaginoscope. Vaginal walls that are pale and dry, have few rugations, and may be friable are estrogen deficient. Low estrogen levels will cause scant cervical mucus. Vaginal cytology for women exhibiting such symptoms will report a maturation index (MI) lacking or low in estrogen.

The bimanual examination can be performed with only an index finger in the vagina if the vaginal vestibule is small. If the hymen is rigid, a rectal bimanual examination may be completed instead of the usual vaginal bimanual examination. On pelvic bimanual examination, enlarged ovaries will be palpated about half the time in patients with PCOS. Assess for position, size, shape, and consistency of the cervix, uterus, and ovaries.

LABORATORY AND DIAGNOSTIC STUDIES

Pregnancy Test: Radioimmunoassay for β-hCG
The pregnancy test is used to identify or rule out pregnancy and is an essential test on all females presenting with amenorrhea.

Thyroid-Stimulating Hormone
A serum TSH test identifies hypothyroidism. When hormonal supplementation is provided, menses usually will resume for these patients. If the amenorrhea is associated with galactorrhea and hyperprolactinemia, the prolactin level will have to be measured again after the thyroid function levels have become normal.

Prolactin Levels
The prolactin level is most reliable when it is a fasting measurement. When the patient's fasting prolactin level is normal (<50 ng/ml), a PCT is indicated. If the patient's level is high (>50 ng/ml) or if she has galactorrhea, a cone-down view of the sella turcica is taken to rule out a pituitary adenoma. An adenoma greater than 10 mm is unlikely if the cone view is normal and the prolactin level is less than 100 ng/ml. A prolactin elevation less than 100 ng/ml but higher than normal is most frequently caused by prescribed or illicit drugs. The hyperprolactinemia usually subsides a few weeks after stopping the offend-ing drug. Microscopic examination of breast discharge will reveal fat globules and no red blood cells (see Chapter 24).

Serum Follicle-Stimulating Hormone Levels
Ovarian failure, which causes a low estradiol secretion, will raise the FSH level higher than 40 mIU/ml. If both the FSH and LH levels are greater than 50 mIU/ml, then primary ovarian failure is established. If the patient is older than 30 years, menopause is diagnosed; if she is younger than 30 years, a karyotype should be done. An FSH measurement of less than 40 mIU/ml denotes a hypothalamic-pituitary dysfunction and secondary ovarian failure.

Serum Luteinizing Hormone Levels
A serum LH level greater than 35 milliunits/ml is frequently seen in patients with PCOS. An LH/FSH ratio higher than 2:1 is suggestive of PCOS, whereas a ratio higher than 3:1 is considered diagnostic of PCOS.

Central Nervous System Imaging
If both FSH and LH levels are low, indicating a problem of the pituitary, imaging of the central nervous system is warranted. Either contrast-enhanced CT or MRI of the sella turcica will determine if there is an abnormality. If the prolactin level is greater than 100 ng/ml or the cone-down view of the sella turcica is abnormal, CT or MRI with contrast enhancement should be obtained.

Pelvic Ultrasound and Vaginal Ultrasound
Pelvic and vaginal ultrasound studies are used to determine the presence of a uterus and its anatomical size and endometrial thickness, and whether there are fibroids or other tumors. Ultrasound is used to measure ovarian size, to identify cysts, and to evaluate follicular development. In primary amenorrhea, ultrasound is helpful in assessing müllerian agenesis and gonadal dysgenesis because there may be internal organs and no conduit to the perineum. One third of these patients also have urinary tract abnormalities; therefore an abdominal ultrasound can be obtained at the same time to evaluate that system.

Progesterone Challenge Test (Progesterone Withdrawal Test)

The PCT consists of the administration of oral medroxyprogesterone acetate 10 mg daily for 5 days or parenteral progesterone in oil 200 mg intramuscularly. The patient will respond to the medication within 2 to 7 days. If there is a positive PCT response, the patient will bleed. This demonstrates that there are sufficient endogenous estrogens to prepare the endometrium and confirms that there is a functioning outflow tract. It substantiates an intact HPO axis.

Estrogen and Progesterone Challenge Test

The estrogen and PCT (E and PCT) consists of the administration of conjugated estrogens 1.25 mg daily for 21 days and medroxyprogesterone acetate 10 mg for the last 5 days of the regimen (days 17 through 21). If there is no menstrual flow, administer the regimen a second time. If there is no flow after both courses of therapy, the cause is either the outflow tract or the uterine endometrium. The E and PCT is positive if there is menstrual flow within 2 to 7 days. A positive test denotes that there is inadequate estrogen production either from inadequate functional ovarian follicles or from inadequate pituitary gonadotropic stimulation.

Chromosome Analysis (Karyotyping)

A buccal smear or vaginal smear of epithelial cells is stained with cresyl violet and examined microscopically. Karyotyping is done to delineate probable chromosomal abnormalities. It is used in the work-up for ambiguous genitalia, primary amenorrhea, oligomenorrhea, delayed puberty, or abnormal development at puberty.

Endometrial Biopsy

Endometrial biopsy may be used to show the hormonal response of the uterine endometrium.

Basal Body Temperature Charting

A woman can take her awakening body temperature each day and chart it to determine if ovulation is occurring. This test is based on the fact that progesterone increases the body temperature by 0.5° F to 0.8° F for 11 days during the luteal phase. If this increase in temperature occurs, ovulation has occurred, and a positive estrogen component is inferred. Digital read-out thermometers are quick and easy to use.

Maturation Index

A vaginal cytological smear (Papanicolaou smear) for evaluation of ovarian function can determine the hormonal status of the vagina.
- Lack of estrogen effect is demonstrated by predominance of parabasal cells.
- Low estrogen effect is demonstrated by predominance of intermediate cells.
- Increased estrogen effect is demonstrated by predominance of intermediate cells.

Both increased and decreased estrogen effects can be reflective of a hormonal imbalance of the HPO axis.

Progesterone Levels

Serum progesterone levels collected at weekly intervals can establish whether ovulation has occurred. A value greater than 3 ng/ml is found with ovulation.

DIFFERENTIAL DIAGNOSIS

Pregnancy

Pregnancy is the most common reason for amenorrhea of the childbearing woman. Determining the pregnancy status of the patient is the first step in the amenorrhea work-up.

Constitutional Problems

Delayed Puberty

A pituitary adenoma must be ruled out for all patients with delayed puberty. Yearly prolactin levels should be performed for those with delayed puberty because of the possibility of occult pituitary adenomas.

Anorexia Nervosa and Bulimia

Anorexia nervosa and bulimia are disorders that are psychiatric in origin. Affected women have such a fear of being fat that they do not eat or they purge after eating. Often these women are overachievers and have low self-esteem. The majority are adolescents, with a mean age of 13 to 14. Amenorrhea is caused by extreme weight loss and/or cachectic state.

Exercise-Induced Amenorrhea

This amenorrhea is common in competitive athletes, but exercise can also cause skipped menses in the casual trainer. Gymnasts, ballerinas, and long distance runners are at high risk, especially if they started their training at a very early age. Body fat of 17% is needed for menarche, whereas 22% body fat is necessary for ovulation. BMI estimates the woman's body fat level.

Congenital or Chronic Disorders

Turner's Syndrome

Turner's syndrome causes primary amenorrhea because of ovarian agenesis. The typical features are short stature, webbed neck, shieldlike chest, and delayed secondary sex characteristics.

Cushing's Syndrome

Cushing's syndrome is caused by an excess secretion of adrenocorticotropic hormone (ACTH) from a pituitary or adrenal adenoma. Classically, patients present with a "moon face," acne, hirsutism, kyphosis, purplish striae of the abdomen, and hypertension. CT may reveal pituitary or adrenal adenoma.

Thyroid Dysfunction

Amenorrhea from thyroid dysfunction will subside as soon as serum thyroid levels return to normal. Hypothyroidism frequently causes amenorrhea and is characterized by fatigue, constipation, cold intolerance, and dry skin.

Polycystic Ovary Syndrome

PCOS typically causes infertility in women ages 15 to 30 years. Half of these women will exhibit hirsutism and obesity. The ovaries are often large and contain multiple fluid-filled cysts. The diagnosis is established by ultrasonography.

Uterine and Outflow Tract Problems

Imperforate Hymen

The woman with an imperforate hymen may present with a painful, bulging perineum. There is lack of an intact outflow tract, which causes the primary amenorrhea.

Cervical Os Stenosis

Stenosis of the cervical os can be the cause for either primary or secondary amenorrhea. Stenosis is often caused by therapeutic procedures of the cervix such as cryotherapy or cone biopsies. These procedures cause scarring and stenosis of the os, obstructing the outflow tract.

Asherman's Syndrome

Asherman's syndrome occurs when the uterine endometrial lining is denuded or scarred, usually by infection or curettage. The patient will not respond to either a PCT or an E and PCT.

Hypothalamic-Pituitary-Ovarian Axis Problem

Menopause

The average age of menopause in the United States is 51 years. The cause is primary ovarian failure. It is a state of hypoestrogenemia. The gonadotropin levels rise (FSH >40 milliunits/ml), and the estradiol levels fall (<15 pg/ml). Clinical symptoms are hot flashes, night sweats, insomnia, mood changes, and amenorrhea for 12 months.

Sheehan's Syndrome

Sheehan's syndrome is activated by severe obstetrical hemorrhage, which causes pituitary ischemia and infarction. The pituitary gland becomes dysfunctional.

Medications

Prescription and illicit drugs may increase prolactin levels, which in turn promote galactorrhea. Offending drugs are primarily the dopamine antagonist agents and estrogens as well as marijuana.

Chest Wall or Nipple Stimulation

Prolactin inhibits the pulsatile secretion of GnRH, unbalancing the HPO axis and possibly causing amenorrhea. The higher the prolactin level, the greater the chance that the patient will be amenorrheic.

Pituitary Adenoma

Pituitary macroadenomas and microadenomas should be suspected if the prolactin level is greater than 100 ng/ml or if there are any abnormalities of the cone-down view of the sella turcica. Patients with pituitary adenomas should be referred to an endocrinologist. Patients with prolactin levels exceeding 1000 ng/ml probably have an invasive tumor.

DIFFERENTIAL DIAGNOSIS OF *Common Causes of Amenorrhea*

CONDITION	HISTORY	PHYSICAL FINDINGS	DIAGNOSTIC STUDIES
Pregnancy			
Pregnancy	Breast tenderness, morning sickness, urinary frequency	Globular, enlarged uterus; soft, bluish color cervix	β-hCG pregnancy test positive; ultrasonography positive
Constitutional Problems			
Delayed puberty	No menstruation at age beyond 16 years; more than 5 years between initiation of breast growth and menarche	Breast stage 1 persists beyond age 13.4; pubic hair stage 1 persists beyond age 14.1	Prolactin normal; TSH, T_4 normal; CBC, U/A normal; chemistry profile normal; bone age normal; skull radiograph normal
Anorexia nervosa/bulimia	Mean age 13-14; fear of being fat; low self-esteem; depression; isolation; overachiever; food is parental battleground; preoccupation; hair loss; abdominal bloating, pain, constipation	Amenorrhea before or after weight loss; cachexia; low body fat; short stature; yellow, dry, cold skin; acrocyanosis: increased lanugo hair; hypotension, systolic murmurs, often mitral valve prolapse	TSH normal; prolactin normal; FSH and LH usually low; glucose normal; ECG: bradycardia, low-voltage changes, T wave inversions, and occasional ST segment depression
Exercise-induced amenorrhea	Began athletic training at young age; more common with long distance runners, ballerinas, gymnasts	BMI <17% body fat	TSH normal; prolactin normal
Congenital or Chronic Disorders			
Turner's syndrome	Congenital; short stature; infantile sexual development	Characteristics: webbed neck, low-set ears, shieldlike chest, short fourth metacarpal	Karyotype (45,X)
Cushing's syndrome	Weight gain; weakness; back pain	Moon face, acne, hirsutism, purple striae of abdomen	Cortisol increased; 17-ketosteroids increased; CT adenoma
Thyroid dysfunction	Hypothyroid: delayed growth, weight gain, fatigue, constipation, cold intolerance; hyperthyroid: weight loss, nervousness, heat intolerance	Hypothyroid: dry skin, fine hair, galactorrhea; hyperthyroid: moist skin, hyperpigmentation over bones, thin hair, goiter	Hypothyroid: TSH high; hyperthyroid: TSH low; T_3 high; T_4 high
Polycystic ovary syndrome	Infertility	Hirsutism; obese; enlarged ovaries	Ultrasonography: enlarged ovaries with multiple fluid-filled cysts; testosterone high

Continued

DIFFERENTIAL DIAGNOSIS OF *Common Causes of Amenorrhea—cont'd*

CONDITION	HISTORY	PHYSICAL FINDINGS	DIAGNOSTIC STUDIES
Uterine and Outflow Tract Problems			
Imperforate hymen/stenotic cervical os	Monthly bloating, cramping, and pelvic pressure; no menses; cryotherapy or other procedure to cervix	Fibrotic hymen without patent opening; stenotic cervical os	Clinical diagnosis by history and findings
Asherman's syndrome	History of uterine infection; tuberculosis, schistosomiasis; uterine iatrogenic scarring; curettage, irradiation	Pelvic examination normal	PCT negative; E and PCT negative; hysteroscopy adhesions
Hypothalamic-Pituitary-Ovarian Axis Problem			
Menopause	Hot flashes, night sweats, insomnia, mood changes	Pale, dry vaginal mucosa; few rugae	FSH and LH high; estradiol low
Sheehan's syndrome	Recent history of postpartum hemorrhage and shock during delivery	Hair loss; depigmentation of skin; mammary and genital atrophy	Pituitary and end-organ hormones low; hemoglobin low
Medications/chest wall or nipple stimulation	Breast nipple discharge; history of dopamine antagonists, estrogens, or illicit drugs; stimulation to nipples: exercise or sexual; history of chest wall surgery or herpes zoster	Nipple discharge: bilateral; multiduct; milky, clear, or yellowish discharge	Wet mount or hemoccult of nipple discharge: negative for RBCs; prolactin high; cone-down view of sella turcica; MRI or CT with contrast
Pituitary adenoma	Delayed puberty; history of visual changes, increasing headaches	Visual field defects; galactorrhea	Prolactin high; cone-down view of sella turcica positive; MRI or CT with contrast positive

CBC, Complete blood cell count; *U/A,* urinalysis; *T₃,* triiodothyronine; *T₄,* thyroxine; *ECG,* electrocardiogram; *RBCs,* red blood cells.

CHAPTER RESOURCES

Bielak KS, Harris S: Amenorrhea, e-Medicine http://www.emedicine.com/ped/topic2779.htm. Last updated December 9, 2005.

Goodman LR, Warren MP: The female athlete and menstrual function, *Curr Opin Obstet Gynecol* 17(5):466, 2005.

Goswami D, Conway GS: Premature ovarian failure, *Hum Reprod Update* 11(4):391, 2005.

Hunter MH, Sterrett JJ: Polycystic ovary syndrome: it's not just infertility, *Am Fam Physician* 62:1079, 2000.

Pletcher JR, Slap GB: Menstrual disorders: amenorrhea, *Pediatr Clin North Am* 46:505, 1999.

Sabatini S: The female athlete triad, *Am J Med Sci* 322:193, 2001.

Wilson GR, Haddad JE, Haddad CJ: Amenorrhea: common causes and evaluation, *Compr Ther* 31(4):270, 2005.

Common Problems of the Breasts

Breast Lumps and Nipple Discharge

From 80% to 90% of all breast lumps are found by the woman or her partner before diagnosis through clinical breast examination (CBE) or mammography. The three most common breast lumps are fibroadenomas, fibrocystic breast changes, and breast carcinoma. Fibroadenomas are benign solid tumors most frequently seen in women younger than 30 years. "Fibrocystic breast changes" refer to a heterogeneous group of nonproliferative changes of stromal and/or glandular elements of the breast tissue that includes benign cysts, diffuse and localized nodularity, nipple discharge, and breast tenderness. Fibrocystic symptoms are seen with great frequency in women ages 30 to 50 years but less often in those who are menopausal.

Breast carcinoma is the most common cancer in women and the second leading cause of cancer-related death. The risk of breast cancer in women rises steadily with age and accelerates rapidly after the age of 50. Although benign conditions that affect the breast are more common, the presence of a lump raises legitimate fears. The goal of the assessment process is to reach a diagnosis that addresses the possibility of breast cancer.

Nipple discharge is a complaint commonly elicited from postmenarchal female clients. It is often related to pregnancy, recent breast-feeding, or estrogenic medications. In women who are not lactating, nipple discharge is most frequently caused by intraductal papilloma, duct ectasia, or cancer. Nipple discharge is more commonly caused by benign lesions than by cancerous ones. Physiological stimulation (e.g., sucking, pregnancy, mechanical stimulation) of the breasts may produce discharge, as can breast trauma and inflammation

(e.g., herpes zoster, mammoplasty), pituitary disorders (e.g., irradiation of pituitary), or tranquilizing drugs (e.g., phenothiazines, methyldopa).

DIAGNOSTIC REASONING: FOCUSED HISTORY FOR BREAST LUMPS

Is This Lump Likely to Be Malignant?

Key Questions
- How long has the lump been present?
- Is the lump changing (e.g., getting bigger, worse, or more painful)?
- Is the lump in one breast only or are there lumps in both breasts?
- When was your last menstrual period?
- Is there any discharge from the nipple?
- Have you recently been treated for a breast infection?

Duration and Growth

The primary presenting complaint of a malignant lesion is that of a single, hard, painless lump in the breast that is unchanged by the cyclic hormonal milieu. A change from the patient's normal physical findings is the most persuasive criterion for considering a diagnosis of breast cancer.

Malignant lumps are more likely to be new lumps that show progressive increase in size. The lump grows until there is an alteration in the contour of the breast tissue. An unchanged lump of long duration (years) is almost always benign. Half of all newly appearing benign cysts resolve within two or three menstrual cycles.

Unilateral Versus Bilateral

Breast lumps found bilaterally in identical quadrants of the breast are more likely to be benign. A solitary unilateral lump, although usually a cyst, fibroadenoma, or lipoma (rare), raises more suspicion for malignancy.

Postmenopausal

Cyclic cysts of the breast are less common after menopause and necessitate diagnostic investigation. A postmenopausal woman with unilateral mastalgia (breast pain) has a greater risk for breast cancer. Perimenopausal and postmenopausal women are also at greater statistical risk for breast cancer because of the higher incidence of breast cancer as they age. A new breast lump in a postmenopausal woman warrants a high degree of suspicion for cancer.

Nipple Discharge With a Lump

The occurrence of nipple discharge with the presence of a lump is worrisome because it may represent a ductal cancer. One example is Paget's disease, which may present as a breast mass with a bloody nipple discharge. This condition demands further investigation, such as mammogram, ductogram, or biopsy.

Infection

Any residual masses in the breast after antibiotic therapy are suspicious for malignancy and require biopsy.

Does the Person Have Additional Risk Factors for Breast Cancer?

Key Questions

- Have you ever had breast cancer?
- Do you have a family history of breast cancer (e.g., first-degree relative)?
- Have you ever had ovarian, endometrial, colon, or thyroid cancer?
- Do you have a family history of ovarian, endometrial, colon, or prostate cancer?
- Have you ever received radiation to the chest or had a malignancy in childhood?

Risk Factors

The presence of risk factors in a woman who has a lump raises the index of suspicion for malignancy. It is important to remember that the absence of such risk factors is not cancer protective. About 70% to 80% of all breast cancer patients have no risk factors for malignancy before their diagnosis. Patients with a personal history of epithelial hyperplasia, ductal carcinoma in situ (DCIS), or lobular carcinoma in situ (LCIS) are usually evaluated every 6 months by a breast specialist because of their increased risk for malignancy. Malignant breast tumors in adolescents are more likely to be metastasis than a primary tumor. Hodgkin's, rhabdomyosarcoma, and neuroblastomas may be the primary tumors. A history of chest wall irradiation is a risk factor. See Box 24-1 for a summary of characteristics that might increase a woman's risk for breast cancer.

Is This Condition More Likely to Be Benign?

Key Questions

- How old are you?
- Have you had lumps before? Do you have a history of cystic breast changes or lumpy breasts?
- Does this lump feel like other lumps you have had?
- Do the lumps come and go or change with your periods?
- Have you ever had a mammogram or ultrasound? Why was it done? What were the results?
- Have you ever had a lump drained or biopsied? What was the diagnosis?
- Have you had breast implants?

Age

Fibrocystic breast changes occur predominantly between the ages of 20 and 30. Fibroadenomas are more frequent in women ages 15 to 39. Intraductal papilloma and ductal ectasia occur in the age range of 35 to 55 years, whereas breast carcinoma is most prevalent in women age 40 to 70 years. Any woman older than 25 years who has a breast lump should be evaluated by CBE, diagnostic mammography, and/or ultrasound. Magnetic resonant imaging may sometimes be used in addition to mammography and

Box 24-1	**Primary Risk Factors for Breast Cancer**

Female Gender

Age
75% of all cases occur after age 50; no plateau effect with age

Personal History of Breast Cancer or Cancer In Situ
DCIS is a precursor of cancer and increases the risk for invasive breast cancer, usually in the same breast

Previous History of Breast Biopsies for Benign Breast Disease
Biopsy-proved proliferative changes or atypical epithelial hyperplasia; fibrocystic histological findings that increase the risk of breast cancer are moderate or severe hyperplasia (1.5-2 times the risk), atypical hyperplasia (5 times the risk), and lobular carcinoma in situ (8-10 times the risk); LCIS is a marker for cancer rather than a precursor; the cancer may occur in either breast

Laboratory Evidence of Specific Genetic Mutation
Increases susceptibility to breast cancer, i.e., mutation in *BRCA1* or *BRCA2* gene

Personal History of Cancer
Ovarian, endometrial, colon, or thyroid cancers

Family History of Breast Cancer
In first-degree relatives (mother, sister, or daughter) or in two or more close relatives

ultrasound. Additional evaluation with tissue biopsy may be required.

Timing, Consistency, and Duration

The most frequent breast complaint is that of a painful, mobile lump that increases in size and tenderness as the menstrual cycle approaches. The lump commonly has discrete borders that allow for measurement of the length, width, and depth of the lesion by the patient (e.g., size of a pea). The lump remains prominent on breast self-examination, is almost always painful to palpate, and frequently causes pain with changes in position of the arm on the affected side. Fibrocystic breast changes exist on a continuum that corresponds with the menstrual cycle. Tenderness and size variations occur throughout the month.

Previous Mammograms or Biopsies

History or documentation of cyclic changes in lumps or the presence of glandular breast tissue on a mammogram or ultrasound supports a clinical diagnosis of benign disease. More convincing evidence of benign disease occurs when there is a clear fluid aspirate from the cyst with no residual or recurring breast lump, with the caveat that benign disease and malignant disease can occur simultaneously.

Breast Implants

With a ruptured implant, augmented breast tissue is pushed away from the chest wall by the implant.

Could This Lump Be Mastitis Related to Lactation?

Key Questions

- Have you recently had a baby?
- Are you currently breastfeeding or breast suckling?
- Are your nipples sore or cracked?
- Have you had pierced nipples?
- Is your breast painful or hot? Are there any areas of redness?
- Have you had a fever?

Childbirth

Engorgement or congestive mastitis begins on day 2 or 3 after delivery and affects both breasts. A breast mass in a lactating woman is usually associated with mastitis, an inflammation of breast tissue, and a blocked duct. It occurs most often in primiparous nursing mothers and is usually caused by coagulase-positive *Staphylococcus aureus*. It can also occur during periods of weaning when the flow of milk is disrupted. Inflammatory breast cancer in lactating women is rare but must be considered.

Sore or Cracked Nipples
Cracked nipples may be a site for the introduction of infection.

Pierced Nipples
Pierced nipples may be a site for the introduction of infection.

Painful or Hot Breast
Mastitis is characterized by a breast that is painful, hot, and red. In lactating women, the most frequent symptom is a painful erythematous lobule in an outer quadrant of the breast. Although mastitis is most common in lactating women, it can also occur in nonlactating women, usually as the result of a generalized dermatitis occurring from insect bites, sunburn, or allergic reactions. However, the most common cause of an inflamed breast in nonlactating women is inflammatory breast cancer. In inflammatory breast cancer, the entire breast is swollen, heavy, and edematous.

Fever
Fever is a sign of infectious mastitis and occurs most often in association with lactation and breastfeeding. High fever does not occur because of simple breast engorgement in the postpartum period. Also, fever does not usually occur in inflammatory breast cancer and is rare in dermatitis reactions.

DIAGNOSTIC REASONING: FOCUSED HISTORY FOR NIPPLE DISCHARGE
A focused history can help sort out the causes of the most frequently presenting cases of nipple discharge. Questioning should address normal lactation, high circulating levels of prolactin, and malignancy.

Is This Normal Lactation?

Key Questions
- When was your last normal menstrual period? How frequent are your cycles?
- Is it possible that you are pregnant? What are you using for birth control?
- When was your last delivery or miscarriage? How long were you pregnant?
- Did you breastfeed? For how long? When did you stop?

- Is the nipple discharge clear or milky?
- How long have you had the nipple discharge?

Menstrual Cycle
Frequently, fibrocystic breast changes are most marked just before menses and manifest as a spontaneous multiple duct discharge that can be either unilateral or bilateral.

Pregnancy and Lactation
Pregnancy is the most common cause of breast tenderness and clear or milky nipple discharge (galactorrhea). A bloody nipple discharge during pregnancy is usually the result of vascular engorgement and clears within weeks. Recent pregnancy and/or breastfeeding (within 8 weeks) may account for a prolonged clear or milky discharge that is successfully suppressed by decreased breast stimulation or by the administration of dopamine agonist therapy (bromocriptine or pergolide). If the patient has had prolonged lactation, there may be milk formation even though prolactin levels are normal.

Color of Discharge
Normal lactation produces a discharge that is milky and nonpurulent. Mastitis associated with breastfeeding may produce purulent discharge. A subareolar abscess may also produce a purulent discharge. Mastitis and abscesses that produce purulent nipple discharge MUST be distinguished from inflammatory breast cancer by evoking remission with antibiotic therapy or by biopsy.

Oral contraceptives may cause a clear, serous, or milky discharge from single or multiple ducts. Ductal ectasia and papillomatosis can produce a greenish or brownish nipple discharge. A serous or serosanguineous discharge from a single duct is usually indicative of an intraductal papilloma, but may be from an intraductal cancer. A bloody nipple discharge can occur with benign or cancerous conditions.

Duration of Discharge
Women who breastfeed sometimes experience a milky discharge long after the termination of nursing. New-onset discharge in a woman who is not pregnant or lactating

requires further investigation (see the following discussion).

Is the Discharge Related to High Prolactin Levels?

Key Questions

- What medications are you taking?
- Do you jog or run? If yes: Do you wear a sports bra? Do your nipples rub on your clothing?
- Are your breasts fondled, squeezed, or suckled during sexual activity?
- Do you have a thyroid condition?
- What medical conditions or health problems do you have?
- If a newborn: Has the discharge been present since birth?

Medicines

Patients taking multiple tranquilizing medications are often found to have nipple discharge. Discontinuation of the medication(s) will eliminate most clear or milky bilateral nipple discharge. However, the condition may not warrant a drug cessation trial. See Box 24-2 for medications that can produce nipple discharge.

Behavioral Activities

Nipple stimulation (sexual or during jogging) increases prolactin levels, as does the use of marijuana. Only about 13% of men with hyperprolactinemia will develop gynecomastia and galactorrhea. Women commonly experience both galactorrhea and amenorrhea.

Other Causes of Galactorrhea

Certain genetic disorders, medical conditions, and central nervous system lesions can be responsible for the production of galactorrhea.

- Genetic disorders: Chiari-Frommel syndrome, Argonz-del Castillo (Forbes-Albright) syndrome
- Medical conditions: chronic renal failure, sarcoidosis, Schüller-Christian's disease, Cushing's disease, hepatic cirrhosis, hypothyroidism

---

Box 24-2	**Drugs That May Produce Nipple Discharge**

Estrogens or Drugs That Increase Estrogen
Digitalis
Marijuana
Heroin

Dopamine Receptor Blockers
Phenothiazines
Haloperidol
Metoclopramide
Isoniazid

Central Nervous System (CNS) Dopamine Depleters
Tricyclic antidepressants
Reserpine
Methyldopa
Cimetidine
Benzodiazepines

- Central nervous system lesions: pituitary adenoma, empty sella, hypothalamic tumor, head trauma

Newborn

The breasts of a newborn may be abnormally enlarged secondary to the effects of maternal estrogens. A discharge that is usually white may be present and is commonly referred to as "witch's milk."

Can the Nipple Discharge Be a Sign of Malignancy?

Key Questions

- Is the nipple discharge spontaneous or must it be expressed?
- Does it come from one or both nipples?
- Does it come from one or multiple nipple ducts?
- Do you also have a breast lump?
- Are you postmenopausal?

Spontaneous Versus Expressed Discharge

Spontaneous discharge is more concerning than expressed discharge. Bilateral spontaneous discharge is likely related to lactation, or systemic causes (e.g., hyperprolactinemia). Unilateral spontaneous discharge is associated with intraductal papilloma or cancer.

Unilateral Versus Bilateral Discharge

Unilateral discharge is usually associated with an intraductal papilloma or cancer. Bilateral breast findings seldom represent cancer.

Single-Duct Versus Multiple-Duct Discharge

Single-duct involvement is more suspicious for intraductal papilloma or cancer. Multiple-duct discharges usually are caused by hyperprolactinemia or duct ectasia.

Associated Mass

An associated mass may be benign or malignant. Further evaluation is mandatory. Ultrasonography is helpful in differentiating solid from cystic lesions and is often the first step in the evaluation of a cyst or a mass in the woman with firm, dense breast tissue.

Postmenopausal

Postmenopausal women have a higher incidence of breast cancer. Other risky signs for a cancerous cause of nipple discharge are

presence of a mass or lump, unilateral nipple discharge, abnormal cytology, and an abnormal mammogram.

Nipple discharge that is spotaneous, unilateral, and from a single duct is suspicious for a cancerous etiology.

DIAGNOSTIC REASONING: FOCUSED PHYSICAL EXAMINATION

Perform a multiposition physical examination of the breasts and nipples. See Box 24-3 on the effectiveness of CBE.

Inspect Breasts and Nipples

Inspect the breasts while the patient is sitting with her arms at her sides, arms pushing down on hips (to contract the pectoralis muscles), and arms elevated above head and while the patient is bending forward from the waist (gravity pulling on breast tissue). Look for changes in breast shape or contour, a lump, or dimpling. Contraction of underlying muscles in the different arm positions will accentuate skin findings caused by a fixed adherent lesion, characteristic of cancer. Look for breasts that are notably asymmetrical. The skin over the lesion may then flatten or dimple inward, or the nipple might be directed differently than the nipple of the

---

Box 24-3	**Evidence-Based Practice: Effectiveness of Clinical Breast Examination in Detecting Breast Cancer**

In a systematic review of the literature, Barton et al. (1999) found that randomized clinical trials demonstrated reduced breast cancer death rates in women screened by both CBE and mammography. Evidence of the effectiveness of CBE alone was less direct. CBE alone detected from 3% to 45% of diagnosed breast cancers that screening mammography missed. The precision of CBE was difficult to determine because of the lack of consistent and standardized examination techniques. The authors estimated CBE sensitivity at 54% and specificity at 94%. The likelihood ratio of a positive CBE result was 10.6 (95% confidence interval [CI], 5.8 to 19.2), whereas the likelihood ratio of a negative test result was 0.47 (95% CI, 0.40 to 0.56). Longer duration of CBE and a higher number of specific techniques used were associated with greater accuracy. The value of inspection was not proved. The authors concluded that indirect evidence supports the effectiveness of CBE in screening for breast cancer. Although the screening clinical examination by itself does not rule out disease, the high specificity of certain abnormal findings greatly increases the probability of breast cancer. The authors' bottom line for the CBE procedure: position the patient properly; use a vertical-strip pattern to cover all breast tissue; make circular motions with the pads of the middle three fingers and examine each breast area with three different pressures; and spend at least 3 minutes per breast.

Barton MB, Harris R, Fletcher SW: Does this patient have breast cancer? The screening clinical breast examination: should it be done? How? *JAMA* 282:1270, 1999.

opposite breast. Normal nipples are everted and point in like directions. Lifelong inversion, either unilateral or bilateral, is also normal, but a new inversion is suspicious. Engorgement (congestive mastitis) involves both breasts, which are enlarged and tense. Infectious mastitis usually involves one lobe or a quadrant of one breast.

Observe Skin of Breasts and Nipples

Observe skin color for erythema and unilateral prominent blood vessels, which may be a presentation of breast cancer. Prominent vessels plus a tender cordlike vein suggest thrombophlebitis of the superficial veins of the breast. Both conditions require a CBE and a mammogram to look for a mass. Paget's disease begins as a scaling eczematoid area on the nipple and progresses to a deep lump behind the nipple well. Paget's disease can produce darkly pigmented lesions that are suspicious for malignant melanoma. An excisional or punch biopsy is recommended to distinguish Paget's disease from malignant melanoma or other ulcerative lesions like Bowen's disease, eczema, or papillomatosis. Observe the condition of the skin of the nipples for cracks or dried exudate or the presence of nipple flattening or retraction.

Palpate Breasts With Patient Sitting

Place the palm of your right hand at the patient's right clavicle at the sternum. Sweep downward from the clavicle to the nipple, feeling for superficial lumps. Repeat the sweep until you have covered the entire right chest wall. Repeat the procedure using your left hand for the left chest wall.

Perform bimanual digital palpation. Place one hand, palmar surface facing up, under the patient's right breast. Position your hand so that it acts as a flat surface against which to compress the breast tissue. With the fingers of the other hand walk across the breast mound, feeling for lumps as you compress the tissue between your fingers and your flat hand. Repeat the procedure for the other breast.

If the woman has augmentation of breast tissue, small masses, including those from ruptured implants, may best be felt with the patient in the sitting position.

Palpate Lymph Nodes

Palpate the supraclavicular, infraclavicular, and axillary lymph nodes (Figures 24-1 and 24-2). The supraclavicular lymph nodes can be accessed by having the patient shrug her shoulders; then feel deep in the supraclavicular hollow. Feel for lymph nodes, noting their size, shape, consistency, and mobility. The presence of a small (<1 cm), single, rubbery, and mobile lymph node can be a sign of inflammation: rarely is it a sign of early malignancy. On the other hand, finding one or more lymph nodes in the same region that are greater than 1 cm, firm, fixed to the chest wall, or of a matted consistency is highly suggestive of metastatic disease.

Palpate Breasts and Nipples With Patient Supine

With the patient supine, ask her to position one arm above her head. Place a small towel behind the scapula to aid in flattening the breast tissue. Palpate all areas of breast tissue, feeling for lumps or nodules. Remember that the breast tissue extends from the second or third rib to the sixth or seventh rib, and from the sternal margin to the midaxillary line. It is essential to include the tail of Spence in palpation. Recall that the greatest amount of glandular tissue lies in the upper outer quadrant of the breast with tissue extending from this quadrant into the axilla to form the tail of Spence.

Palpate using your finger pads because they are more sensitive than your fingertips. Palpate systematically, pushing gently but firmly, toward the chest with your fingers rotating in a clockwise or counterclockwise pattern. At each point press inward, using three depths of palpation: light, then medium, and finally deep palpation. Strip, concentric circle, or wedge methods are commonly used for ensuring palpation of the entire breast. Any method is acceptable, as long as every part of the breast is palpated. Regardless of the method, glide your fingers from one point to the next. Avoid lifting your fingers off the breast tissue because doing so makes it easy to miss tissue.

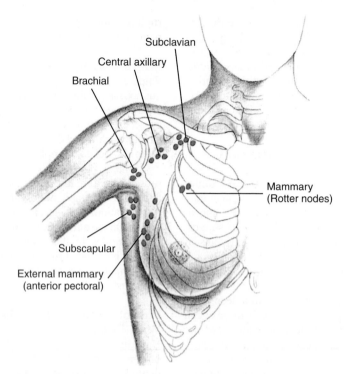

FIGURE 24-1 Six groups of lymph nodes may be distinguished in the axilla. (From Seidel HM et al: *Mosby's guide to physical examination,* ed 6, St Louis, 2006, Mosby.)

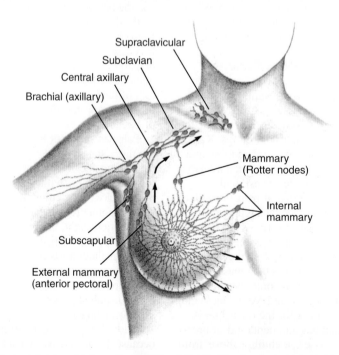

FIGURE 24-2 Lymphatic drainage of the breast. (From Seidel HM et al: *Mosby's guide to physical examination,* ed 6, St Louis, 2006, Mosby.)

Assess Nipple Well

At the completion of the examination return to the nipple and with two fingers gently depress the tissue inward into the well behind the areola. Your fingers and tissue should move easily inward. A normal nipple well is a smooth concave structure. Most lumps in this area will be found at the areola border. Repeat with the other breast.

Examine Nipple for Discharge

Palpate for discharge only if the patient presents with a complaint of nipple discharge. Place the thumb and first finger 1 to 2 cm outside the border of the areolar complex and gently compress, sliding the fingers toward the nipple in a milking fashion. Repeat this maneuver twice, cephalocaudally and laterally. Determine if the discharge is unilateral or bilateral. Look closely to determine if the discharge is from a single duct or multiple ducts. Palpation of a single site on the areola border may reproduce the discharge and reveal the responsible duct. Specimen collection is often easier and of a larger quantity when the patient is sitting.

Inflammatory symptoms and a purulent nipple discharge are suggestive of a breast abscess.

Transilluminate Breast Masses

Transillumination of a breast mass (best performed in a darkened room) may sometimes provide diagnostic clues. A fluid-filled cyst will transilluminate whereas a solid mass will not. A solid lump is more frequently a malignant mass, whereas a cystic, fluid-filled lump is more commonly benign.

Characterize Lumps

Accurately measure any lumps by marking the edges with a pen and measuring the width and length with a centimeter ruler. Estimate the depth of the lesion, contour, shape, fluctuation, firmness, and mobility.

Fluctuation can be determined by holding the edges of the mass against the chest wall and pressing the center with finger pads. Fluctuation ("bouncy" consistency) occurs with cysts, lipomas, and abscesses. Cysts are frequently tender, especially premenstrually.

Reexamination in 1 or 2 weeks will usually demonstrate cyclic hormonal changes of the tissue, and lump size and tenderness will have changed. In the postmenopausal woman, hormone replacement therapy may stimulate similar symptoms of breast lumps and pain (mastodynia). A single, firm, asymmetrical, immobile mass in a postmenopausal woman will, when biopsied, prove to be cancerous 75% of the time.

LABORATORY AND DIAGNOSTIC STUDIES

The diagnostic accuracy of ultrasound, mammography, and aspiration biopsy ranges from about 70% to 80% and varies with the training and skills of the clinician or technician. Therefore a high degree of suspicion for cancer and excellent patient follow-up should be sustained for a breast lump or nipple discharge.

Ultrasound

Ultrasound is helpful in differentiating solid from cystic lesions. In women under age 30 years ultrasound is often the first step in the evaluation of a cyst or a mass. The ultrasound finding of a cystic lesion may be followed by aspiration of the cyst, eliminating it to make sure it is not concealing another abnormal breast finding. The ultrasound identification of a solid mass may be followed by tissue biopsy.

Mammography

Screening mammography (conventional film or digital) is used to identify nonpalpable breast lesions. It consists of two views—craniocaudal (CC) and medial lateral oblique (MLO). In the presence of a palpable mass or nipple discharge, a diagnostic mammogram, which involves additional views, spot compression, and magnification views, is necessary.

Mammography is of less diagnostic value in women younger than 30 years because of the density of the breast tissue.

Magnetic Resonance Imaging (MRI)

MRI is used primarily to evaluate abnormal areas that are seen on a mammogram and to assess breast implants for leaks or ruptures. MRI is sometimes useful in viewing breast abnormalities that can be felt but are not visible with mammography or ultrasound. It may also be used to image dense breast tissue, which is often found in younger women. Contrast is used to enhance the vascularity of malignant lesions. Although MRI is highly sensitive (85% to 100%), it lacks specificity. MRI is inferior to mammography in detecting in situ cancers and cancers smaller than 3 mm.

Fine-Needle Aspiration (FNA) and Cytological Examination

Fine-needle aspiration biopsy uses a small-gauge needle to obtain fluid and cellular material. FNA is a routinely performed office procedure that is both diagnostic and therapeutic. It immediately determines if the lump is a cyst or a solid tumor. The aspirate is sent for cytological evaluation to determine the presence or absence of malignant cells. If the aspirate is negative for cytology, the mass completely goes away and is not present on follow-up examinations; no further treatment is necessary.

Stereotactic or Needle Localization Biopsy

FNA can also be used with ultrasonography or stereotactic imaging to further assess and obtain adequate sampling in poorly defined palpable masses. The lesion is located, marked, and verified by imaging to assist in the identification of the tissue to be sampled.

Core-Needle Biopsy (CNB)

Core-needle biopsy uses a large-gauge needle to obtain several cores of tissue. It produces a larger tissue sample than FNA. It may be used in conjunction with ultrasonography or stereotactic imaging for small or difficult to palpate lesions. Local anesthesia is required.

Excisional Biopsy

Excisional biopsy is the gold standard for evaluating breast masses. It is performed in an operating room using local or general anesthetic, and the entire lesion is removed. Excisional biopsy is indicated if there is a large breast mass or for those lesions in which more conservative biopsy has produced equivocal results. The surgical specimen is evaluated histologically.

Microscopy

Microscopy of nipple discharge can reveal "fat cells" of galactorrhea, leukocytes of infection, or red blood cells. Care must be taken to prevent the slide from drying out. Place a coverslip on the slide immediately after obtaining the specimen and review the slide shortly after it is prepared.

Cytological Smear

A cytological specimen of discharge is placed directly from the nipple onto the slide, or, if there is only a small amount of discharge, it can easily be collected with a saline-saturated cotton-tipped applicator and spread onto the slide. The slide is then fixed in the same manner as a cervical specimen. This technique may expose cancerous cells. However, a negative smear is not conclusive, and additional work-up is mandated.

Ductography (Ductogram)

A ductogram is useful in evaluating the cause of nipple discharge. Contrast medium is injected by the radiologist into the discharging duct, and a mammogram is taken, which can show a filling defect (commonly an intraductal papilloma), a dilated or cystic appearance (duct ectasia or fibrocystic disease), or an abrupt obstruction (malignancy).

Serum Prolactin Level

Elevated serum prolactin levels can produce nipple discharge. Hyperprolactinemia should be suspected when the prolactin level exceeds 20 to 25 ng/ml. Prolactin elevation secondary to medications is generally less than 100 ng/ml. Prolactinomas are found when the prolactin level exceeds 150 ng/ml.

Thyroid Function Testing

Thyroid-stimulating hormone (TSH) is high in hypothyroidism. About 20% of patients with hyperprolactinemia have hypothyroidism. TSH testing is done to rule out primary hypothyroidism as a cause of the hyperprolactinemia and associated nipple discharge.

DIFFERENTIAL DIAGNOSIS
Single Breast Mass
Cancer

Breast cancer can occur at any time after puberty but it occurs more frequently with increasing age. Classically, breast cancer is a single lump that is hard, nontender, and immobile with borders that are not clearly delineated from the rest of the breast tissue. It occurs most commonly in the upper outer quadrant of the breast. Malignant tumors will eventually affix to the skin, ligaments, or chest wall and cause retractions. Cancers infrequently cause pain or tenderness on palpation, but some do. The tumors continually increase in size (although at varying rates) and do not come and go. Other suspicious signs of cancer include nipple inversion, dimpling of the breast, bloody nipple discharge, and axillary lymphadenopathy. Occasionally, breast cancer presents as diffuse swelling, pain, or breast erythema. Unilateral breast pain in a postmenopausal woman is suggestive of cancer. A mammographic finding of a nonpalpable mass or preinvasive lesion associated with macrocalcifications may be the only evidence of a malignant breast mass. Benign lumps are usually smooth, round, and freely movable. However, colloid, medullary, and expansive intraductal cancers can feel like benign tumors.

Fifteen percent of women younger than 40 years who have breast cancer are diagnosed during pregnancy or the postpartum period. Pregnant and postpartum breast cancer patients make up about 2% of total breast cancer patients. The normal physiological changes of the breast tissue during these times necessitate a thorough history and physical examination. A breast lump during pregnancy or lactation is more difficult to sample for a biopsy because of the increased vascularity of the breasts. Additionally, the lactating breast can act as an ideal medium for bacterial infection and is slower to heal.

Cysts

Benign cysts occur with higher frequency than any other type of breast lump. They are typically round or elliptical, soft or fluctuant, and mobile. Cysts are not attached to the surrounding breast, nipple, or chest wall, so there is no dimpling of breast tissue or nipple retraction. There are often multiple cysts, frequently in the upper outer quadrants of each breast. Cysts vary in size throughout the menstrual cycle and are usually at their smallest and least tender stage at the end of menses (end of the secretory phase). Transillumination of a cyst allows light to pass through the lump and supports the clinical diagnosis.

Fibroadenoma

Fibroadenoma usually occurs as a single, nontender, rubbery, firm, ovoid, or lobulated mass that measures 1 to 5 cm in diameter. This lump is freely mobile; thus there is no dimpling or retractions. It also does not vary in size with the menstrual cycle. Fibroadenomas can be multiple or bilateral about 25% of the time. They are the most commonly occurring breast mass in adolescence. Only biopsy can distinguish them from dysplasia, cancer, or cystosarcoma phyllodes.

Cystosarcoma phyllodes is a type of fibroadenoma in which the tumor grows rapidly and reaches a large size. Surgical removal of the tumor with a margin of normal breast tissue or simple mastectomy is sometimes necessary to prevent recurrence. The tumor is rarely malignant.

Abscess

Abscesses often follow systemic signs of mastitis. If mastitis is not treated early with antibiotics, it can progress to an abscess. A peripheral abscess is found more than 1 cm away from the areola and is usually caused by *S. aureus* or streptococcal organisms. A subareolar abscess is located in the nipple complex and may be associated with duct ectasia. Anaerobic organisms are the likely cause for subareolar abscesses. A chronic abscess can be encapsulated by fibrous tissue, causing the mass to be an irregularly shaped, firm mass that is nontender. An abscess should be incised and drained, and breastfeeding stopped.

Fat Necrosis

Fat necrosis occurs as the result of thickened and retracted scar tissue from an injury and subsequent hematoma. A biopsy alone can differentiate this single, fixed, often irregular tumor from carcinoma.

Lipoma

A lipoma is a fatty tumor of the breast with borders that are smooth and well-defined. The mass has a fluctuant consistency and is usually nontender and mobile.

Tuberculosis

Tuberculosis is an uncommon breast finding but should be considered, especially in immunocompromised patients. In early stages, tuberculosis may appear as a solitary, firm, irregular, nontender mass.

Ruptured Implant

With a ruptured implant, augmented breast tissue is pushed away from the chest wall by the implant. Masses found in these patients often are best palpated with the patient in the sitting position. The definitive diagnosis is made by mammogram, ultrasound, or magnetic resonance imaging.

Inflammatory Breast Mass
Mastitis and Acute Abscess

An acute abscess typically follows lactational mastitis. It is exquisitely tender on palpation and is very warm to the touch. The breast is erythematous and swollen, and the abscess usually involves only one fourth of the breast. The mass has a fluctuant consistency. Chills and fever may be present. Axillary lymphadenopathy suggests an abscess, but inflammatory breast cancer must be considered.

Inflammatory Breast Cancer

Inflammatory breast cancer presents similar to acute mastitis but differs from mastitis in that the entire breast is swollen and fever is rarely present. Axillary lymphadenopathy is present. Inflammatory breast cancer is a rapidly progressing disease; therefore close follow-up and prompt referral are necessary.

Multiple or Bilateral Breast Lumps
Fibrocystic Breast Changes

Fibrocystic breast changes usually present as multiple, bilateral painful masses, which frequently intensify premenstrually during the luteal phase of the menstrual cycle. The masses often rapidly fluctuate in size, are transient in appearance, and cause cyclic mastodynia (see Chapter 25). They occur most often in women ages 30 to 50 and are rare in postmenopausal women. Fibrocystic histological findings that increase the risk of breast cancer are moderate or severe hyperplasia (1.5 to 2 times the risk), atypical hyperplasia (5 times the risk), and lobular carcinoma in situ (8 to 10 times the risk).

Nipple Discharge
Intraductal Papilloma

Intraductal papillomas are the most common benign lesions to cause a bloody nipple discharge. They usually are unilateral, subareolar lesions occurring in perimenopausal women. Solitary papillomas do not increase breast cancer risk.

Duct Ectasia

Mammary duct ectasia occurs most frequently in menopausal women. The subareolar ducts become blocked with desquamating secretory epithelium, necrotic debris, and chronic inflammatory cells. This condition is frequently bilateral and is characterized by pain, tenderness, periods of inflammation, and a nipple discharge that is spontaneous, sticky, multicolored, and from multiple ducts. Nipple retraction may occur. There is no known association with malignancy.

Neonatal Discharge ("Witch's Milk")

Newborns may have breast enlargement and a white nipple discharge secondary to maternal estrogens. This condition will disappear within 1 to 2 weeks after birth.

Hyperprolactinemia

Hyperprolactinemia can cause nipple discharge in both men and women. The nipple discharge is usually bilateral and milky and from multiple ducts. Additional symptoms may include amenorrhea, decreased libido, or gynecomastia. Approximately 75% of women presenting with galactorrhea and amenorrhea have hyperprolactinemia. A prolactin-secreting tumor may produce additional symptoms such as headaches and visual disturbances. Normal serum fasting prolactin levels are generally less than 30 ng/ml. A prolactinoma is likely if the prolactin level is greater than 250 ng/ml and less likely if the level is less than 100 ng/ml.

Male Breast Disease
Acute Mastitis

Acute mastitis in males occurs from trauma (e.g., nipple chafing from jogging) and pres-

ents as previously discussed in the preceding section on mastitis.

Cancer

Male breast cancer is extremely rare and represents about 1% of all breast cancers. It begins as a painless induration, retraction of the nipple, and an attached mass. It progresses to include lymphadenopathy and skin and chest wall lesions.

DIFFERENTIAL DIAGNOSIS OF *Common Causes of Breast Lumps and Nipple Discharge*

CONDITION	HISTORY	PHYSICAL FINDINGS	DIAGNOSTIC STUDIES
Single Breast Mass			
Cancer	Usually older than 35; unilateral new lump	Single, hard, nontender, fixed lump; borders irregular or not discrete; may be erythema, dimpling, increased vessel patterns; may have nipple discharge	Diagnostic mammogram; ultrasound; tissue biopsy
Cysts	Younger age, often younger than 35; often multiple	Round or elliptical; soft or fluctuant; mobile	Clinical examination; FNA: clear aspirate; mammogram; ultrasound: cyst(s)
Fibroadenoma	Common in adolescence	Single, sharply circumscribed, mobile lump	Diagnostic mammogram; ultrasound; biopsy
Abscess	History of mastitis	Single mass; irregular shape; chronic abscess may be nontender	Biopsy
Fat necrosis	May have history of injury at site	Single, fixed, and often irregular tumor	Biopsy
Lipoma	May have others on arms, trunk, buttocks, or back; usually nontender	Single tumors; smooth, well-defined; fluctuant consistency	Biopsy
Tuberculosis	History of tuberculosis, positive PPD, or chest radiography; immunocompromised patient status	Single; irregular shape; nontender	Biopsy
Ruptured implant	History of augmentation; change in size or shape of breast	Nodule palpated best when patient is sitting	Diagnostic mammogram; ultrasound; MRI
Inflammatory Breast Mass			
Mastitis and acute abscess	Primigravidas more often than gravidas; >1 wk after delivery; breastfeeding; tender nipples	Red, warm, tender; usually unilateral, one fourth of breast, or one lobule; breast engorgement; fever; nipple discharge: pus	Culture positive for *S. aureus, Escherichia coli, Streptococcus*; elevated WBCs

Continued

DIFFERENTIAL DIAGNOSIS OF *Common Causes of Breast Lumps and Nipple Discharge—cont'd*

CONDITION	HISTORY	PHYSICAL FINDINGS	DIAGNOSTIC STUDIES
Inflammatory breast cancer	History of mastitis or inflammatory process of breast	Entire breast swollen; fever rarely present; axillary lymphadenopathy	Biopsy
Multiple or Bilateral Breast Lumps			
Fibrocystic breast changes	Multiple breast lumps of both breasts; cyclic changes that worsen at time of menses	Bilateral nodularity, dominant lumps; tender, mobile	FNA; ultrasound; mammogram
Nipple Discharge			
Intraductal papilloma	Bloody nipple discharge; usual age is 40-50 yr	Unilateral, subareolar	Diagnostic mammogram; ductogram
Fibrocystic breast changes	Milky nipple discharge; cyclic changes that worsen at time of menses	Spontaneous, clear or milky, bilateral, multiduct nipple discharge; multiple breast lumps of both breasts	Diagnostic mammogram; ductogram
Duct ectasia	Green nipple discharge	Greenish or brownish nipple discharge	Diagnostic mammogram; ductogram
Neonatal discharge (witch's milk)	Milky discharge 1-2 wk after birth	Enlarged breast tissue, milky discharge lasting 1-2 wk after birth	None
Hyperprolactinemia	Milky or clear nipple discharge; amenorrhea; history of medications: estrogenic, dopamine blockers, or dopamine depleters; hypothyroidism; pregnancy; postabortion; nipple stimulators; visual changes	Spontaneous, unilateral or bilateral, multiduct; clear or milky nipple discharge	Serum prolactin levels; MRI if indicated
Male Breast Disease			
Acute mastitis	History of clothing rubbing nipple (e.g., jogging); swelling or lump of chest wall; tenderness of site	Red, warm, tender; usually unilateral, one fourth of breast, or one lobule; breast engorgement; fever; nipple discharge/pus	Culture: positive for *S. aureus, E. coli, Streptococcus*; elevated WBCs
Cancer	Family history of male breast cancer; painless lump of chest wall	Induration, retraction of nipple or mass in nipple well; fixed, nontender; lymphadenopathy	Mammogram; FNA; tissue biopsy

PPD, Purified protein derivative (tuberculin).

CHAPTER RESOURCES

Apantaku LM: Breast cancer diagnosis and screening, *Am Fam Physician* 62:596, 2000.

Arca MJ, Caniano DA: Breast disorders in the adolescent patient, *Adolesc Med Clin* 15(3):473, 2004.

Barton MB, Harris R, Fletcher SW: Does this patient have breast cancer? The screening clinical breast examination: should it be done? How? *JAMA* 282:1270, 1999.

Kerlikowske K, Smith-Bindman R, Britt-Marie Ljung BM et al: Evaluation of abnormal mammography results and palpable breast abnormalities, *Ann Intern Med* 139(4):274, 2003.

Klein S: Evaluation of palpable breast masses, *Am Fam Physician* 71(9):1731, 2005.

Pena KS, Rosenfeld JA: Evaluation and treatment of galactorrhea, *Am Fam Physician* 63:1763, 2001.

Pruthi S: Detection and evaluation of a palpable breast mass, *Mayo Clin Proc* 76:641, 2001.

Santen R, Mansel R: Benign breast disorders, *N Engl J Med* 353(3):275, 2005.

Templeman C, Hertweck SP: Breast disorders in the pediatric and adolescent patient, *Obstet Gynecol Clin North Am* 27:19, 2000.

Breast Pain

Nearly 70% of women experience breast pain during their lives; it is the most common breast-related complaint among women. A common problem in women who are still menstruating, breast pain is less common in older women. The pain may be mildly annoying or severe, and it may be periodic or nearly constant. Breast pain may occur in one or both breasts or in the underarm (axilla) region of the body.

Because of awareness about breast cancer, many women worry that mastalgia may indicate malignancy. The cause of breast pain is not known. Its relationship to the menstrual cycle and its occurrence in premenopausal women suggest a hormonal etiology. Mastalgia is rarely associated with breast cancer and is usually related to fibrocystic changes in premenopausal women.

Breast pain associated with gynecomastia is seen in some young males. An abnormal ratio of estrogen to androgen causes the breast tissue to grow and become tender. It is also seen with Klinefelter's syndrome, a sex chromosomal disorder (XXY) that occurs in males.

DIAGNOSTIC REASONING: FOCUSED HISTORY

Is This Cyclic or Noncyclic Mastalgia?

Key Questions

- Are you still menstruating?
- What is the relationship of the pain to your menstrual cycle?
- When is the pain most severe?

Pre/Post Menopause

Cyclic pain occurs premenopausally and is associated with the menstrual cycle. Postmenopausal pain is not cyclic.

Relationship to Menstrual Cycle/Severity

Cyclic pain occurs in relation to the menstrual cycle. Typically it is most severe before the menses and goes away spontaneously with or after the menses. Premenstrual water retention in the breasts has also been proposed as a cause of mastalgia.

What Characteristics of the Pain Will Help Me With a Diagnosis?

Key Questions

- Describe the pain.
- Is the pain in one breast or both? Where in the breast(s) is it?
- Does the pain radiate?

Pain Description

Cyclic pain is usually described as a heaviness most likely caused by hormonal changes that affect the breast tissue, resulting in edema and increased nodularity. Noncyclic pain is described as sharp and burning.

Location and Radiation

Cyclic pain is usually bilateral and poorly localized. Women often describe it as radiating to the axillae and arms. Noncyclic pain is often unilateral and well localized.

Could Age Help Explain the Cause?

Key Question

- How old are you?

Breast tissue changes with age. Women under the age of 25 have more stromal and lobular breast characteristics, and fibroadenomas are more frequently seen in this kind of tissue. Women ages 25 to 40 years are more likely to have cyclic mastalgia and nodularity. After age 40, women's breasts begin to involute and they are more likely to have cysts and duct ectasia. Women over the age of 50 have an increased risk for breast cancer.

In adolescent males, an abnormal ratio of estrogen to androgens can occur, causing breast tissue to grow and become tender.

Is the Pain Associated With a Lump or Discharge?

Key Questions

- Have you felt a lump?
- Do you have a history of cystic breast changes or lumpy breasts?
- Do the lumps come and go or change with your periods?
- Have you ever had a mammogram or ultrasound? Why was it done? What were the results?
- Have you ever had a lump drained or biopsied? What was the diagnosis?
- Do you have any nipple discharge?

Lumps

Noncyclic pain is occasionally secondary to the presence of a fibroadenoma or cyst. Fibrocysts that increase in size and tenderness as the menstrual cycle approaches can contribute to breast pain. Cyclic cysts of the breast are less common after menopause and necessitate diagnostic investigation. A postmenopausal woman with unilateral breast pain has a greater risk for a diagnosis of breast cancer.

Previous Mammograms or Biopsies

History or documentation of cyclic changes in lumps or the presence of cystic or glandular breast tissue on a mammogram or ultrasound supports a clinical diagnosis of benign disease.

What Else Could Be Causing the Pain?

Key Questions

- When was your last period? Have you missed any periods? Could you be pregnant?
- Is your breast hot or red?
- Does the pain get worse with deep inspiration?
- What medications are you taking?
- Have you had any trauma to your chest?

Missed Periods/Pregnancy

Pregnancy is the most common cause of breast tenderness.

Hot or Red Breast

Mastitis is characterized by a breast that is painful, hot, and red. In lactating women, the most frequent symptom is a painful erythematous lobule in an outer quadrant of the breast. Although mastitis is most common in lactating women, it can also occur in nonlactating women, usually as the result of a generalized dermatitis occurring from insect bites, sunburn, or allergic reactions. However, the most common cause of an inflamed breast in nonlactating women is inflammatory breast cancer. In inflammatory breast cancer, the entire breast is swollen, heavy, and edematous.

Pain With Deep Inspiration

Pain with deep inspiration suggests a musculoskeletal etiology. Costochondritis especially affects the second and third ribs.

Medications

In postmenopausal women, hormone therapy may stimulate symptoms of breast lumps and pain. Many herbal products, especially ginseng and dong quai, may also cause some women to experience an onset of breast pain, as do soybean products or tofu. Women on liquid diet supplements that have a soy base may experience breast changes and discomfort.

Gynecomastia can occur as a result of medications such as corticosteroids, hormonal medications, diazepam, and illicit drugs.

Trauma to Chest

Chest trauma, whether by accident or from abuse, can cause breast pain. In female adolescents, breast pain has been linked to sexual abuse.

Key Questions
- Have you ever had any chest pain or shortness of breath?
- Have you ever had any abdominal pain with this breast pain?

Chest Pain or Shortness of Breath
See Chapter 9 for a discussion of chest pain. It is important to rule out cardiac disease when assessing any type of chest pain, including breast pain. The major cause of death in American women is heart disease with atypical presenting symptoms.

Abdominal Pain
See Chapter 13 for a discussion of abdominal pain. Gallbladder disease and hiatal hernia may also refer pain to the breast region. These conditions must be ruled out when evaluating breast pain.

DIAGNOSTIC REASONING: FOCUSED PHYSICAL EXAMINATION
Perform a Breast Examination
Perform a multiposition physical examination of the breasts, nipples, and regional lymph nodes as described in Chapter 24. In the vast majority of women with breast pain, the physical examination is negative. In addition in children, assess for breast development using the Tanner Sexual Maturity Rating scale of breast development (see Chapter 23).

Characterize Lumps
If you find a mass on physical examination, determine its size, depth, contour, shape, fluctuation, firmness, and mobility. Fluctuation can be determined by holding the edges of the mass against the chest wall and pressing the center with finger pads. Fluctuation ("bouncy" consistency) occurs with cysts, lipomas, and abscesses. Cysts are frequently tender, especially premenstrually. Reexamination in 1 or 2 weeks will usually demonstrate cyclic hormonal changes of the tissue, and lump size and tenderness will have changed.

A single, firm, asymmetrical, immobile mass in a postmenopausal woman will, when biopsied, prove to be cancerous 75% of the time.

Examine Chest Wall
Palpate the intercostal spaces for costochondral margin tenderness and swelling. Palpation that reproduces the pain, especially affecting the second and third ribs, suggests costochondritis.

Examine the Genital Area in the Male
Sexual maturation should be assessed by using the Tanner Sexual Maturity Rating scale (see Figure 25-1). Boys with Klinefelter's syndrome will have sparse or absent pubic hair and small testes and penis. Testicular palpation should be performed to estimate the size of the testicles.

LABORATORY AND DIAGNOSTIC STUDIES
Urine for Human Chorionic Gonadotropin (hCG)
Test the urine for hCG to rule out pregnancy.

Mammography
In the absence of a mass on physical examination, women 40 years of age and older should have a screening mammogram unless one was obtained in the previous 10 to 12 months. The purpose of the mammogram is to look for concurrent breast pathology in women whose age places them at risk for breast cancer. Screening mammography (conventional film or digital) is used to identify nonpalpable breast lesions. It consists of two views: craniocaudal (CC) and medial lateral oblique (MLO). When the physical examination is normal, mammograms are not indicated in women younger than 30 years. In the vast majority of women with breast pain, mammography shows no evidence of breast pathology. If a mass is found on a screening mammogram, additional views and imaging may be ordered.

Ultrasound
If a mass is found on mammography, ultrasound is helpful in differentiating solid from

FIGURE 25-1   Tanner stages of penis, testis, and scrotal development in boys. (Photographs from Van Wieringen JC: *Growth diagrams 1965 Netherlands Second National Survey on 0- to 24-year-olds,* Groningen, The Netherlands, 1971, Wolters-Noordhoff; reprinted with permission of Kluwer Academic Publishers.)

cystic lesions. In women under age 30 years, ultrasound is often the first step in the evaluation of a cyst or a mass. The ultrasound finding of a cystic lesion may then be followed by aspiration of the cyst, eliminating it to make sure it is not concealing another abnormal breast finding. The ultrasound identification of a solid mass should be followed by tissue biopsy.

Fine-Needle Aspiration and Cytological Examination

Fine-needle aspiration biopsy uses a small-gauge needle to obtain fluid and cellular material if a mass is present. It immediately determines if the lump is a cyst or a solid tumor. The aspirate is sent for cytological evaluation to determine the presence of absence of malignant cells.

Karyotyping

Chromosomal testing determines the presence of the XXY chromosomal disorder or related chromosomal variants.

DIFFERENTIAL DIAGNOSIS

Cyclic Breast Pain

Cyclic mastalgia—pain that corresponds to changes in the menstrual cycle—is the most common type of mastalgia and can account for as much as two thirds of breast pain. Cyclic breast pain is usually bilateral, is often greatest in the upper outer breast quadrant, and is described as dull, heavy, and aching, often radiating to the axilla and arm. The pain has a variable duration and is often relieved after the menses. Typically for several days preceding the menstrual flow, the breasts of these women enlarge, become lumpy and tender to touch, and produce a generalized aching. The nipples may become extremely sensitive and very uncomfortable. Cyclic pain is usually bilateral and poorly localized. Compared with noncyclic mastalgia, cyclic breast pain occurs more often in younger women.

Cyclic breast pain is attributed to the fluctuations of hormones during the menstrual cycle. As the breasts prepare for pregnancy each month by increasing the number of milk-producing cells, as much as 15 to 30 ml of fluid may be stored in each breast. This fluid can cause breast enlargement and the possibility of tenderness and pain. Additional factors that contribute to cyclic pain include caffeine intake, high-sodium diets, and high-fat diets. Thyroid conditions have also been shown to be a cause of cyclic breast pain.

Noncyclic Breast Pain

Noncyclic mastalgia is most common in women 40 to 50 years of age. It accounts for about one fourth of breast pain cases. The duration of symptoms tends to be shorter than that of cyclic pain, and noncyclic breast pain resolves spontaneously in 50% of cases. The pain is localized to a specific area in the breast and is described as sharp, stabbing, burning, and throbbing. Noncyclic mastalgia is occasionally secondary to the presence of a fibroadenoma or cyst, and the pain may be relieved by treatment of the underlying breast lesion.

Noncyclic mastalgia has no relationship to the menstrual cycle. It may be constant or intermittent with irregular exacerbations, and increased nodularity is often noted on physical examination. Cysts, fibroadenomas, duct ectasia, mastitis, breast injury, and breast abscesses have been associated with noncyclic pain. Additional causes include referred pain from infected teeth, medication-induced pain, and musculoskeletal pain.

Mastitis/Abscess

Mastitis is inflammation and infection of the breast tissue characterized by sudden onset of swelling, tenderness, erythema, and heat, which is usually accompanied by chills, fever, and increased pulse rate. Most infections are staphylococcal, often *Staphylococcus aureus*. Mastitis is most common in lactating women after milk is established, usually the second to third week after delivery; however, it may occur at any time. Mastitis is not an indication to discontinue breastfeeding. Abscess formation can result, which presents as discharge of pus (suppuration) and a large hardened mass with an area of fluctuation, erythema, and heat. The underlying pus-filled abscess may impart a bluish tinge to the skin.

Mammary Duct Ectasia

Mammary duct ectasia occurs most frequently in menopausal women. The subareolar ducts become blocked with desquamating secretory epithelium, necrotic debris, and chronic inflammatory cells. This condition is frequently bilateral and is characterized by pain, tenderness, periods of inflammation, and a nipple discharge. Nipple retraction may occur. There is no known association with malignancy. Mammogram and ultrasound can show ectasia.

Pregnancy

Pregnancy is the most common cause of breast tenderness. Test the urine for β-hCG to rule out pregnancy.

Costochondritis

A common musculoskeletal cause of breast pain is Tietze's syndrome or costochondritis, which is inflammation of the cartilage of the ribs. This pain, which originates in the area of the sternum and the ribs, is localized close to the sternum and causes tenderness on palpation when moving the rib cage or when taking a deep breath.

Klinefelter's Syndrome

This sex chromosomal disorder (XXY) occurs in males and is characterized by gynecomastia and prepubertal testes. In some adolescent boys, the first sign of Klinefelter's syndrome is breast pain and gynecomastia. Patients may lack secondary sexual characteristics because of a decrease in androgen production. This results in sparse facial, body, pubic and axillary hair, a high-pitched voice, and a female type of fat distribution. By late puberty, 30% to 50% of boys with Klinefelter's syndrome manifest gynecomastia, which is secondary to elevated estradiol levels and increased estradiol/testosterone ratio. The risk of developing breast carcinoma is at least 20 times higher than normal.

Breast Lumps Associated With Breast Pain

See Chapter 24 for a discussion of breast lumps and nipple discharge.

◆ DIFFERENTIAL DIAGNOSIS OF *Common Causes of Breast Pain*

CONDITION	HISTORY	PHYSICAL FINDINGS	DIAGNOSTIC STUDIES
Cyclic breast pain	Corresponds to changes in menstrual cycle Bilateral; pain often greatest in upper, outer breast quadrant Dull, heavy, and aching pain; radiates to axilla and arm; varying duration	Often no physical findings; breasts may be tender	None; history and clinical examination
Noncyclic breast pain	Women 40-50 years No relationship to menses Pain localized to specific area in breast; described as sharp, stabbing, burning, throbbing	Often no physical findings; breast may be more nodular; lump may be present	Mammogram/ultrasound

Continued

DIFFERENTIAL DIAGNOSIS OF *Common Causes of Breast Pain—cont'd*

CONDITION	HISTORY	PHYSICAL FINDINGS	DIAGNOSTIC STUDIES
Mastitis/abscess	Sudden onset of swelling, tenderness, erythema, and heat, which is usually accompanied by chills, fever, and increased pulse rate Lactating women after milk is established, usually second to third week after delivery	Swelling, redness, tenderness Possible abscess formation with hardened mass, area of fluctuation, erythema, and heat Underlying pus-filled abscess may impart bluish tinge to skin	None; clinical examination
Mammary duct ectasia	Menopausal women Bilateral or unilateral pain, tenderness; periods of inflammation; nipple discharge	Often no physical findings Nipple retraction may occur; lump may be present	Mammogram; ultrasound
Pregnancy	Missed period; contraceptive use failure	Breast tenderness and swelling	Urine for hCG
Costochondritis	Pain in area of sternum and ribs; pain with deep inspiration	Tenderness on palpation, when moving rib cage, or when taking a deep breath	None; trial of NSAIDs
Klinefelter's syndrome	Adolescent boy with breast tenderness and enlargement	Testes prepubertal, gynecomastia, decreased body hair	Karyotyping
Breast lumps associated with breast pain	See Chapter 24 for discussion on breast lumps and nipple discharge		

NSAIDs, Nonsteroidal antiinflammatory drugs.

CHAPTER RESOURCES

Amory JK, Anawalt BD, Paulsen CA et al: Klinefelter's syndrome, *Lancet* 356:333, 2000.

Hamed H, Fentiman IS: Benign breast disease, *Int J Clin Pract* 55:461, 2001.

Johnson C: Benign breast disease, *Nurse Pract Forum* 10:137, 1999.

Morrow M: The evaluation of common breast problems, *Am Fam Physician* 61:2371, 2000.

Neinstein LS: Breast disease in adolescents and young women, *Pediatr Clin North Am* 46:607, 1999.

Padden DL: Mastalgia: evaluation and management, *Nurse Pract Forum* 11:213, 2000.

Santen R, Mansel R: Benign breast disorders, *N Engl J Med* 353(3):275, 2005.

Smith RL, Pruthi S, Fitzpatrick LA: Evaluation and management of breast pain, *Mayo Clin Proc* 79(3):353, 2004.

Templeman C, Hertweck SP: Breast disorders in the pediatric and adolescent patient, *Obstet Gynecol Clin North Am* 27:19, 2000.

X

Common Problems of the Musculoskeletal System

26

Limb Pain

Complaints of pain in a limb present a diagnostic challenge because of the many possible pathophysiological causes. Because of the broad range of differential diagnoses, it is best to use a framework of differentiating the pain as a symptom of musculoskeletal injury, musculoskeletal or joint disease, systemic disease, or a mixture of factors. Pain can be the result of a direct reaction in tissues, secondary reaction in adjacent tissues, or referral from a proximal or distal lesion or from organs such as the heart or kidney. In children, aches and pains in limbs are common; however, the presence, location, and intensity of the pain are often difficult to assess. Interpretation of pain is often made by the parents.

It is helpful to distinguish between limb pain that affects the bones, muscles, and tendons and injury/inflammation of a joint that can affect surrounding musculature, nerves, and blood vessels. For example, lower extremity pain is often referred from the low back and emanates from irritated nerve roots or is secondary to myofascial syndromes of the low back, pelvic, and hip musculature.

DIAGNOSTIC REASONING: FOCUSED HISTORY

Is the Pain Related to an Urgent Problem That Needs Immediate Treatment to Avoid Disability or Death?

Key Questions

- Have you had a recent injury?
- Describe exactly how the injury occurred.
- Do you have any other symptoms, such as fatigue, fever, or swollen joints?

- What is the severity of the pain? Does it occur with exercise or rest?

Injury

Injuries to the musculoskeletal system can range from simple muscular strain to a significant fracture associated with nerve or vascular injury. Therefore when a patient presents with a history of trauma, the priority is to assess the vascular integrity of the limb. Neurological integrity is next. Symptoms of coldness, severe pain, or paresthesia are signals that physical examination should begin immediately to assess the extent of injury and the need for emergency treatment. Acute pain and swelling that follow trauma usually indicate injury to a previously normal structure.

If the injury does not warrant urgent attention, obtain further history. Ask questions that specify the mechanism of injury, such as a direct blow or impact, landing position after a fall, twisting, jumping, running, overstretching, or overuse. When discussing the precipitating event, ask the patient to describe any noise such as snapping, popping, or breaking that may have occurred with the injury.

Constitutional Symptoms

The presence of generalized symptoms such as fever, weight loss, general malaise, or hot swollen joints suggests the presence of a systemic disorder such as infection or rheumatic disease. In addition infection in a child causes systemic illness and the child appears ill.

Fever related to joint problems can be the result of hematogenous seeding by an organism, direct invasion as a result of trauma or puncture, or migration from an adjacent area of infection. In rheumatic fever, a β-hemolytic

351

streptococcal infection precedes the initial joint pain by 1 to 3 weeks. Often the hip joint may be the first of many joints affected before polyarticular migratory involvement occurs. The fever is sustained, not intermittent. Fever spikes are seen with chronic forms of arthritis in children.

Other systemic infections associated with polyarthritis include bacterial endocarditis, Lyme disease, syphilis, and viruses such as hepatitis B, rubella, cytomegalovirus, human immunodeficiency virus (HIV), Epstein-Barr virus, and varicella zoster.

Severity of Pain

Unrelenting diffuse pain, often occurring at night, is an indication of bone involvement, either through an infection such as osteo-myelitis, septic hip, or bone cancer. Claudication and neurogenic pain increase with activity and decrease with rest, more immediately for vascular causes and more slowly for neurogenic causes.

Lack of spontaneous movement of a limb in a child indicates pain and is often called "pseudoparalysis."

What Does the Location of the Pain Tell Me?

Key Questions

■ Where does it hurt?
■ Is the pain local or generalized?

Location

Location of pain provides a clue for identifying the site where the pain originates. Local pain receptors signal the site of irritation, and an increase in sensitivity (hyperesthesia) results. Referred pain generally involves the muscle chains, nerve pathways, and vessels. Unilateral, circumscribed limb or quadrant pain involves autonomic nerve fibers. Bilateral pain is more likely to originate from systemic involvement. Diffuse pain with inconsistent distribution may be the result of psychosomatic conditions such as depression and anxiety. Diffuse pain over trigger points is indicative of fibromyalgia. Collagen

diseases and connective tissue diseases can affect one or more joints. The more vaguely defined the boundaries of the pain, the deeper or more central is the location of the somatic irritation. The obturator nerve has sensory branches that innervate the hip and skin on the medial aspect of the thigh, causing pain that comes from the hip to feel as though the pain is in the knee.

Could This Be Caused by a Sprain or Strain?

Key Questions

■ Describe how the injury occurred.
■ Did you hear a noise with the injury, such as a ripping or cracking sound?
■ Were you able to use the limb after the injury?

Strain

A strain involves injury to muscles and tendons, whereas sprains involve injury to ligamentous structures. Both types of injuries can produce a ripping or tearing sound and range in severity from minor damage to a complete tear. Injuries are generally classified as mild, moderate, or severe. A moderate to severe strain/sprain may involve some loss of joint or ligament stability. Strains may be acute or chronic. Injury commonly occurs when lateral stress is applied while the joint is plantar flexed. This position is the least stable position of the ankle, and the over-stretched ligaments are more susceptible to eversion or inversion forces.

Sprain

Sprains cause minimal to moderate pain increasing 1 to 2 days after the trauma when the inflammatory process begins. A complete disruption that severs the sensory nerve fibers within the structure will cause little pain, whereas a partial injury irritates sensory fibers and may produce intense pain.

In children, ligaments and joint capsules are two to five times stronger than the epiphysis; therefore growth plate injuries are more common than sprains.

Fracture

A fracture produces diffuse swelling around the injured bone soon after injury. Deformity will be present if the fracture is displaced. A patient may report hearing a crack and being disabled by the increased severity of pain with weight bearing or movement of the limb. With stress fracture, there may be mild swelling and tenderness and pain with weight bearing.

If There Is No History of Trauma or a Precipitating Event, What Else Is Causing the Pain?

Key Questions

- Describe your usual daily activities at home, work, and with hobbies.
- How does the pain affect your activities?
- Do you have other illnesses?

Overuse

Repetitive microtrauma results from cumulative injury or overuse. This type of trauma most often affects the fingers, wrists, and upper extremities. Persons who work on keyboards for long periods may complain of paresthesia of the fingers and pain and soreness of the wrists and fingers. Weekend hobbies or participation in sports may result in overuse of certain muscle groups associated with those activities.

Activities

A person may adapt to chronic musculoskeletal problems by using an assistive device such as a cane or by limiting activities. Rheumatic disorders produce symmetrical discomfort and pain with inactivity. Noninflammatory conditions are often associated with asymmetrical pain after extended use. Children will often not walk on a limb that causes pain. Infants will have lack of movement of the limb as well as irritability and fussiness when the limb is moved passively.

Other Illnesses

The presence of coronary artery disease increases the risk of arterial insufficiency and associated claudication pain. Peripheral neu-ropathy associated with diabetes can produce a burning pain or "pins and needles" sensation, especially in the lower extremities.

In Joint Pain With Injury, What Do I Need to Know About the Specific Joints Involved?

Upper Extremity: Shoulder, Wrist, Elbow
Key Questions

- Is the pain in your dominant limb?
- Did you fall on an outstretched hand or arm?
- Did you overuse a joint?

Pain in the dominant hand may indicate repetitive microtrauma or overuse. Breaking a fall with an outstretched arm is a common mechanism of injury for a fracture or dislocation of the hand or wrist.

Lower Extremity: Knee, Ankle
Key Questions

- How is the pain affected by weight bearing or activity?
- Did you feel a sense of "giving way"?
- Did you hear a pop, tear, or other sound?
- What position was your leg in when you hurt your knee?

Continuing with an activity means the injury did not totally disrupt any ligamentous structures. An inability to straighten or bend the knee suggests a mechanical blockage, such as a patellar dislocation or meniscus tear. In chondromalacia, the patient can bend the knee, but the movement is usually painful.

A loud pop is virtually diagnostic of an anterior cruciate ligament (ACL) tear. A ripping sound suggests a meniscus injury. A cracking sound may signify a bony injury or dislocation of the patella.

A sudden change in direction or sudden stop may put more force on the ligaments than they can dissipate, resulting in acute rupture. A sudden twisting injury is likely to represent a meniscus tear and a serious ligament disruption. Running or jumping activities are commonly associated with knee and ankle injuries.

In children, 10% to 20% of knee symptoms are the result of a problem in the hip joint.

Could This Be Musculoskeletal or Joint Disease?

Key Question

■ Describe the pain.

In general, sharp, piercing, stabbing, cutting, pinching, gnawing pain is most common with lesions of the nerves and skin. Dull, tearing, boring, burning, and cramping are common terms used to describe pain arising from deeper structures such as muscles, joints, and internal organs. Pulsating, pounding, throbbing, and hammering are common descriptions of vascular pain. Gradually increasing sensations of pressure, tension, heaviness, and calf pain indicate venous obstruction. Severe pain that develops over 1 to 4 days is typical of osteomyelitis or septic arthritis in children, which is an emergency condition.

Muscle pain is caused by receptors located in bursa, muscle fibers, ligaments, and tendon attachments. It is a diffuse, dull, gnawing, boring, or tearing pain that increases with use and decreases with rest.

Intraarticular pain arises from receptors of the synovial membrane, joint capsule, or the fibrochondral layers of the articular surfaces. Joint pain is either inflammatory or degenerative. Inflammatory joint pain radiates diffusely to surrounding tissues. It is intense, sharp, burning, boring, or pulsating (effusion) pain. It persists during rest and is evident especially at night, worsening in the morning with morning stiffness that lasts more than 45 minutes, and then improves throughout the day.

Degenerative joint pain radiates to the soft tissue structures around the joint (i.e., muscles, ligaments, tendons). It is dull, boring, and gnawing when associated with muscle pain, or it can be a sharp, acute pain that increases with overuse.

Bone lesions cause a dull ache; periosteal pain is sharp and not well localized, and increases in intensity with dependency of the extremity.

Neuralgic pain occurs in the distribution of a peripheral nerve or nerve root. The pain is stabbing or cutting and can also present as pricking or lacerating.

What Does the History of Swelling Tell Me?

Key Questions

■ Is there any swelling?
■ When did the swelling begin?

Swelling

Swelling around a joint is always abnormal. Children do not always recognize swelling; they often report that they cannot squat down or flex their knee fully because it feels "full or tight."

Generally, swelling that develops immediately or within 2 hours after an injury is the result of a fracture or hemarthrosis and indicates a severe injury. Swelling 6 to 24 hours after an injury is usually of synovial origin, such as a meniscal tear, subluxation, dislocation, or ligamentous damage. Swelling after 24 hours suggests an inflammatory response.

Is This an Acute or a Chronic Problem?

Key Questions

■ When did the pain first occur?
■ When did you first notice a problem?

Pain experienced hours after an injury or physical activity is usually caused by acute extensor injury or overuse. Severe ligament sprain is manifested as an immediately disabling pain at the moment of the injury.

Determining if the complaint is acute or chronic helps to differentiate the cause. Chronic joint problems compound each other, whereas intermittent or episodic pain is characteristic of diseases of the musculoskeletal system. In children, limping or not using the extremity may be a signal that the child is experiencing pain. Parents will often note the loss of motion in an extremity or an awkward gait; they often report that the child is unable to perform routine activities.

Patients may report noticing pain, weakness, or difficulty in activities of daily living, such as using a hair dryer, opening jars, holding a pen, or handling eating utensils.

How Is Activity Affected?

Key Questions

- What are your usual activities?
- What activity makes the pain worse?
- What movements make the pain worse?

A large percentage of musculoskeletal injuries are caused by repetitive motion that leads to microtrauma and eventually cumulative damage. Repetitive microtrauma in the lower extremities from inappropriate rate and intensity of training, shoe wear, or playing surfaces can cause stress fractures of the weight-bearing bones of the lower limbs. Pain is worse over the site of the fracture.

In children, pain in the groin or referred to the knee and anterior thigh, occurring intermittently after activity and gradually becoming constant, may indicate Legg-Calvé-Perthes disease (LCPD).

Intraarticular lesions usually worsen with joint motion and sports activities. Intraosseous tumors are less sensitive to joint motion.

In children with a septic hip, pain increases with movement.

What Does Joint Stiffness or Locking Tell Me?

Key Questions

- Have you had any joint stiffness?
- Does activity make the stiffness worse or better?
- Do you have locking of the knee?

Joint Stiffness or Locking

Stiffness is felt after being in one position for a long time. This complaint gets confused with locking of the knee, which is an abrupt occurrence where the patient complains that something "gets in the way" and is unable to fully extend the knee. Manipulation of the leg often results in an equally abrupt unlocking. This is usually a sign of a chronic unstable meniscus tear.

Stiffness is a common feature of any inflammatory arthropathy. It is important to know whether it is localized or generalized. The length of time the stiffness lasts in the morning is a useful index of active synovitis in disease states such as rheumatoid arthritis (RA) or systemic lupus erythematosus (SLE). With most inflammatory arthropathies, stiffness and pain are alleviated by activity, whereas mechanical problems are aggravated by activity. Musculoskeletal tumors commonly present with mild joint stiffness because of muscle involvement but rarely demonstrate instability.

What Does the History of a Limp Tell Me?

Key Questions

- Is there pain with the limp?
- Did the limp develop suddenly?
- Is the limp constant or intermittent?
- What is the effect of running or climbing stairs?

Limp

Limping is a pathological alteration of a smooth, regular gait pattern and is never normal. Gait can be divided into two phases: stance and swing. The stance phase starts with the foot in contact with the ground and ends with the toe being lifted off the ground; the limb supports all the body weight. The swing phase begins with the toe elevated from the ground and ends with the heel strike. During the swing phase, the foot is not touching the ground; the pelvis rotates forward and tilts slightly while the trunk maintains a neutral position. Limp after strenuous running may indicate a stress fracture.

Quadriceps weakness causes difficulty in climbing stairs. During ambulation, this weakness causes the knee to be unstable on heel strike, and assistance is needed to push the knee manually into an extended position.

Neuromuscular diseases can result in progressive and painless muscle weakness or spasticity that affects ambulation in a variety of ways.

Symptoms of pain and limping in children may often be incorrectly attributed to trauma instead of indicating a more serious problem such as neoplastic tumors or bone infections.

Could This Be Caused by Systemic Disease?

Key Questions

- Have you been treated with antibiotics recently?
- Have you had any recent immunizations?
- Does the pain awaken you at night?
- Is the pain worse at night?

Medications

Certain antibiotics can cause serum sickness in children, producing joint pain and fever.

Transient arthralgia may occur 6 to 8 weeks after receiving MMR (measles, mumps, rubella) immunization. Recurrent or permanent arthritis may follow rubella vaccination, especially in adult females.

In adults, fluoroquinolone antibiotics can produce tendinitis or tendon rupture.

Night Pain

Intense pain may occur at rest and during the night. At first the pain may occur only when the patient changes position while sleeping; however, as the pain increases, it will disrupt sleep. Report by an adolescent of night pain is a red flag for the intraosseous pain of a bone tumor. Pain in the lower limbs in children 6 to 12 who are in a rapid linear growth period may awaken a child at night. The cause of these "growing pains" is unknown, but they are thought to result from muscle structures that have to catch up with bone growth. They are usually bilateral, and no objective findings are found.

Could the Pain Be Caused by Lyme Disease?

Key Questions

- Have you been camping or spending time in wooded areas?
- Have you noticed any skin rash?

Lyme Disease

Lyme disease is an infection caused by the tick-borne spirochete *Borrelia burgdorferi*. Early symptoms include diffuse arthralgias, myalgias, fever, chills, and a characteristic targetlike rash. Although the arthralgia may involve multiple joints, usually the knee is the affected joint. Joint manifestations occur 1 week to 2 years following the initial illness. Patients may or may not recall the antecedent tick bite or exposure.

What Does the Past Medical History Tell Me?

Key Questions

- Have you had anything like this before?
- Do you have a chronic disease?
- Could you have been exposed to any sexually transmitted infection?
- Have you been treated with cortisone?
- Have you had a recent upper respiratory tract infection?

Chronic diseases, such as sickle cell anemia, inflammatory bowel disease, Crohn's disease, hypothyroidism and hyperthyroidism, or collagen vascular diseases, are frequently associated with skin rashes, psoriasis, and limb and joint pain.

Gonorrhea may disseminate to the musculoskeletal system in 1% to 3% of individuals with the disease. Of these, more than 80% develop arthritis.

Patients with chronic illness that requires long-term administration of corticosteroids are at risk for cortisone-induced necrosis of the hip. Sickle cell anemia can cause hip pain during a sickle cell crisis. Viral infections may cause diffuse myalgia.

Is This a Mixed Condition?

Consider the possibility that a patient may have a condition that is a mix of factors, such as a systemic disorder that has resulted in an acute injury. Clues to mixed etiology might include an injury that seems out of proportion to the extent of the precipitating activity or the presence of a chronic condition or other symptoms that might point to an undetected chronic condition. It is important to evaluate the limb pain in the context of the whole person.

DIAGNOSTIC REASONING: FOCUSED PHYSICAL EXAMINATION

Evaluation of musculoskeletal injuries should include examination of joint stability, deformity, and function. Examination should be done as soon after an injury as possible for an accurate diagnosis. Always observe for symmetry, and then functionally assess limbs and joints bilaterally, beginning with the unaffected side. Order the examination so that the most painful tests will be done last. See Figures 26-1 through 26-4 for anatomical landmarks of the shoulder, elbow, knee, and ankle.

Observe Patient Walking, Removing Coat/Jacket, Getting Into a Sitting Position

Subtle clues of child abuse must be considered when the patient history is not consistent with the type or extent of injury. Abuse should always be considered in an infant within the first year when symptoms and history suggest a fracture, multiple injuries, rotational injuries, or multiple bruises in different states

of healing. Radiographs may show previous fractures.

Persons who have septic joints appear ill, and movement of the joint will increase the pain. Inspect the patient with minimal clothing obstructing your view of movements. A child with a septic hip lies with the thigh in a position of flexion, abduction, and external rotation and cries when a lower limb is moved.

In adults, an internally rotated abducted leg is the posture assumed with a posterior hip dislocation. An externally rotated hip and shortened lower extremity are signs of hip fracture.

General stiffness or limitation of motion of a single joint forces the surrounding joints to accommodate by moving with greater excursion or range of usual movement. This makes the gait appear irregular or jerky.

Look for Limp

Pain, weakness, and deformity cause limping. Limping will be accentuated if the patient is asked to walk on the heels or tiptoes.

Common abnormal gaits related to limping are Trendelenburg gait, antalgic gait, and circumduction gait. Trendelenburg gait is a ducklike gait that reflects unilateral weakness of the gluteus medius muscle. The pelvis drops on the unaffected side during weight bearing on the affected side. In antalgic gait,

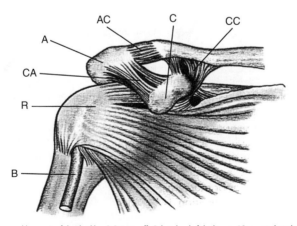

FIGURE 26-1 Bones and ligaments of the shoulder. *R,* Rotator cuff; *B,* long head of the biceps; *AC,* acromioclavicular joint capsule; *CC,* coracoclavicular ligaments; *A,* acromion; *C,* coracoid process; *CA,* coracoacromial ligaments. (From Mercier LR: *Practical orthopedics,* ed 5, St Louis, 2000, Mosby.)

FIGURE 26-2 Bony and ligamentous anatomy of the elbow. *R,* Radial collateral ligament; *O,* orbicular ligament; *B,* biceps insertion; *U,* ulnar collateral ligament; *C,* capitellum; *T,* trochlea. (From Mercier LR: *Practical orthopedics,* ed 5, St Louis, 2000, Mosby.)

there is an acute one-sided limp because the patient takes quick soft steps to shorten the period of weight bearing on the involved extremity. Stance time on the affected limb is decreased while stride length of the opposite side is shortened, allowing a quicker return of weight bearing to the unaffected limb. This is a reflex response to weight bearing on a painful limb.

Circumduction gait is seen with pathology of the foot or ankle and reduces discomfort by limiting movement of the ankle. The gait is characterized by a circular outward swing of the leg and external rotation of the foot that requires less ankle movement. External rotation of the entire extremity is seen with slipped capital femoral epiphysis.

Have the patient stand on one foot, and then the other. When standing on one leg, the gluteus medius on that side maintains the opposite side of the pelvis level, balancing the trunk over the weight-bearing hip. If the hip abductors are weak or painful, the opposite side of the pelvis dips down during the stance phase. With each step, the trunk shifts toward the side of a painful or weak extremity to decrease the force transmitted through the extremity to the hip.

Assessment of gait is best done either before or after examination, when patients are less aware that they are being observed.

FIGURE 26-3 Basic anatomy of the right knee joint. (From Mathers LH et al: *Clinical anatomy principles,* St Louis, 1996, Mosby.)

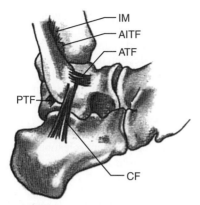

FIGURE 26-4 The lateral ankle ligaments—anterior and posterior talofibular (ATF and PTF, respectively) and calcaneofibular (CF). Also shown are the anterior inferior tibiofibular (AITF) ligament and the beginning of the interosseous membrane (IM). (From Mercier LR: *Practical orthopedics*, ed 5, St Louis, 2000, Mosby.)

Ankle plantar flexion and dorsiflexion are necessary for normal gait. If plantar flexion is restricted, there is no push-off and the forefoot and heel come off the floor at the same time. The result is a higher knee lift and the forefoot may slap against the floor. This condition is seen with weakness from peroneal nerve injury or with painful dorsiflexors associated with shin splints.

Observe the patient walking with and without shoes. If a child walks without difficulty with shoes off, the shoes are probably the problem. Inadequate shoe width is a common source of foot pain in children.

Have Patient Locate the Pain

Have the patient point to the area of pain. Location of pain and actual area of pathology may not be consistent. Hip pain often is referred to the knee area because the anterior branch of the obturator nerve passes close to the hip joint and, if irritated, provides a painful sensation to the medial side of the knee. True hip joint pain arises in the trochanteric bursa and is perceived in the groin area.

Shoulder pain from rotator cuff tendinitis is felt over the lateral aspect of the deltoid.

Swelling of the elbow may compress the ulnar nerve, producing a tingling sensation in the fourth and fifth fingers.

Pain in the groin, lateral hip, or knee in a child may indicate LCPD.

Pain in the groin, buttocks, or lateral hip in a child may indicate slipped femoral capital epiphysis.

Vague, nebulous discomfort in the front of the thighs, in the calves, and behind the knees located outside of the joints in a child may indicate growing pains.

Note Any Deformities

Fractures generally produce unilateral deformities or swelling in the extremities. Inflammatory and degenerative joint disease produce observable joint swelling and deformity that usually occurs bilaterally.

Osteoarthritis typically involves the distal interphalangeal (DIP) and proximal interphalangeal (PIP) joints, spine, hips, knees, and first metatarsophalangeal (MTP) joints. Joints are enlarged with Heberden's (DIP joints) and Bouchard's (PIP joints) nodes.

Joints affected by RA include PIPs, metacarpophalangeal (MCP), wrists, knees, elbows, cervical spine, and MTPs. Joints are swollen with a fusiform-shaped swelling of the PIP joints. Subluxation, ankylosis, and ulnar deviation may be observed as a result of joint destruction from chronic inflammation.

Assess Vital Signs

Elevated temperatures are seen with neoplastic, systemic, and infectious processes such as osteomyelitis, septic arthritis and septic hip in children, and rheumatic disease. Neonates may not exhibit a fever with a septic hip but may refuse to feed and will exhibit other symptoms of septicemia, such as lethargy and subnormal temperature. Palpate for quality and presence of pulses in any injured limb and compare to the opposite side. Assess peripheral pulses for presence, rate, regularity, strength, and equality.

Inspect the Skin and Nails

Inspect the skin for redness and inflammation. Chronic venous obstruction in the lower extremities causes a brownish coloring of the skin. Trophic skin changes from arterial insufficiency cause thin, shiny skin with an absence of hair and brittle nails.

Lyme disease usually presents with a rash before joint involvement; however, rash may occur concurrently. The rash, often characteristically found on the trunk, is an erythematous papule that develops into an annular lesion with a clear center. Concentric rings may develop, giving it a bull's-eye appearance (erythema migrans).

Look for a puncture or an abscess that could be the source of infection and seeding if a septic joint or osteomyelitis is suspected. Swelling and redness in a joint or in the midshaft of the tibia may be caused by osteomyelitis.

Look for an ingrown toenail that may alter gait. When the nails are trimmed by rounding off the edges, the hypertrophied and inflamed soft tissue fold can overlap the nail, and ingrowth at the distal margin will occur. Ingrown toenail is enhanced when tight-fitting shoes compress the soft tissues around the nail.

Look for ecchymosis and bruising. These indicate trauma as a source for pain as well as raise a suspicion of abuse. Ecchymosis indicates underlying bleeding and disruption of soft tissue or bone. Ecchymosis changes color over a period of days. Initially the color is dark red or violet, and in 1 to 3 days the bruise is blue-brown; in 1 week, it is yellow-green; and after 1 week, it is light brown. Ecchymosis resolves within 2 to 4 weeks.

Ecchymosis in the popliteal fossa after dislocation of the knee may be a sign of arterial disruption. Hemarthrosis, or bleeding into a joint, usually occurs within 1 to 2 hours of an injury and can occur secondary to hemophilia or other bleeding disorders, or it can be associated with visible ecchymoses caused by blood leaking into soft tissues.

Swelling and redness of a joint indicate underlying infection or inflammation. Edema will present as an asymmetrical area of swelling. Effusion, or fluid in the joint capsule, always distends the joint in a smooth symmetrical manner.

Observe the muscles around the painful limb area. Decreased muscle tone or atrophy from disuse begins immediately after injury; however, it will not be clinically apparent for approximately 1 week.

Asymmetrical gluteal folds may indicate a congenital dislocated hip (Figure 26-5).

Measure Limb Circumference and Length

Use a tape measure to locate points at which to measure and compare limb circumference. Differences may be the result of muscle atrophy or edema. To measure leg length, have the patient lie supine with legs in comparable positions and measure the distance from the anterior iliac spines to the medial malleoli of the ankles. If a discrepancy is found, ask the patient to lie supine with knees flexed 90 degrees and feet flat on the table. If one knee is higher, the tibia of that extremity is longer. If one knee projects further anteriorly, the femur of that extremity is longer.

Palpate Extremities and Joints

Always palpate those areas that are suspected to be painless first and then compare with the affected limb.

A   **B**

FIGURE 26-5 Ortolani's sign for congenital dislocation of the hip. A "click" is palpable or audible as the hip is reduced by abduction. If the test is negative, the examination should always be repeated in 2 to 4 months. (From Mercier LR: *Practical orthopedics,* ed 5, St Louis, 2000, Mosby.)

Determine if there is edema (e.g., presence of interstitial fluid). Induration is interstitial swelling that has progressed and is now firm. An effusion is a collection of fluid in the joint capsule, which can be the result of rupture of a vascular structure or a synovial secretory response to an inflammatory process. The consistency of the fluid is noteworthy. Pus has a thick consistency and is less fluctuant than synovial fluid. Hematoma has a more gel-like consistency. Swelling in an ankle sprain is diffuse and nonfluctuant. Knee ligament sprain is much more fluctuant. To assess for fluid in the knee joint, press above the knee and watch the concave or shallow areas of the joint become distended and bulge on either side of the kneecap. Note that swelling can extend above and below the point of pathology.

In severe knee trauma, rupture of the capsule allows fluid to escape into surrounding tissues, and less distention may be apparent than with lesser injuries.

Palpate for fluid bulge if the knee is painful. Milk the fluid up into the suprapatellar pouch and then bring the hand down the lateral aspect of the knee looking for a medial fluid bulge. Palpate deeply to detect muscle fibrillation, fasciculation, or tumors.

Feel for heat in the affected joint, which can indicate an inflammatory or infectious process. Evaluate the joint for crepitus, both palpable and auditory. Tendinitis can produce a grating sensation on palpation of the ligament or a grating sound with movement.

Perform Passive/Active Range of Motion of All Limbs

Range of motion (ROM) may be limited because of pain, weakness, or deformity.

If pathology is in the joint, pain will be the same with active and passive motion. If the disease is outside the joint or extraarticular, passive motion may be painless while active motion produces pain. During passive tests, move the joint until an end point or end range is felt to help determine the affected structure and the severity of the injury.

There are six end points to note when assessing joint movement: (1) bone-to-bone sensation, felt with an osteophyte or abnormal bone development; (2) spasm, which can indicate severe ligamentous injury; (3) capsular feel or a firm arrested movement, with some give to it, which can indicate chronic joint effusion, arthritis, or capsular scarring; (4) spring block, or joint rebound at the end of range of movement, caused by an articular derangement or an intraarticular body; (5) tissue approximation, a normal end feel caused by tissue limiting further movement, such as the biceps muscle limiting elbow flexion; and (6) empty end feel, present when there is no tissue resistance, but the patient stops the movement because of pain. This last condition indicates bursitis, extraarticular abscess, or tumor.

Test for Muscle Strength

Test for flexor and extensor strength against resistance of both the proximal and distal muscle groups. Proximal muscle weakness is seen in myopathic disorders. Distal muscle weakness is seen secondary to a neuropathic process. Generally, if the opposite side is normal, strength should be compared to it. A scale of 0 to 5 is used to rate muscle strength (Table 26-1).

In the presence of significant pain, muscle strength may be unreliable. If the contraction is strong and painful, the pathology is caused by mild musculotendinous damage. If the contraction is weak and painful, the pathology is the result of severe musculotendinous damage. If the contraction is weak and painless, the pathology results from a neurological lesion (paresis).

Perform a Neurological Examination

A complete assessment of sensory and motor function and deep tendon reflexes should be done on the affected and contralateral limbs. If systemic illness is suspected, perform a complete neurological examination. A referral is indicated if initial treatment does not adequately control pain, if function loss is progressing, or if the patient is immunocompromised.

Table 26-1	**Muscle Strength Test**		
GRADE	MUSCLE STRENGTH		TERM
0	No palpable contraction		Zero
1	Muscle contracts but part does not move		Trace
2	Muscle moves part but not against gravity		Poor
3	Muscle moves part through range against gravity		Fair
4	Muscle moves part even with resistance		Good
5	Normal strength against resistance present		Excellent

LABORATORY AND DIAGNOSTIC STUDIES

Complete Blood Cell Count

A complete blood cell count (CBC) is obtained to evaluate for anemia associated with chronic disease, infection, or neoplasm. An altered white blood cell (WBC) count may indicate infection or leukemia.

Erythrocyte Sedimentation Rate

An erythrocyte sedimentation rate (ESR) is elevated when inflammation is present. It is a nonspecific test.

Joint Aspiration

Joint aspiration is performed to assess synovial fluid for elevated WBC count, Gram stain, culture and sensitivity, crystal analysis, presence of glucose, and consistency or "string test." This procedure is performed using local anesthesia under sterile technique. Synovial fluid will flow easily when the joint capsule is penetrated.

Radiography

Obtain at least two radiographic views, anteroposterior and lateral, because injuries are not always apparent on a single view. Any evidence of fracture or dislocation will require orthopedic attention. Sometimes radiographic comparisons with the opposite limb may be useful. Traumatic knee injuries should include four radiographic views: anteroposterior, lateral, tunnel (intracondylar notch) view, and a 30-degree sunrise (patella) view. Other diagnostic imaging techniques such as magnetic resonance imaging (MRI), computed tomography (CT), or bone scanning are usually ordered by a specialist. MRI is usually used in spine, joint, and soft tissue imaging. CT scans are usually used for bone visualization.

Antinuclear Antibodies

Antinuclear antibody (ANA) tests are positive with high titers in RA and SLE; however, other conditions, such as aging, medications, and other connective tissue disease, can produce positive antibody titers.

Rheumatoid Factor

Rheumatoid factor (RF) is the single most useful test to confirm a diagnosis of RA and is positive in 80% of patients with this disease.

C4 Complement

C4 complement determines serum hemolytic complement activity, a protein that binds antigen-antibody complexes for the purpose of lysis. Complement is increased in active inflammatory disease and in autoimmune disorders such as juvenile RA.

C-Reactive Protein

C-reactive protein (CRP) indicates the presence of abnormal plasma protein or a nonspecific response to inflammation caused by both infectious and noninfectious processes. CRP is elevated in RA and infection.

Lyme Titer Enzyme-Linked Immunosorbent Assay Serology

Enzyme-linked immunosorbent assay (ELISA) detects antibodies against *B. burgdorferi,* which causes Lyme disease. However, the ELISA may not detect antibodies for several weeks after the onset of infection.

DIFFERENTIAL DIAGNOSIS
Musculoskeletal Inflammation
Tenosynovitis (Tendinitis)

Soft tissue disorders of tendinitis, bursitis, and fibrositis tend to co-occur. Tenosynovitis is a term that refers to inflammation of the tendon and tendon sheath. In an acute inflammation, usually caused by trauma related to recreational or occupational activities, effusion may accumulate and result in swelling; with chronic inflammation, ROM will be limited by fibrosis of the tendon sheath.

The patient's chief complaint will be pain that is worse with movement and swelling around the affected area. Occupational and recreational history will provide vital clues to a traumatic or overuse cause of pain. Persons with arthritis may have tendinitis secondary to joint disease. Crepitus may be felt on palpation of the tendon.

Bursitis

Bursitis is inflammation of a sac lined with synovial fluid, most often secondary to traumatic tenosynovitis of the shoulder, hip, knee, and elbow. Numerous bursae lie over bony prominences and reduce friction from motion of fascial planes. Bursitis is caused by overuse and trauma and may be associated with RA. If isometric contraction of a group of muscles causes pain, the muscles or tendons, or both, may be involved. Bursitis causes an aching pain that radiates to points of tendon insertion or further along the limb. Muscle weakness may also be present. Palpation reveals local tenderness and swelling without full range of joint motion.

Fibrositis (Myofascitis, Fibromyositis)

Fibromyositis is a response to underlying conditions, such as polymyalgia rheumatica, RA, ankylosing spondylitis, hypothyroidism, neuritis, and viral infection, that generate major muscle tension around a large, weight-bearing proximal joint. Fatty and fibrous nodules may be palpable, and painful trigger sites can be located throughout the shoulder and pelvic girdles or lower extremities. Patients complain of stress and anxiety, sleep disturbance, painful trigger points, and joint stiffness.

Osteomyelitis

The presentation of osteomyelitis, a pyogenic infection of bone, depends on the age of the patient as well as the bone involved. This condition should be suspected in any patient who complains of pain in long or flat bones and walks with an antalgic limp. Fever, chills, and vomiting are usually present in acute osteomyelitis but may not occur in the neonate or young infant. Chronic osteomyelitis is characterized by relapse of pain, erythema, swelling, or evidence of purulent discharge. The hallmark is a constant local pain that progressively worsens. The slightest motion of the limb aggravates the pain. The child keeps the limb motionless. Laboratory findings show increased WBCs, ESR, and CRP. Radiographs may show bone destruction or deep soft tissue swelling at the site of infection.

Joint Inflammation
Osteoarthritis

Osteoarthritis (OA) is a degenerative disease of joint cartilage that results in osteophyte (spur) development and synovial inflammation. It is the most common form of arthritis and is present to some extent in all elderly persons. Patients will complain of joint stiffness, pain, and limited movement, most often of the spine (cervical and lumbar), large proximal joints (e.g., knee, hip), and PIP joints. Symptoms may be asymmetrical. Heberden's nodes develop on the DIP joints. Patients at increased risk have a history of performing repetitive weight-lifting tasks, have sustained some form of joint trauma, are obese, or have been diagnosed with diabetes mellitus. Acute arthritis is associated with an increased ESR, and radiographs will show spurs, joint deformity, and erosive changes.

Rheumatoid Arthritis

RA is a systemic polyarthritis with a wide spectrum of clinical presentation. Symptoms of RA include morning stiffness of symmetrical small joints in the hands and feet, swelling, and progressive fatigue. Other symptoms may include fever, weight loss, anorexia, and diaphoresis. Rheumatoid nodules are soft and spongy and appear on the elbows, forearms, and hands. Pericarditis, pleuritis, and vasculitis are associated conditions. Laboratory data may disclose a normochromic, normocytic anemia, an elevated ESR, and a positive rheumatoid factor in 75% to 90% of patients. Radiographs may show bony erosion at the joint margins and joint deformities. Box 26-1 lists criteria for the diagnosis of RA.

Juvenile Rheumatoid Arthritis

Juvenile rheumatoid arthritis (JRA), the most common connective tissue disease in children, presents with fatigue, low-grade fever, weight loss, and failure to grow. Night pain and morning stiffness that improve with activity are common symptoms. Younger children may present with irritability, refusal to walk, or guarding of a joint. The disease may be systemic, affect fewer than four joints (pauciarticular), or affect more than four joints (polyarticular). Laboratory findings show anemia, leukocytosis, and thrombocytosis. Rheumatoid factor and ANA may be negative. ESR is elevated.

Septic Arthritis

Septic arthritis is a sudden pain and inflammation of a single joint, sometimes associated with systemic signs such as fever, malaise, and diaphoresis. The hip is a common site of blood-borne joint infection in neonates, infants, and young children. The presentation depends on the age of the child. A neonate may be afebrile but irritable, refusing to feed and failing to gain weight. In the older child, the onset of pain and fever is acute, and the child refuses to bear weight. ROM of the hip is markedly restricted and very painful.

In adults, migratory joint pain and tenosynovitis may follow 2 to 4 weeks after a mucosal site infection with *Neisseria gonorrhoeae*. Knee, wrist, ankle, and hand joints are most commonly affected. Joint aspiration shows increased WBCs, and culture of fluid or pus may reveal bacterial, tubercular, fungal, syphilitic, and viral organisms. The ESR and CRP are also elevated. With hip involvement, ultrasound shows marked distention of the hip joint, with varying degrees of femoral hip displacement. Septic arthritis is an emergency situation, and treatment must be initiated immediately.

Gout

Gout is a joint inflammation caused by deposits of urate crystals and is associated with an inborn error of uric acid secretion or with metabolic disorders (e.g., hemolytic anemia, renal insufficiency, sarcoidosis). Males older than 30 years and persons with a family history of gout are most often affected. The patient reports a recurrent, sudden onset of pain early in the morning that subsides over several days, especially of the first MTP joint. The joint is warm, tender, and red; tophi—chalky subcutaneous deposits of sodium urate—may be present on extensor surfaces. Gout can be differentiated from pseudogout by the presence of calcium pyrophosphate crystals, involvement of large joints, and secondary osteoarthritis. Laboratory findings during an acute attack show elevated serum uric acid levels, ESR, and

Box 26-1	**Diagnostic Criteria for Rheumatoid Arthritis (Four Criteria Must Be Present)**

Morning stiffness at least 1 hour before improvement for more than 6 weeks
Arthritis of three or more joints for more than 6 weeks
Arthritis of hand joints for more than 6 weeks
Symmetrical arthritis of same joint
Rheumatoid nodules
Positive serum rheumatoid factor
Radiographic changes showing erosions or bony decalcification

Modified from Arnett FC, Edworthy SM, Bloch DA et al: The American Rheumatism Association 1987 revised criteria for the classification of rheumatoid arthritis, *Arthritis Rheum* 31(3):315, 1988.

WBC levels. The joint may be aspirated for fluid to observe uric acid crystals and cultured to exclude septic arthritis.

Musculoskeletal Pain Related to Trauma or Overuse
Shoulder

Dislocation (Glenohumeral Joint Instability). A patient with shoulder dislocation presents with anterior and/or posterior joint pain, periarticular muscle spasm, anxiety, and limited movement. An anterior dislocation causes inability to internally rotate and abduct the humerus. Posterior dislocation causes limitation of external rotation, arm abduction, and hand supination with the shoulder flexed forward. Radiographs of the shoulder (anteroposterior, lateral, and axillary views) will exclude fracture of surrounding bones.

Acromioclavicular Joint Injury. Acromioclavicular joint injuries usually result from sports injuries or motor vehicle accidents. Injury occurs when the acromion, scapula, and upper extremity are driven inferiorly, and the supporting ligamentous structures are sprained or torn. The severity of injury is classified into three grades: partial tear (dislocation) of the acromioclavicular ligament (I); partial tear of the acromioclavicular and coracoclavicular ligaments (II); and complete rupture of the acromioclavicular and coracoclavicular ligaments and joint separation (III). History will reveal the nature of the injury. The patient will have pain and limited shoulder movement and may present with obvious deformity if there is a severe injury.

Bicipital Tendinitis. Bicipital tendinitis is an overuse syndrome of the biceps brachii muscle that ends in two tendons—one attached to the radial tuberosity (arm adduction) and one to the forearm fascia (arm abduction and internal rotation). The syndrome may be associated with other shoulder disorders, such as impingement syndrome. Children may have anomalies of the intertubercular groove, and younger individuals report repeated trauma from swimming, volleyball, baseball, or golf. Pain is localized to the intertubercular

groove, is aggravated by the offending movement, and subsides with rest. Yergason's test can indicate bicipital tendinitis. A positive test is characterized by pain in the intertubercular groove with resistance to supination of the forearm while the elbow is flexed 90 degrees. A Fisk radiographic view enables the examiner to determine the size of the intertubercular groove.

Rotator Cuff Tear. Rotator cuff tears are acute injuries in children and young adults but occur as chronic injuries in older adults. In acute tears, the shoulder pain is severe, and the patient is unable to raise the arm sideways because of pain. In a complete tear, attempts to raise the arm laterally will produce a shoulder shrug. In a partial tear, the patient can raise the arm but cannot maintain the position with any resistance. Inflammation secondary to injury can cause rotator cuff tendinitis that produces shoulder pain, weakness, and a grating sound with movement.

Chronic rotator cuff tears are most common in persons older than 50 years, the result of cumulative and repeated impingement processes. The onset of pain is insidious and is made worse with the arm in an overhead position. Patients experience shoulder pain with sleep and tenderness over the acromioclavicular joint. Examination may reveal minimal restriction in movement, crepitus, and weakness in external rotation of the shoulder. Radiographs will show any bony abnormality such as an acromial spur.

Elbow

Olecranon Bursitis. Olecranon bursitis is commonly seen in patients who engage in contact sports, repetitive motion, rubbing or pressure to the elbow, or overuse. Pain is localized over the bursae, and swelling may be the result of hemorrhage in a traumatic injury. Range of joint motion is usually normal. The joint may be warm and red. When these signs are present, carefully examine the skin over the elbow to ensure intactness, because a penetrating injury may cause a septic bursitis. Radiography will exclude underlying bone infection and show the plane of soft tissue swelling.

Lateral Humeral Epicondylitis (Tennis Elbow). Epicondylitis is an aseptic inflammation of the bone-tendon junction, resulting from repetitive concentric contractions that transmit force via the muscles to the origin on the lateral epicondyle. Persons most at risk for tennis elbow are the nonathletes who have occupations that require repeated contractions of extensor and supinator muscles. Athletes at risk are tennis players, bowlers, and hockey players. Patients present with gradual onset of pain and tenderness over the lateral epicondyle that progresses in intensity. Palpation over the lateral epicondyle produces point tenderness, although elbow movement is not limited. Resisted forearm supination with the elbow flexed at 90 degrees will intensify symptoms.

Subluxation of the Radial Head (Nurse-Maid's Elbow). Subluxation of the radial head is caused by a rapid upward pulling of the child's hand or wrist. The radial head is pulled out of the annular ligament. This ligament then becomes caught between the radial head and the joint, causing the elbow to be flexed and pronated. The child cries at the event and then refuses to move the arm and may complain of pain in the elbow. Radiographs are normal.

Wrist and Hand

Wrist Fracture. Wrist fractures usually are the result of falling on an outstretched hand and may involve a number of types of fracture. Patients present with a painful, swollen distal forearm and wrist and may complain of numbness if the median nerve is involved. Gently palpate to locate the site of maximal pain, particularly the navicular ("snuffbox") area located between the extensor pollicis longus and the extensor pollicis brevis tendons when the mechanism of injury is hyperextension of the wrist. Pain localized here indicates a scaphoid (navicular) fracture. Assess pulses, pain sensation, and motor function (range and strength). Radiographic views (posteroanterior, lateral, and oblique) will reveal the bone involved. In a Colles' fracture, the distal radius is displaced

dorsally and shows up as a "silver fork" deformity on lateral view radiographs.

Finger Fracture. The most common fractures of the fingers are those of the metacarpals and phalanges, commonly seen in sports injuries. Older persons usually sustain fractures as a result of falls. Correct diagnosis of a fractured finger is important in preventing long-term disability of use. Patients will present with a history of trauma or injury. Physical examination includes assessment of vascular and neurological function, tenderness and swelling, ROM of each joint, and signs of joint instability or deformity. Three radiographic views (posteroanterior, lateral, and oblique) are needed for a complete evaluation.

Ganglion. Ganglions are cysts that contain a gelatinous fluid formed by outpouching of a joint capsule or tendon sheath. They most often occur on the dorsum of the wrist. A ganglion can be distinguished from a tumor by its soft consistency and transillumination.

Hip

Slipped Capital Femoral Epiphysis. In children undergoing a rapid growth spurt, the onset of knee pain, an antalgic limp, and leg weakness may indicate a slipped capital femoral epihysis (SCFE). Pain may be of several weeks' or months' duration and is exaggerated by strenuous physical activity. Examine the child in a prone position and assess the symmetry of medial rotation of the hip. A reduction of medial rotation may indicate SCFE. A widening of the epiphyseal plate can be visualized in a lateral view radiograph.

Transient Synovitis of the Hip. A nonspecific inflammatory condition of the hip, transient synovitis is the most common cause of a painful hip in children younger than 10 years. History may reveal a recent upper respiratory tract infection or minor injury. The child complains of pain in the anteromedial aspect of the thigh and knee and walks with an antalgic limp; there is tenderness on palpation over the anterior aspect of the hip joint. Movement of the hip causes pain and is limited. There may be a low-grade fever. Ultrasound should be used for diagnosis, comparing it with the good hip. WBC count is usually normal, although the ESR may be elevated.

Legg-Calvé-Perthes Disease. This disease occurs as osteochondritis of the femoral head epiphysis and is characterized by a period of avascular necrosis of the femoral head, followed by revascularization and bone healing. It occurs most commonly in boys between the ages of 3 and 11 years. The child has groin or medial thigh pain and a limp. The pain may be recurring, and the child may have been limping for several months. The loss of medial hip motion is an early sign. There is a high incidence of hernia, undescended testicles, and kidney abnormalities in children with this condition. Radiographs show the ossific nucleus of the femoral head combined with the widened articular cartilage space compared with the opposite hip.

Iliopsoas Tendinitis. This tendinitis is caused by frequent repetitive flexions of the hip joint and is common in weight lifters, oarsmen, and football players. The patient complains of mildly intense groin pain on the anterior hip, which worsens with movement. An acute injury involves forced extension of a flexed leg, and in younger age-groups, radiographic evaluation is done if evulsion of the epiphysis is suspected. Test for iliopsoas tendinitis by having the seated patient place the heel of the affected leg on the knee of the other leg. This movement will create pain and a tense iliopsoas muscle.

Knee
Chondromalacia Patellae. Chondromalacia of the patella is a change in the patellofemoral joint cartilage, which most often occurs in adolescent females. The condition can be caused by trauma, anatomical anomalies, and misalignment of the patella. Softening of joint cartilage, tufts of patellar cartilage, fissures, or ulcers occur. Patients present with anterior knee pain that is worse while climbing stairs or biking. Radiographic

studies of the knee, including tangential and sunrise views, show irregularities of the patellofemoral joint.

Patellar Tendinitis (Jumper's Knee). This overuse syndrome is characterized by inflammation in the distal extensors of the knee joint. Patellar tendinitis is more common in athletes who habitually place excessive strain on their knees from jumping or running. Determine the quadriceps (Q) angle by measuring the angle between the center of the patella to the anterior superior iliac spine and from the center patella to the tibial tubercle. An angle greater than 10 degrees in males and 15 degrees in females suggests patellar tendinitis. Persons affected complain of dull, achy knee pain that may have associated clicking or popping. Associated malalignment from femoral anteversion or ankle varus may be present.

Medial Collateral Ligament Sprain. Medial collateral ligament injuries are common and are the result of valgus stress to the knee. The patient limps soon after the injury and may or may not have pain. On physical examination, there is mild effusion and point tenderness over the medial collateral ligament. To test for stability of the medial collateral ligaments, the knee is flexed about 30 degrees with the patient supine, and one hand is placed over the lateral knee with the other around the ankle. Apply medial pressure to the knee while pulling the ankle outward. An instability of the medial collateral ligament produces a sensation of opening the medial aspect of the joint. Applying lateral pressure in the same knee position tests for lateral ligament sprain. A radiograph is obtained to rule out fracture.

Medial Meniscus Tear. Medial meniscus injuries, more common than lateral meniscus injuries, occur after a twisting injury to the knee. The patient has pain, difficulty flexing the knee, and difficulty bearing weight. There often is a clicking or catching in the knee joint, and the joint may be swollen and tender. To examine for medial meniscus injury, perform the McMurray test to assess for clicking, locking, or a springy end point of motion. With the patient supine, place one hand under the heel and flex the knee 90 degrees with slight abduction. Apply a lateral and medial force to the knee while extending and adducting it. A palpable or audible click indicates medial meniscus injury.

Anterior Cruciate Ligament Tear. Ligaments may be stretched or torn if the knee is twisted or hyperextended. The ACL, located in the center of the knee, is one of the most common ligaments damaged in knee injuries. An ACL injury is often associated with an audible pop and a giving-way sensation in the knee, often with swelling from hemarthrosis. Physical examination reveals a positive Lachman's test. With the patient supine and the knee flexed 20 to 30 degrees, anchor the patient's foot to the table; then pull the tibia forward. Anterior motion is a sensitive test for ACL laxity.

Osgood-Schlatter Disease. This condition, most common in adolescent males, is a painful swelling of the anterior aspect of the tibial tubercle. It is caused by strenuous activity, especially of the quadriceps muscles. The patient will often limp, and the pain will be worse with activities such as stair climbing and kneeling. Examination will reveal a warm, swollen, tender tibial tubercle, and flexion and extension will increase pain intensity. Joint examination of the knee is normal.

Baker's Cyst (Popliteal Cyst). A popliteal cyst occurs when fluid from the knee joint enters the connecting bursa and becomes trapped. Patients complain of a fullness or swelling of the posterior knee and calf pain aggravated by walking and alleviated by rest. Examination of the knee focuses on assessment of a change in consistency of the mass on extension (hardening) and flexion (softening), called Foucher's sign. Foucher's sign is negative with a Baker's cyst and positive with a tumor or popliteal aneurysm. The cyst can rupture and cause edema and tenderness of the lower extremity with a positive Homans' sign. Ultrasound will detect the cyst or recently ruptured cyst.

Ankle and Foot

Ankle Sprain (Inversion or Eversion). The most common mechanism of ankle injury is an inversion force that stresses the lateral ligamentous support of the joint. The lateral ligaments are of greater length than the medial ligaments and are more predisposed to injury. An audible pop or tear implies a rupture or tear of the ligament. Swelling of the ankle within minutes of injury indicates bleeding and soft tissue trauma. Patients with a ligamentous injury will generally be able to walk and bear weight on the injured foot, even though it may be uncomfortable. Examine the injured joint by palpating the course and attachment points of the ligaments and perform joint ROM to test for ligamentous integrity.

Shin Splints (Medial Tibial Stress Syndrome). Shin splints are an inflammation of the origin of muscles on the shaft of the tibia caused by overuse, often by running athletes. Patients report achy pain and tenderness over the medial tibia that increases with exercise, especially running, and improves with rest. A radiograph of the tibia will exclude fracture.

Achilles Tendinitis. The gastrocnemius and soleus muscles conjoin to form the Achilles tendon. Inflammation of this tendon creates pain and swelling where the tendon inserts into the calcaneus, and a patient will report a tightness of the tendon that makes walking or running difficult. Tendinitis may be caused by overuse, especially running, or by decreased vascularity to the tendon sheath. Examination reveals tenderness over the Achilles tendon with palpation and ankle ROM, especially with dorsiflexion, crepitus over the tendon with motion, and weakness of the calf muscles.

Plantar Faciitis. Plantar faciitis, which affects women twice as often as men, is caused by chronic weight-bearing stress when laxity of foot structures allows the talus to slide forward and medially, the calcaneus to drop, and plantar ligaments and fascia to stretch. Persons who are obese or who engage in excessive standing are at greatest risk. Pain is worse on awakening and is relieved with non–weight-bearing activity. Tendons and joints become inflamed, and muscles spasm because of the misalignment of structures. Patients often complain of heel pain.

Muscle Pain (Myalgia)
Viral Infections
Viral infections can produce diffuse myalgias that are usually associated with fever, chills, upper respiratory tract symptoms, and malaise. A patient with influenza will have intense myalgia and high fever, and appear quite ill. Since viral illnesses are highly contagious, epidemics in both children and adults in a community may be a useful clue to diagnosis. A paraviral IgM titer is diagnostic of an acute parvovirus B19 infection.

Psychogenic
Pain that is diffuse, varies in pattern, and is unaffected by activity or rest may be psychogenic in origin. A careful history may reveal any secondary gain the patient may derive from the pain and suggest the presence of an anxiety or depression disorder. On examination, the patient may display facial expressions and descriptions of discomfort to palpation and movement that are inconsistent. This diagnosis involves excluding other causes.

Fibromyalgia
Fibromyalgia is a syndrome characterized by chronic fatigue, generalized musculoskeletal pain, and multiple trigger points of pain on physical examination. It affects primarily women between 20 and 50 years of age. Other symptoms associated with this syndrome include stage IV sleep disturbance, anxiety or depression, obsessive-compulsive behavior, and irritable bowel syndrome. Symptoms are exacerbated by stress. Physical examination shows focal tenderness without signs of synovitis.

Systemic Disorders
Acute Leukemia
Leukemia is the most common cancer in children, and bone and joint pain is the most common presenting complaint. The bone pain is diffuse and nonspecific, and may extend to adjacent joints. Laboratory findings may show the WBC count as elevated, depressed, or normal. Severe anemia is common as is a depressed platelet count. Radiographs of the limb at the distal end of the femur and the proximal end of the tibia show abnormal areas of radiolucency.

Sickle Cell Disease
Sickle cell disease is a genetic disorder characterized by production of hemoglobin S, an anemia secondary to short erythrocyte survival, and sickle-shaped erythrocytes. It affects mainly African American, Mediterranean, and Southeast Asian population groups. Sickle cell disease manifests itself after the first 6 months of life. The child presents with painful or vaso-occlusive crises characterized by symmetrical, painful swelling of the hands and feet. Older persons report pain in long bones and joints, abdominal pain, decreased appetite, fever, and malaise. The laboratory findings reveal a hemoglobin S genotype and anemia, but findings can vary depending on the hemoglobin genotype, age, gender, and presence of other organ involvement.

Systemic Lupus Erythematosus
SLE is a systemic inflammatory condition that occurs most often in women. It is characterized by arthritis that commonly involves the small joints of the hands, wrists, ankles, and knees, as well as malar rash, oral ulcers, glomerulonephritis, hematological disorders, and psychological symptoms. The pain is transient but severe. Laboratory findings show leukopenia with neutrophils predominating the peripheral count, and the ANA is positive.

Lyme Arthritis
The bite of the deer tick transmits the spirochete *B. burgdorferi*. Patients may not recall a tick bite but will have been in an endemic area. The presenting complaints in Lyme disease are diffuse joint pain and swelling, a targetlike skin rash (erythema migrans), fever, and chills. These symptoms may be present for weeks before the spirochete spreads via blood and lymph tissue to the myocardium and central nervous system. A chronic arthritis may appear months after the initial infection. The arthritis is asymmetrical and occurs in the

large joints. The knee is a commonly affected joint. The patient has an antalgic limp with diffuse swelling and warmth of the knee joint anteriorly as well as local synovial thickening. Laboratory diagnosis reveals elevation of immunoglobulin M (IgM) titers and IgG antibodies against the spirochete. The ESR is elevated.

Neuroblastoma

Neuroblastoma is a malignant tumor that usually occurs in children under 5 years of age. It originates from cells in the sympathetic ganglia and adrenal medulla but can arise from any part of the sympathetic nervous system and metastasize to the bone. The presenting complaint may be varied, but bone pain, limp, pallor, and fatigue may be present. CT or MRI is used to identify the primary location of the tumor. In the urine, 3-methoxy-4-hydroxymandelic acid and homovanillic acid levels are elevated.

Osteogenic Sarcoma

Osteogenic sarcoma is a tumor that occurs in persons 10 to 25 years old, with the most common site being the distal femur or the proximal tibia. The patient initially complains of local intermittent pain that quickly progresses to a constant and severe pain, and an antalgic limp may develop. Palpation reveals tenderness over the area affected. Laboratory findings show an increase in serum alkaline phosphatase level; radiograph shows a "sunburst" image.

Nerve Entrapment Syndromes
Thoracic Outlet Syndrome

Thoracic outlet syndrome is the result of compression of nerve and vascular structures in the neck area. Arterial compression creates pallor and decreased pulses and weakness, with eventual skin and nail atrophy in the affected extremity. Nerve compression creates paresthesias, dysesthesias, and pain. History may disclose that the patient sleeps with the arm extended against the head, causing morning symptoms of pain and paresthesias. Reaching, working with the arm raised, and lifting exacerbate pain. Other risk factors include a rounded, sagging shoulder posture

and shoulder muscle deformities. A common compression occurs with the cervical rib compressing the subclavian artery. A bruit may be heard over the supraclavicular fossa. Electromyographic studies help to delineate the specific nerve involvement; however, they may not identify the vascular involvement.

Carpal Tunnel Syndrome

Carpal tunnel syndrome involves entrapment of the median nerve in the dominant hand, resulting from repeated strain that causes thickening of the flexor tendon sheath. A dull, achy pain is felt across the wrist and forearm with paresthesia, weakness, or clumsiness of the hand; atrophy; dry skin; and skin color changes of the hand secondary to impaired nerve innervation. Symptoms are often worse at night. History reveals repetitive activity of the upper extremity. Carpal tunnel syndrome most often occurs in women and in persons older than 30 years. Examination discloses dry skin on the thumb, index finger, and middle finger (median nerve distribution). Thenar atrophy may be present. Tinel's sign and Phalen's test are positive (Table 26-2).

Peroneal Nerve Compression

Peroneal nerve compression can be caused by a cast, sports injury, or trauma. Pain is felt across the head of the fibula and can result in footdrop.

Tarsal Tunnel Syndrome

The posterior tibial nerve is involved, and pain is felt across the ankle and proximal foot. Tarsal tunnel syndrome is occasionally associated with motor weakness of the proximal toe flexors. Patients may not remember a specific onset but report pain and weakness of the foot muscles. Tapping the posterior tibial nerve posterior and inferior to the medial malleolus elicits pain. Ask the patient about shoe fit and use of any orthotic devices.

Neuritis

Vascular metabolism affected by systemic disorders such as diabetes mellitus can cause a nerve to become ischemic, producing toxins that can directly damage the nerve. Inflammation can be of the nerve axon, myelin sheath,

Table 26-2	Selected Tests Used to Assess for Musculoskeletal Disorders	

TEST	DESCRIPTION	FINDINGS
Shoulder		
Yergason's test	Patient supinates forearm against resistance.	A positive test produces pain in bicipital groove and is suggestive of bicipital tendinitis.
Rotator cuff tear	Ask patient to externally rotate and abduct shoulder.	In a partial tear, patient can raise arm but cannot maintain position against resistance; in a complete tear, attempts to abduct arm will produce a shoulder shrug.
Elbow		
Tennis elbow	Have patient resist forearm supination with elbow flexed 90 degrees.	Pain with this movement indicates lateral humeral epicondylitis.
Wrist		
Finkelstein's test	Have patient flex fingers over a clenched thumb; then passively deviate wrist ulnarly.	Movement produces pain in de Quervain's disease (first dorsal compartment tenosynovitis).
Tinel's sign	Tap over median nerve (palmar surface of wrist) to assess for compression neuropathy.	In a positive test, patient reports a tingling or prickling sensation distal to site tapped along first three digits, wrist pain, and weak grip.
Phalen's test	Ask patient to maintain palmar flexion for 1 minute with dorsal surfaces of each hand pressed together.	Test is positive if maneuver produces numbness and paresthesia in fingers innervated by median nerve.
Leg/Hip		
Iliopsoas	Have seated patient place heel of affected leg on knee of other leg.	Pain with this movement indicates muscle iliopsoas tendinitis.
Knee		
Foucher's sign	Look for change in consistency of a mass in popliteal fossa that hardens with extension and softens with flexion.	A positive sign indicates a popliteal tumor or aneurysm; a negative sign indicates a Baker's cyst.
Bulge sign	Apply lateral pressure to area adjacent to patella.	Medial bulge will appear if fluid is in knee joint.
Drawer sign	With patient supine, flex knee 90 degrees and hip 45 degrees with foot on table; apply slow, steady anterior pull, and in same position gently push tibia back.	Tests for cruciate ligament stability; abnormal anterior or posterior movement of tibia on femur is a positive drawer sign and indicates ligamentous instability.
McMurray's maneuver	With patient supine, maximally flex knee and hip; externally and internally rotate tibia with one hand on distal end of tibia; with other hand, palpate joint.	Pain and a palpable or audible click are positive findings and indicate a meniscus injury.
	Extend knee with slight lateral pressure with tibia internally rotated.	Positive finding in this position indicates a lateral meniscus injury.
	Extend knee with slight internal pressure on tibia externally rotated.	Positive finding in this position indicates a medial meniscus injury.
Collateral ligament test	Apply medial or lateral pressure when knee is flexed 30 degrees and when it is extended.	Medial or lateral collateral ligament sprain will show laxity in movement and no solid end points, depending on degree of sprain.
Lachman's test (cruciate ligaments)	With knee flexed 30 degrees, pull tibia forward with one hand while other hand stabilizes femur.	Positive test is a mushy or soft end feel when tibia is moved forward, indicating damage to anterior cruciate ligament.

or both. Soft tissue inflammation contributing to neuropathy can be caused by collagen disorders (e.g., SLE, scleroderma).

Diabetes mellitus is commonly associated with sensory peripheral neuropathy and results in pain and sensory loss that is more intense in the lower extremities.

Alcoholism is associated with distal, demyelinating neuropathy that may resolve with cessation of alcohol ingestion.

DIFFERENTIAL DIAGNOSIS OF *Common Causes of Limb Pain*

CONDITION	HISTORY	PHYSICAL FINDINGS	DIAGNOSTIC STUDIES
Musculoskeletal Inflammation			
Tenosynovitis (tendinitis)	Repetitive trauma activities; pain with movement	Swelling over tendon, crepitus	None
Bursitis	History of overuse; aching pain over affected bursae that radiates along limb	Local tenderness, swelling; limited joint motion; muscle weakness	None
Fibrositis	Pain in trigger sites throughout body, joint stiffness, disturbed sleep	Fatty, fibrous nodules in muscles; palpation of trigger points elicits pain	None
Osteomyelitis	Presentation depends on age, location of infection; history of infection, trauma, penetration, invasive procedure; refusal to bear weight (hip); constant pain	Fever, chills, vomiting; pain localized over affected area but progressively worsens; soft tissue injury or abscess	Increased WBCs, ESR, C-reactive protein; radiographs
Joint Inflammation			
Osteoarthritis	Older adults; asymmetrical joint pain and stiffness that improves throughout day; history of repetitive joint trauma; obesity	DIP, PIP joints enlarged; Heberden's nodes; limited cervical spine ROM	ESR; radiograph may reveal osteophytes, loss of joint space
Rheumatoid arthritis	Morning stiffness of small joints; symmetrical involvement; anorexia, weight loss	Fever, rheumatoid nodules, ulnar deviation of wrists	Increased ESR, positive rheumatoid factor, anemia on CBC; radiograph shows bony erosion
Juvenile rheumatoid arthritis	Fatigue, weight loss, failure to thrive, refusal to walk, joint pain and stiffness	Fever, rash, guarding of joints, limited ROM; joint swelling, nodules	Elevated WBCs, ESR; positive rheumatoid factor and antinuclear antibody
Septic arthritis	History of systemic infection, malaise, diaphoresis, refusal to bear weight (hip), acute joint pain	Fever; red, swollen joint; limited range of motion	WBCs, culture of joint aspirate, ESR, C-reactive protein, ultrasound of joint
Gout	Acute pain of large joint, asymmetrical; males over 30 years, history of gout	Inflamed, swollen joint; tophi; sodium urate crystals	Increased serum uric acid level, ESR, WBCs
Musculoskeletal Pain Related to Trauma or Overuse			
Shoulder dislocation	History of trauma, pain	Limited rotation, arm abduction, and hand supination	Radiograph of shoulder
Acromioclavicular joint injury	History of trauma, pain	Limited shoulder movement; obvious deformity	Radiograph of shoulder
Bicipital tendinitis	History of overuse of biceps; pain worse with movement	Positive Yergason's test; pain localized over intertubercular groove	Radiograph (Fisk view)

DIFFERENTIAL DIAGNOSIS OF *Common Causes of Limb Pain—cont'd*

CONDITION	HISTORY	PHYSICAL FINDINGS	DIAGNOSTIC STUDIES
Rotator cuff tear	Acute: younger persons, history of trauma, severe pain; chronic: older, pain worse with overhead movement, sleep disturbance	Acute: inability to raise arm laterally, shrug shoulders; chronic: tenderness over AC joint, crepitus, weakness in external shoulder rotation	Radiograph may reveal humeral displacement or spurs
Olecranon bursitis	Repetitive motion of or pressure to elbow; localized pain	Warmth, redness, and swelling over joint; full ROM	Radiograph to rule out fracture of olecranon process
Lateral humeral epicondylitis	History of repetitive contraction of extensor and supinator muscles; pain over lateral epicondyle that progresses	Tenderness over lateral epicondyle; palpation produces pain, motion does not; supination against resistance worsens pain	None
Subluxation of radial head	Occurs in children; pain in elbow or arm	Affected arm is flexed; child cries when attempts are made to move joint	Radiograph of elbow
Wrist fracture	History of fall on an outstretched hand; pain and swelling of forearm and wrist	Palpation of snuffbox increases pain; observe for joint deformity	Three-view radiographs to determine scaphoid or Colles' fracture
Finger fracture	History of trauma or fall, joint tenderness	Joint swelling, instability	Three-view radiographs (PA, lateral, and oblique)
Ganglion	Noticeable lump on dorsal surface of wrist	Gelatinous filled nodule, soft, transilluminates	None
Slipped capital femoral epiphysis	Children: during rapid growth spurts; knee pain worse with activity	Limitation of medial hip rotation, limp	Radiograph of epiphyseal plate
Transient synovitis of hip	Children less than 10 yr; history of upper respiratory tract infection; limp, pain in anteromedial thigh and knee	Tenderness on palpation over anterior hip; hip movement increases pain and is limited; low-grade fever	Ultrasound, ESR
Legg-Calvé-Perthes disease	Boys 3-11 yr; groin or medial thigh pain, limp	Decreased hip ROM	AP and frog lateral radiographs of hip; LCPD may show increased density of femoral head
Iliopsoas tendinitis	History of repetitive flexion of hip; pain worse with movement	With patient sitting, place heel of affected leg on knee of other; test is positive if pain is elicited	None
Chondromalacia patellae	Adolescent females; history of knee trauma or misalignment, knee pain worse with activity	Tenderness to palpation over knee	Four-view radiographs of knees to rule out arthritis
Patellar tendinitis	History of overuse, especially running or jumping; dull, achy knee pain; click	Q angle >10 degrees in males, 15 degrees in females; clicking or popping with knee movement	None
Medial collateral ligament sprain	History of valgus stress to knee; limp; pain	Effusion and point tenderness over knee; valgus and varus pressure to assess instability	AP and lateral radiographs may reveal a ligament avulsion of femoral origin
Medial meniscus tear	History of twisting injury to the knee, pain, difficulty flexing, bearing weight, clicking or catching of knee with movement	Positive McMurray's test, clicking or locking during joint movement	Four-knee view radiographs to rule out bony abnormality

DIFFERENTIAL DIAGNOSIS OF *Common Causes of Limb Pain—cont'd*

CONDITION	HISTORY	PHYSICAL FINDINGS	DIAGNOSTIC STUDIES
Anterior cruciate ligament tear	History of twisting or extension knee injury; audible "pop"	Swelling; positive Lachman's test	Radiograph to rule out fracture
Osgood-Schlatter disease	Adolescent males; knee pain and swelling aggravated by activity, limp	Tenderness, warmth, swelling over anterior tibial tubercle	Radiograph with knee rotated inward may show soft tissue swelling
Baker's cyst	Fullness or swelling of posterior knee, aggravated by walking	Negative Foucher's sign; normal joint examination; positive Homans' sign in ruptured cyst	None
Ankle sprain	History of inversion stress with audible "pop," immediate swelling	Swelling, soft tissue trauma, able to perform active ROM with ligament sprain	Radiograph needed only with tenderness over the lateral malleolus to rule out fracture
Shin splints	Ache or pain over medial tibia that is worse with exercise, history of running	Tenderness over medial tibia	AP and lateral radiographs may show a stress fracture; a bone scan will be positive with increased uptake along the medial tibia
Achilles tendinitis	Pain and tightness over Achilles tendon, especially with walking or running	Tenderness over Achilles tendon; pain worse with dorsiflexion of ankle; calf weakness	Lateral ankle radiograph reveals enlarged posterosuperior tuberosity of the calcaneus
Plantar fasciitis	History of chronic weight bearing; aching feet, muscle spasms, obesity	Misalignment of foot structures, especially talus, calcaneus, and plantar ligaments	None
Muscle Pain (Myalgia)			
Viral infections	History of upper respiratory tract infection; malaise, chills, cold symptoms, general muscle aches	Fever, ill-appearing adult or child	Viral serum titer
Psychogenic	Pain is diffuse; varies in pattern of activity, setting; history of depression or anxiety	Normal examination or patient response to examination maneuvers disproportionate to physical findings or subjective complaints	None
Fibromyalgia	Female 20-50 yr; history of depression, sleep disturbance, chronic fatigue, general muscle and joint aches	Palpation of trigger points will produce pain; normal physical examination	None
Systemic Disorders			
Acute leukemia	Hip pain in children, refusal to walk	Fever, hepatosplenomegaly, bruising	CBC
Sickle cell disease	African American, family history; appears after 6 mo of age; acute pain with swelling of hands and feet, abdominal pain, decreased appetite, malaise	Normal examination	Hemoglobin S genotype
Systemic lupus erythematosus	Female; transient arthritis of small joints, malar rash	Normal examination may have joint tenderness on palpation	Kidney function tests, antinuclear antibody, CBC

DIFFERENTIAL DIAGNOSIS OF *Common Causes of Limb Pain—cont'd*

CONDITION	HISTORY	PHYSICAL FINDINGS	DIAGNOSTIC STUDIES
Lyme arthritis	History of exposure to endemic areas of deer tick; chills, diffuse joint pain and swelling; often knee is affected	Asymmetrical swelling, warmth of joint; erythema migrans; may have myocardial involvement	Serum IgM and IgG antibodies, ESR
Neuroblastoma	Under 5 yr; pain in bones	Unexplained fever	Urine for vanillylmandelic or homovanillic acid; CT scan
Osteogenic sarcoma	Persons 10-25 yr; intermittent pain of lower femur, upper tibia; limp	Tenderness over affected area	Radiograph, serum alkaline phosphatase
Nerve Entrapment Syndromes			
Thoracic outlet syndrome	History of sleeping with arm against head; morning shoulder pain; pain worse with lifting; paresthesia, weakness, or clumsiness of hand; symptoms worse at night	Bruit over supraclavicular fossa; pallor, decreased pulses of upper extremity, weakness, skin and nail atrophy	None
Carpal tunnel syndrome	History of repetitive upper extremity motion; paresthesia, weakness, or clumsiness of hand; symptoms worse at night	Positive Phalen's and Tinel's signs; weakness of hand; dry skin over distribution of median nerve	None
Peroneal compression	History of pressure to knee from a cast, sports injury, or trauma; pain over head of fibula; clumsy gait	Unilateral footdrop	None
Tarsal tunnel syndrome	Pain in ankle and proximal foot; weakness of toe flexors; ill-fitting shoes	Tapping posterior tibial nerve elicits pain	None
Neuritis	Pain and sensory loss, usually of lower extremities; history of alcohol ingestion, diabetes	Decreased sensory and pain sensation	Liver function tests, hemoglobin A_{1c} to rule out diabetes

CHAPTER RESOURCES

Fagan H: Approach to the patient with acute swollen/painful joint, *Clin Fam Pract* 7:305, 2005.

Garbez R, Puntillo K: Acute musculoskeletal pain in the emergency department: a review of the literature and implications for the advanced practice nurse, *AACN Clin Issues* 16:310, 2005.

Goolsby MJ: Evaluating acute musculoskeletal complaints, *J Acad Nurs Pract* 13:193, 2001.

Goroll AH, Mulley AG: *Primary care medicine*, ed 5, Philadelphia, 2006, Lippincott Williams & Wilkins.

Gutierrez K: Bone and joint infections in children, *Ped Clin North Am* 52:779, 2005.

Leet AI: Evaluation of the acutely limping child, *Am Fam Physician* 61:1011, 2000.

Leung A, LeMary F: The limping child, *J Pediatr Health Care* 18:219, 2004.

Roberts DM: Emergency department evaluation and treatment of knee and leg injuries, *Emerg Med Clin North Am* 18:67, 2000.

Solomon DH, Simel DL, Bates DW et al: The rational clinical examination. Does this patient have a torn meniscus or ligament of the knee? Value of the physical examination, *JAMA* 286:1610, 2001.

Acute Low Back Pain

A report of acute low back pain (ALBP), although quite common, requires a thorough evaluation. The underlying pathophysiology of back pain is frequently multifactorial and includes both physiological and psychological components. The most common causes of ALBP relate to musculo-ligamentous injuries and age-related degenerative processes. About 90% of ALBP episodes in adults are related to mechanical causes that resolve within 4 weeks without serious sequelae. A smaller percentage of patients will continue to have chronic symptoms without organic pathology or will have underlying disease.

In children, the prevalence of back pain increases with age and with involvement in sports. Anthropometric variations in children place them at risk for excess strain on the spine, producing back pain. These variations include reduced hip mobility, decreased lumbar extension and increased lumbar flexion, poor abdominal muscle strength, tight hamstring muscles, and lumbar hyperlordosis.

ALBP is defined as activity intolerance producing lower back or back-related leg symptoms of less than 3 months' duration. The Agency for Health Care Policy and Research (AHCPR), now the Agency for Healthcare Research and Quality (AHRQ), guidelines provide the following framework for causes of ALBP:

- Potentially serious conditions (e.g., spinal fracture, tumor or infection, or cauda equina syndrome)
- Sciatica, or leg pain and numbness of the lateral thigh, leg, and foot, suggesting nerve root compression (Figure 27-1)
- Nonspecific back problems such as musculoskeletal strain, diskogenic pain, or bony deformity secondary to inflammatory disease
- Nonspinal causes secondary to abdominal involvement (e.g., gallbladder, liver, renal, pelvic inflammatory disease; prostate tumor; ovarian cyst; uterine fibroids; aortic aneurysm; or thoracic disease)
- Psychological causes such as stress, work environment (e.g., disability, Worker's Compensation, secondary gains)

When evaluating ALBP, the goal of the clinician is first to identify signs of potentially serious conditions through a careful history and physical examination. A holistic approach to the patient is needed to appreciate the extent to which pain affects the patient's daily routine or work-related activities. Because ALBP is a common occupation-related complaint and a cause of disability and lost productivity, the clinician must gain insight into the psychosocial and economic situation of the patient to help arrive at a correct diagnosis.

DIAGNOSTIC REASONING: FOCUSED HISTORY

Is This a Potentially Serious Cause of ALBP?

Key Questions

- Do you have a fever?
- Have you experienced any trauma to the spine or back?
- Do you have any other health problems? Have you been treated for cancer?
- What is your age?
- Have you had loss of control of your bowels or bladder?
- Are you taking any medications?

Nerve root	L4	L5	S1
Pain			
Numbness			
Motor weakness	Extension of quadriceps	Dorsiflexion of great toe and foot	Plantar flexion of great toe and foot
Screening exam	Squat and rise	Heel walking	Walking on toes
Reflexes	Knee jerk diminished	None reliable	Ankle jerk diminished

FIGURE 27-1 Testing for lumbar nerve root compromise. (From Bigos S et al: *Acute low back problems in adults, clinical practice guidelines,* Quick Reference Guide Number 14, Rockville, Md, 1994, Department of Health and Human Services, U.S. Public Health Service, Agency for Health Care Policy and Research, AHCPR Publication No. 95-0643.)

Fever

The presence of a fever indicates an inflammatory condition such as spondyloarthropathy or systemic infection. Infection is a likely diagnosis when there are chills and fever, weight loss, a recent history of bacterial infection, intravenous drug use, or an immunosuppressed patient. Ewing's sarcoma is a malignant tumor and can mimic spinal infection, occurring as back pain that can be accompanied by fever. Children with diskitis will have a fever and refuse to walk because of back pain.

Trauma

Acute trauma to the spinal cord can result in fracture, dislocation, or misalignment of muscles, ligaments, and intervertebral disks. Trauma may be caused by a blunt impact, repetitive injury, or sudden stress caused by lifting or pulling. Low back pain is the most common occupational injury reported. Injury to the back usually results in contusions and abrasions but can also cause spinal fracture if the force is major, such as that sustained in a motor vehicle accident or fall. In the elderly, an acute spinal fracture might result from strenuous lifting when osteoporosis is present. Injuries to the posterior structures of the spine account for most cases of low back pain in adolescents who are athletically active.

Injury to the spinal column should be suspected in anyone whose level of consciousness is impaired after an accident. Cervical spine fractures are sustained during flexion, extension, compression, rotation, or a combination of forces.

Age

In the absence of trauma, the sudden onset of severe low or middle back pain in persons older than 30 years might suggest a dissecting aortic aneurysm. The pain will not be alleviated by rest. Patients older than 50 years are at increased risk for compression fracture as well as cancer.

Systemic Disease

Metabolic disease, inflammatory disorders, and fibromyalgia can lead to back pain. Patients with a history of cancer may have increased risk of a spinal tumor. Neuroblastoma is common in young children, and although it occurs in the abdomen, metastases to the spine may produce back pain. Systemic disease may also be accompanied by unexplained weight loss. Persons younger than 20 years and older than 50 years are at increased risk for tumor, as are those with a history of cancer.

Bowel and Bladder Symptoms

Loss of urinary or stool continence indicates cauda equina or S1-S2 nerve root compromise secondary to a herniated disk, nerve root entrapment, spinal stenosis, infection, or tumor. Constant lumbar puncture with saddle anesthesia, urinary retention, and fecal incontinence are symptoms of cauda equina syndrome, which is considered a surgical emergency.

Children are embarrassed to talk about urinary or bowel habits and changes. Hidden spinal cord tumors might have a relationship to developmental delays in bladder and bowel control. Children under 4 years of age who have back pain should be evaluated for serious diseases, such as intraspinal tumors, dermoid cysts, and malignant astrocytomas.

Medications

Long-term use of corticosteroids can lead to compression fractures of the vertebrae. Use of intravenous drugs may suggest infection as a cause.

What Does the Location of Pain Tell Me?

Key Question

■ Where does it hurt?

Location of Pain

In general, children are less specific than adults when describing location of pain. Traumatic lesions are more likely to occur in the cervical and lumbar portions of the spine, where there is more motion and less protection. Generalized pain or pain over a fairly wide anatomical area is frequently seen with overuse problems and inflammatory conditions.

Sciatica pain is a sharp, burning pain that radiates down the posterior and lateral leg to the foot or ankle. Back pain with neck stiffness can indicate cervical osteomyelitis. Rheumatoid arthritis produces pain in the upper back and neck. Localized pain is seen with spondylolysis and tumors. Flank pain in adults may indicate a kidney infection. Pain of gallbladder disease radiates to the subscapular areas. Compression fractures of vertebrae associated with osteoporosis or malignancy may produce pain over the midthoracic area.

Children with traumatic low back derangement will have pain and muscle spasm in the lumbar area from the pressure and shock of an impact injury collision.

What Does the Pattern of Pain Tell Me?

Key Questions

■ When did the pain start?
■ How long have you had this pain?
■ What does the pain feel like?
■ Does it interfere with sleep?
■ Have you had this pain before?

Onset

The onset of ALBP is sudden, and more than half of patients with this symptom do not associate it with a specific precipitating event or injury. The vast majority of cases of ALBP resolve with conservative treatment in 4 weeks, and radiographic or further diagnostic studies are not recommended until then.

Children are frequently poor historians and parents may have a difficult time remembering when the pain started. Association with events such as birthdays, holidays, and activities is helpful in establishing the onset of the pain. Pain that is mild and of short duration (1 to 2 weeks) is rarely serious.

Back pain lasting longer than 4 weeks needs to be reevaluated for further diagnostic studies.

Duration

Subacute back pain is of 6 to 12 weeks' duration. Chronic back pain is pain of more than 3 months' duration. In persons under 40 years of age, the cause may be postural or may indicate congenital spinal deformity, such as scoliosis or ankylosing spondylitis. In older persons, chronic back pain is more likely to indicate degenerative disease such as spinal stenosis or disk herniation. In children, back pain present for more than 3 weeks is often due to organic and serious causes.

Pain Characteristics

In children, expression of pain depends on the child's ability to put feelings of pain into behavior; observing for these behaviors is important. Ask children to rate the pain using a pain scale from 1 to 10 or use happy to sad faces rated from 0 to 5. Ask adults to rate pain from 0 (no pain) to 10 (worst pain ever) and assess how much the pain interferes with daily activities. Intractable back pain, especially night pain with constitutional findings, is likely to indicate neoplastic disease. Painful scoliosis and stiffness are common presenting symptoms of a spinal tumor.

Night Pain

Night pain is a worrisome symptom that often signals a serious problem such as tumor, infection, or inflammation. Generally, muscle pulls, overuse injuries, spondylolysis, spondylolisthesis, and Scheuermann's disease (an exaggeration of the normal posterior convex curvature of the thoracic spine) produce less pain at night. Morning stiffness that improves

as the day progresses suggests ankylosing spondylitis.

Nighttime back pain is unusual and indicates the need for a complete and thorough work-up.

Recurring Pain

Back pain in young children who have had previous injuries or fractures may be a symptom of child abuse. In the older adult, it may be an indication of compression fractures of the spine. As with young children, it may also signal abuse by a caregiver.

What Does the Pain in Relation to Activity Tell Me?

Key Questions
- What makes the pain worse?
- What makes the pain better?

Aggravating Factors

Pain experienced in the lumbar area occurring after strenuous sporting activities is usually the result of trauma to the muscles and tendons, causing contusions and sprain. It occurs when the patient pushes the muscles and ligaments past the normal level of tolerance. Repeated injury can cause soft tissue scarring and shortening.

Stress and fatigue fractures of the pars interarticularis, the region between the superior and inferior articulating facets of the vertebra, occur when lumbar lordosis places more stress on the pars, such as in gymnastics and tennis.

Pain that is aggravated by activity is usually musculoskeletal in origin. Pain of ankylosing spondylitis is relieved with exercise. Spinal stenosis is associated with increased pain with standing, sneezing, or coughing.

Any child who has voluntarily given up a pleasurable activity because of back pain has a severe symptom.

Alleviating Factors

Back pain not associated with any activity and not relieved by rest may indicate tumor. Back pain relieved with aspirin or nonsteroidal anti-inflammatory drugs in children may indicate an inflammatory cause. Pain that is alleviated by rest and heat indicates a musculoskeletal cause. Pain of spinal stenosis is relieved on flexion of the spine.

Suspect spondylolisthesis, or forward slippage of one vertebra over another, if the onset of pain is during hyperextension, such as with a back handspring, butterfly stroke in swimming, or a tennis serve. The defect arises from a stress fracture or stress reaction of the isthmus of the pars interarticularis in the area of L5-S1. The pain localizes to the low back and occurs during a growth spurt and after engaging in sporting events. The pain improves with rest and is worse with standing.

What Does Radiation of Pain Tell Me?

Key Questions

■ Does the pain travel?
■ Show me where the pain travels.

Radiation of Pain

Referred pain is of two types: (1) pain referred from the spine into areas lying within the lumbar and upper sacral dermatomes; and (2) pain referred from the pelvic and abdominal viscera to the spine. Pain from the upper lumbar spine usually radiates to the anterior aspects of the thighs and legs, and that of the lower lumbar spine radiates to the gluteal regions, posterior thighs, and calves.

Pain from visceral disease is usually felt within the abdomen or flanks. Gallbladder pain radiates around the trunk to the right scapula. Position does not affect the pain.

Persons with spondylolysis, a destruction of vertebral structure, or spondylolisthesis, an anterior displacement of a vertebra, complain of hamstring tightness and buttock discomfort as well as low back pain.

Pain that is sharp and burning and radiates down the lateral or posterior aspect of the leg to the lateral ankle or foot is called sciatica, and is a classic symptom of nerve root irritation most often caused by disk displacement.

Are There Signs of Neurological Damage?

Key Questions

■ Have you been stumbling?
■ Have you noticed any change in your balance or coordination?
■ Does the child frequently stumble or fall?
■ Do you have numbness or tingling in your extremities?

Stumbling

Spinal cord tumors such as astrocytoma or ependymoma may present as a disturbance of movement, posture, or strength in the spine or extremities. Impairment of proprioception or sensation from an upper motor neuron lesion, exhibited by footdrop or ataxia, may produce stumbling.

Numbness and Tingling

Radiculopathy (nerve root pain) is sharp pain felt in a dermatomal pattern and is sometimes associated with numbness and tingling.

Is There a Family History of Back Pain?

Key Question

■ Does anyone in your family have scoliosis or a crooked spine?

Family History

Spondylolysis and scoliosis are often seen in families, with a 40% familial occurrence in Alaskan Eskimos.

Could This Pain Be Caused by a Systemic Disease?

Key Question

■ Have you been ill?

Illness

Pharyngitis or upper respiratory tract infections such as pneumonia can be the precursor to diskitis in children. The intervertebral disk in children receives its blood supply from the surface of the adjacent vertebral bodies, providing the mechanism necessary for infection. Uveitis and iritis may be associated with juvenile rheumatoid arthritis or juvenile ankylosing spondylitis.

A female patient with pelvic inflammatory disease may have mild to moderate dull, aching, lower abdominal, pelvic, or possibly back pain. With pyelonephritis, the patient may complain of fever, nausea and vomiting, headache, and back or flank pain.

DIAGNOSTIC REASONING: FOCUSED PHYSICAL EXAMINATION

Observe the Patient's General Appearance

Any person appearing ill with a fever, limp, or unwillingness to walk is highly suspect for having an infectious cause of back pain.

Observe for symmetry of posture and movement from a direct anterior, posterior, and lateral view of the patient. Note the amount of thoracic kyphosis (anteroposterior curve) and lumbar lordosis (anterior convexity) and the alignment of the head and neck above the center of gravity. Children with diskitis often protect their back by sitting in a hyperextended position, using the arms as support, and may lie down and cry if they are made to sit.

Observe Gait

Shifting or leaning to one side (listing) and atypical scoliosis may indicate a tumor. Listing is caused by asymmetrical sustained muscle contraction. The spinal curvature serves to relieve the discomfort and reduce pressure on a nerve root.

Severely affected gait in spondylosis is caused by hamstring tightness and results in uneven stride length with a persistently fixed knee to prevent hip flexion, which would stretch the tight hamstring muscles and increase pain.

Assess Vital Signs

Fever may indicate systemic infection as well as diskitis. Unexplained weight loss may suggest neoplasm, infection, or depression.

Examine Skin

Dermal cysts and/or a hairy patch over the spine may indicate spinal anomaly or tumor.

A doughy, fatty mass in the midline of the back (sometimes covered with hair [Faun's beard]) is evidence of a lipoma, which may extend into the spinal cord and produce neurological symptoms.

Examine Eyes, Ears, Nose, and Mouth

Uveitis iritis is seen in juvenile rheumatoid arthritis and ankylosing spondylitis. Pharyngitis, otitis media, or infection of hematogenous origin may be the cause of diskitis in children.

Inspect the Back and Extremities

Observe for spinal alignment and symmetry of the tips of the scapula, iliac crests, and gluteal crease. If indicated, measure and compare leg lengths from the anterosuperior iliac crest to the medial malleolus. Measurements can be performed with the patient standing or supine. Legs should be of equal length or have less than 1-cm difference in length. Leg length differences are associated with sacroiliac, facet joint, and disk pathology.

From posterior and lateral viewpoints, observe the patient bending forward with feet together to detect scoliosis, kyphosis, or stiffness and guarding.

Percuss and Palpate Back and Spine

Painful scoliosis and stiffness are common in osteoid osteoma. Idiopathic scoliosis is usually painless without functional limitation. Point tenderness over the affected area is a finding associated with compression fracture of vertebrae or an infection of the spine.

Palpate and percuss the back to determine if tenderness is in the paravertebral muscular or midline spinous processes, which may indicate diskitis in children or osteomyelitis. To rule out the sacroiliac joint as the site of origin of low back pain, apply pressure over the joint with the patient's hip flexed 90 degrees and the leg adducted across the midline. This position places stress on the sacroiliac joint and will aggravate the pain if this is the site of origin.

Use fist percussion over the costovertebral angles to discriminate flank pain caused by renal disease from spinal pathology. Apply fist percussion over the costovertebral angles and over the spine to localize tenderness.

Perform Range of Motion of the Spine

Ask the patient to flex, extend, rotate, and bend the spine laterally. Decreased mobility and back pain along the spine may indicate muscle spasm, neoplasm, or bony deformity. Pain with forward flexion usually indicates a mechanical cause. Back extension pain increases with spinal stenosis.

Look for compensating effects of hip motion on the spine. The absence of lumbar flexion may be totally masked by a normal range of hip flexion when the patient bends forward. Test lumbar flexion by placing a mark over the fourth lumbar vertebra and another over the sacrum. Lumbar flexion is demonstrated by an increased distance between these two marks when the patient bends forward.

Observe for limitation of motion on forward bending caused by hip flexion contracture. Lumbar lordosis does not flatten with forward bending and is an organic cause for back pain. In children, Scheuermann's kyphosis, an exaggeration of the normal posterior convex curvature of the thoracic spine, produces pain with forward flexion, and spondylolysis produces pain with hyperextension.

Perform Straight Leg Raising

The straight leg raising (SLR) test can assess sciatic (L5 and S1) nerve root tension. With the patient supine, place one hand above the knee, the other cupping the heel, and slowly raise the limb. Instruct the patient to say when to stop because of pain. Observe for pelvic movement and the degree of leg elevation when the patient tells you to stop. Ask the patient to tell you the most distal point of pain sensation, such as the back, hip, thigh, or knee. While holding the leg at the limit of elevation, dorsiflexing the ankle and internally rotating will add tension to the neural structures and increase the pain if nerve root tension is present.

Pain below the knee at less than 70 degrees of elevation that is aggravated by dorsiflexing the ankle or hip rotation is a sign of L5 or S1 nerve root tension, suggestive of a herniated disk. This test can also be performed with the patient sitting. In a positive test, the patient will resist extension or will compensate with hyperextension of the spine.

Lift each leg in succession to detect contralateral pain in patients with nerve root compression.

An SLR test in children might be unremarkable with a tumor.

Check Hip Mobility

With the patient prone and supine, check active hip flexion, extension, internal and external rotation, and strength against resistance. Weakness of the gluteus maximus is associated with lumbar or referred pain from L5 nerve roots or gluteal nerve injury. In small children, check for congenital hip dysplasia with the child supine, abducting the hips (see Chapter 26). The knees should appear of equal height and should externally rotate equal degrees. The presence of a hip click, joint instability, uneven hip-to-knee length with hips and knees flexed, and uneven gluteal skinfolds suggests congenital hip dislocation.

Examine Feet

Perform active range of motion of the ankle, feet, and toes against resistance. Weakness, pain, or limitation of dorsiflexion movement indicates an L4 nerve root injury. Similar symptoms produced by plantar flexion indicate S1, S2 involvement. Deformities of the foot, such as talipes equinovarus (clubfoot) or hallux malleus (claw toes), may aggravate misalignment of back structures because of asymmetry.

Evaluate Muscle Strength

Evaluate strength against resistance of the lower extremity muscle groups. Test the patient's ability to stand on toes and heels and to squat. A person with S1 nerve root involvement may have little motor weakness but may demonstrate difficulty in toe walking. Difficulty heel walking or squatting indicates involvement of L5 and L4 nerve roots. Leg extension at the knee against resistance tests L4 root function. In young children who are unable to cooperate for measurement of muscle strength, use measurements of like limb-girths as an estimate of the bilateral symmetry of muscle strength.

Measure Muscle Circumference
Differences in muscle circumference greater than 2 cm in two opposite limbs may signify atrophy secondary to neurological impairment.

Test Sensory Function
All neurological test results are evaluated by comparing the symmetry of responses or perceptions. Bilateral comparison is the simplest, most efficient way to determine the presence, location, and extent of any abnormality. A sensory examination is a general guide in determining the level of spinal cord involvement. Test for light touch and pain sensation in the sensory areas of L3-S1 dermatomes (see Figure 27-1). Dermatomes overlap and vary greatly in individuals; thus only gross changes can be detected by pinprick. Test 5 to 10 pinpricks in each dermatomal area if the patient reports numbness and tingling. Disk lesions rarely produce bilateral symptoms. It is sometimes difficult to distinguish numbness from cutaneous nerve versus dermatomal origin. Numbness from cutaneous nerve lesions does not occur in a dermatomal pattern. Numbness and tingling are uncommon symptoms in most children with back pain. When these symptoms are present, it suggests a serious problem.

Assess Deep Tendon Reflexes
Normal deep tendon reflexes (DTRs) are symmetrical. DTRs are increased when an upper motor neuron lesion is present and decreased with a lower motor neuron lesion. A positive Babinski's sign indicates a disorder of upper motor neurons, affecting the motor area of the brain or corticospinal tracts, caused by spinal tumors or demyelinating disease. DTRs are decreased if a tumor is pressing on a peripheral nerve. Asymmetrical abdominal reflexes are seen in tumors of the spine.

An absent or a decreased ankle jerk reflex suggests an S1 nerve root lesion. An L3-4 disk herniation is the most common cause of a diminished knee-jerk reflex.

Palpate the Abdomen
Palpation of the abdomen is performed to detect possible visceral causes of back pain. In an elderly person, a ruptured aortic aneurysm can cause acute, severe, midthoracic back pain. If an aortic aneurysm is suspected, immediate surgical referral is critical.

Check Rectal Sphincter Tone
In cauda equina syndrome, the compression of S1-S2 nerve roots results in decreased sphincter tone and decreased sensation in the perianal area. This syndrome is a surgical emergency.

LABORATORY AND DIAGNOSTIC STUDIES
According to national practice guidelines, no diagnostic tests are warranted within the first 4 weeks for acute onset of low back pain without neurological signs.

Plain Radiographs
Radiographs are useful in localizing the area of discomfort and ruling out fracture, tumor, osteophytes (bone spurs), or vertebral infection.

Standing Anteroposterior and Lateral Views of the Spine
These views of the spine accentuate any deformity, such as scoliosis, and demonstrate vertebral integrity.

Oblique and Flexion Views of the Spine
These views increase the sensitivity for determining instability.

Spine Radiograph
A flat lumbosacral spinal radiograph is obtained when there is a history of trauma or in persons older than 50 years who have ALBP with signs of neurological deficit. Older persons may have a history of straining or lifting.

Bone Scan

Bone scan is a radioisotope technique indicating blood flow and bone formation or destruction and can reveal inflammatory and infiltrative processes and occult fractures. The distal wrist and lumbosacral spine can be scanned to assess bone mineral density and risk of osteoporosis.

Electromyography

Electromyography (EMG) is performed to assess the extent of nerve root compression and function of the peripheral nerves.

Diagnostic Imaging

Magnetic resonance imaging (MRI) is useful in evaluating soft tissue detail, such as disk herniations and spinal cord pathology, especially in vertebral osteomyelitis. Computed tomography (CT) scans are usually used for bone visualization.

Urinalysis

Urinalysis is performed to assess kidney and metabolic function, including infectious processes, to rule out a visceral cause of back pain, such as the pain of pyelonephritis.

Erythrocyte Sedimentation Rate

The erythrocyte sedimentation rate (ESR) will be elevated in about 90% of patients with a serious musculoskeletal infection; however, there is no direct relationship between ESR and the severity of infection. The test is nonspecific.

Complete Blood Cell Count

The complete blood cell count (CBC) will detect anemia as well as other conditions that might manifest as back pain, such as tumor or infection. The anemia of chronic disease is usually hypochromic or normochromic with low iron indices.

DIFFERENTIAL DIAGNOSIS

Potentially Serious Causes of Acute Low Back Pain

Spinal Fracture

The patient may relate a history of major trauma to the back from an impact or fall or, if elderly, a history of strenuous lifting or a minor fall. Pain is felt near the site of injury. Any suspicion of spinal fracture should be treated as an emergency. The patient is immobilized to prevent further damage and transported by emergency personnel for radiographs of the suspected area of fracture.

Tumor (Osteoblastoma, Spinal Metastasis, Osteoid Osteoma)

Primary tumors are a more common cause of back pain in children, whereas metastasis is a more common cause in adults. The lower thoracic and upper lumbar vertebrae are the most common sites of bony metastatic disease from marrow tumors. A health history and diagnostic tests may reveal other signs of general poor health such as weight loss, fatigue, weakness, and anemia.

Infection (Osteomyelitis, Diskitis)

The spine is the most common site of osteomyelitis in adults, secondary to adjacent infection or following invasive instrumentation that results in bacterial seeding of the bone via the arterial blood. *Staphylococcus aureus* is the most frequently identified organism. Vertebral osteomyelitis causes stiffness and pain, usually localized over the site of infection. A tender spinous process, positive SLR test, and paravertebral muscle spasm may be seen in vertebral osteomyelitis or septic diskitis. Patients may have hip pain secondary to involvement of L2-S1.

Diskitis is usually a benign disorder in children that results in intervertebral disk inflammation. Children will be reluctant to walk, sit, or stand. Pain will be aggravated by motion and relieved by rest. History will reveal a recent bacterial infection, often secondary to pharyngitis or otitis media, intravenous drug use, diabetes mellitus, or immunosuppression. A small percentage of adults will report an acute onset of fever, weight loss, and general malaise; however, the majority may only have the symptom of back pain present from 2 weeks to years.

Cauda Equina Syndrome

Compression of the S1 nerve root produces a constant back pain with saddle distribution anesthesia (buttock and medial and posterior thighs), fecal incontinence, bladder dysfunction, motor weakness of the lower limbs, and radiculopathy. The patient may limp and guard lumbar spine movement, will not be able to heel walk or toe walk, and will have abnormal or asymmetrical knee and ankle deep tendon reflexes. SLR test will be positive. This syndrome is a surgical emergency.

Sciatic Problems
Sciatica
The most common cause of sciatica is herniated disk. History may disclose repetitive motion strain or strenuous lifting, twisting, and bending. Low back pain is associated with pain and burning that radiates along the lateral thigh, leg, and foot, sometimes associated with numbness along the dermatomal areas. SLR and sitting knee extension produce radicular pain below the knee at less than 60 degrees of limb elevation, and pain may be felt in the buttocks or posterior thigh. Bowel and bladder functions are normal.

Nonspecific Back Problems
Musculoskeletal Strain (Postural, Overuse)
Back structures such as muscles and ligaments can become inflamed from overuse or strain. History often reveals no precipitating event for the onset of pain. Patients may report that pain is alleviated by rest, especially in the supine position with hips and knees flexed, and by the application of heat or cold. Pain is aggravated by sitting, walking, standing, and with certain motions. On physical examination, palpation will localize the pain, and muscle spasms may be felt. Range of motion of the spine will increase the pain, especially forward flexion. Neurological examination shows no abnormalities.

Spondylolisthesis
Pain can be the result of a disruption of the vertebral spinous process, where the disruption results in subluxation of the vertebral body onto adjacent structures. This usually occurs between L5 and S1. Pain is usually chronic. Examination of the spine may disclose a palpable, prominent spinous process. Forward flexion may be limited.

Ankylosing Spondylitis
Ankylosing spondylitis is a systemic inflammatory condition of the vertebral column and sacroiliac joints. Peak incidence is in persons 20 to 30 years old; males are most often affected. Patients report chronic low back pain, which is worse on morning rising and lessens as the day progresses. Examination shows an excessive thoracic kyphosis and rounding of the posterior thoracic spine with forward flexion of the head, neck, and lower back. About 30% of patients will have arthritis of other joints. Radiographs may reveal fusion of vertebrae, and ESR is elevated.

Spinal Stenosis
Spinal stenosis is a bony encroachment on the nerve roots of the lumbar spine and is the most common cause of low back pain in adults older than 50 years. Patients report low back pain associated with lumbosacral radiculopathy, pain with walking or standing, and pain relief with sitting. Neurogenic (pseudo) claudication pain of the lower extremities is made worse with prolonged standing, walking, bending, or hyperextending the back.

Scheuermann's Disease
Adolescent males develop this disease as a result of anterior disk protrusion, causing wedging of the thoracic vertebrae and an exaggeration of the normal posterior convex curvature of the thoracic spine. The cause is unknown but may develop from excessive lifting or spinal flexion. The patient complains of mild to moderate pain, worsening toward the end of the day or after physical activity but relieved by rest. Physical examination demonstrates an increase in thoracic kyphosis on lateral view, made sharper by forward bending.

Osteoporosis
Osteoporosis is a loss of mineralized bone mass that can result in a compression fracture of the vertebral body, usually occurring in the thoracic area. Back pain is often chronic and poorly localized. Multiple compression fractures may produce dorsal kyphosis and

cervical lordosis. Persons at greatest risk are postmenopausal Caucasian women, especially those slight in build who have a history of inactivity. It is also common in persons older than 70 years who have age-related reduction in vitamin D synthesis. Osteoporosis can also be secondary to endocrine imbalance (such as hyperthyroidism), organ disease, drugs (such as corticosteroids), or excessive intake of alcohol.

Nonspinal Causes
Aortic Aneurysm (Dissecting)
Sudden onset of severe low or middle back pain that is not alleviated by rest in persons older than 30 years might suggest a dissecting aortic aneurysm. The patient may exhibit pallor, diaphoresis, and confusion. Pulses and blood pressure measured on each upper extremity will be asymmetrical. Emergency surgery is indicated.

Gallstones
The presence of gallbladder problems increases with age. A gallbladder attack often follows the ingestion of a fatty meal. A crampy right upper quadrant (RUQ) pain, following the ingestion of a fatty meal, is produced by spasms of the cystic duct that is obstructed with a stone. Gallbladder pain radiates around the trunk to the right scapula. Position does not affect the pain. Patients complain of belching, bloating, and an acidic stomach. Attacks may increase in frequency and severity and cause nighttime wakening. During an attack, palpation will show RUQ tenderness. Physical findings between attacks may be normal or there may be tenderness to palpation of the RUQ on inspiration (Murphy's sign) if the gallbladder is inflamed. An RUQ mass may be felt if the gallbladder is obstructed. Obstruction is an emergency surgical situation.

Pyelonephritis
With pyelonephritis, the patient will appear ill and diaphoretic and may complain of nausea and vomiting, headache, and back or flank pain. The patient may have a fever. Severe lumbar tenderness will be found on fist percussion for costovertebral angle (CVA) tenderness. Urinalysis will show cloudy, malodorous urine, and microscopy will show the presence of casts and cells (i.e., red blood cells, white blood cells, and epithelial cells).

Pleuritis
Inflammation of the pleural lining of the lungs often follows an upper respiratory tract infection. Pleuritic pain is sharp, worsens on inspiration or with coughing, and is lessened by lying on the affected side. Physical examination of the lungs will be normal, or crackles and bronchial breath sounds will be heard on auscultation. A chest radiograph will provide information on the condition of the lungs.

Pelvic Inflammatory Disease
The symptoms of pelvic inflammatory disease (PID) depend on the extent of infection. Infection usually begins in the lower urinary tract or cervix and spreads to the endometrium, fallopian tubes, and peritoneum. The sexually active female patient may have mild to moderate dull, aching, lower abdominal, pelvic, or possibly back pain. She will report tenderness during cervical motion, uterine motion, or palpation of the adnexa. History may be positive for sexually transmitted infections (usually *Neisseria gonorrhoeae* and *Chlamydia trachomatis*), vaginal symptoms, or use of an IUD for contraception.

Psychogenic Causes
Psychological Back Pain
A careful history is needed to gain insight into the psychosocial and economic issues surrounding report of back pain. The patient may have a history of recent life stressors, be involved in a legal injury or Worker's Compensation action, or have a history of depression or alcohol abuse. The clinician should be aware of exaggerated signs of pain such as moaning, grimacing, or overreaction. A patient who is a malingerer pretends to suffer, but when distracted will show inconsistent and variable results on examination, such as SLR, or will describe radiation of pain inconsistent with dermatome distribution.

◆ DIFFERENTIAL DIAGNOSIS OF *Common Causes of Acute Low Back Pain*

CONDITION	HISTORY	PHYSICAL FINDINGS	DIAGNOSTIC STUDIES
Potentially Serious Causes			
Spinal fracture	Trauma to spine or back; pain is felt near site of injury	Palpable tenderness over site of fracture	Considered an emergency; immobilize patient and transport for radiographs
Tumor	History of cancer; progressive pain is unremitting; occurs at night and at rest	Weight loss, fever, tenderness near tumor	ESR; bone scan
Osteoblastoma	Neck or back pain not relieved by aspirin; occurs in older adolescents and young adults	Localized tenderness; may have scoliosis with muscle pain	Plain film shows an expansive osteolytic lesion surrounded by thin peripheral rim of bone; bone scan; CT scan
Osteoid osteoma	Occurs primarily in adolescents; rare in patients over age 40; well-localized pain that may be more severe at night and relieved by aspirin or other prostaglandin inhibitors	Painful, well-localized scoliosis may be present	Bone scan
Infection (vertebral osteomyelitis)	History of infection, invasive procedure; continuous, dull back pain; chronic back pain	Acute onset presents with fever, diaphoresis; tenderness over affected disk; positive SLR	ESR; blood culture; bone biopsy; CT scan; MRI
Diskitis	Pain aggravated by movement; more common in children	Tenderness over-affected disk	ESR
Cauda equina syndrome	Constant pain in a saddle distribution; urinary retention, fecal incontinence, radiculopathy	Positive SLR, abnormal DTRs, motor weakness	Surgical emergency
Sciatica Problems			
Sciatica	Acute back pain with radiculopathy; history of strain or trauma, relief with sitting	Paravertebral tenderness and spasm; positive SLR; sitting knee extension, sensory findings	EMG if chronic
Nonspecific Back Problems			
Musculoskeletal strain	Pain in back, buttocks; history of new activity or exertion; relief of pain with sitting	Paravertebral tenderness, scoliosis, or loss of lumbar lordosis; no neurological signs	None
Spondylolisthesis	Young person in a sport that demands rapid movement between hyperflexion and hyperextension or requires excess loading in hyperextension	No neurological signs; pain localized to low back, just below level of iliac crest; tight hamstrings	Lumbar spine radiographs

Continued

DIFFERENTIAL DIAGNOSIS OF *Common Causes of Acute Low Back Pain* *—cont'd*

CONDITION	HISTORY	PHYSICAL FINDINGS	DIAGNOSTIC STUDIES
Ankylosing spondylitis	Persons under age 40: insidious onset; progressive morning back pain relieved with exercise	Painful sacroiliac joints, reduced spine mobility; may have uveitis	ESR; spinal radiographs
Spinal stenosis	Pain worse throughout day; aggravated by standing, relieved by rest; pseudoclaudication	Signs of osteoarthritis of joints; may have neurological signs	Spinal radiographs
Scheuermann's disease	Affects mostly adolescent males; mild to moderately severe pain, worse at end of day, relieved by rest	Normal examination; may show an exaggerated thoracic kyphosis that is fixed in attempted hyperextension	Thoracic spine radiographs
Osteoporosis	Chronic, poorly localized back pain; postmenopausal; slight build; history of inactivity or endocrine disorder	Palpable tenderness over area of compression fracture; kyphosis or lordosis; loss of height	Bone densiometry; spinal radiograph to assess fracture
Nonspinal Causes			
Aortic aneurysm	Severe, acute-onset pain not related to activity or movement; increased risk in persons over age 30; pallor, diaphoresis, anxiety, confusion	Intact aneurysm will be a visible pulsatile midline upper quadrant abdominal mass; in a dissected aneurysm, upper extremity pulse and pulse pressures are asymmetrical; posterior thoracic pain may be felt	Emergency surgical referral
Gallstones	Increased incidence with age; steady, intense pain in RUQ with radiation to right scapula or shoulder; belching, bloating, fatty food intolerance	Normal physical examination or positive Murphy's sign on palpation of abdomen	Surgical referral
Pyelonephritis	Ill-appearing; sweating, nausea, back or flank pain, headache	Fever: cloudy, malodorous urine; CVA tenderness on percussion	Urinalysis; urine culture
Pleuritis	History of recent URI; pleuritic pain	Normal examination or crackles and bronchial breath sounds	PPD; chest radiograph
Pelvic inflammatory disease	Sexually active female; low back and abdominal pain; history of urinary or vaginal symptoms, sexually transmitted disease, IUD, multiple sex partners	Cervical and uterine motion tenderness, adnexal tenderness; cervicitis, fever	Gonorrhea, *Chlamydia* cultures; ESR
Psychogenic Causes			
Psychological back pain	History of psychosocial stressors, depression, exaggerated expressions of pain	Exaggerated or inconsistent reactions to testing; normal examination	None

CHAPTER RESOURCES

Balagué F: Low-back pain in children, *Lancet* 361:1403, 2003.

Deyo RA, Rainville J, Kent DL: What can the history and physical examination tell us about low back pain? *JAMA* 268:760, 1992.

Deyo RA, Weinstein JN: Low back pain, *N Engl J Med* 344:363, 2001.

Koes BW, van Tulder MW, Ostelo R et al: Clinical guidelines for the management of low back pain in primary care: an international comparison, *Spine* 26(22):2504, 2001.

Kraft DE: Low back pain in the adolescent athlete, *Pediatr Clin North Am* 49:643, 2002.

XI

Common Problems of the Neurological System

CHAPTER 28

Headache

Headache is a subjective feeling of pain caused by a variety of intracranial and extracranial factors. It is one of the most common complaints in adults and children, with most headaches being self-treated with an over-the-counter analgesic. Most headaches are acute and self-limited and are not life threatening. Less than 1% of cases of headache are due to serious intracranial disease. The goals for the practitioner in evaluating a headache are to (1) identify life-threatening causes of headache, (2) diagnose treatable disease associated with some headaches, and (3) provide symptom relief. To accomplish these goals, the practitioner needs to conduct a careful history and physical examination, even though physical findings will be normal for the majority of patients with a headache.

Pain from headache arises from stimulation of pain-sensitive structures of the head and brain caused by traction, inflammation, vascular dilation, muscle contraction, or dysregulation of ascending brainstem serotonergic systems (Figure 28-1). Headaches can be categorized as primary or secondary. Primary headaches are characterized by the absence of structural pathology or systemic disease; they account for more than 90% of all headaches. Secondary headaches are attributed to an underlying disorder. Primary headaches are of five major types: migraine, tension-type headache (TTH), cluster headache and other trigeminal autonomic cephalalgias, and other primary headaches. Generally, pain arising from disordered function, damage, or inflammation of structures located anterior to and above the tentorium is felt in the front of the head, whereas pain felt in the back of the head arises from structures located below the tentorium. Extracranial structures that are sensitive to pain include the skin, scalp, blood vessels, facial muscles, eyes, ears, teeth, nasal cavity, mucous membranes of the mouth and pharynx, and the temporomandibular joint (TMJ). The substance of the brain itself is not sensitive to pain, but sensitive structures include the blood vessels, sensory nerves, and ganglia.

Cranial structures project pain to the surface close to the source of pain. Pain from extracranial structures is usually felt in the immediate region affected (Figure 28-2). The head is innervated extensively from the first branch of the trigeminal nerve (cranial nerve V). It has significant anatomical connections to the upper cervical roots C1-C3, which supply the posterior fossa and neck structures.

Headache has been divided by symptomatology into types using the diagnostic criteria revised in 2004 by the Headache Classification Committee of the International Headache Society.

Of the types classified, only a few are common (Box 28-1). Headaches can also be categorized into acute (new onset), subacute, or chronic. Acute headaches warrant close attention. The headache associated with subarachnoid hemorrhage (SAH) has an intense sudden onset. Subacute headaches are localized headaches preceding neurological findings, often caused by a vascular disorder or a space-occupying lesion. Headaches of greatest concern to clinicians are those that are persistent, severe, sudden in onset, and different from the patient's usual headache. The major clue to assessment of chronic headache is a change in the usual pattern of occurrence. Clinicians can ask patients to keep a

FIGURE 28-1 Mechanisms of cranial pain. (From Noble J et al: *Textbook of primary care medicine,* ed 3, St Louis, 2001, Mosby.)

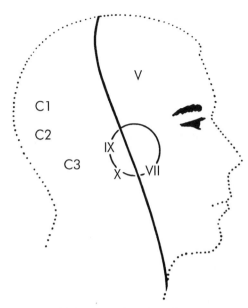

FIGURE 28-2   Sensory pathways for cranial pain.

headache diary that includes notes on timing, frequency, and association with sleep, diet, emotional episodes, and other potentially contributing factors.

DIAGNOSTIC REASONING: FOCUSED HISTORY

What Clues Indicate This Is a Potentially Serious, Life-Threatening Headache?

The clinician may first need to assess whether the patient is fully oriented before proceeding with further history. A mental status screening can be performed using the Mini-Mental State Examination (see Chapter 30). If the patient shows a mental status deficit, immediate emergency treatment is indicated. Box 28-2 summarizes warning signs of a potentially serious cause for headache.

Key Questions

- How did the headache begin?
- What is your age? Have you had this type of headache before?

Box 28-1	First Level of the International Classification of Headache Disorders

Primary Headaches
1. Migraine
2. Tension-type headache (TTH)
3. Cluster headache and other trigeminal autonomic encephalalgias
4. Other primary headaches

Secondary Headaches
5. Headache attributed to head/neck trauma
6. Headache attributed to cranial or cervical vascular disorder
7. Headache attributed to nonvascular intracranial disorder
8. Headache attributed to substance or its withdrawal
9. Headache attributed to infection
10. Headache attributed to disorder of homeostasis
11. Headache or facial pain attributed to disorder of cranium, neck, eyes, ears, nose, sinuses, teeth, mouth, or other facial or cranial structures
12. Headache attributed to psychiatric disorder

Cranial Neuralgias, Central and Primary Facial Pain, and Other Headaches
13. Cranial neuralgias and central causes of facial pain
14. Other headache, cranial neuralgia, central or primary facial pain

From the Headache Classification Committee of the International Headache Society: The International Classification of Headache Disorders, *Cephalalgia* 24 (suppl 1):9, 2004.

- On a scale from 0 (no pain) to 10 (worst pain ever), how severe is the pain?
- Is there a history of recent trauma to the head?
- Was there a loss of consciousness?
- Do you notice any other symptoms associated with the headache pain?
- Do you have any chronic health problems?

Onset and Severity

Sudden onset of a severe headache without a history of chronic headache suggests an intracerebral hemorrhage (ICH) secondary to a ruptured aneurysm or vascular anomaly. Severity of headache is a very subjective measure and can sometimes be difficult to interpret. Headache of an ICH without a history of trauma is rare in children and adolescents, but the prevalence increases with age, especially in persons older than 50 years or in someone who is being treated with anticoagulation therapy.

Onset of sudden severe headache with neurological signs is an emergency; the patient needs immediate emergency treatment.

Subarachnoid hemorrhage (SAH) is often precipitated by physical activity and is described as the "worst headache ever." Patients also complain of a stiff neck and may have a transient loss of consciousness, nausea and vomiting, photophobia, pupillary dilation, and seizure. Some patients who have a leaking aneurysm may complain of headache for several days but will subsequently have a worsening headache with neurological findings.

If SAH is suspected, the patient needs transport to an emergency center for a computed tomography (CT) scan and possible surgical intervention because early diagnosis and treatment improve prognosis.

History of Trauma

Trauma to the head may cause subdural or epidural bleeding. The patient may have a brief loss of consciousness followed by a period of lucidity that can last for minutes to days, with subsequent relapse and appearance of neurological signs. Epidural hematomas are often associated with skull fracture.

Minor head trauma may result in headache because of soft tissue or extracranial injury. Pain is often localized to the site of injury and is self-limiting. Anyone who has experienced head trauma should be carefully observed for at least 24 hours for signs of neurological damage.

Associated Symptoms

The entry of infectious organisms, chemical agents, and drugs into the subarachnoid space causes inflammation of meningeal structures and associated blood vessels, resulting in a headache. Headache associated with infection presents with fever and possibly meningismus (stiff neck), which can indicate meningitis or encephalitis. Unilateral upper or lower extremity weakness with loss of manual dexterity is seen in children with hemiplegic migraine.

An ICH presents as a sudden and severe "thunderclap" headache associated with confusion, vomiting, lethargy, and focal neurological signs; it is caused by a ruptured vascular anomaly or an aneurysm. Drowsiness or confusion can be produced by increased intracranial pressure secondary to meningitis or metabolic disorders.

Brain tumors in children, especially young children, are difficult to diagnose because of the child's inability to describe headache or diplopia until about 4 years of age. Signs are vague, and the developing skull in the infant may accommodate a pathological condition for some time. However, headache as the initial manifestation of brain tumor is followed quickly by neurological signs such as vomiting, recurrent morning headaches, reflex asymmetry, and papilledema.

Presence of Chronic Disease

Persons with AIDS are at increased risk for cryptococcal meningitis, encephalitis, or generalized sepsis. Persons being treated with anticoagulation therapy or the elderly are at increased risk for headache from a serious cause, such as an ICH or acute glaucoma. Headaches secondary to metabolic disorders can be the result of hyponatremia, uremia, hypoglycemia, and hypercapnia.

After Determining the Headache Is Not Serious, How Can I Narrow Down the Causes?

Key Questions

- What does it feel like?
- Where does it hurt?
- What makes it worse?
- How long have you had this headache?
- Can you tell when a headache is developing?

Characteristics of the Pain

A moderately intense, constant throbbing headache is associated with dilation of the cervical arteries. Severe pain indicates an expanding lesion, such as a tumor or hematoma, edema, or enlargement of the ventricles secondary to hydrocephalus.

Migraine headache pain is caused by the production of various substances on dilated arteries that sensitize those arteries to pain. The pain is steady or throbbing and is usually limited to the same side. Migraine headaches are thought to result from an initial phase of intercranial or extracranial vasoconstriction, followed by a longer interval of vasodilation. Frequently the headache takes 3 to 4 hours to reach peak pain levels.

Cluster headaches (uncommon in children) are the result of an unknown vascular change that occurs within a period of 5 minutes.

Tension (muscle contraction) headaches usually occur at school or work and often disappear on weekends and vacations or during periods of relaxation.

Location

Pain secondary to trauma or inflammation is perceived as near the site of insult, such as the occipital area, nape of neck, bifrontal area, or generalized to the head. Noxious stimulation from any type of disease of the eye, ear, nose, or paranasal sinuses may spread to cause pain in the head.

Adults describe tension-type headaches (TTHs) as a "hatband" distribution of pain, whereas children describe a generalized headache or discomfort.

Orbital pain is seen with increased intraocular pressure. Periorbital pain may be present with sinusitis, migraine, or trigeminal neuralgia, or it may be a sign of ocular disease. TMJ pain is located in the frontotemporal or temporal regions and may be unilateral or bilateral. Nonpulsatile headache in the occipital and paracervical regions is often caused by contraction of muscles of the head and neck.

Aggravating Factors

Triggers are present in many patients with migraine and include sound, odor, or estrogen fluctuations associated with the menstrual cycle. The most common food triggers are red wine, chocolate, and ripe cheese—foods high in tyramine or tryptophan. Migraine is usually worse with activity, whereas patients with TTHs are able to continue their usual routine. Stress can trigger any type of primary headache and must be considered a comorbid condition.

Duration

Most TTHs last less than 24 hours, a similar duration as migraine headaches. Cluster headaches usually last less than 3 hours and tend to occur in clusters. A subacute headache persists for days and weeks.

Aura and Prodrome

In migraine with aura, visual symptoms predominate and range from nonspecific blurring to scintillating scotomata with zigzag patterns, diplopia, and stars or flashes. Aura often precedes the onset or is simultaneous with headache. Prodromal symptoms include fatigue, depressed or euphoric mood, increased or decreased appetite, constipation or diarrhea, and yawning.

What Does the Chronicity of Pain Suggest?

Key Questions

- How often do you get a headache?
- Can you describe any pattern to the headache?
- How long does the headache last?
- Have you had this kind of headache before?

- Do you drink alcohol? Do you take any medications?

Frequency

As a rule, a patient with a persistent headache for more than 3 months may demonstrate physical findings such as papilledema, bilateral or unilateral cranial nerve VI (abducens) palsies, gait or balance disturbances, or spasticity of the lower extremities. However, in the absence of such symptoms, a recurrent headache of more than 3 months' duration is rarely related to structural or systemic findings. If a headache has been present continuously for more than 4 weeks, without accompanying neurological signs or symptoms, it is most likely psychogenic in origin, especially if coupled with prolonged school or work absences, increased stress, and depression.

Pattern and Duration of Headache

Headaches that occur throughout the day suggest a tension type. Sinus headaches occur after arising and worsen as the day progresses, especially when the person bends forward, but are less painful in the evening. Headaches associated with severe hypertension are not common and occur only with a diastolic blood pressure reading of 130 mm Hg or greater. They are occipital, worse on arising, and lessen as the day progresses. Meningeal inflammation produces a pain that fluctuates throughout the day and night with no clear pattern. Migraine pain is episodic, occurring from several times a week to once a year. Cluster headache pain demonstrates a pattern of attacks that occur daily for several weeks with long periods of remission. The pain is short, often lasting less than 1 hour, but is intense.

Prior History of Headache

Headaches can be described as acute (new onset), subacute, or chronic. Acute-onset headaches must be evaluated for organic causes. Subacute and chronic headaches are usually caused by vascular inflammation or muscle tension. Chronic headaches are usually described as dull, bilateral, or bandlike. Chronic daily headaches may be mixed,

produced by a combination of vascular and muscular causes.

Organic lesions may initially produce pain that is intermittent, but as the lesion progresses the duration and frequency of the attack will increase.

Psychogenic headache pain is daily, constant, diffuse, and difficult to describe.

Age of Patient at First Onset

The age of onset of migraines can be from 5 to 8 years old. Usually migraine headaches begin at ages 10 to 30 years. New onset of migraine headaches in adults older than age 50 is unusual. Tension headaches have a usual first-onset age of 8 to 12 years. Cluster headaches have a usual first-onset age of 20 to 40 years.

Lifestyle Habits and Medications

Alcohol is an important trigger for migraine and cluster headaches although it may relieve a TTH. Smoking is a risk factor for cardiovascular and respiratory disease. Patients may be experiencing side effects of medications with headache.

What Associated Symptoms Does the Patient Have?

Key Questions

- Do you have any nausea or vomiting?
- Do you notice any vision changes?
- Does light bother you?
- Are you dizzy?

Nausea and Vomiting

Nausea and abdominal pain are more common in children with migraines, whereas nausea and vomiting are more common in adults. Vomiting can be a sign of increased intracranial pressure. Headaches from tumors in the midline, cerebellar, and ventricular areas of the cranium obstruct the normal flow of the cerebrospinal fluid, producing hydrocephalus and headache and early morning vomiting that occurs usually without nausea.

Vision Changes

Migraine headaches may have an aura that precedes them. A frequently reported visual aura is a scintillating scotoma or twinkling spots of brightly colored lights. In children, visual scintillation is the most common aura of migraine, often limited to one eye.

Cluster headaches are associated with ipsilateral conjunctival injection, lacrimation, and edema of the eyelid.

Photophobia

Photophobia is often present with migraine headaches but is not present with tension headaches. Patients with meningitis often complain of photophobia.

Dizziness

Approximately one third of patients with migraine headaches experience vertigo. The vertigo may appear as an aura, occur during the headache, or occur separately.

What Do the Aggravating and Alleviating Factors Suggest?

Key Questions

- Does anything make the headache better?
- Does anything make the headache worse?

Alleviating Factors

Patients with meningeal irritation obtain partial relief from being recumbent and lying quietly. Headaches that respond to mild analgesics are more likely to be tension headaches. Children obtain complete relief after a brief period of rest with a migraine headache, although rest does not affect a tension headache in children. Some adults experience migraine headache relief with sleep or rest, particularly in a dark, quiet environment.

Aggravating Factors

Increased headache with sneezing or coughing may indicate a benign headache or may be due to a lesion at the level of the foramen magnum, long before clinical signs are present. Migraine headaches are made worse with exertion. Patients with cluster headaches have worse pain when lying down. Headaches that are much worse in the early morning and improve on arising may indicate tumor. Benign exertional headaches can occur

during coitus. Trigeminal neuralgia pain can be triggered by stimulation of the affected nerve, produced by rubbing the face or chewing.

What Does Family History Indicate?

Key Question

- Does anyone else in the family have headaches?

Family History

TTHs have no family history. Migraines have a positive family history.

Is There Anything Else That Would Help Narrow the Cause or Causes?

Key Questions

- Have you been ill recently?
- Have you taken any medications or vitamins?
- Could you have been exposed to carbon monoxide?

Recent Health History

Any substance introduced iatrogenically into the ventricular and lumbar fluid spaces can lead to chemical meningitis. Radiographic contrast media, antibiotics, and steroids can cause headache. Lumbar puncture (LP) can cause a severe headache in 25% of patients. The headache is eased by lying down and aggravated by sitting or standing. Chronic infection, including otitis media, mastoiditis, sinusitis, dental or pulmonary infection, cardiovascular lesions with shunting, or endocarditis, predisposes to development of a brain abscess. Half of all brain abscesses occur in children with cyanotic congenital heart disease. Penetrating skull fractures can also be a portal of entry for bacteria and contribute to the occurrence of brain abscess. Melanomas may metastasize years after excision and may first be indicated by neurological changes.

History of Ingestion

Outdated tetracycline use can cause pseudotumor cerebri (increased intracranial pressure without any intracranial mass or hydrocephalus), as can excessive intake of vitamin A and substances found in some topical acne preparations.

Withdrawal from certain substances, such as caffeine or nitrates, can also produce headache.

Exposures

Exposure to carbon monoxide (CO) may cause a severe, throbbing, generalized headache. Hemoglobin values less than 10 g/dl may cause headache as a result of hypoxia.

Occupational exposure to other toxins should be assessed through an occupational history. Winter headaches may be caused by a faulty kerosene or gas heater.

DIAGNOSTIC REASONING: FOCUSED PHYSICAL EXAMINATION

Observe the Patient

Assess level of alertness and orientation to person, place, and time. Any patient who complains of headache and exhibits an ataxic gait, uncoordinated movements, or reduced mental alertness should be immediately transported to an emergency center for neurological evaluation.

A patient who appears ill or toxic is a suspect for meningitis. The patient is usually lying down with the lights off (photophobia) and may complain of chills. Most toddlers cannot communicate the characteristics of a headache but instead become irritable and cranky and rub their eyes and head.

Muscle spasm may cause tilting of the head or lifting of the shoulder when there is a posterior fossa tumor, cervical spine disease, or whiplash injury. Ptosis of the eyelid may accompany a cluster headache or brain tumor. Blinking and squinting of the eyes indicate photophobia.

Take Vital Signs and Obtain Growth Parameters

Take temperature, blood pressure, and pulse measurements. Fever may be the only sign of infection. Bradycardia and narrowing of pulse pressure are signs of increased intracranial pressure. In children, if the plotted

height and weight chart is significantly below average, consider a hypothalamic neoplasm. Plot head circumference to assess for normal skull growth. Macrocephaly may indicate hydrocephalus or brain tumor.

Palpate and Percuss the Skull

Palpate for symmetry of contour, tenderness, and lesions on the scalp, face, and neck. Palpate the temporal arteries for quality of pulse and tenderness. Focal tenderness and induration are seen in TTHs. Tenderness over nodular temporal arteries is a sign of temporal arteritis.

Brain abscesses cause pain by localized traction and produce tenderness on skull percussion over the area involved.

Auscultate the Cranium

Intracranial arteriovenous malformations may mimic migraine. Auscultate the orbit and skull to evaluate for cranial bruits.

Inspect the Ears, Eyes, Nose, Mouth, and TMJ

A thorough examination of the face, head, and neck structures is needed to detect organic disease. Examine the ears for signs of infection.

Ipsilateral lacrimation, ptosis, and pupillary constriction are seen with cluster headache. Test extraocular movement (EOM) in all fields of gaze. If a patient cannot look completely to the right or the left (lateral gaze), suspect a cranial nerve VI palsy, possibly the result of increased intracranial pressure. If EOMs are painful, consider optic neuritis.

Observe nasal mucosa for redness and swelling. Rhinorrhea and congestion are seen with sinus headaches. Observe teeth and oral mucosa because upper molar disease and poor dentition can cause headache. Tapping on the teeth or biting down on a tongue blade can elicit pain from sinusitis.

TMJ instability can cause headache pain. See Chapter 2 for a discussion of examination techniques.

Enlarged pupils seen during a headache indicate migraine; however, if they outlast a headache, then organic disease should be suspected.

Upper motor neuron facial weakness may be present in hemiplegic migraine.

Perform Ophthalmoscopy

On opthalmoscopic examination, note contour of optic disc and clarity of margins. Note papilledema and inspect vasculature for hemorrhage or exudate, venous pulsations, and arterial spasm.

Papilledema is often caused by an expanding intracranial mass and increased intracranial pressure. Optic disc atrophy suggests a chronically increased intracranial pressure or a lesion in the optic chiasm.

Meningitis does not produce fundus changes. Retinal hemorrhage in children may indicate abuse.

Assess Cranial Nerve Function

A complete assessment of cranial nerve function may provide evidence for more serious causes of headaches secondary to inflammation, traction, or metabolic imbalance.

- Cranial nerve I—Assess for smell. The sense of smell may be lost when the olfactory nerve is damaged by head injury or by a tumor in the vicinity of the olfactory groove.
- Cranial nerve II—Check visual acuity. Rarely does poor vision contribute to a headache. Poor vision may contribute to eye pain, but children equate this with headache. Double vision may be the presenting ocular symptom of increased intracranial pressure caused by a unilateral cranial nerve VI palsy or a posterior fossa lesion.
- Cranial nerves III, IV, and VI—Check visual fields. Unilateral or homonymous hemianopsia, a loss of the same half of the visual field of both eyes, can occur with migraines or brain tumor headaches when the tumor is in the occipital lobes or adjacent to the visual pathways. A half-field defect is seen with parietal lobe tumor. Cranial nerve III palsy can cause an enlargement of the pupil from compression of the nerve by an expanding lesion. The dilated pupil is always on the side of the expanding lesion. Cranial nerve VI palsy (inability to move eyes in a lateral direction) may be

found with acute hydrocephalus or cerebral edema. Nystagmus suggests a brainstem or cerebellar lesion and is usually ipsilateral. Lateral gaze nystagmus is also present with an elevated blood alcohol level. Vertical and rotatory nystagmus suggests central posterior fossa abnormality.

- Cranial nerve V—Test jaw strength, pain, and touch sensation to face. Trigeminal neuralgia pain can be triggered by stimulation of the affected nerve.
- Cranial nerve VII—Ask the patient to frown, raise eyebrows, show teeth, close eyes against resistance, and puff out cheeks. Test taste on the anterior two thirds of the tongue for sweet and salt discrimination. Salivary and lacrimal glands are innervated by cranial nerve VII.
- Cranial nerve VIII—Test hearing acuity. Unilateral deafness should be investigated to rule out acoustic neuroma.
- Cranial nerve IX, X—Observe swallowing; uvula rise.
- Cranial nerve XI—Test trapezius strength and sternocleidomastoid strength against resistance.
- Cranial nerve XII—Test tongue strength. An intracranial vascular event may cause a hemiplegia or hemiparesis that may be assessed by observing the protruded tongue drift laterally or by the inability to hold position against resistance.

Examine the Neck

Ask the patient to perform full range of motion (ROM) of the neck to observe for stiffness or difficulty with movement, which may indicate muscle tension or meningismus.

Test for Meningismus

Normally the chin can be flexed passively to touch the chest. If neck stiffness (nuchal rigidity) is present, this maneuver is not possible. With the patient supine, attempts to flex the neck cause involuntary hip flexion, and the hips rise (Brudzinski's sign). Attempts to extend the knee joint when the hip joint is flexed may cause the other limb to flex at the hip (Kernig's sign).

Assess Motor Strength and Coordination of Extremities

Asymmetrical increase in muscle tone on the affected side, contralateral to the hemisphere lesion, suggests a cerebral lesion.

Patients who exhibit forearm drift with arms extended and eyes closed may have a motor neuron or cerebellar disturbance with an expanding intracranial lesion.

Test Balance and Gait

Midline cerebellar abnormalities cause marked ataxia. The patient has difficulty standing on the ipsilateral leg and has a tendency to fall or stumble toward the side of the lesion. The gait is also wide-based and halting, and the patient turns with jerky movements. Minimal disturbance is observed when the patient hops on either foot or stands tandem (one foot behind the other).

Assess Deep Tendon Reflexes

Note asymmetry, absence, or hyperactive responses. Increase in or asymmetry of reflexes is seen with cerebral lesions. The plantar or Babinski response is often present with cerebral lesions.

Have Children Draw a Picture of Their Headache

Having a child draw a headache is an inexpensive and accurate way to help diagnosis headaches. The child is given a plain piece of paper and asked to draw a picture of how his or her headache felt before any history of the headache is taken. These drawings help to diagnose migraine headaches. Drawings for migraines include visual images such as flashing. Photophobia is depicted by showing the lights out, a dark room, or a blanket over the head. The need to lie down is also associated with migraine headache. Images for nonmigraine headaches show pictures of pounding or tight headbands. Even very young children (age 4) are able to draw stick figures with significant detail.

LABORATORY AND DIAGNOSTIC STUDIES

Complete Blood Cell Count

Complete blood cell count (CBC) is obtained to detect major blood dyscrasias. Hypoxia secondary to severe anemia can cause headache.

Blood Cultures

Blood cultures should be drawn in a patient who has a fever, headache, nuchal rigidity, and altered mental status.

Computed Tomography Scan

CT scan is the most common noninvasive initial diagnostic tool used to detect intracranial disease and should be done with new-onset severe headache or headache associated with abnormal neurological signs. A CT is done when brain abscess is suspected.

Lumbar Puncture

LP can directly measure cerebrospinal fluid pressure and be analyzed for normal values of components that are altered by disease, such as lymphocytes, glucose, protein, and presence of bacteria. An LP is performed when a central nervous system infection is suspected but is contraindicated if there is suspicion of increased intracranial pressure.

Erythrocyte Sedimentation Rate

Erythrocyte sedimentation rate (ESR) is a nonspecific test that is elevated in the presence of inflammation. An ESR should be performed when temporal arteritis is suspected.

Skull Radiograph

A radiograph of the skull is useful in post-traumatic headache. Specific views must be obtained to better observe intracranial structures, such as the pituitary gland or paranasal sinuses.

DIFFERENTIAL DIAGNOSIS

Primary Headaches

Tension-Type Headache (Muscle)

TTH is the most common type of headache in adults and occurs most often in women. The mechanism of tension headache is uncertain, but is thought to be related to sustained muscle contraction. Tension headache produces a bilateral pain, general or localized, often described as a frontotemporal bandlike distribution. The discomfort is described as a mild to moderate, nonthrobbing pain, tightness, or pressure with a gradual onset. It may last for hours or days, and recurrences may extend over weeks or months. It is associated with hunger, depression, or stress.

Migraine Without Aura (Common)

About 20% of adults experience migraines, and episodes are not uncommon in a child as young as 5 years old. The headache is unilateral and throbbing, and most often accompanied by nausea, photophobia, and exacerbation from physical activity. The headache is usually frontal or periorbital. Onset is rapid and crescendo is within hours. Migraines may recur daily, weekly, or less often, and are rare in persons more than 50 years old and during pregnancy. Chronic migraine is present when attacks occur more than 15 days in a month.

Migraine With Aura (Classic)

Classic migraine headaches are preceded by neurological signs that indicate cortical and/or brainstem involvement. Headaches may be precipitated by bright lights, noise, or tension. Auras may include visual disturbances (e.g., scintillating scotoma—a pattern of twinkling colored lights), ascending paresthesias or numbness, weakness, and aphasia. The pain may be associated with photophobia, phonophobia (noise sensitivity), nausea, and vomiting. Aura usually precedes but may accompany a headache or occur without headache.

Mixed Headache

Mixed headaches are a combination of muscular contraction and vascular dysfunction. The headache is experienced as a throbbing, constant pain during waking hours with symptoms of tightness, pressure, and muscle contraction. Family history of migraine is not uncommon.

Cluster Headache

Cluster headaches are of vascular origin and are less common than migraines. The onset is abrupt, often during the night, and the severity increases steadily. The pain is unilateral, ocular, or periocular and described as burning, piercing or neuralgic. Cluster headaches occur more often in men and last 15 minutes to 2 hours. The episodic recurrences are "clustered" in cycles of days or weeks, with remission lasting months to years. Associated symptoms include ipsilateral rhinorrhea, conjunctival injections, facial sweating, ptosis, and eyelid edema. Alcohol ingestion, stress, or vasodilation secondary to wind or heat exposure may precipitate the pain.

Benign Exertional Headache

These headaches occur suddenly and are related to coughing, sneezing, straining, running, or orgasm. Headache is the result of stretching the pain-sensitive structures in the posterior fossa. They are more common in men. The onset is sudden and "splitting," and pain may last from seconds up to 30 minutes. They should be distinguished from headache of SAH or arterial dissection.

Secondary Headaches
Infectious Origin
Sinusitis

Sinusitis is frequently associated with a sore throat irritated by postnasal discharge, facial or tooth pain, or a headache over the affected sinus that increases in intensity with coughing or bending forward. There also frequently is a cough that worsens in a lying position, morning periorbital swelling, fever, malaise, and recent upper respiratory tract infection. The maxillary sinuses are the most frequently affected. Pain in the temporal and periorbital area suggests frontal sinusitis, whereas maxillary sinusitis produces pain below the eye, in the upper teeth, or both. Ethmoid sinusitis produces medial orbit pain.

Dental Disorders

Patients with dental abscess, nerve root dysfunction, or infection may have headache and facial pain located near the site of the lesion. Tenderness elicited by tapping on the maxillary teeth with a tongue blade may indicate dental root infection or maxillary sinusitis. Inspection of the mouth may reveal ulceration or infection of pain-sensitive structures in the oral mucosa and gingiva.

Pharyngitis

Bacterial infection may irritate pain-sensitive structures in the oropharynx, leading to headache.

Otitis Media

Recurrent otitis media with sequelae of mastoiditis or chronic infection may result in headache. Signs of otitis will be seen on examination of the tympanic membrane.

Meningitis

Bacterial meningitis begins as bacteria colonize in the nasopharynx and enter the central nervous system through the dural venous sinuses or choroid plexus into the subarachnoid space. Common causal organisms in adults are *S. pneumoniae* and *meningitidis.* In children, common organisms are *S. pneumoniae* and *Haemophilus influenzae;* in neonates, group B *Streptococcus* and *Escherichia coli.* Bacterial meningitis is usually accompanied by severe systemic toxicity and mental status changes (encephalitis). In contrast, aseptic meningitis caused by enteroviruses or mumps virus produces a mild illness sometimes without fever. Photophobia and stiff neck are present in varying degrees. The person usually appears ill with a severe headache, fever, chills, myalgias, photophobia, and stiff neck. The Brudzinski and Kernig signs may be positive. A petechial skin rash may be suggestive of meningeal disease. Patients may progress to coma and have seizures.

Neurogenic Origin

Trigeminal Neuralgia

The pain associated with malfunction of the trigeminal nerve (cranial nerve V) is characterized by episodes of a series of bursts or jabs of sharp electrical, stabbing pain lasting seconds that occur repeatedly over minutes or hours with a minute or so of relief between episodes. The pain is limited to the distribution of the three branches of cranial nerve V. Headaches caused by trigeminal neuralgia are stimulated by sensory stimuli to the involved nerves, produced by rubbing or touching the face or swallowing. Trigeminal neuralgia usually occurs in women and persons more than 55 years old. In younger patients, episodes may suggest multiple sclerosis.

Optic Neuritis

Optic neuritis refers to a variety of conditions that affect the optic nerve and reduce visual function. Disorders include demyelinating disease (such as multiple sclerosis), inflammation, viral illness, metabolic disorders, and toxin exposure. The patient has an acute onset of blurred vision with extraocular motion pain that precedes the visual changes by several days. Opthalmoscopic examination reveals a slightly elevated (hyperemic) disc and a blurred disc margin. Treatment is focused on the underlying disease.

Cervical Spine Disorders

The three upper cervical nerves are sensory pathways for pain sensation felt in the posterior head and ipsilateral temporal and eye areas (see Figure 28-2). Disturbances in the neck may cause muscle spasms and pressure on other neck structures. Patients with neck-related headache have pain associated with motion of the neck. Downward pressure on the head makes the pain worse and may cause it to travel down the arms.

Temporal Arteritis (Giant Cell Arteritis)

Temporal arteritis is a vasculitis of the ophthalmic and posterior ciliary branches of the internal carotid artery. It almost always afflicts persons more than 50 years old. It produces a sharp, localized pain over a tender, nodular temporal artery. Other symptoms include fever, malaise, anorexia, weight loss, and/or polymyalgia rheumatica. Ischemic jaw pain and face pain are rare but highly suggestive. Headaches precede the major danger of temporal arteritis—blindness—by weeks. Unilateral blindness may occur suddenly and is not reversible. Left untreated, blindness may occur in the other eye. An ESR >50 mm/hr is almost always present. Suspected temporal arteritis is an emergency, and the patient needs referral to an emergency center for immediate evaluation and treatment.

Metabolic Origin

Carbon Monoxide Poisoning

CO is a colorless, odorless gas with an affinity for binding with hemoglobin to produce carboxyhemoglobin (COHb), which impairs oxygen transport. Symptoms are nonspecific and are dose related. Low COHb levels may produce mild dyspnea and tightness across the head; however, as COHb concentration increases, the headache becomes more severe and is associated with dizziness, nausea, fatigue, and dimmed vision. As COHb levels rise, symptoms increase in severity and lead to loss of consciousness and seizures. Blood gases and COHb blood levels are diagnostic. History may suggest recent smoke inhalation or similar symptoms in multiple family members.

Severe Hypoglycemia

Hypoglycemia is more likely to occur in persons with type 1 diabetes but can occur in anyone taking oral hypoglycemic agents, in younger persons who experience reactive hypoglycemia, or in persons who have ingested excessive amounts of alcohol. A dietary and medication history may lead to a specific causative factor. Headache is generalized and bilateral and is associated with dizziness and a sense of not feeling well. Some persons with diabetes may have nocturnal hypoglycemia and report nightmares and vivid dreams, night sweats, and a headache on awakening. Blood glucose levels can confirm the presence of hypoglycemia.

Drug Withdrawal

Withdrawal from prolonged use of steroids may cause migrainous headaches. Nitrites may precipitate headache. Other drugs causing cranial dilation and an aftereffect of rebound vasoconstriction include hydralazine, alcohol, histamine, nicotinic acid, and caffeine.

Dietary Ingestion

A mild to moderately severe generalized headache may occur after ingestion of tyramines (e.g., aged cheese, red wine), monosodium glutamate, and nitrites in smoked meats. A headache diary will help identify the pattern of headache related to specific foods.

Cerebrovascular Origin
Intracranial Tumor

Intracranial tumors are more common in children. Brain metastases from primary sites in the lung, breast, or kidney are more common in adults. Pain is constant and progressive, is felt in a discrete location, changes with head position, and awakens the person from sleep. Objective neurological signs are present in 98% of all children with brain tumors.

Hydrocephalus

Hydrocephalus is a collection of cerebrospinal fluid (CSF) in the ventricles of the brain and can be caused by tumors or cysts. If fontanels are still open, hydrocephalus will cause an enlargement of the head on measurement. Headache will be progressive and may be associated with neurological findings and mental status changes similar to those observed with dementia. Radiographic techniques are diagnostic, and LP may detect increased CSF pressure.

Subdural Hematoma

Subdural hematoma produces a sudden, severe headache that is associated with a history of head trauma, exertional physical activity, or pharmacological anticoagulation. There is transient loss of consciousness, stiff neck, nausea, vomiting, photophobia, pupillary dilation, and pain over the eye. A thorough history of trauma is essential to obtain. Posttrauma headache can occur hours or a day after injury.

Pseudotumor Cerebri. Teenagers being treated with topical acne preparations, menopausal women, and persons ingesting large amounts of vitamin A are at increased risk for pain from pseudotumor cerebri. Papilledema will be present in many cases, but, without it, the headache may be diagnosed as mixed type. A neurology referral is indicated to ensure that no local obstruction is present before an LP is done to assess for increased intracranial pressure. LP sometimes leads to herniation of the brainstem.

Brain Abscess

Pain is of gradual onset, deep and aching in nature, often worse in morning, and aggravated by coughing or straining. Other signs of increased intracranial pressure may be present, such as papilledema and widening pulse pressure. There may be a recent history of head injury, infection, or assault to the central nervous system.

Intracerebral Hemorrhage

ICH may result in a stroke or sudden coma and is associated with neurological findings defined by the site of bleeding. A person may present with a sudden-onset, severe head-ache, with or without a history of trauma. The severity of symptoms from bleeding intra-cranial aneurysms is correlated to the rate of hemorrhage and graded from I (asymptomatic to minimal headache with nuchal rigidity) to V (deep coma, decerebrate rigidity). Elderly persons with AIDS and persons prescribed anticoagulation therapy are at increased risk for ICH. CT scan is diagnostic.

DIFFERENTIAL DIAGNOSIS OF *Common Causes of Headache*

CONDITION	HISTORY	PHYSICAL FINDINGS	DIAGNOSTIC STUDIES
Primary Headaches Without Structural or Systemic Pathology			
Tension-type headache (muscle)	Common in adults; bilateral pain, general or localized in bandlike distribution; history of anxiety, stress, or depression	Normal physical examination; neck muscle tightness or fasciculations may be palpated	None
Migraine without aura (common)	More common in children; unilateral, throbbing pain; nausea	Photophobia and phonophobia	None
Migraine with aura (classic)	Pain precipitated by environmental stimuli; visual disturbances (scintillating scotoma) precede pain	Nausea and vomiting, photophobia and phonophobia	None
Mixed headache	Throbbing, constant pain during waking hours; muscle tightness; family history of migraine	Mix of findings related to tension and migraine headache pain	None
Cluster headache	Rare in children; abrupt, nighttime onset; unilateral periorbital pain that is severe	Ipsilateral rhinorrhea, nasal stuffiness, conjunctival injection, sweating, ptosis	None
Benign exertional headache	Sudden onset related to physical exertion, Valsalva, or coitus	Normal physical examination	May need to distinguish from subarachnoid hemorrhage with CT scan
Secondary Headaches With Structural or Systemic Pathology **Infectious Origin**			
Sinusitis	Frontal, upper molar, or periorbital pain; cough, rhinorrhea	Low to no fever; pain on palpation of frontal, maxillary sinuses; purulent nasal or postnasal discharge	Radiographs (Waters view)
Dental disorders	Localized pain in jaw and top of head	Malocclusion, caries, abscesses of teeth present, gum disease	Dental referral
Pharyngitis	Sore throat	Fever; infection of posterior pharynx	Throat culture
Otitis media	Ear pain, pain with swallowing	Fever; red, bulging tympanic membrane	None

Continued

DIFFERENTIAL DIAGNOSIS OF *Common Causes of Headache—cont'd*

CONDITION	HISTORY	PHYSICAL FINDINGS	DIAGNOSTIC STUDIES
Meningitis	Severe headache, chills, myalgias, stiff neck; toxic child or adult	Positive Kernig's and Brudzinski's signs; fever, photophobia, petechial rash may be present; mental status changes	Lumbar puncture
Neurogenic Origin			
Trigeminal neuralgia	Persons >55 yr; bursts of sharp pain over face innervated by affected nerve; triggered by stimulus to affected nerve	Normal physical examination; stimulation of triggers may provoke pain	None
Optic neuritis	Acute onset of pain with extraocular movement (EOM), followed by blurred vision	Diminished visual acuity, decreased papillary reflex, hyperemia of optic disc; pain with EOM	Ophthalmology referral
Cervical spine disorders	May have history of trauma; occipital pain, muscle stiffness	Normal physical examination or pain associated with neck motion	Cervical spine radiographs
Temporal arteritis	Age >50 yr; sharp, localized temporal pain; malaise, anorexia; history of polymyalgia rheumatica	Fever, weight loss; tender over a nodular temporal artery	Elevated ESR (>50); immediate referral for treatment
Metabolic Origin			
Carbon monoxide poisoning	History of exposure; throbbing headache, mild dyspnea	Nausea, vomiting, change in mental status, lethargy, loss of consciousness	Blood gases and carboxyhemoglobin level
Severe hypoglycemia	History of diabetes or medication, alcohol, and food ingestion; generalized headache, dizziness, sense of not feeling well	Normal physical examination or pallor, sweating, and weakness	Blood glucose level; may need self-monitoring of blood glucose to establish pattern
Drug withdrawal	Pattern of headache associated with stopping medication or substance use	Normal physical examination	Blood chemistry
Dietary ingestion	Mild to moderately severe headache after ingestion of foods or medication	Normal physical examination	Blood chemistry
Cerebrovascular Origin			
Intracranial tumor	Sudden-onset headache that is progressive, exacerbated by coughing or exercise; worse in morning; history of trauma increases risk	Papilledema, vomiting, asymmetrical reflexes, weakness, sensory deficit, or other neurological deficit	CT scan
Hydrocephalus	Progressive headache, vomiting, irritability	Rapid enlargement of head, bulging fontanels	CT scan and referral

DIFFERENTIAL DIAGNOSIS OF *Common Causes of Headache—cont'd*

CONDITION	HISTORY	PHYSICAL FINDINGS	DIAGNOSTIC STUDIES
Subdural hematoma	History of head trauma, bleeding disorders, child abuse; adult >35 yr; sudden onset of "worst ever" headache, often over eye; transient loss of consciousness	Unequal pupils, photophobia, neurological changes, seizure	CT scan and neurosurgical referral
Pseudotumor cerebri	Teens, menopausal women; history of vitamin A or tetracycline ingestion; progressive headache	Papilledema may be present	CT scan, neurology referral to assess risk related to lumbar puncture
Brain abscess	History of chronic ear infection or cyanotic heart disease	Fever, seizures, focal neurological deficits	CT scan
Intracerebral hemorrhage	Risk factors: persons >50 yr, with AIDS, taking anticoagulation therapy, or with hypertension	If conscious, abnormal neurological findings correlated with extent of lesion	Emergency transport for immediate evaluation (CT scan) and possible surgical treatment

CHAPTER RESOURCES

American College of Emergency Physicians: Clinical policy: critical issues in the evaluation and management of patients presenting to the emergency department with acute headache, *Ann Emerg Med* 39:108, 2002.

Kaniecki R: Headache assessment and management, *JAMA* 289:1430, 2003.

Lewis DW: Headaches in children and adolescents, *Am Fam Physician* 65:625, 2002.

Lipton RB, Bigal ME, Steiner TJ et al: Classification of primary headaches, *Neurology* 63:427, 2004.

Purdy RA: Clinical evaluation of a patient presenting with headache, *Med Clin North Am* 85:847, 2001.

Smetana GW: The diagnostic value of historical features in primary headache syndromes, *Arch Intern Med* 160:2729, 2000.

Stafstrom CE: The usefulness of children's drawings in the diagnosis of headache, *Pediatrics* 109:460, 2002.

Dizziness

Dizziness is a symptom that patients report to account for a variety of conditions, including vertigo, lightheadedness, and loss of balance. In children the symptom is frequently a new sensation, and the complaint is usually poorly defined. The young child may not have words to explain the symptom; family members may state that the child has trouble walking or is irritable or that the child's behavior is different. Older children, like adults, tend to categorize everything from lightheadedness and unsteadiness to spinning and falling as dizziness. This chapter is limited to the discussion of vertigo. Patients with vertigo have the sensation of either their body moving (subjective vertigo) or their environment moving around them (objective), usually described as a spinning or rotary motion.

The sensation of balance depends on interconnections among the visual, vestibular, and sensory systems. Vertigo may be thought of as a disruption of one of these three systems. Vertigo may be central, involving the brainstem or cerebellum; be peripheral, involving the inner ear or vestibular apparatus; or result from systemic causes.

Central vertigo is generally either neoplastic or vascular in origin, although any central nervous system disorder, such as multiple sclerosis, that disrupts the pathway between the vestibular apparatus and the brain may result in dizziness. Common vascular causes include recurrent intermittent vascular insufficiency, transient ischemic attack, or stroke. Migraine headache is a special vascular-related central cause of vertigo.

Peripheral vertigo is typically produced by disruption of the inner ear or vestibular apparatus. Common causes include idiopathic etiologies, vestibular nerve inflammation, inner ear inflammation or infection, or tumor.

Systemic origins include psychogenic, cardiovascular, and metabolic causes. Mixed or other causes include trauma and ototoxicity.

DIAGNOSTIC REASONING: FOCUSED HISTORY

What Does the Patient Mean by Dizziness?

Key Questions

- Describe how you feel when you are dizzy.
- Do you feel as though you or the room is spinning?
- Do you feel your balance is off?
- Do you feel like you are about to faint?

Sensation

Vertigo produces the sensation of either the patient spinning or the environment spinning around the patient. Some patients describe a sensation of their body moving forward or accelerating.

Patients may also complain of loss of equilibrium accompanying the vertigo. Neoplasms and progressive vestibule loss typically produce a change in vestibular function that is slow in onset and manifested as imbalance.

Loss of balance and lack of coordination in the absence of vertigo may be the result of degenerative, neoplastic, vascular, or metabolic disorders. With these symptoms, look for other nervous system abnormalities. Imbalance may also occur in adults as a result of impaired sensory input, either visual or kinetic, such as occurs with peripheral neuropathy.

Children who have a vague sense of unsteadiness may have peripheral neuropathy or a dysfunction of the vestibular or cerebellar system, whereas children who complain of a feeling of motion are more likely to have an abnormality of the vestibular system.

In contrast to dizziness and imbalance, lightheadedness is the feeling that one is about to faint (near syncope). Some patients describe it as a generalized weakness and the feeling that they are about to pass out if they do not lie down. True syncope, or a sudden transient loss of consciousness with concurrent loss of postural tone, always has a spontaneous recovery (see Chapter 10).

Orthostatic hypotension is a frequent cause of lightheadedness and is most common in elderly persons, occurring as a result of abnormal regulation of blood pressure. Neurological causes of orthostatic hypotension are less common and are usually accompanied by neurological findings.

In both children and adults, a complaint of lightheadedness may accompany anemia, hypoglycemia, or hyperventilation syndrome.

Does the Vertigo Result From a Systemic Cause?

Key Questions

- What other medical problems do you have?
- Would you describe yourself as anxious or nervous?
- Do the episodes occur with any specific activity or movement?

Other Medical Problems

Cardiovascular problems are a common cause of vertigo that is systemic in origin. The mechanism of vertigo may include vasomotor instability that decreases systemic vascular resistance, venous return, or both; severe reduction in cardiac output that obstructs blood flow within the heart or pulmonary circulation; or cardiac dysrhythmia that leads to transient decline in cardiac output. Patients with hypertension may experience vertigo while taking antihypertensive or potassium-depleting medications or as a result of postural hypotension.

Anxiety

Psychogenic dizziness is one of the most common causes of vertigo. Symptoms tend to be vague and may include other symptoms such as fatigue, fullness in the head, lightheadedness, and a sense of feeling apart from the environment. Patients may describe themselves as anxious or nervous. Patients may also have other psychiatric diagnoses. Stresses and tensions affecting children, such as divorce, custody battles, and day care, can cause vertiginous-like symptoms in the older child. Anxiety with hyperventilation may cause lightheadedness in a child, who then reports the symptom as dizziness.

Relationship to Activity or Movement

Dizziness when turning, especially when rolling over in bed, is usually due to vertigo. However, unsteadiness while walking is often considered to be disequilibrium, which can be caused by many factors. Dizziness on standing may be the result of decreased cerebral perfusion.

In children, attacks that occur with sudden changes of posture may be the result of hypotension, vascular disease, or positional vertigo.

Is the Vertigo Central (Brainstem or Cerebellar) or Peripheral (Vestibular) in Origin?

Key Questions

- Do you have migraine headaches?
- Do you have other symptoms that bother you?
- Do you have nausea and vomiting?
- When do the episodes occur?

Headaches

Headache is a vascular-related cause of central vertigo. Approximately one third of patients with migraine headaches experience vertigo. The vertigo may appear as an aura, occurring during the headache, or may occur separately. Some of these persons will have additional symptoms that are consistent with vertebrobasilar circulation abnormalities. Migraine both with and without headache is being recognized as a source of dizziness in children.

Other Symptoms

Patients with central vertigo nearly always have neurological symptoms such as double vision, facial numbness, and hemiparesis.

Cerebellar causes may produce other symptoms, such as loss of balance, that closely resemble those of a peripheral disorder; therefore neurological examination findings are important in differentiating the two. Pay particular attention to complaints of motor dysfunction or lack of coordination.

Vertigo that is peripheral in origin does not produce additional neurological symptoms or signs. If the patient has nausea and vomiting, suspect a peripheral vestibular apparatus problem rather than a central cause. Nausea and vomiting are common with vestibular neuronitis and labyrinthitis and occur less often with brainstem lesions.

Timing

Vertigo that occurs on first arising in the morning is usually the result of a vestibular disorder. Vertigo that occurs while turning over in bed is characteristic of benign paroxysmal positional vertigo (BPPV) (peripheral).

What Do Characteristics of the Episodes Tell Me?

Key Questions

- How long do the episodes of dizziness last?
- Is the onset sudden or gradual?
- Do you have any hearing loss?
- Do you have ringing in your ears?

Duration of Episodes

Episodes that last a few seconds are typically caused by BPPV and are usually elicited by a rapid head movement. Episodes lasting minutes to hours may be caused by Meniere's disease or recurrent vestibulopathy.

Episodes that last days or weeks are commonly produced by vestibular neuronitis. Patients may feel better when they lie completely still. Stroke can also produce long-lasting episodes. The two can be differentiated based on medical history and physical examination findings.

Sudden onset of prolonged dizziness (lasting ≥60 minutes) suggests central causes such as infection, brainstem infarction, inflammation, or vestibular hemorrhage. Trauma can also produce prolonged dizziness.

The child with chronic recurrent dizziness (episodes lasting <30 minutes) may have

central causes such as seizure problems or migraine headache. The cause may also be peripheral, such as BPPV. Chronic persistent episodes may indicate brainstem lesions, anemia, diabetes, thyrotoxicosis, or a psychosomatic disorder.

Onset

A gradual onset of dizziness is typical of an acoustic neuroma or other neoplastic process that is slow growing. BPPV can also have a gradual onset.

Acute or sudden onset of vertigo is characteristic of labyrinthitis, Meniere's disease, stroke, or vertebrobasilar causes.

Recurrent episodes are typical of BPPV, vertebrobasilar causes, and Meniere's disease.

Hearing Loss and Tinnitus

A classic triad of symptoms—vertigo, hearing loss, and tinnitus—defines Meniere's disease. Patients may also complain of a sensation of fullness in the ears. The hearing loss may be unilateral or bilateral. Patients with secondary or early tertiary syphilis may have symptoms identical to those of Meniere's disease. Tinnitus, hearing loss, and pain in the ear point to lesions in the inner ear or cranial nerve VIII.

Patients with labyrinthitis and perilymphatic fistulas may also experience hearing loss but without tinnitus. An acoustic neuroma will produce unilateral hearing loss with tinnitus. Patients with recurrent vestibulopathy usually do not complain of hearing loss.

What Else Should I Consider?

Key Questions

- What medications are you taking?
- Are you now or have you recently been ill?
- Have you had any recent injury to your head? Did you have dizziness before the head injury?
- Have you had any previous ear surgery?

Medications

Mediations that are salt-retaining or ototoxic may produce vertigo, lightheadedness, or unsteadiness. Salt-retaining drugs include steroids and phenylbutazone. Ototoxic medications include ethacrynic acid, strepto-mycin, gentamicin, aminoglycosides, aspirin, and furosemide.

Psychotropic drugs may also produce vertigo. Antihypertensive drugs may cause hypotension leading to lightheadedness. Sedatives, alcohol, and anticonvulsants may cause a sense of disequilibrium.

Current or Recent Illness

Vestibular neuronitis is associated with recent viral infection, often an upper respiratory tract infection. If a patient is currently ill, consider labyrinthitis because it is frequently associated with concomitant bacterial and viral infection. Current ear or sinus infection can produce dysfunction of the vestibular apparatus, resulting in vertigo. Recent abnormalities of middle ear ventilation and middle ear effusion are the most common cause of balance disturbance in childhood. In balance disturbance, transmission of pressure gradients through the labyrinthine windows to the inner ear fluids and the vestibular sensory receptors is altered.

History of Head Trauma

Trauma to the head or ear can cause disturbance of both peripheral and central balance mechanisms. Certain traumas can cause acute destruction of the inner ear and produce vertigo. Direct trauma can occur to the labyrinth from a temporal bone fracture. A blow to the head or a whiplash injury can also produce a concussive effect on the labyrinth. Children who have a history of head trauma can present with vertigo caused by labyrinthine damage.

Vertigo often occurs as a residual symptom and usually gradually improves over the course of a year. Trauma can also produce a fistula between the middle and inner ear, causing tympanic membrane (TM) damage and ossicle disruption.

Previous Otology History and Procedures

Patients with cholesteatoma usually have a history of chronic middle ear infection, otorrhea, and conductive hearing loss. Prior surgical procedures of the ear can produce

peripheral vertigo through disruption of the vestibular apparatus or through formation of a perilymph fistula.

DIAGNOSTIC REASONING: FOCUSED PHYSICAL EXAMINATION

Take Vital Signs and Note Blood Pressure

Assess orthostatic blood pressure to rule out postural hypotension as the cause of vertigo. Assessment is made by measuring the blood pressure in both the supine and standing positions. A drop in arterial blood pressure of at least 30 systolic and 20 diastolic mm Hg when the patient changes from the supine to the standing position indicates orthostatic hypotension.

Note General Appearance

In a patient who is currently ill, suspect labyrinthitis. In a patient who is acutely nauseated and vomiting, suspect vestibular neuronitis.

Have Patient Hyperventilate and Perform Valsalva Maneuver

Perform this testing if you suspect psychogenic vertigo because the maneuver may reproduce the vertigo in these patients. Ask the patient to perform a Valsalva maneuver and to breathe in and out or blow vigorously for 1 to 3 minutes.

Perform Vision Examination

A recent change in visual acuity or new corrective lenses may cause transient episodes of imbalance.

Perform Ear Examination

Look for the presence of effusion or infection that signals serous otitis or otitis media. Look for the presence of a cholesteatoma. It will appear as a shiny white irregular mass; foul-smelling discharge may also be present. Note the integrity of the TM; trauma may sometimes cause its disruption. Perform pneumatic otoscopy (see Chapter 2), which will enable you to determine whether changes in pressure trigger an episode of vertigo. If the patient has a fistula, changes in pressure transmitted directly to the inner ear will cause a sudden episode of vertigo.

Perform Screening Hearing Tests

Perform Rinne (AC:BC) and Weber (lateralization) tests. Expect sensorineural loss with Meniere's disease, labyrinthitis, perilymph fistula, and acoustic neuroma. In sensorineural loss, the sound lateralizes to the unaffected ear. With sensorineural hearing loss, bone and air conductions are both reduced in Rinne tests, but the ratio remains the same (AC:BC). Patients with a cholesteatoma, serous otitis, or otitis media may demonstrate a conductive hearing loss (see differential diagnosis table).

Perform Positional Nystagmus Testing/Provoking Maneuvers

A test for nystagmus assesses the function of the vestibular branch of the acoustic nerve (cranial nerve VIII). The presence and characteristics of nystagmus are important in determining central versus peripheral causes of vertigo. Nystagmus is defined by the axis on which it occurs (horizontal, vertical, rotary, or mixed) and by the direction in which it occurs. Nystagmus is composed of quick and slow components that can be observed. With the eye fixated, a slow drift away from the position of fixation is corrected by a quick movement back to the original position. The direction of the nystagmus is determined by the quick component because it is easier to see. The quick component depends on the interaction between the vestibular system and the cerebral cortex and represents the compensatory response to vestibular stimu-

lation. The slow component moves in the direction of the movement of the endolymph, a clear fluid within the membranous labyrinth of the inner ear.

Fixed nystagmus, which always beats in the same direction, occurs with peripheral disorders of BPPV, Meniere's disease, vestibular neuronitis, or labyrinthitis. Vestibular nystagmus typically consists of a horizontal-rotary, jerk motion of both the slow and fast components. The nystagmus associated with central causes may be horizontal, vertical, rotary, or inconsistent. Pronounced rotary, unidirectional upgaze or downgaze nystagmus always arises from central processes. Nystagmus that is equally rapid in both directions is characteristic of central causes. In vertigo of peripheral origin, nystagmus generally resolves on fixation within 24 to 48 hours, whereas nystagmus associated with central vertigo does not. See Table 29-1 for a comparison of characteristics.

Positional Maneuvers (Barany or Dix-Hallpike Maneuvers)

To determine the origin of vertigo and accompanying nystagmus, seat the patient on the table with the patient's head turned to the left or right. Quickly lower the patient to a lying position with the head lower than the table edge so that the ear faces the floor. Repeat with the head turned to the other side and then again with the head in the midline. The maneuver produces intense vertigo in patients with vestibular problems and may cause mild vertigo in patients with central causes. Watch for nystagmus during this

Table 29-1	Comparison of Nystagmus in Central and Peripheral Vertigo	
CHARACTERISTICS	**CENTRAL**	**PERIPHERAL**
Severity	May be disproportionate to vertigo	Proportionate to vertigo
Axis	Horizontal, vertical, rotary; unidirectional upgaze or downgaze	Horizontal, rotary
Consistency of direction	May be inconsistent	Consistent; always beats in same direction
Type	Irregular or rapid in both directions	Has both slow and quick components

maneuver. The patient's eyes should be kept open to observe the duration and direction of the nystagmus. The nystagmus associated with peripheral causes has a 3- to 10-second delay in onset, lessens with repetition, and is in a fixed direction. In contrast, the nystagmus associated with central causes begins immediately, does not fatigue with repetition, and may be in any and changing directions. With inner ear damage, the rapid phase of nystagmus is always in the same direction regardless of the direction of gaze (Box 29-1).

Provocation Maneuvers

In patients who experience vertigo associated with position changes or rapid movement of the head, provoke nystagmus and vertigo by having the patient assume the positions that cause the vertigo. Provocation assists in the diagnosis of BPPV. If you suspect a perilymph fistula, perform pneumatic otoscopy. The pressure applied to the middle ear may provoke nystagmus and vertigo.

Perform Neurological Examination

Look for brainstem or cerebellar dysfunction, which could cause abnormal neurological findings. Specifically test cranial nerves, looking for sensory and/or motor deficits. With the exception of hearing loss, cranial nerve function should be normal in patients with peripheral vertigo. Patients with brainstem

Box 29-1	**Evidence-Based Practice: Dix-Hallpike Maneuver**

The Dix-Hallpike maneuver has a positive predictive value of 83% and a negative predictive value of 52% for the diagnosis of BPPV. After the initial test, the induced symptoms are typically less intense in perhiperal vertigo; the intensity stays about the same in central vertigo. The combination of a positive Dix-Hallpike maneuver and a history of vertigo or vomiting suggests a peripheral vestibular disorder. Laboratory tests identify the etiology of vertigo in less than 1% of patients with vertigo

Data from Labuguen RH: Initial evaluation of vertigo, *Am Fam Physician* 73(3):244, 2006.

dysfunction typically have diplopia as well as changes in sensory and motor function.

Test cerebellar function. Testing gait differences while blindfolded may be helpful. Ataxia from bilateral vestibular loss is worsened by loss of visual input, whereas ataxia from cerebellar disease remains about the same. The sensitivity of gait testing is increased by watching tandem gait (heel to toe). When trying to walk a straight line, the patient with a cerebellar lesion will tend to fall toward the side of the lesion. However, gait disturbances may also be present with peripheral vertigo.

Test the patient's ability to perform rapid alternating movements (RAMs) either through pronation-supination or through touching thumb to fingers sequentially. Movements should be smooth and rhythmic, and the patient should be able to gradually increase speed. Stiff, slowed, or jerky movements indicate cerebellar dysfunction.

Perform the past-pointing test. Have the patient sit with arm extended forward and index finger pointed while you sit in the same position facing the patient. The tips of your fingers should touch. Then ask the patient to close the eyes, raise the arm above the head, and bring the arm and finger back to the same position. In patients with central lesions or unilateral vestibular abnormalities, the arm will deviate toward the side of the lesion.

Test sensory and motor function. Look for focal deficits that may occur with central vertigo. Many patients with vertigo also complain of generalized weakness; therefore it is important to distinguish between generalized weakness and focal motor impairment caused by brainstem disorder.

Perform Cardiovascular Evaluation

Note the heart rate and rhythm and attempt to detect dysrhythmias. Auscultate carotid and temporal arteries for bruits that may alert you to a cardiovascular cause for the vertigo.

Congenital heart disease can produce episodes of syncope that might be falsely interpreted as vertiginous episodes (see Chapter 10).

LABORATORY AND DIAGNOSTIC STUDIES

Audiometry

Audiometry is used to quantify hearing loss. The patient is tested at specific frequencies (pure tones) and specific intensities. Hearing loss is measured in decibels. Audiometry is used anytime the patient presents with both vertigo and hearing loss (i.e., Meniere's disease, acoustic neuroma, labyrinthitis, perilymph fistula, or use of ototoxic medications) (see Chapter 2).

Electronystagmography

Electronystagmography (ENG) electronically detects nystagmus that may not be detected visually. Vestibular function is evaluated using gaze testing, positional changes, and caloric stimulation. Eye movements are recorded electronically. Caloric stimulation is produced by ear irrigation with warm and then cool water.

ENG is most useful in diagnosing chronic peripheral disorders (i.e., Meniere's disease and persistent BPPV) to determine the degree and progression of the vestibular deficit. It may also be useful in patients with psychogenic vertigo to provide reassurance that no organic disease is present.

Magnetic Resonance Imaging

Magnetic resonance imaging (MRI) of the brain is indicated when the history and physical examination point to acoustic neuroma or a central cause of the vertigo. Consider urgent MRI if vertigo is of sudden onset or is accompanied by severe headache, direction-changing nystagmus, or neurological signs or if the patient has risk factors for stroke.

Computed Tomography

Computed tomography (CT) scanning of the brain is indicated whenever there is persistent vertigo and in all cases with additional signs of neurological disturbance. In patients with medical conditions such as renal failure, hypertension, or a hematological malignancy who have sudden onset of vertigo, CT scan is used to look for hemorrhage into the cerebellum, brainstem, or labyrinth.

Electroencephalography

An electroencephalogram (EEG) should be obtained for patients who have vertigo associated with alterations of consciousness.

Cardiac Monitoring

An electrocardiogram (ECG) or Holter monitoring can provide confirmatory information on cardiovascular causes of vertigo.

Hematology and Urinalysis

Complete blood cell count (CBC) may reveal anemia, which can cause presyncopal lightheadedness. Urine or serum glucose levels will detect diabetes mellitus, which can produce vertigo. Urine testing and blood urea nitrogen (BUN) level may reveal renal failure, which can also be associated with vertigo.

Serological Testing for Syphilis

Because secondary syphilis or early tertiary syphilis can produce the same symptoms that occur in Meniere's disease, screening is advocated by some to rule out syphilis as a cause.

DIFFERENTIAL DIAGNOSIS

Central Causes

Brainstem Dysfunction and Cerebellar Dysfunction

Central vertigo produced by disorders of the brainstem and cerebellum is usually caused by neoplastic or vascular processes, including recurrent intermittent vascular insufficiency, transient ischemic attack, and stroke. Neoplasms are usually slow growing; therefore vestibular dysfunction is of gradual onset and usually manifests as a problem with equilibrium.

Vascular causes are more common and may produce acute-onset, long-lasting, or recurrent transient episodes of vertigo. Patients usually manifest other neurological deficits. With brainstem disorders, patients may have complaints of diplopia, dysarthria, dysphagia, and paresthesia. They may demonstrate sensory and motor deficits. Cerebellar dysfunction usually results in difficulties in fine-motor coordination, including RAM, finger-to-finger testing, and gait disturbance.

Multiple Sclerosis

Multiple sclerosis can produce a wide range of neurological symptoms. Vertigo occurs in up to 50% of patients with multiple sclerosis. Disease onset is usually in the third and fourth decades of life. MRI shows characteristic demyelinating plaques.

Migraine Headache

Approximately 30% of persons with migraine headaches have vertigo. It may be present before the headache begins, during the headache, or independent of the headache. Patients may have other symptoms consistent with vertebrobasilar vascular abnormalities such as visual changes, tinnitus, decreased hearing, ataxia, or paresthesia. Diagnosis is usually made on the basis of the history.

Peripheral Causes

Benign Paroxysmal Positional Vertigo

Episodes of BPPV are characterized by acute onset of vertigo associated with rapid head movement or position changes. Many women complain of dizziness with position change around the time of their menses. The episodes are brief, lasting a few seconds. Nystagmus may be elicited by positional testing. Testing positional changes may provoke the vertigo. There is no hearing loss. Diagnosis is made on the basis of the history and clinical findings. This is one of the most common causes of vertigo, especially in older adults.

Benign Paroxysmal Vertigo of Childhood

BPV of childhood occurs most often in preschoolers. The disorder tends to be recurrent with one to four attacks per month. The episodes occur suddenly, and the child cries out for help. Vomiting, pallor, sweating, and nystagmus are common during the episode. The neurological and audiological examinations are entirely normal. Some children may have a hypoactive or absent response to caloric testing (ear irrigation with warm and then cool water).

Meniere's Disease

Meniere's disease is characterized by a classic triad of symptoms—vertigo, hearing loss, and tinnitus. A sensation of ear fullness may also be present. The attacks are abrupt and recurrent and last for minutes to several hours. The interval between attacks may be weeks or months. Between episodes, the patient is asymptomatic. On physical examination, sensorineural hearing loss is present in the affected ear, or it may be bilateral.

Vestibular Neuronitis

Vestibular neuronitis is frequently preceded by an acute viral infection. These patients usually present with severe vertigo, nausea, and vomiting. The vertigo lasts for days to weeks. Remaining completely motionless may help the symptoms. Auditory function is not affected. Physical examination reveals nystagmus that intensifies in amplitude when the gaze is directed away from the affected ear. Visual fixation minimizes the nystagmus.

Labyrinthitis

Frequently associated with a concurrent viral or bacterial illness, labyrinthitis produces severe vertigo that lasts for several days. Labyrinthitis may be a complication of otitis media or meningitis. This condition is distinguished from vestibular neuronitis by the accompanying hearing loss that occurs as a result of destruction of the inner ear.

Acoustic Neuroma

Also called a vestibular schwannoma, acoustic neuroma is a benign tumor that originates most often in the vestibular portion of cranial nerve VIII (acoustic). It usually causes unilateral sensorineural hearing loss, tinnitus, and loss of equilibrium. The neuroma grows slowly; therefore loss of equilibrium is more often a symptom than is vertigo. Acoustic neuroma can also occur in cranial nerve V (trigeminal) with symptoms of paresthesia consistent with the nerve distribution. Large tumors of cranial nerve VI (abducens) may compress the brainstem.

Perilymph Fistula

Fistula formation can occur as a result of ear trauma, from a direct blow, secondary to otologic surgery, or indirectly from straining, coughing, or pressure changes. In this condition there is leakage of perilymph from either the round or the oval window into the middle ear. Sensorineural hearing loss is frequently present as well as vertigo. The fistula will often heal spontaneously but sometimes may require surgery.

Sinusitis and Otitis

Serous otitis, otitis media, and sinusitis can cause disruption of the vestibular apparatus, producing vertigo. History and physical examination findings will be consistent with the specific disorder (see Chapters 2 and 4).

Cholesteatoma

Collection of squamous debris often associated with chronic middle ear infection can form a cholesteatoma, which enlarges and destroys structures in its way. On physical examination, the cholesteatoma will appear as a shiny white irregular mass. Foul-smelling discharge may be evident, and there may be visible bone destruction. A conductive hearing loss may be present.

Systemic Causes
Psychogenic

Psychogenic causes of vertigo are common. Patients often describe themselves as anxious or nervous and may have psychiatric diagnoses (see Chapter 32). Their symptoms are vague and imprecise. Neurological examination is normal. No nystagmus is present or elicited. The vertigo may be reproduced with hyperventilation. MRI may be useful to provide reassurance.

Cardiovascular

Orthostatic hypotension and cardiac dysrhythmias can produce vertigo. The diagnosis of postural hypotension can be made by taking orthostatic blood pressure readings. The diagnosis of cardiac conditions may involve CBC, blood chemistry, ECG, cardiac stress testing, and echocardiography.

Neurosyphilis

Secondary or early tertiary syphilis can present with symptoms similar to those of Meniere's disease. The patient demonstrates various clinical symptoms, including papilledema, aphasia, monoplegia or hemiplegia, cranial nerve (CN) palsies, pupillary abnormalities, or focal neurological deficits. The Argyll Robertson pupil, which occurs almost exclusively in neurosyphilis, is a small irregular pupil that reacts normally to accommodation but not to light. Serological testing will be positive for syphilis.

Other Causes
Ototoxic Drugs and Drugs Causing Salt Retention

Medications that are ototoxic or cause salt retention may produce vertigo, lightheadedness, or unsteadiness. Drugs causing salt retention include steroids and phenylbutazone. Ototoxic medications include aspirin, ethacrynic acid, streptomycin, gentamicin, aminoglycosides, and furosemide. Psychotropic drugs may also produce vertigo. Ototoxic drugs may produce a sensorineural hearing loss. Audiometry should be performed with any noted hearing loss.

Trauma

Injury to the head or ear can produce disturbance of the vestibular apparatus and result in vertigo, resulting from labyrinthine concussion, temporal bone fracture, or perilymph fistula. Head trauma can also produce cerebral concussion involving the anterior tip of the temporal lobe. Trauma from otologic procedures can also cause vertigo.

DIFFERENTIAL DIAGNOSIS OF *Common Causes of Dizziness*

CONDITION	HISTORY	PHYSICAL FINDINGS	DIAGNOSTIC STUDIES
Central Causes			
Brainstem dysfunction/ cerebellar dysfunction	Elderly; acute-onset; recurrent vertigo; tinnitus; hearing OK	Symptoms of brainstem/vertebrobasilar vascular abnormality: ataxia, double vision; lack of coordination; sensory/motor deficits; vertical, lateral, rotary nystagmus; hearing normal; cerebellar: impaired RAM, finger-to-finger testing	MRI
Multiple sclerosis	Often in third to fourth decade of life	May have no other findings or may have other neurological symptoms	MRI
Migraine headache	Headache history; other migraine symptoms	May have symptoms of vertebrobasilar vascular abnormalities, as above	None
Peripheral Causes			
Benign paroxysmal positional vertigo (BPPV)	Adults: associated with positional changes; recurrent episodes; lasts seconds to minutes; some relief if motionless	Lateral or rotary nystagmus; no tinnitus or hearing loss	Provoke nystagmus and vertigo by position that causes response; ENG
Benign paroxysmal vertigo of childhood	Children: usually preschoolers, sudden onset with crying by child	Vomiting, pallor, sweating, and nystagmus common; no loss of consciousness; neurological and audiological examination may be normal	May have hypoactive or absent response to caloric testing
Meniere's disease	Sudden onset; lasts hours, recurrent; tinnitus and fullness in ears	Lateral or rotary nystagmus; fluctuating hearing loss: low tones; sensorineural	Positional maneuvers, audiometry, ENG
Vestibular neuronitis	Sudden onset; antecedent viral infection	Nausea and vomiting; nystagmus; no hearing loss	Positional maneuvers
Labyrinthitis	Sudden onset, lasts hours to days	May currently be ill; lateral nystagmus; hearing loss; rarely tinnitus; nausea and vomiting may be present	Positional maneuvers, audiometry
Acoustic neuroma	Adults; gradual onset; mild vertigo; persistent tinnitus; facial numbness, weakness	Unilateral hearing loss, poor speech discrimination	MRI; audiometry
Perilymph fistula	History of trauma; hearing loss	Nystagmus and vertigo with pneumatic otoscopy; sensorineural hearing loss	Audiometry
Otitis/sinusitis	Pain in ear or face; history of ear or sinus infections; gradual onset of vertigo	Serous otitis, otitis media; tenderness over sinuses; purulent nasal discharge; no nystagmus	See Chapters 2 and 4

Continued

DIFFERENTIAL DIAGNOSIS OF *Common Causes of Dizziness—cont'd*

CONDITION	HISTORY	PHYSICAL FINDINGS	DIAGNOSTIC STUDIES
Cholesteatoma	History of chronic middle ear infections	Shiny white irregular mass on otoscopic examination; foul-smelling discharge may be present; bone destruction may be visible; conductive hearing loss may be present	Audiometry
Systemic Causes			
Psychonegic	Vague symptoms; recurrent; may describe self as anxious; may have other psychiatric diagnoses	Normal neurological and auditory examinations	Hyperventilation to reproduce the vertigo
Cardiovascular	CV history; antihypertensive medications	Orthostatic blood pressure; dysrhythmias; carotid or temporal bruits	Depends on client condition and symptoms
Neurosyphilis	Vertigo, tinnitus, fullness in ears	Various clinical symptoms; papilledema, aphasia, monoplegia or hemiplegia, central nervous palsies, pupillary abnormalities, Argyll-Robertson pupil; focal neurological deficits	Serology for syphilis
Other Causes			
Ototoxic and salt-retaining drugs	Medication history: steroids, phenylbutazone, ethacrynic acid, aspirin, streptomycin, gentamicin, aminoglycosides, furosemide, psychotropic drugs	Sensorineural hearing loss	Audiometry
Trauma	History of trauma to head or ear	Depends on nature and location of injury; may exhibit peripheral or central symptoms	MRI/CT

CHAPTER RESOURCES

Casselbrant M, Mandel E: Balance disorders in children, *Neurol Clin* 23(3):805, 2005.

Clark MM: How to sort out a complaint of dizziness, *Patient Care Nurse Pract* May:7, 2003.

Fetter M: Assessing vestibular function: which tests, when? *J Neurol* 247(5):335, 2000.

Koelliker P, Summers RL, Hawkins B: Benign paroxysmal positional vertigo: diagnosis and treatment in the emergency department—a review of the literature and discussion of canalith-repositioning maneuvers, *Ann Emerg Med* 37:392, 2001.

Labuguen R: Initial evaluation of vertigo, *Am Fam Physician* 73:245, 2006.

Lawson J et al: Diagnosis of geriatric patients with severe dizziness, *J Am Geriatr Soc* 47:12, 1999.

MacGregor D: Vertigo, *Pediatr Rev* 23:10, 2002.

Sloane PD, Coeytaux RR, Beck RS et al: Dizziness: state of the science, *Ann Intern Med* 134(9 Pt 2):823, 2001.

Weisleder P, Fife TD: Dizziness and headache: a common association in children and adolescents, *J Child Neurol* 16:727, 2001.

XII

Common Problems in Mental Status

Confusion in Older Adults

Confusion is a symptom rather than a disease state. It is the inability to think quickly or coherently. A confused patient is disoriented to time, person, or place and may demonstrate impaired cognitive function. Older adults are far more likely to experience an acute confusional state as a result of hospitalization or surgery, systemic or electrolyte imbalance, organ failure, excessive medication, nutritional deficiency, systemic infection, or cerebral insufficiency, such as stroke or transient ischemic attacks. When an older patient presents with confusion, the differential diagnosis includes delirium, dementia, or depression.

Delirium, caused by alteration in brain metabolism, is characterized by abrupt onset, reduced level of acute consciousness, and sleep/wake cycle disturbance. **Delirium is a medical emergency** and can occur as a result of medications, alcohol use or alcohol withdrawal, narcotic reaction or narcotic withdrawal, Wernicke's syndrome (vitamin B_{12} deficiency), hepatic encephalopathy, acute illness, chronic illness, interacting diseases, or trauma (e.g., head injury).

Dementia, a chronic generalized impairment of brain function, affects thinking but not level of consciousness. A common early complaint in dementia is forgetfulness, with loss of concentration and loss of memory. Causes of dementia can be classified as reversible (or partially reversible), modifiable, or irreversible (Box 30-1).

Depression as a cause of confusion, especially in the elderly, is considered a reversible cause of dementia. When anxiety symptoms are also present, depression may manifest as mild delirium (see Chapter 32).

DIAGNOSTIC REASONING: FOCUSED HISTORY

Obtaining an appropriate history from a confused patient involves the use of another person as the historian. Preferably that person is someone who has had consistent contact with the patient and can report about usual behavioral patterns and the conditions involved with this episode.

Is This a Condition That Requires Immediate Intervention?

Key Questions
- How suddenly did the confusion start?
- Is the patient alert and aware of time, person, and place?
- Has the patient expressed thoughts of suicide (in words or actions)?
- Does the patient use alcohol or other drugs?

Confusion that is acute in onset and persistent may indicate delirium, a cerebrovascular event, cerebral infection, subdural hematoma, or neoplasm. A history of altered level of consciousness and the patient's current state indicate a medical condition that requires immediate intervention. Acute-onset confusion may produce paranoia and aggression. Suicidal ideation may accompany depression and is also an indication for immediate intervention and further evaluation. If the patient has been abusing alcohol or other chemical substances, acute withdrawal may require immediate medical intervention.

If the onset is gradual and the patient is not seriously ill, consider depression or dementia. Remember that depression and

Box 30-1 | Causes of Dementia

Reversible Causes of Dementia
D Drugs/medications
E Emotional illness/depression
M Metabolic/endocrine disorders
E Eye/ear involvement/environmental
N Nutritional/neurological
T Tumors/trauma
I Infection
A Alcoholism/anemia/atherosclerosis

Modifiable Causes of Dementia
Normal pressure hydrocephalus
Hepatic encephalopathy
HIV encephalopathy (AIDS dementia complex)

Irreversible Causes of Dementia
Alzheimer's disease
Multi-infarct dementia
Huntington's chorea

dementia can coexist. Unless the patient is suicidal or seriously ill, both depression and dementia can be handled in a more temperate manner.

What Distinguishing Characteristics of Confusion Does This Patient Exhibit?

Key Questions

- Was the onset of the confusion abrupt (i.e., over a period of minutes or hours) or gradual (i.e., a few days, weeks, or months)?
- Does the confusion change within a 24-hour period (stable or fluctuating)?
- Is there a change in the sleep pattern?
- Is the patient alert and aware?
- Has the patient experienced seeing, hearing, or feeling things that are not there?
- Is there any history of head trauma?

Onset and Duration

Confusion that is abrupt in onset but short-lived may indicate a transient ischemic attack (TIA). Sudden onset, usually over a period of hours, is characteristic of delirium. In delirium, the condition is persistent but has been present for no longer than 1 month. In an acute confusional episode, the symptoms are less severe than with delirium with a less sudden onset. The onset in depression is usually gradual, over a period of weeks, and is persistent over time. In dementia, the onset is insidious and gradual; the condition has often been present for many weeks or months.

Fluctuation in Symptoms

With delirium, the symptoms may fluctuate over the course of a day and frequently are worse at night and with fatigue. The course is more stable with both depression and dementia, with little variation over a 24-hour period.

Disturbance in Sleep/Wake Cycle

The sleep/wake cycle in delirium is always impaired. Either the wakefulness is abnormally increased and the patient gets little or no sleep, or the patient has night insomnia and is drowsy and tired during the day. Thus the sleep/wake cycle is usually fragmented, and the patient tends to be restless and agitated and has hallucinations while awake during the night.

Level of Consciousness

In both dementia and depression, the individual is likely to be both alert and aware, although the mood may be depressed. With delirium, the patient will have a decreased level of consciousness, be less alert and aware, and may be difficult to arouse. With an acute confusional state, the person will demonstrate impaired concentration and make errors in thinking.

Hallucinations

Visual, tactile, and auditory hallucinations are common with delirium, especially at night when changes in environment or activity occur. Hallucinations are uncommon in both depression and dementia, although hallucinations may occur in late-stage dementia.

Head Trauma

Head trauma can produce confusion and disorientation. In older adults, common causes of head trauma include motor vehicle crashes, physical abuse, and falls.

Key Questions

- Has the patient shown any tremor, especially at rest?
- Has the patient had any trouble walking?
- Has the patient complained of severe headache and/or nausea?
- Has the patient had a fever?
- Has the patient gained or lost weight?
- Does the patient engage in his/her usual activities?

Tremor and Gait Disturbance

Tremors are associated with parkinsonism, human immunodeficiency virus (HIV) encephalopathy, and liver disease. Gait disorder is associated with parkinsonism, medication reactions, and head trauma.

Headache, Nausea, and Fever

Headache and nausea are associated with head trauma, stroke, and tumor. Fever is usually present with HIV infection, systemic infections, or acute alcohol withdrawal.

Change in Weight and Usual Activities

Patients with depression may exhibit vegetative symptoms (e.g., cessation of talking, eating, dressing, and toileting; insomnia; weight loss or gain; diminished interest in most activities or former pleasures) and feelings of worthlessness.

What Does the Pattern of Cognitive Losses Tell Me?

Key Questions

- What specific problems with mental abilities or thinking have you noticed?
- What behavioral changes or personality changes have you noticed?

Changes in Mental Abilities and Behaviors

Patients with delirium have global cognitive losses that involve memory, thinking, perception, and judgment. These patients may become completely disoriented, irritable, and fearful. They may be difficult to arouse or conversely have insomnia. Families sometimes note visual hallucinations.

Patients in an acute confusional state may be disoriented—especially for time, less for place, and almost never for self. They show impaired concentration, experience sensory misperceptions, and make errors in thinking.

Dementia, particularly early in the disorder, presents with more selective cognitive losses. Family members complain that patients cannot remember recent events, are disoriented, are irritable or depressed, have poor hygiene, show poor judgment, make financial errors, are socially withdrawn, have difficulty finding or saying the right words, are clumsy or fall, have urinary incontinence, have deteriorating interpersonal relationships, and show personality changes.

Fewer cognitive losses occur with depression. These persons may exhibit cognitive losses consistent with confusion—apathy and drowsiness, impaired concentration, and errors in thinking. The most common cognitive symptoms are severe negative thinking, guilt, and remorse.

Is the Confusion Caused by a Concurrent Health Problem?

Key Questions

- Does this patient have any chronic health conditions?
- Has the patient been hospitalized recently, and if so, for what reason?
- Has the patient been acutely ill recently?
- Is there a history of mental illness or similar thought disturbance?

Current and Past Health Status

You may need to obtain past medical records to obtain a complete medical history. Most likely you will have to use a relative or close friend to determine current and past health status. Many systemic conditions and disorders can produce alteration in mental status, particularly in older patients (Box 30-2). Chronic health problems such as alcoholism, renal failure, liver disease, severe

---

Box 30-2	**Systemic Conditions Associated With Confusional States**

Endocrine
Hypo/hyperthyroidism

Metabolic
Anemia (severe)
Hypo/hypercalcemia
Hypo/hypercortisolism
Hypo/hyperglycemia
Hypomagnesemia
Hypo/hypernatremia
Wilson's disease (copper disorder)
Porphyria

Infectious
AIDS
Cerebral amebiasis
Cerebral cysticercosis
Cerebral toxoplasmosis
Cerebral malaria
Fungal meningitis
Lyme disease
Neurosyphilis
TB meningitis

Cardiovascular
Congestive heart failure
Hyperviscosity

Cerebrovascular
Cerebral insufficiency (TIA, CVA)
Postanoxic encephalopathy

Pulmonary
COPD
Hypercapnia
Hypoxemia

Renal
Renal failure
Uremia

Neurological
Hepatic encephalopathy
Hypertensive encephalopathy
Limbic encephalitis
Head trauma

Other
Alcoholism
Anemia (severe)
Leukoencephalopathy
Metastatic cancer to brain
Sarcoidosis
Sleep apnea
Vasculitis (e.g., SLE)
Vitamin deficiencies (B_{12}, folate, niacin, thiamine)
Whipple's disease

---

anemia, chronic obstructive pulmonary disease, severe cardiovascular disease, and HIV predispose individuals, especially the elderly, to the development of confusion. Patients with multiple chronic health problems are particularly at risk.

Could the Confusion Be Caused by Medication?

Key Questions

- What medications is the patient taking?
- Is the patient taking the medications correctly?

Medications

Drugs that can produce altered mental status include the following:
- Alcohol
- Antibiotics (e.g., isoniazid, aminoglycosides)
- Anticholinergic agents
- Anticonvulsants
- Antidepressants
- Antihypertensive agents (e.g., reserpine, β-blockers, methyldopa, clonidine, hydralazine)
- Antiparkinsonian agents
- Cardiac drugs (e.g., digitalis, lidocaine, β-blockers, vasodilators, diuretics)
- Chemotherapeutic agents (e.g., methotrexate)
- Gastrointestinal drugs (e.g., H_2 blockers, metoclopramide)
- Illicit drugs (e.g., amphetamines, cocaine, opiates)
- Narcotics
- Over-the-counter cold/allergy preparations

- Sedatives
- Tranquilizers

Taking Medication Correctly
Combinations of these medications increase the probability of medication-induced confusion. People who are confused may be taking medications improperly, which compounds the problem. Further, older adults may need lower doses or a gradual increase in dosages of medications used to treat both acute and chronic conditions.

What Risk Factors Do I Need to Consider?

Key Questions
- How old is the patient?
- How many medications is the patient taking?
- Is the patient HIV positive?
- Has the patient experienced recent life losses?

Age
Older adults are at risk for the development of confusion, delirium, dementia, and depression. Factors that place them at risk include the use of multiple medications, the existence of multiple medical conditions, and the physiological changes associated with aging. Dementia occurs in approximately 5% to 10% of adults ages 65 to 80 years, 20% of those older than 80 years, and almost half of those older than 85 years.

Polypharmacy
Older adults who are taking multiple medications are at risk for medication interactions and resulting confusion (see also the preceding list of medications that can produce altered mental status).

Human Immunodeficiency Virus
Patients with HIV infection or those who are immunocompromised are at increased risk for the development of HIV encephalopathy (AIDS dementia complex) or dementia caused by central nervous system (CNS) opportunistic infections.

Recent Bereavement
Recent loss and the lack of a social network place an individual at risk for depression. Both cause profound biopsychosocial stress that can easily exceed the person's resources and skills. Extreme mourning or isolation can be physically and emotionally draining.

DIAGNOSTIC REASONING: FOCUSED PHYSICAL EXAMINATION

Take Vital Signs
The presence of a fever may indicate infection or alcohol withdrawal. A diastolic blood pressure greater than 120 mm Hg suggests hypertensive encephalopathy, whereas a systolic blood pressure less than 90 mm Hg may indicate impaired cerebral perfusion.

Note Level of Consciousness
In both dementia and depression, the individual is likely to be alert and aware, although the mood may be depressed. With delirium, the patient will have a decreased level of consciousness, be less alert and aware, and may be difficult to arouse. With an acute confusional state, the patient will demonstrate impaired concentration and have difficulty thinking.

Perform a Mental Status Examination
A thorough mental status examination is essential. Administer the Mini Mental State Examination (MMSE) (see Figure 30-1 for sample items from the MMSE). Patients with delirium may be unable to cooperate or answer questions. Patients with dementia are cooperative and willing to try but make mistakes and give incorrect or "near miss" answers. Patients with depression are less cooperative and are more likely to give "don't know" answers, refuse to answer questions, or be less willing to try.

Global cognitive loss is consistent with delirium. Losses occur in the following areas: memory, thinking, perception, information acquisition, information retention, information processing, information retrieval, and information use. Thus the MMSE score

> Orientation to Time
> "What is the date?"
>
> Registration
> "Listen carefully, I am going to say three words. You say them back after I stop. Ready? Here they are. . .
> HOUSE (pause), CAR (pause), LAKE (pause). Now repeat those words back to me."
> [Repeat up to 5 times, but score only the first trial.]
>
> Naming
> "What is this?" [Point to a pencil or pen.]
>
> Reading
> "Please read this and do what it says." [Show examinee the words on the stimulus form.]
>
> CLOSE YOUR EYES

FIGURE 30-1 Sample items from the MMSE. For a full copy of the MMSE, administration instructions, and scoring guidelines, contact Psychological Assessment Resources. Reproduced special permission of the Publisher, Psychological Assessment Resources, Inc., 16204 North Florida Avenue, Lutz, FL 33549, from the Mini Mental State Examination, by Marshal Folstein and Susan Folstein, Copyright 1975, 1988, 2001 by Mini Mental LLC, Inc. Published 2001 by Psychological Assessment Resources, Inc. Further reproduction is prohibited without permission of PAR, Inc. The MMSE can be purchased from PAR, Inc., by calling (800) 331-8378 or (813) 968-3003.

will be very low with inability to perform most or all of the items.

Dementia, particularly early in the disorder, presents with selective cognitive losses that may occur in one or more of the following areas. Specific losses include the following:

- Apraxia: cannot draw simple geometric figures
- Visuospatial problems: cannot draw intersecting pentagons
- Cannot perform commands
- Selective cognitive loss
- Loss of abstract reasoning
- Problems with orientation
- Problems with recent memory
- Problems with number retention

Fewer cognitive losses occur with depression than with dementia. Loss of concentration is an important symptom of depression. The individual is aware of losses and may highlight disabilities, especially memory loss. Along with loss of memory, impaired concentration and errors in judgment are common.

In older persons, also administer the Geriatric Depression Scale (Figure 30-2). The test is positive for depression if the score is above 5.

Perform a Complete Neurological Examination

Normal neurological findings are typical of early dementia and depression. Abnormal findings suggest other organic involvement.

Cranial Nerves

Check vision, hearing, and sensory impairment as contributing factors in confusion. Dilated pupils suggest alcohol withdrawal; pinpoint pupils may indicate narcotic excess or use of eye drops. Changes in pupil size may also indicate neurological changes such as those that occur with stroke or neoplasm. The sense of smell is often impaired in dementia. Patients with parkinsonism may exhibit a typical facial presentation: masked facial expression, poor blink reflex, and drooling. Speech is slowed, slurred, and monotonous.

Proprioception and Cerebellar Function

Test coordination through rapid alternating movements (RAMs), accuracy of movement, balance (Romberg's test), and gait. Slowed RAMs are characteristic of early HIV encephalopathy. Tremor and restlessness are associated with alcohol intoxication or

Geriatric Depression Scale (short form)

Choose the best answer for how you felt over the past week.

1. Are you basically satisfied with your life?   yes/no

2. Have you dropped many of your activities and interests?   yes/no

3. Do you feel that your life is empty?   yes/no

4. Do you often get bored?   yes/no

5. Are you in good spirits most of the time?   yes/no

6. Are you afraid that something bad is going to happen to you?   yes/no

7. Do you feel happy most of the time?   yes/no

8. Do you often feel helpless?   yes/no

9. Do you prefer to stay at home, rather than going out and doing new things?   yes/no

10. Do you feel you have more problems with memory than most?   yes/no

11. Do you think it is wonderful to be alive now?   yes/no

12. Do you feel pretty worthless the way you are now?   yes/no

13. Do you feel full of energy?   yes/no

14. Do you feel that your situation is hopeless?   yes/no

15. Do you think that most people are better off than you are?   yes/no

This is the scoring for the scale. One point for each of these answers. Cut-off: normal (0-5), above 5 suggests depression.

1. no	6. yes	11. no
2. yes	7. no	12. yes
3. yes	8. yes	13. no
4. yes	9. yes	14. yes
5. no	10. yes	15. yes

FIGURE 30-2 Geriatric Depression Scale (short form). (From Sheikh JI, Yesavage JA: Geriatric Depression Scale: recent evidence and development of a shorter version, *Clin Gerontol* 5:165, 1986.)

withdrawal. Tremor (especially resting), rigidity, and bradykinesia indicate parkinsonism. Asterixis, sometimes referred to as "liver flap" or "liver tremor," is an involuntary tremor of the hands, tongue, and feet that is characteristic of hepatic or metabolic encephalopathy. Postural tremor is present with HIV encephalopathy. Writhing movements (chorea) typify Huntington's disease.

Gait abnormalities are found with multiinfarct dementia, normal pressure hydrocephalus, and HIV encephalopathy.

Sensation (Primary and Cortical)

Agnosia (failure to identify or recognize objects despite intact sensory function) is present with dementia.

Reflexes

Test deep tendon reflexes (DTRs) and the superficial plantar reflexes. Hyperreflexia and primitive reflexes are present in late dementia. Hyperreflexia is also present in multiinfarct dementia, HIV encephalopathy, and costovertebral angle (CVA).

A positive Babinski's sign on testing the plantar reflex is present in multi-infarct dementia, CVA, and head injury. Cogwheeling (resistance to a passively stretched hypertonic muscle resulting in a rhythmical jerk similar to a ratchet) suggests parkinsonism.

Motor Tone and Function

Apraxia (impaired ability to carry out motor activities despite intact motor function) indicates dementia. Motor weakness, especially of the legs, loss of coordination, and impaired handwriting are consistent with early HIV encephalopathy.

Language

Aphasia (language disturbance) is often present in dementia and may also occur with CVA and head injury.

Localizing and Lateralizing Signs in Central Nervous System

Focal neurological signs (i.e., exaggerated DTRs, positive Babinski's sign, gait abnormalities, and hemiparesis) are consistent with multi-infarct dementia. Focal deficits also occur with cerebrovascular injury.

Patients with late HIV encephalopathy demonstrate weakness that is greater in the legs than in the arms, ataxia, spasticity and hyperreflexia, positive Babinski's sign, myoclonus, and bladder and bowel incontinence.

Psychomotor agitation or retardation is consistent with depression. An agitated confusional state without focal signs may occur with head trauma.

Perform a Respiratory Examination

Monitor the rate and effort of respirations. Auscultate the lung fields. Tachypnea suggests hypoxia. Bibasilar crackles indicate congestive heart failure (CHF) with hypoxia. Asymmetrical crackles suggest pneumonia with hypoxia. Patients with dementia or depression in the absence of concomitant lung disease will have normal findings.

Evaluate the Cardiovascular System

Perform a careful cardiovascular examination. Tachycardia suggests sepsis, hyperthyroidism, hypoglycemia, agitation, anxiety, or alcohol withdrawal. Be alert for indicators of cardiovascular problems that can produce hypoxia, such as CHF or myocardial infarction (MI).

Examine the Abdomen

Examine the abdomen and percuss for CVA tenderness. Specific findings may indicate a local or systemic cause for the confusion. For example, urinary retention suggests urinary tract infection, CVA tenderness points to pyelonephritis, and an enlarged liver may indicate hepatic encephalopathy.

LABORATORY AND DIAGNOSTIC STUDIES

Diagnostic testing is aimed at detecting or confirming a metabolic/organic cause of the confusion. If dementia seems likely, these same tests can rule in or rule out reversible or modifiable causes of the dementia. Most tests will be normal when the diagnosis is depression.

Complete Blood Cell Count

Leukocytosis suggests infection. Anemia as a cause of confusion in chronic illness can also be detected.

Blood Chemistry

High or low potassium or sodium levels, dehydration, or acidosis can all produce confusion. Elevated or depressed magnesium and calcium levels, hypoglycemia, and hyperglycemia can also cause confusion. Elevated blood urea nitrogen (BUN) and creatinine levels or an elevated BUN/creatinine ratio may indicate renal failure. Elevation in liver enzymes suggests liver dysfunction.

Thyroid Function Tests

Abnormal levels of thyroid-stimulating hormone (TSH) may indicate thyroid dysfunction, either thyroid toxicosis or a hypothyroid state. An elevated TSH level is related to chronic symptoms of depression.

Serum B$_{12}$ and Folate

Deficiencies of vitamin B$_{12}$ and folate are reversible causes of dementia.

Serology for Syphilis

A positive test can indicate neurosyphilis as the cause of confusion.

Arterial Blood Gases

Arterial blood gases (ABGs) are used to determine the presence or degree of hypoxia.

Toxicology Screen and Blood Alcohol Level

These tests can be used to determine alcohol or drug intoxication as a cause of confusion.

Urinalysis

Urinalysis is used to detect infection and may point to renal indicators of systemic disease. See Chapter 18 for a complete discussion of urinalysis.

Chest Radiograph

A chest radiograph is used to detect infection, CHF, chronic pulmonary disease, pneumonia, or other respiratory-associated causes of hypoxia.

Lumbar Puncture

Lumbar puncture is used to rule out bacterial, fungal, or tumor meningitis (see Chapter 28).

Electrocardiography

Electrocardiography (ECG) is used to rule out certain cardiovascular causes of hypoxia, such as MI or dysrhythmias.

Electroencephalography

Electroencephalography (EEG) can be used to identify a seizure disorder as a cause of or a contributing factor to confusion.

Computed Tomography or Magnetic Resonance Imaging

Computed tomography (CT) or magnetic resonance imaging (MRI) is used to diagnose cerebrovascular bleeding, injury, abscess, or tumor or if focal neurological signs are present. These imaging tests usually do not yield useful information related to the diagnosis of dementia.

Positron Emission Tomography (PET Scan)

PET is useful in confirming the diagnosis of Alzheimer's disease. PET images demonstrate the metabolic activity of organs and other tissues. A radiopharmaceutical, which includes both sugar (glucose) and a radionuclide (a radioactive element) that releases signals, is injected into the patient and its emissions are measured by a PET scanner. Using the gamma ray signals discharged by the injected radionuclide, PET measures the amount of metabolic activity at a site in the body and a computer reassembles the signals into images. PET highlights areas with increased, diminished, or no metabolic activity, thereby pinpointing problems. A distinctive image appears in the area of the brain affected by Alzheimer's disease. It can be seen in early disease. PET also is useful in differentiating Alzheimer's disease from other forms of dementia such as vascular dementia, and from other memory disorders such as clinical depression.

DIFFERENTIAL DIAGNOSIS
Delirium

The incidence of delirium increases progressively after the fourth decade of life. Because delirium is associated with an increased risk of death, it should always be considered first in patients who exhibit cognitive impairment or behavioral changes.

Delirium is characterized by reduced ability to maintain attention to external stimuli, disorganized thinking, decreased level of consciousness (LOC), perceptual disturbances, disturbed sleep/wake cycle, disorientation, and memory impairment. The patient will evidence a decreased LOC and impaired arousal, increased or decreased psychomotor activity, and irritability. The onset is rapid, and the condition can last from hours to weeks. Fluctuations over the course of the day are common, with lucid intervals during the day and worse symptoms at night. The thought process is disorganized, and the patient is usually disoriented, most commonly to time. There is a tendency for the patient to mistake the unfamiliar for familiar places and people. Hallucinations, usually visual, are common. Physical examination findings depend on the underlying cause of the delirium. The patient often exhibits asterixis or tremor. Speech is incoherent, hesitant, slow, or rapid. Box 30-3 gives *DSM-IV-TR* criteria for the diagnosis of delirium.

Confusion

Confusion is less abrupt and less severe than delirium, with less severe disorientation and more subtle motor signs. The diurnal variation is less severe than in delirium. The person may be apathetic and drowsy and will show disorientation—especially for time, less for place, and almost never for self. Concentration is impaired, and the person lacks direction and selectivity and is easily distracted. Errors in thinking are common. The person may exhibit tremor and difficulty in motor relaxation.

Dementia

Dementia is characterized by acquired persistent and progressive impairment of intellectual function, with compromise in at least two of the following areas:
- Language (aphasia)
- Memory
- Visuospatial skills (apraxia, agnosia)
- Emotional behavior or personality
- Cognition

- Calculation, abstraction, judgment, for example

Boxes 30-4 and 30-5 give *DSM-IV-TR* diagnostic criteria for dementia and Alzheimer-type dementia.

The onset of symptoms is insidious, with the course stable through the day and night. The condition can be present for months or years, with progressive deterioration. Recent and remote memory is impaired. The patient is alert and attention is relatively unaffected, although orientation is usually impaired. Hallucinations are usually absent until late in the course of the disease. Speech is usually unimpaired although the person has difficulty finding words. Sleep is often fragmented. On mental status examination, the patient tries hard and provides "near miss" answers. Physical findings are often absent. The olfactory sense may be impaired. Box 30-6 lists common presentations of dementia, Box 30-7 lists phases of Alzheimer-type dementia, and Box 30-8 describes a staging system for Alzheimer's disease.

Alzheimer-type dementia can sometimes be distinguished from vascular or multi-infarct dementia (MID) by obtaining a cardiovascular history, determining the progression of symptoms, and detecting the presence or absence of focal neurological signs and symptoms (Table 30-1).

Depression

Depression can produce confusion, especially in the elderly. The onset of the confusion is often abrupt, with some diurnal variation. Generally, depression is more consistent over

---

Box 30-3	*DSM-IV-TR* **Criteria for Diagnosis of Delirium**

A. Disturbance of consciousness (i.e., reduced clarity or awareness of the environment) with reduced ability to focus, sustain, or shift attention.
B. Change in cognition (i.e., memory deficit, disorientation, language disturbance) or the development of a perceptual disturbance that is not better accounted for by a preexisting, established, or evolving dementia.
C. Disturbance develops over a short period of time (usually hours to days) and tends to fluctuate during the course of the day.
D. History, physical examination, or laboratory evidence indicates that the disturbance is a direct physiological consequence of a general medical condition, substance intoxication, or medication side effect.

Reprinted with permission from the *Diagnostic and Statistical Manual of Mental Disorders, Fourth Edition, Text Revision*, Copyright 2000, American Psychiatric Association.

Box 30-4	*DSM-IV-TR* Criteria for Diagnosis of Dementia

A. The development of multiple cognitive defects manifested by both:
  1. Memory impairment (cannot learn new or recall previous information)
  2. One or more of the following cognitive disturbances:
     a. Aphasia (language disturbance)
     b. Apraxia (impaired ability to carry out motor activities despite intact motor function)
     c. Agnosia (failure to identify or recognize objects despite intact sensory function)
     d. Disturbance in executive functioning (planning, organizing, sequencing, abstracting)
B. The cognitive deficits in A1 and A2 cause considerable impairment in social or occupational functioning and represent substantial decline from a previous level of functioning.

Reprinted with permission from the *Diagnostic and Statistical Manual of Mental Disorders, Fourth Edition, Text Revision,* Copyright 2000, American Psychiatric Association.

Box 30-5	*DSM-IV-TR* Criteria for Diagnosis of Alzheimer-Type Dementia

Criteria as outlined in Box 30-4 for dementia plus:
C. The course is characterized by gradual onset or continuing cognitive decline.
D. The cognitive defects in criteria A1 and A2 are not the result of any of the following:
  1. Other CNS conditions that cause progressive deficits in memory and cognition (e.g., CVD, parkinsonism, Huntington's chorea, brain tumor)
  2. Systemic conditions that are known to cause dementia (e.g., hypothyroidism, vitamin B_{12} or folic acid deficiency, niacin deficiency, hypercalcemia, neurosyphilis, HIV infection)
  3. Substance-induced conditions
E. The deficits do not occur exclusively during the course of a delirium.
F. The disturbance is not better accounted for by an Axis 1 disorder (e.g., major depressive disorder, schizophrenia).

Reprinted with permission from the *Diagnostic and Statistical Manual of Mental Disorders, Fourth Edition, Text Revision,* Copyright 2000, American Psychiatric Association.

Box 30-6	Common Presentations of Dementia

Memory loss	Language difficulty
Depression	Social withdrawal
Irritability	Behavioral change
Poor hygiene	Urinary incontinence
Insomnia	Hallucinations (late)
Paranoia	Anxiety
Weight loss	Failure to thrive
Poor work performance	Falls, clumsiness
Financial errors	Deteriorating interpersonal relationships
Poor judgment	Personality changes
Delirium	

Box 30-7   **Phases of Alzheimer-Type Dementia**

Progression of symptoms corresponds with the progression of underlying nerve cell degeneration. Damage typically begins with cells involved in learning and memory and gradually spreads to cells that control thinking, judgment, and behavior. The damage eventually affects cells that control and coordinate movement.

Limbic
2 to 3 years after onset
Olfactory system involved
Memory loss
Can perform tasks

Parietal
3 to 6 years after onset
Loss of comprehension of spoken language
Cannot name common objects
Apraxia: cannot perform motor skills although motor system intact
Agnosia: failure to identify or recognize objects despite intact sensory function
Misinterprets visual and auditory stimuli
Delusions

Late Frontal
6 to 8 years after onset
Motor disturbances: walking, swallowing, moving
Primitive reflexes
Seizures
Sensation remains intact

Box 30-8   **Stages of Alzheimer's Disease**

Staging systems for Alzheimer's disease vary. The Alzheimer's Association uses seven stages to describe the progression of Alzheimer's disease.
Stage 1: No impairment (normal function)
Stage 2: Very mild cognitive decline (may be age-related changes or earliest signs of Alzheimer's disease)
• Memory lapses, especially in forgetting familiar words or names or the location of everyday objects.
• Symptoms not evident during a medical examination or apparent to friends, family or co-workers.
Stage 3: Mild cognitive decline
• Problems with memory or concentration; may be measurable in clinical testing or apparent during a detailed medical interview.
• Friends, family, or co-workers begin to notice deficiencies.
• Common difficulties include:
  1. Word- or name-finding problems noticeable to family or close associates
  2. Decreased ability to remember names when introduced to new people
  3. Performance issues in social or work settings
  4. Reading a passage and retaining little material
  5. Losing or misplacing a valuable object
  6. Decline in ability to plan or organize
Stage 4: Moderate cognitive decline (Mild or early-stage Alzheimer's disease)
• The affected individual may seem subdued and withdrawn, especially in socially or mentally challenging situations.
• Clear-cut deficiencies in the following areas:
  1. Decreased knowledge of recent occasions or current events
  2. Impaired ability to perform challenging mental arithmetic; e.g., counting backward from 100 by 7s
  3. Decreased capacity to perform complex tasks, such as marketing, planning dinner for guests, or paying bills and managing finances
  4. Reduced memory of personal history

Continued

Box 30-8	**Stages of Alzheimer's Disease—cont'd**

Stage 5: Moderately severe cognitive decline (Moderate or mid-stage Alzheimer's disease)
- Major gaps in memory and deficits in cognitive function emerge. Some assistance with day-to-day activities becomes essential.
- Individuals may:
  1. Be unable during a medical interview to recall such important details as their current address, their telephone number, or the name of the college or high school from which they graduated
  2. Become confused about where they are or about the date, day of the week, or season
  3. Have trouble with less challenging mental arithmetic; e.g., counting backward from 40 by 4s or from 20 by 2s
  4. Need help choosing proper clothing for the season or the occasion
  5. Usually retain substantial knowledge about themselves and know their own name and the names of their spouse or children
  6. Usually require no assistance with eating or using the toilet

Stage 6: Severe cognitive decline (Moderately severe or mid-stage Alzheimer's disease)
- Memory difficulties continue to worsen, significant personality changes may emerge, and affected individuals need extensive help with customary daily activities.
- Individuals may:
  1. Lose most awareness of recent experiences and events as well as of their surroundings
  2. Recollect their personal history imperfectly, although generally able to recall their own name
  3. Occasionally forget the name of their spouse or primary caregiver but generally can distinguish familiar from unfamiliar faces
  4. Need help getting dressed properly; without supervision, may make such errors as putting pajamas over daytime clothes or shoes on wrong feet
  5. Experience disruption of their normal sleep/wake cycle
  6. Need help with handling details of toileting (flushing toilet, wiping and disposing of tissue properly)
  7. Have increasing episodes of urinary or fecal incontinence
  8. Experience significant personality changes and behavioral symptoms, including suspiciousness and delusions, hallucinations, or compulsive, repetitive behaviors
  9. Tend to wander and become lost

Stage 7: Very severe cognitive decline (Severe or late-stage Alzheimer's disease)
- This is the final stage of the disease when individuals lose the ability to respond to their environment, the ability to speak, and, ultimately, the ability to control movement.
  1. Lose capacity for recognizable speech, although words or phrases may occasionally be uttered
  2. Need help with eating and toileting and there is general incontinence of urine
  3. Lose the ability to walk without assistance, and then the ability to sit without support, the ability to smile, and the ability to hold their head up
  4. Reflexes become abnormal and muscles grow rigid; swallowing is impaired

From Alzheimer's Association: *Stages of Alzheimer's disease;* accessed April 20, 2006, from http://www.alz.org/AboutAD/Stages.asp.

time than delirium. The confusion is of short duration compared with dementia. A past history of psychiatric problems, including undiagnosed depressive episodes, is common. During mental status examination, the patient tends to highlight disabilities, especially memory loss. The memory loss is equal for recent and remote events. The cognitive losses, however, are fluctuating rather than stable over time. The patient manifests a depressed or anxious mood, including sleep and appetite disturbance. Hallucinations are usually absent, although the patient may have suicidal thoughts. Depression as a cause of confusion can be easy to miss because it is often associated with anger, anxiety, and unclear thinking as well as denial (see Chapter 32).

DIFFERENTIAL DIAGNOSIS OF *Common Causes of Delirium, Confusion, Dementia, and Depression*

CONDITION	HISTORY	PHYSICAL FINDINGS	DIAGNOSTIC STUDIES
Delirium	Onset abrupt; fluctuations over course of day common with lucid intervals during day and worst symptoms at night; lasts hours to weeks; unable to maintain attention to external stimuli; disorganized thinking, perceptual disturbances, disturbed sleep/wake cycle; hallucinations, usually visual, common	Decreased LOC, impaired arousal, decreased psychomotor activity; disoriented, most commonly to time; physical examination findings depend on underlying cause of delirium; patient often exhibits asterixis, tremor, and difficulty in motor relaxation; speech incoherent, hesitant, slow, or rapid	CBC, electrolytes, glucose, BUN, creatinine, LFTs, TFTs, serum B_{12}, folate, serology for syphilis, ABGs, toxicology screen, blood alcohol level, U/A, ECG, EEG, chest radiograph, lumbar puncture, CT or MRI (when CVA or injury suspected)
Confusion	Less abrupt, less severe than delirium; diurnal variation less severe than delirium; concentration impaired, easily distracted; errors in thinking common	Apathetic, drowsy; disoriented especially for time, but less for place, almost never for self; less severe disorientation, more subtle motor signs than in delirium	CBC, electrolytes, glucose, BUN, creatinine, LFTs, TFTs, serum B_{12}, folate, serology for syphilis, ABGs, toxicology screen, blood alcohol level, U/A, ECG, EEG, chest radiograph, lumbar puncture, CT or MRI (when CVA or injury is suspected)
Dementia	Onset insidious, course stable through day and night; present for months or years, with progressive deterioration; recent and remote memory impaired; hallucinations usually absent until late in course of disease; sleep often fragmented	Alert, attentive; orientation usually impaired; on mental status examination, patient tries hard, provides "near miss" answers; demonstrates one or more of following cognitive disturbances: asphasia (language disturbance); apraxia (impaired ability to carry out motor activities despite intact motor function); agnosia (failure to identify or recognize objects despite intact sensory function); disturbance in executive functioning (planning, organizing, sequencing, abstracting); physical findings often absent in Alzheimer type; olfactory sense may be impaired; speech usually unimpaired although difficulty with finding words;	CBC, electrolytes, glucose, BUN, creatinine, LFTs, TFTs, serum B_{12}, folate, serology for syphilis, ABGs, toxicology screen, blood alcohol level, U/A, ECG, EEG, chest radiograph, lumbar puncture, CT or MRI (when CVA or injury suspected; does not yield useful information for dementia); PET scan

Continued

◆ DIFFERENTIAL DIAGNOSIS OF *Common Causes of Delirium, Confusion, Dementia, and Depression—cont'd*

CONDITION	HISTORY	PHYSICAL FINDINGS	DIAGNOSTIC STUDIES
		findings in multi-infarct dementia include focal neurological signs/symptoms: exaggerated DTRs, positive Babinski's sign, gait abnormalities, hemiparesis	
Depression	Onset of confusion often abrupt, with some diurnal variation, generally more consistent over time than delirium; confusion of short duration compared to dementia; past history of psychiatric problems common, including undiagnosed depressive episodes; cognitive losses fluctuating rather than stable over time; sleep/appetite disturbance; hallucinations usually absent although person may have suicidal thoughts	Depressed or anxious mood; tends to highlight disabilities, especially memory loss; memory loss equal for recent and remote events; physical examination often normal	Geriatric Depression Scale in elderly; CBC, electrolytes, glucose, BUN, creatinine, LFTs, TFTs, serum B_{12}, folate, serology for syphilis, ABGs, toxicology screen, blood alcohol level, U/A, ECG, EEG, chest radiograph, lumbar puncture, CT or MRI (when CVA or injury suspected)

LFTs, liver function tests; *TFTs,* thyroid function tests; *U/A,* urinalysis.

CHAPTER RESOURCES

Adelman AM, Daly MP: Initial evaluation of the patient with suspected dementia, *Am Fam Physician* 71:745, 2005.

American Psychiatric Association: *Diagnostic and statistical manual of mental disorders, ed 4, text revision: DSM-IV-TR,* Washington, DC, 2000, American Psychiatric Association.

Author: Altered mental status, *Clin Rev* 15:56, 2005.

Bostwick JM: The many faces of confusion: timing and collateral history often hold the key to diagnosis, *Postgrad Med* 108:60, 2000.

Espino DV, Jules-Bradley AC, Johnston CL et al: Diagnostic approach to the confused elderly patient, *Am Fam Physician* 57:1358, 1998.

Foreman MD, Mion LC, Tryostad L et al: Standard of practice protocol: acute confusion/delirium: NICHE Faculty, *Geriatr Nurs* 20:147, 1999.

Gleason OC: Delirium, *Am Fam Physician* 67:1027, 2003.

Thibault JM, Steiner RW: Efficient identification of adults with depression and dementia, *Am Fam Physician* 70:1101, 2004.

Sleep Problems

Each year more than 10 million Americans seek medical help about sleep problems. Patients report a subjective condition of insufficient or nonrestorative sleep despite adequate opportunity to sleep. Insomnia is prevalent in 30% to 40% of the adult population, with 10% to 15% reporting that it is chronic, severe, or both. More than 40% of parents report sleep problems with their children, and 20% of these are considered significant. The consequences of chronic sleep problems include difficulty with concentration, fatigue, lack of energy, and irritability. Sleep disturbances in the elderly can result in increased falls and accidents. In children, sleep disturbances can produce problems in learning and behavior as well as affect physical development. Further, sleep problems in children can affect family functioning. Sleep has two separate stages: rapid eye movement (REM) sleep, which is linked with dreaming, and non–rapid eye movement (NREM) sleep, which is a deeper sleep state. NREM is further divided into four sleep stages. In each stage the sleep is progressively deeper. Generally an individual moves from stage 1 (NREM) sleep to stage 4. Stages 3 and 4 are the deepest sleep stages. At the end of stage 4, a person then goes backward in the stages toward the progressively lighter sleep of stage 1. The pattern is then followed by the first REM sleep stage. Movement from stage 1 to the end of REM is termed a sleep cycle. This cycle usually lasts 90 minutes in adults and approximately 50 minutes in infants. In one night generally five cycles are completed. As sleep cycles, the REM period increases in length from 10 minutes to occupying most of the 90-minute cycle. Also the proportion of stage 2 increases, with stages 3 and 4 decreasing in length.

The total amount and composition of sleep change throughout life. Sleep quality is often judged by the amount of time spent in stage 4 sleep. People who do not have adequate REM sleep feel they have had too little sleep.

Newborns fall directly into REM sleep. This REM sleep in infancy is thought to provide the brain stimulation for maturation. At age 5 REM sleep decreases to that of the adult, approximately 20% of total sleep. The REM portion of sleep is constant through all age ranges; however, NREM sleep stages 3 and 4 begin to decline in adolescents, and in the elderly, stages 3 and 4 disappear. The elderly may experience more frequent awakenings during the night; some need to compensate for this with rest periods during the day. Some elderly clients view their pattern of diminished sleep with frustration, whereas others accept it as an opportunity to have more time for other activities.

Sleepiness is regulated by two primary processes: the body's circadian rhythm, which causes an increase in sleepiness twice during a 24-hour period (usually between midnight and 7 AM and for a brief period in the mid-afternoon), and the physiological need for sleep, which is increased by sleep loss and sleep disruption.

DIAGNOSTIC REASONING: FOCUSED HISTORY

Define the Nature of the Problem

Key Questions
- What kind of sleep problem are you (the child) having?
- Are you having difficulty falling asleep?
- Are you having difficulty staying asleep?

- Are you having difficulty staying awake during the day?
- What medications have you taken for the sleep problem?
- How long has the problem existed?

Nature of the Problem

Sleep disorders include sleeplessness (insomnia), episodic disturbance of behavior associated with sleep (parasomnias), and excessive sleepiness (hypersomnia). Most childhood sleep disorders are night awakening, inability to fall asleep, going to bed problems, circadian rhythm problems, and parasomnias. Often it is the caregiver, not the child, who perceives sleep to be a problem.

Difficulty Falling Asleep

Difficulty in falling asleep is often related to poor sleep hygiene practices, the use of medications or stimulants, or disruption in circadian rhythms. Difficulty falling asleep can occur as a result of pain or as a symptom of anxiety.

Difficulty Staying Asleep

Difficulty staying asleep occurs when the sleep cycle is disrupted; this may be related to physiological factors, illness, depression, pain, or use of medications or alcohol.

Daytime Sleepiness

Nighttime insomnia and daytime sleepiness are not isolated symptoms. Daytime sleepiness may be related to increased need for sleep because of nighttime sleep loss, or it may represent narcolepsy.

Medications

Over-the-counter and prescription medications used to promote sleep can all have short-term side effects such as daytime sleepiness and headaches. Long-term use of sleep medications often produces tolerance and a need for increased doses to achieve sleep. Some of the agents, particularly the benzodiazepines, are habituating with long-term use, and stopping them may cause withdrawal symptoms. Use of sleep medications by persons with sleep apnea may be dangerous.

Duration of Problem

Sleep disorders can be transient (lasting a few days), short term (lasting weeks), or chronic (lasting months to years). An acute problem, lasting a few days to a few weeks, can be caused by stress, acute illness, environmental disturbance, or jet lag. A chronic problem may be due to a specific sleep disorder, a mood disorder, or the use of medications or stimulant substances. Primary insomnia is diagnosed when no underlying cause can be identified.

Is This a Specific Sleep Disorder?

Key Questions

- Do you have a creeping, crawling, or uncomfortable feeling in the legs that is relieved by moving the legs?
- Does your bed partner report that your arms or legs jerk during sleep?
- Do you (the child) snore loudly, gasp, choke, or stop breathing during sleep?
- Do you (the child) have difficulty staying awake during the day or do you fall asleep during routine tasks (for adults, especially driving)?
- Do you have episodes of muscle weakness?

Limb Sensation

Restless legs syndrome includes the sensation of crawling, pulling, and tingling with an irresistible urge to move the legs. Symptoms increase in the evening, especially when the person is lying down and remaining still. Patients often have coexisting periodic limb movements in sleep.

Limb Jerking

Periodic leg movements during sleep are common in persons older than 65 years. Bilateral repeated, rhythmic jerking or twitching movements, primarily in the legs, characterize periodic limb movement disorder. Less frequently, movement occurs in the arms.

Snoring

Obstructive sleep apnea (OSA) is characterized by loud snoring and restless sleep patterns. The patient may report insomnia but more commonly notes excessive daytime sleepiness.

Passive parental smoking can be a risk factor for snoring in children. Passive smoke can provoke mucosal edema and inflammation, resulting in a narrowing of the pharynx and causing snoring.

Daytime Dozing, Excessive Sleepiness During the Day, and Muscle Weakness

Excessive daytime sleepiness may be caused by narcolepsy. Adults with narcolepsy report falling asleep while driving or while performing routine tasks. Initially, children with narcolepsy have great difficulty getting up in the mornings. When awakened, the child may appear to be confused or may be aggressive or verbally abusive. The child may fall asleep during school, in the automobile on the way home from school, or while watching television. Cataplexy is common in adults. This disorder is identified as episodes of sudden muscular weakness and atonia generally instigated by an emotional trigger. The patient will have to lean against a wall for support because his or her legs feel rubbery.

The degree of daytime sleepiness can be quantified using the Epworth Sleepiness Scale (Box 31-1).

Could the Sleep Problem Be Secondary to an Illness?

Key Questions

- Have you been ill recently?
- Do you have a chronic health condition?
- What medications (prescription and over the counter) do you take?
- Do you have depression or anxiety?

Box 31-1 | The Epworth Sleepiness Scale

One tool that may be used in evaluating daytime sleepiness is the Epworth Sleepiness Scale. The scale is a simple questionnaire that measures general level of daytime sleepiness by gauging the probability of falling asleep in a variety of situations. The patient rates on a scale of 0 to 3 the likelihood that he or she would doze in each of eight different situations as part of his or her "usual way of life in recent times."

The patient's responses are added together, and the total score can range from 0 to 24. A normal range of scores is from 2 to 10, with a modal score of 6. Scores increase linearly in obstructive sleep apnea syndrome (OSAS) patients according to the severity of the apnea. Any score higher than 10 is considered significant.

The Epworth Sleepiness Scale has high test-retest reliability in normal subjects ($r = .82$, $p < .001$). It is a unitary scale with high internal consistency (Cronbach's coefficient alpha = .88). Strengths of the tool are that it is simple, easy to understand, and a very inexpensive measurement of daytime sleepiness.

On a scale of 0 to 3, indicate the likelihood that you would fall asleep in the following situations, taking into account your usual way of life in recent times. Using the scale below, choose the most appropriate number for each situation:

0 = would never doze
1 = slight likelihood of dozing
2 = moderate likelihood of dozing
3 = high likelihood of dozing

Situation—Likelihood of Dozing:

Situation	
Reading while seated	_____
Watching TV	_____
Sitting, inactive, in a public place such as a theater or meeting	_____
As a passenger in a car for an hour without a break	_____
Lying down to rest in the afternoon when circumstances permit	_____
Sitting and talking to someone	_____
Sitting quietly after a lunch during which you did not drink alcohol	_____
In a car, while stopped for a few minutes in traffic	_____
Total:	_____

Modified from Johns MW: Daytime sleepiness, snoring and obstructive sleep apnea, The Epworth Sleepiness Scale, *Chest* 103:30-36, 1993.

Illness: Acute or Chronic

Acute illness can be a cause of sleep disturbance. In children, otitis media and chronic serious otitis, even without acute infection, can disturb sleep. Some authors believe that middle ear pressure rises when the child is supine at night and have seen sleep improve with treatment of otitis. In children, enlarged adenoids and upper airway obstruction may cause awakening.

Gastroesophageal reflux (GERD) may cause night awakening with few symptoms during the day. GERD, chronic obstructive pulmonary disease (COPD), peptic ulcer disease, and congestive heart failure are associated with paroxysmal nocturnal dyspnea (PND), which frequently disturbs sleep and is often interpreted by the patient as insomnia. Prostatic hypertrophy may cause nocturia and thus disturb sleep.

Medications

Many medications can have stimulating effects and cause sleep disruption. Common offenders include antidepressants, decongestants, bronchodilators, β-blockers, thyroid preparations, phenytoin, methyldopa, and corticosteroids. The potential sedating effects of medications should also be considered in patients who report excessive daytime sleepiness. Medications such as antihistamines often cause sleep disturbances.

Pain

Pain may interfere with sleep onset or contribute to early awakenings. Patients with chronic pain may have mood and cognitive disturbances that contribute to insomnia and early morning awakening.

Psychological Causes

Conditions causing insomnia include depression, anxiety disorder, panic disorder, mania, and acute psychosis. People with depression tend to have early morning awakening, whereas those with anxiety disorder have trouble falling asleep (see Chapter 32).

Could This Be Related to Sleep Hygiene?

Key Questions

- What is your bedtime routine?
- What else do you do in your bedroom?
- Do you consume alcohol, nicotine, or caffeine before bedtime?
- Do you exercise before bedtime?
- How do you put your child to sleep?
- Where does your child sleep?

Bedtime Routine

Sleep hygiene is related to health practices and environmental influences on sleep. It is important to have a consistent bedtime and waking-up time.

Environment

Using the bedroom for other activities such as work or watching television can produce an environment that disrupts sleep. Lights and a television that are on produce awakening cues. Routinely using the bedroom for other activities may also condition the patient to an arousal state while in the bedroom. Noise may affect sleep by leading to increasing amounts of wakefulness, increase in light sleep, and decrease in REM sleep, causing daytime sleepiness. Individual differences occur, but generally sleeping at temperatures above and below normal disrupts the ability to stay asleep.

Consumption of Stimulants

Caffeine (coffee, tea, chocolate), diet pills (with ephedrine), and nicotine are stimulants that can cause sleep disruption. Although the consumption of alcohol before bedtime promotes sleep onset, alcohol tends to shorten total sleep time and exacerbate other conditions such as GERD and sleep apnea. Alcohol withdrawal in a heavy drinker may be associated with restlessness and sleep disturbance that can continue for a prolonged period after alcohol cessation.

Exercise

Vigorous exercise before bedtime is a stimulant; it should be avoided for 1 to 2 hours before bedtime.

Child's Routine

A child who is put to bed still awake and learns to fall asleep using self-comforting measures is often able to calm himself or herself and to return to sleep when he or she rouses in the middle of the night, as do most children and adults. Toddlers are fearful of separation, and routines need to be established before bedtime. This routine allows the toddler a sense of predictability and security; having a nightly routine is helpful.

Infant Sleeping Environment

Sleeping with parents is done in many cultures. However, some infants who sleep with parents have sleep problems. As parents arise or move from the bed, the infant awakens because of the lighter sleep state. Infants in waterbeds or on very soft bedding, on couches with pillows, or in any situation in which their heads may slip between a wall or bedpost are at risk of suffocation. The sleep environment should be quiet and dark, and the room temperature should be comfortable.

Could This Be Lifestyle Related?

Key Questions

- Are you a shift worker?
- Do you sleep in the same bed each night?
- Do you travel frequently?

Shiftwork

Shiftwork, particularly periodic shiftwork, has been a reported cause of sleep disruption. It may interrupt the usual circadian rhythm or alter usual sleeping patterns and habits.

Sleep Environment

Sleeping in unfamiliar surroundings affects the quality of sleep and increases sleep latency. It is associated with more wakefulness, an increased amount of light sleep, and a shorter REM sleep stage.

Travel

Jet lag is a common cause of sleep disruption. It may interrupt the usual circadian rhythm or alter usual sleeping patterns and habits. Even 1 to 2 hours of time zone change can disrupt the usual sleep/wake pattern.

Could This Be Age Related?

Key Questions

- How old is the patient (e.g., a child, adolescent, older adult)?
- What age was the child when the problem began?
- Does your child have problems going to bed?
- Does your child refuse to go to sleep?
- Does your child wake up screaming at night?

Age: Child

Newborns wake every 20 minutes to 4 hours during a 24-hour period, reflecting their sleep/wake cycle. This cycle changes between 3 and 6 months with the establishment of a diurnal sleep/wake rhythm. During this time, an initial "settling" period that typically takes 10 to 20 minutes begins to occur. Daytime sleep decreases over the next 3 years and consolidates at night. At age 4, most children no longer nap. School-age children sleep approximately 8 hours a night.

Problems Going to Sleep/Sleep Refusal

Toddlers have a strong attachment to their caregiver, and separation from this person at bedtime causes distress and sleep problems. Further, older toddlers who are in the preoperational stage are developing a sense of autonomy and use going to bed as an issue of control and/or a general pattern of oppositional behavior. Examination of the child's naptime is important. In the school-age child and adolescent, problems going to sleep may be caused by anxiety, negative conditioning, delayed sleep phase (often due to caffeine), or a bedtime that is too early. Vigorous activity before bedtime may delay sleep onset.

Wake Up Screaming at Night

Night terrors are nocturnal episodes in which the child sits straight up in bed, screams, and is inconsolable for up to 30 minutes before relaxing and falling back to sleep. These actions occur within the first few hours of sleep. The child is not readily awakened, although he or she may seem to be awake. The child is not able to be consoled and has no recollection of the event the next day.

Nightmares are bad dreams that awaken the dreamer. They occur later at night than night terrors. Unlike night terrors, the dream is remembered, and the child is awake and may be consoled by the caregiver.

Age: Adolescent

Adolescents have an increase in the amount of sleep required. However, a concomitant decrease in the amount of sleep obtained leaves most adolescents with a sleep debt. To recover from the debt, the adolescent sleeps later on the weekends.

Age: Menopausal Women

Menopause-related changes may contribute to or cause sleep disturbance. Hot flashes promote arousal from sleep. Menopause is associated with reduced total sleep time, prolonged time to initiate sleep, and reduced REM sleep.

Age: Older Adult

Older adults achieve less total nighttime sleep. They may take longer to initiate sleep, spend more time in the lighter stages of sleep, and experience increased fragmentation of the entire sleep cycle.

Older adults have more nighttime arousals and awakenings. Sleep is shorter in duration, more shallow, and more fragmented. Older persons tend to awaken earlier in the morning. If the onset of sleep is not correspondingly earlier, excessive daytime sleepiness may result. Daytime napping may compound the probe by reducing the drive for sleep at the usual bedtime hour.

Could This Be Conditioned Insomnia?

Key Questions

- Are you able to fall asleep easily in places other than the bedroom?
- If a child: What does the child do when he or she awakens at night?
- If a child: What actions do you take to get the child back to sleep?

Sleep Location

Most cases of insomnia develop initially in response to a psychosocial stressor. As sleeplessness persists, the patient begins to associate the bed with wakefulness and heightened arousal rather than sleep. The patient may fall asleep easily outside the bedroom (e.g., while watching television or reading in another room) but feel wide awake in bed.

Child's Need for Comfort or Food

Infants who are soothed and cuddled and placed in bed when they are asleep do not learn how to settle themselves; when these infants are aroused at night, they require the same routine to fall back asleep. Children who do not have self-comforting behaviors will be unable to fall asleep on their own. These criers awaken, cry, and want to be held or rocked before they can go back to sleep. An infant older than 6 months who continues to wake during the night is considered a trained night crier.

Children who need to be fed after they are awakened at night are trained night feeders. The child does not need the additional nutrition but becomes conditioned to a feeding to go back to sleep. Caregivers often bottle-feed or breastfeed the child until the child falls back to sleep. The intake of nighttime feeding after 7 or 8 months of age may prevent the development of a more mature circadian rhythm. This rhythm is a digestive-endocrine-sleep/wake cycle that adjusts to a day/night cycle, resulting in a consolidation of sleep.

Could This Be Somnambulism?

Key Question
- Do you (the child) sleepwalk?

Sleepwalking usually occurs only once a night and lasts about 15 minutes. The person gets out of bed and moves about slowly and in an automatic manner with a blank facial expression. The person may mumble. After a great deal of effort, the person can be awakened with little or no memory of the episode.

DIAGNOSTIC REASONING: FOCUSED PHYSICAL EXAMINATION

Obtain Growth Parameters
Children who have OSA may present with failure to thrive. In adults, obese middle-age men and older men with hypertension are most often affected by sleep apnea.

Inspect the Ears
Otitis media and serous otitis may cause wakefulness in infants and children because of the pressure of fluid accumulation in the middle ear, especially when in the supine position.

Inspect the Nose
Obstruction of the nose by secretions may cause sleep apnea in infants younger than 6 weeks. In children older than 6 weeks or in adults, nasal obstruction may cause OSA.

Inspect the Mouth, Throat, and Neck
Look for a narrow pharyngeal space, a long or edematous uvula, and enlarged tonsils and adenoids. Enlarged tonsils may cause obstruction while the person is sleeping. In adults, a heavy or thick neck is a risk factor for sleep apnea.

Auscultate the Lungs
Nighttime wheezing in patients with asthma often causes sleep disturbances. Congestive heart failure is a risk factor for sleep apnea.

Palpate the Abdomen
GERD may elicit upper abdominal pain on palpation.

LABORATORY AND DIAGNOSTIC STUDIES

Sleep Diary
A sleep diary should be kept for 1 to 2 weeks. Have the patient record bedtime, total sleep time, time until sleep onset, number of awakenings, use of sleep medications, time out of bed in the morning, a rating of quality of sleep, daytime symptoms, daytime naps, number and time of alcoholic drinks, and life stresses.

Sleep Studies
Objective assessment of sleep uses polysomnography (PSG) to assess sleep apnea, specific sleep stage abnormalities, nocturnal myoclonus, and unusual nocturnal behaviors. PSG includes an electroencephalogram (EEG), electro-oculogram (EOG), electromyelogram (EMG), electrocardiogram (ECG), measures of oxygen saturation, carbon dioxide values, nasal and oral airflow, thoracic and abdominal respiratory movements, and leg muscle activity. The PSG is taken during sleep, usually for the entire night. A multiple sleep latency test (MSLT) is a series of four or five nap opportunities, each separated by a 2-hour interval. The 15- to 20-minute naps are used to assess sleep disorders such as obstructive sleep apnea and narcolepsy.

Actigraphy
Actigraphy is a technique to record activity during waking and sleeping without application of any electrodes. An actigraph is worn on the wrist and is about the size of a watch. It records movement and nonmovement data plotted against time for 1 or 2 weeks. The patient wears the device continuously during sleep and daily routine activities. Actigraphy is suitable for extended examination of the sleep/wake cycle.

DIFFERENTIAL DIAGNOSIS

Restless Legs Syndrome
Restless legs syndrome includes the sensation of crawling, pulling, and tingling with an irresistible urge to move the legs. Symptoms increase in the evening, especially when the person is lying down and remaining still. The symptoms occur before sleep, causing a delay in sleep onset. Patients often have

coexisting periodic limb movements in sleep. Renal failure with uremia or iron or folate deficiency sometimes underlies restless legs syndrome.

Periodic Leg Movement
Periodic leg movements during sleep are common in people older than 65 years. Bilateral repeated, rhythmic jerking or twitching movements, primarily in the legs, characterize periodic limb movement disorder. Less frequent movement can occur in the arms. The movements occur every 20 to 90 seconds and can cause brief arousal that disrupts sleep and decreases the amount of time in the deep stages of sleep. The patient may not report waking up but complains that sleep was not refreshing. The condition commonly coexists with restless legs syndrome.

Obstructive Sleep Apnea
OSA is characterized by loud snoring, restless sleep patterns, and decreased oxygenation of circulating blood. When OSA has signs of right-sided heart failure, it is labeled obstructive sleep apnea syndrome (OSAS). During sleep, the normal tone of the airway muscles is relaxation, especially during REM sleep cycles. However, the diaphragm during this time is active. The activity of the diaphragm unchecked by the airway muscles leads to the collapse of the upper airway. Associated with this is any anatomical barrier such as enlarged adenoids, with resulting obstruction.

Risk factors for sleep apnea include male sex and obesity (especially a heavy or thick neck). The condition may be associated with hypothyroidism, neurodegenerative disorders, and cardiovascular disorders. Generally in children, OSA is the result of enlarged tonsils and adenoids after age 6 weeks. Children ages 4 to 6 years are most prone to this condition. Most children presenting with OSA have failure to thrive and may also exhibit nocturnal enuresis, hyperactivity, learning problems, and morning headaches.

The patient may report insomnia but more commonly notes excessive daytime sleepiness. Hundreds of apneic episodes occur during the night. The frequent interruptions coupled with repeated drops in blood oxygen saturation may cause a marked decline in daytime alertness and performance. The patient should be evaluated in a sleep laboratory.

Narcolepsy
Narcolepsy is a disorder of excessive daytime sleepiness. It is characterized by sudden, irresistible attacks of daytime sleepiness that last 10 to 30 minutes. Most adults with narcolepsy also experience cataplexy, a sudden loss of muscle tone, that occurs in response to sudden emotional stimuli. Although the episodes are typically brief, the person is at risk for falls or other accidents because he or she cannot move or speak. Cataplexy is not commonly seen in children. Sleep paralysis usually occurs once or twice a week at the time of sleep onset. There is a period of mental alertness, but the person is paralyzed except for respiratory and eye musculature. Hypnagogic (brief, vivid, dreamlike) hallucinations typically occur at sleep onset. Involuntary daytime sleep attacks may begin in adolescence or young adulthood. People with this problem may have symptoms for years before the disorder is diagnosed. Not all persons with the disorder experience all symptoms. Narcolepsy is fairly uncommon in children.

Secondary to Illness or Medications
GERD, COPD, peptic ulcer disease, and congestive heart failure are associated with paroxysmal nocturnal dyspnea. The sleep disturbance is often interpreted by the patient as insomnia. Prostatic hypertrophy may cause nocturia and thus disturb sleep.

Many medications can have stimulating effects and cause sleep disruption. Common offenders include antidepressants (activating selective serotonin reuptake inhibitors), decongestants, bronchodilators, β-blockers, thyroid preparations, phenytoin, methyldopa, and corticosteroids.

Pain may interfere with sleep onset or contribute to early awakenings. Patients with chronic pain may have mood and cognitive disturbances that contribute to insomnia and early morning awakening.

Psychological conditions that cause insomnia include depression, anxiety disorder, panic disorder, mania, and acute psychosis.

Poor Sleep Hygiene

Sleep hygiene is related to health practices and environmental influences on sleep. Bedtime routines or environmental distracters or stimulants affect the ability to fall asleep. Lights and a television that are on produce awakening cues. Routinely using the bedroom for other activities may also condition the patient to an arousal state while in the bedroom. Noise may reduce the amount of REM sleep and lead to daytime sleepiness.

Caffeine, diet pills, and nicotine are stimulants that can cause sleep disruption. Alcohol consumed before bedtime tends to shorten total sleep time and exacerbate other conditions such as GERD and sleep apnea.

A child who is put to bed still awake and learns to fall asleep using self-comforting measures is often able to calm himself or herself and return to sleep when he or she rouses in the middle of the night, as do most children and adults. Toddlers are fearful of separation and routines need to be established before bedtime.

Infants who sleep with parents may have sleep problems. As parents arise or move from the bed, the infant awakens because of the lighter sleep state. There have been reports of alcohol abuse, obesity, and a deeply sleeping parent rolling over onto the child. The American Academy of Pediatrics recommends that all infants sleep on their backs for the first 6 months of life to decrease the risk of sudden infant death syndrome (SIDS). The sleep environment should be quiet and dark and the room temperature should be comfortable.

Lifestyle

Shiftwork, particularly periodic shiftwork, has been a reported cause of sleep disruption. It may interrupt the usual circadian rhythm or alter usual sleeping patterns and habits.

Sleeping in unfamiliar surroundings affects the quality of sleep and increases sleep latency. It is associated with more wakefulness, an increased amount of light sleep, and a shorter REM sleep stage.

Jet lag is a common cause of sleep disruption. It may interrupt the usual circadian rhythm or alter usual sleeping patterns and habits. Even 1 to 2 hours of time zone change can disrupt the usual sleep/wake pattern.

Age Related
Night Awakening

Newborns wake every 20 minutes to 4 hours during a 24-hour period, reflecting their sleep/wake cycle. This cycle changes between 3 and 6 months with the establishment of a diurnal sleep/wake rhythm. During this time an initial "settling" period that typically takes 10 to 20 minutes begins to occur. The infant drifts from stage 1 NREM sleep into stage 3 or 4. The infant may return to stage 1 and cycle again. After one or two cycles of NREM sleep, REM is entered at about 60 to 90 minutes. The initial one third of the night is mostly deep sleep (NREM stages 3 and 4). The last half of the night is predominantly stage 2 NREM and REM. Daytime sleep decreases over the next 3 years and consolidates at night. At age 4, most children no longer nap. School-age children sleep approximately 8 hours a night. Stage 4 sleep decreases to 75 to 80 minutes. This decline is associated with an increase in stage 2 sleep. The onset of REM sleep decreases from about 140 minutes in the 6- to 7-year-old to 124 minutes in the 10- to 11-year-old.

Sleep Refusal

Toddlers are emerging from a sensory motor period to a preoperational period. They have a strong attachment to their caregiver, and separation from this person at bedtime causes distress and sleep problems. Further, older toddlers who are in the preoperational stage are developing a sense of autonomy and use going to bed as an issue of control and/or a general pattern of oppositional behavior. Examination of the child's naptime is important. In the school-age child and adolescent, anxiety, negative conditioning, delayed sleep phase (often caused by caffeine), or a bedtime that is too early may be the cause. Also, vigorous activity before bedtime may delay sleep onset.

Night Terrors

Night terrors are nocturnal episodes in which the child sits straight up in bed, screams, and is inconsolable for up to 30 minutes before relaxing and falling back to sleep. These actions occur within the first few hours of sleep. Children at around the age of 3 years have NREM occurring more in the first part of the night; this may account for the night terror. The child is not readily awakened, although he or she seems to be awake. It is not possible to console the child, and the child has no recollection of the event the next day. Night terrors occur between the ages of 3 and 10 years.

Nightmares

Nightmares are bad dreams that awaken the dreamer. They occur later at night than night terrors and occur during REM sleep, which in children is near the end of the sleep cycle. Unlike night terrors, the dream is remembered and the child is awake and may be consoled by the caregiver. Nightmares occur at any age.

Adolescent Patterns

Adolescents have an increase in slow-wave sleep with an increase in the amount of sleep required. However, most adolescents are in a sleep debt because they tend to leave less time for sleep. Repeated changes in the sleep cycle (short sleep periods followed by occasional long sleep periods) may disrupt the circadian rhythm, causing a delayed sleep phase syndrome.

Menopausal Women

Menopause-related changes may contribute to or cause sleep disturbance. Evidence that sleep difficulties are related to the hormonal changes of menopause is mixed. Hot flashes and night sweats promote arousal from sleep.

Older Adult Patterns

Sleep in older adults is characterized by more nighttime awakenings and reduced or nonexistent deep states of NREM sleep. However, REM sleep tends to be preserved. That older adults sleep less than younger adults may reflect their ability to sleep, not their need to sleep. Although a mild deterioration in sleep quality may be normal in the aging process, significantly disrupted nighttime sleep or excessive daytime functioning is not considered part of normal aging. Older persons have a circadian rhythm disruption and tend to awaken earlier in the morning. If the onset of sleep is not correspondingly earlier, excessive daytime sleepiness may result. Daytime napping may reduce the drive for sleep at the usual bedtime hour. A night owl pattern is delayed bedtime until early morning hours, and the condition may progress to day-night reversal, where sleep does not begin until dawn and continues until midday.

Conditioned Insomnia
Trained Night Crier

Children who do not have self-comforting behaviors will be unable to fall asleep on their own. These criers awaken, cry, and want to be held or rocked before they can go back to sleep. An infant older than 6 months who continues to wake during the night is considered a trained night crier.

Trained Night Feeder

A child who needs to be fed once awakened at night is noted as a trained night feeder. The child does not need the additional nutrition but becomes conditioned to requiring a feeding to go to sleep. Caregivers often bottle-feed or breastfeed the child until the child falls back to sleep. The intake of nighttime feeding after 7 or 8 months of age may prevent the appearance of a more mature circadian rhythm. This rhythm is a digestive-endocrine-sleep/wake cycle that adjusts to a day/night cycle, resulting in a consolidation of sleep. Continued nocturnal feeding keeps the infant in a recurrent interruption pattern and prevents consolidation of sleep and frequent night awakenings.

Somnambulism

Sleepwalking occurs during NREM stages 3 and 4, which occur in the initial one third of the night. Sleepwalking usually occurs only once a night and lasts about 15 minutes. The person gets out of bed and moves about slowly and in an automatic manner with a blank look on the face. Sometimes the person is mumbling; after a great deal of effort, the person can be awakened but will have little to no memory of the episode. Providing a safe environment is important because genuine risk of injury exists during the sleepwalking episode. Sleepwalking in an elderly person may be a sign of dementia.

DIFFERENTIAL DIAGNOSIS OF *Common Causes of Sleep Disorders*

CONDITION	HISTORY	PHYSICAL FINDINGS	DIAGNOSTIC STUDIES
Specific Disorders			
Restless legs syndrome	Irresistible urge to move legs while in bed	Normal	Sleep studies
Periodic limb movement	Older than 65 years; reports of rhythmic jerking of legs or arms while asleep	Normal	Sleep studies
Obstructive sleep apnea	Apneic episodes, loud snoring, restless sleep patterns	Decreased O_2; enlarged adenoids, tonsils	Sleep studies: polysomnography
Narcolepsy	Excessive sleepiness, cataplexy		Referral to sleep specialist
Secondary to illness or medications	GERD, COPD, PND, CHF, enlarged prostate/nocturia; depression or anxiety Medications: antidepressants, decongestants, bronchodilators, β-blockers, thyroid preparations, phenytoin, methyldopa, corticosteroids	Consistent with medical condition	Consistent with underlying medical condition; trial off or change of medication(s)
Poor sleep hygiene	Routine, habits, environment not conducive to sleep; use of alcohol, caffeine, diet pills, nicotine	Normal	Sleep diary
Lifestyle	Shift work, travel, jet lag	Normal	Sleep diary
Age Related			
Night awakening	Single to repeated awakening at night	Initial physical examination to eliminate medical associated illness	As directed by examination
Sleep refusal	Refusal of child to go to sleep	Normal	None
Night terrors	Inconsolable awakening occurring early in sleep, lasting 15 minutes, no memory of event	Normal	None
Nightmares	Occur later in sleep cycle; dream is remembered	Normal	None
Adolescent patterns	Decrease in amount of sleep obtained	Normal	Sleep diary
Menopausal women	Hot flashes	Consistent with menopause	Sleep diary

Continued

DIFFERENTIAL DIAGNOSIS OF *Common Causes of Sleep Disorders—cont'd*

CONDITION	HISTORY	PHYSICAL FINDINGS	DIAGNOSTIC STUDIES
Older adult patterns	Nighttime arousals and awakenings; night owl pattern; early wakening; daytime napping	Physical examination to rule out underlying medical condition	Sleep diary
Conditioned insomnia	Identify initial trigger with persistent problem	Physical examination to rule out underlying medical condition	Sleep diary
Trained night crier	Child unable to soothe self	Normal	None
Trained night feeder	History of frequent feedings on awakening at night	Normal	None
Somnambulism	Sleepwalking in early sleep cycle	Normal	None

CHAPTER RESOURCES

Anders T, Eiben L: Pediatric sleep disorders: a review of the past 10 years, *J Am Acad Child Adolesc Psychiatry* 36:9, 1997.

Bower CM: Pediatric obstructive sleep apnea syndrome, *Otolaryngol Clin North Am* 33:49, 2000.

Capp P, Pearl P, Lewin D: Pediatric sleep disorders, *Prim Care Clin Office Pract* 32(3): 549-562, 2005.

Culpepper L: Insomnia: a primary care perspective, *J Clin Psychiatry* 66(suppl 9):14, 2005.

Davis KF, Parker KP, Montgomery GL: Sleep in infants and young children: part two: common sleep problems, *J Pediatr Health Care* 18(3):130, 2004.

Doghramji PP: Detection of insomnia in primary care, *J Clin Psychiatry* 62(suppl 10):18, 2001.

Doghramji K, Neubauer DN: Insomnia: waking up to a significant problem, *Consultant* 45(suppl 13):53, 2005.

Hajak G: Insomnia in primary care, *Sleep* 23(suppl 3):S54, 2000.

Hoban TF: Sleep and its disorders in childhood, *Semin Neurol* 24(3):327, 2004.

Howard B, Wong J: Sleep disorders, *Pediatr Rev* 22:327, 2001.

Roth TY, Roehrs T: Sleep organization and regulation, *Am Acad Neurol* 54:52, 2000.

Shaver JL, Zenk SN: Sleep disturbance in menopause, *J Womens Health Gend Based Med* 9:109, 2000.

Thiedlke C: Sleep disorders and sleep problems in childhood, *Am Fam Physician* 63:277, 2001.

Zunkel GM: Insomnia: overview of assessment and treatment strategies, *Clin Rev* 15(7):38, 2005.

Mood Changes, Behavior Changes, and Psychosocial Concerns

A large percentage of primary care visits have psychological or psychosocial origins. A practitioner must first rule out organic causes for symptoms, mood changes, and behavior changes. Some patients are able to express that their symptoms may be related to situational stress or a psychosocial cause. Others may be able to identify that psychological or emotional difficulties are causing worrisome symptoms or symptoms that interfere with their ability to function. Often the practitioner suspects an underlying psychological or psychosocial disturbance that the patient may not be able to articulate. This chapter focuses on some commonly encountered psychological conditions and psychosocial concerns, and provides an approach to elicit more information, determine suicidal risk, and evaluate for a diagnosable psychological disorder (Figure 32-1).

Do not assume that an emotional symptom has a psychosocial cause until physical causes have been fully explored. Anxiety and depression are both prevalent in the primary care setting. Although they are distinct and separate diagnoses, they often co-occur. Substance use is encountered either as a primary condition or as a co-morbid condition and may be a consequence of a psychological or psychosocial condition, or the cause of a psychosocial concern.

DIAGNOSTIC REASONING: FOCUSED HISTORY

Is This a Psychosocial Problem?

Key Questions (to self)
- Does the presenting concern provide any clues?
- Are there behavioral cues present?

Presenting Concern

Fatigue, lack of energy, sleep disturbance, and an inability to concentrate are symptoms that may bring a patient to the primary care setting. These symptoms are common in patients experiencing situational stress, depression, anxiety, or substance use problems. Prolonged somatic symptoms that have not been diagnosed, such as headache, chest pain, abdominal pain, low back pain, or dizziness, may suggest a psychosocial or psychological cause. It is imperative that you consider these clues as you rule out an organic cause. Also see specific chapters that address these symptoms.

Behavioral Cues

A history of frequent primary care or emergency department visits for unexplained symptoms may point to a psychosocial cause. Sometimes the patient's affect and general appearance do not match the presenting concern. An emotional response that is not consistent with the severity of the presenting problem or situation may point to a psychosocial problem.

Agitation and restlessness reported or observed by others are a common manifestation of depression, anxiety, and/or substance abuse. Changes in personality or in relationships are associated with substance use, depression, and anxiety.

Could This Be a Result of a Physiological Problem?

Key Questions
- History and review of systems (ROS) questions based on the presenting concern
- Have you had a major illness recently?
- How long have you had these symptoms?

FIGURE 32-1 A suggested approach to the visit. There are areas of overlap.

History and ROS for Presenting Concerns

See specific chapters that discuss the presenting concern: Chapter 9, Chest Pain; Chapter 13, Abdominal Pain; Chapter 28, Headache; Chapter 29, Dizziness; Chapter 30, Confusion in Older Adults; Chapter 31, Sleep Problems; Chapter 34, Fatigue.

Chronic Conditions

Mood disorders can occur secondary to a physiological condition. Patients who have had a major health event such as a myocardial infarction, stroke, or trauma or who have chronic symptoms such as pain are at risk for the development of depression.

The mnemonic THINC MED is useful when evaluating for underlying organic causes for changes in mood or behavior. Box 32-1 identifies conditions that are commonly associated with anxiety and depression.

Could This Be Caused by Medication?

Key Questions

- What prescribed medications are you currently taking?
- What over-the-counter (OTC) and/or herbal medicines do you take?
- What dietary supplements are you taking?

Medication History

Many medications can cause psychiatric symptoms and mood changes. Box 32-2 lists medications that can produce symptoms of depression, anxiety, and mania.

Box 32-1 **THINC MED**

Major categories of medical conditions that mimic psychological conditions are as follows:

T: Tumors

H: Hormones (e.g., thyroid, adrenal, gonads, insulin)

I: Infections and immune diseases (e.g., AIDS, lupus, syphilis, Lyme disease)

N: Nutrition

C: Central nervous system (e.g., head trauma, seizures, multiple sclerosis, Parkinson's disease, dementia)

M: Miscellaneous (e.g., sleep apnea, anemia, congestive heart failure)

E: Electrolyte abnormalities and toxins (e.g., hypercalcemia, hypo/hyperphosphatemia, hypo/hypernatremia)

D: Drugs (including nicotine, caffeine, prescribed medications, illicit drugs, and alcohol)

From Goolsby MJ, Grubbs L: *Advanced assessment: interpreting findings and formulating differential diagnoses,* Philadelphia, 2006, FA Davis.

OTC Medications, Herbal Medicines, and Dietary Supplements

Some OTC medications, herbal preparations, and dietary supplements may contribute to psychiatric symptoms. A complete list of all preparations that the patient is taking is a starting point for evaluating side effects and interactions.

Is This a Domestic Violence Situation?

Key Questions

- Have you been hit, kicked, punched, or otherwise hurt by someone within the past year?
- Do you feel safe in your current relationship?
- Is there a partner from a previous relationship who is making you feel unsafe now?

A positive response to any one of these three questions constitutes a positive screen for partner violence (Feldhaus, et al, 1997). The first question, which addresses physical violence, has been validated in studies as an accurate measure of 1-year prevalence rates. The latter two questions evaluate the perception of safety and provide estimates of the short-term risk of further violence and the

---

Box 32-2 **Medications Associated With Changes in Mood**

Medications That Can Cause Symptoms of Depression
Antivirals
Anticonvulsants
Barbiturates
Benzodiazepines
Beta-adrenergic blockers
Antiparkinsonian medications
Calcium-channel blockers
Antabuse
Estrogens
Fluoroquinolone antibiotics
Statins
Interferon alfa
Accutane
Narcotics

Medications That Can Cause Symptoms of Anxiety
Thyroid hormones
Theophylline
Albuterol

Medications That Can Cause Symptoms of Mania
Anticholinergics
Cogentin
Corticosteroids
Cyclosporine
Antiparkinsonian medications
Capoten
Tagamet
Antabuse
Thyroid hormones
Monoamine oxidase inhibitors (MAOIs)
Opioids

---

need for counseling, but reliability and validity evaluations have not yet been established. A positive screen requires further assessment and clinical follow-up, including ascertaining patient safety.

Could This Be Situational Stress or Normal Grief?

The BATHE model provides a framework for understanding the patient in the context of his/her total life situation (Lieberman, 1997).

Key Questions

Background—ascertains the context of the visit
- What is going on in your life?
- What is going on right now?
- Has anything changed recently?

Affect—elicits the emotional response and allows the patient to label the feeling
- How do you feel about that?
- What is your mood?

Trouble—determines the symbolic meaning of the situation for the patient
- What about the situation troubles you most?
- What worries or concerns you?

Handling—helps to assess patient resources and responses to the situation
- How are you handling that?
- How are you coping?

Empathy—reflects an understanding that the patient's response is reasonable under the circumstances
- That must be very difficult for you.
- I can understand that you would feel that way.

BATHE Model

This model provides a patient-centered technique that helps establish a relationship with the patient, that serves as a rough screening test for anxiety, depression, or situational stress disorders, and that takes minimal time.

Could This Be a Result of Substance Abuse?

Key Questions

- In the past year, have you used alcohol or drugs more than you meant to?
- Have you wanted or needed to reduce your drinking or drug use in the past year?

A positive response to one question indicates a substance use concern. When the screen is positive, the CAGE questions can be used to detect alcoholism. Other substances can be substituted for alcohol in the CAGE questionnaire (Box 32-3, CAGE). Other questionnaires for alcohol use are also available (Box 32-4, TACE; and Box 32-5, RAFFT).

Box 32-3 CAGE Questionnaire

A framework for detecting alcoholism*

C: Concern, Cut down	Have you ever felt you should Cut down on your drinking?
A: Annoyed	Have people Annoyed you by criticizing your drinking?
G: Guilt	Have you ever felt bad or Guilty about your drinking?
E: Eye-opener	Have you ever had an Eye-opener drink first thing in the morning to steady your nerves or get rid of a hangover?

From Ewing JA: Screening for alcoholism using CAGE. Cut down, annoyed, guilty, eye opener, *JAMA* 280:1904, 1998.
*Answering "yes" to one or more of the four questions raises a high index of suspicion for alcohol abuse and dependence. The CAGE questionnaire has been used and tested extensively in many populations. It is considered to be a reliable method of screening for alcohol abuse in adults. It has reported sensitivities of 43% to 94% and specificities ranging from 70% to 97%.

Box 32-4 TACE Questionnaire

A framework for prenatal detection of risk drinking*

T: Tolerance	How many drinks does it Take to make you feel high? (Positive = more than 2)
A: Annoyed	Have people Annoyed you by criticizing your drinking?
C: Cut down	Have you felt you ought to Cut down on your drinking?
E: Eye-opener	Have you ever had an Eye-opener drink first thing in the morning to steady your nerves or get rid of a hangover?

From Sokol RJ, Martier SS, Ager JW: The TACE questions: practical prenatal detection of risk-drinking, *Am J Obstet Gynecol* 160:863, 1989.
*A positive answer to T alone or to two of A, C, or E may signal a problem with a high degree of probability, and positive answers to all four indicates great certainty of a problem.

Box 32-5	**The RAFFT Questionnaire**

A framework for detecting substance use disorders in adolescents
R: Relax   Do you drink or take drugs to Relax, feel better about yourself, or fit in?
A: Alone   Do you ever drink or take drugs while you are Alone?
F: Friends   Do any of your closest Friends drink or use drugs?
F: Family   Does a close Family member have a problem with alcohol or drugs?
T: Trouble   Have you ever gotten into Trouble from drinking or taking drugs?

From Bastiaens L, Francis G, Lewis K: The RAFFT as a screening tool for adolescent substance use disorders, *Am J Addict* 9:10, 2000.

How Can I Narrow My Diagnosis?

Begin with broad screening questions. If the patient's response to the screening question(s) is positive, proceed to elicit more specific symptoms. While a negative response to a given screening question decreases the likelihood of a disorder, the sensitivity of such screening is not perfect, and answers should be interpreted within the context of the patient's entire history and physical examination.

Key Questions

- Is there a personal or family history of mental illness?
- Over the past 2 weeks, have you felt down, depressed, or hopeless?
- Over the past 2 weeks, have you had little interest or pleasure in your daily activities?
- Do you tend to be an anxious or nervous person?
- Have you had periods of feeling so happy or energetic that your friends told you were talking too fast or that you were too "hyper"?

Prior Mental Illness, Family History

A personal or family history of prior mental illness increases the likelihood of a current mental illness. Studies support the influence of both behavioral and biological factors in the development of mental health conditions.

Down, Depressed, Hopeless, Loss of Interest or Pleasure

These are cardinal symptoms for depression, and the presence of at least one of these symptoms is required to diagnose clinically significant depression. Research suggests that

Box 32-6	**SIG E CAPS**

Neurovegetative signs in depression
S : Sleep disorder (either increased or decreased sleep)
I : Interest deficit (anhedonia)
G : Guilt (worthlessness, hopelessness, regret)
E : Energy deficit
C : Concentration deficit
A : Appetite disorder (either decreased or increased)
P : Psychomotor retardation or agitation
S : Suicidality

From Carlat DJ: The psychiatric review of symptoms: a screening tool for family physicians, *Am Fam Physician* 58:1617, 1998.

these two questions (Over the past 2 weeks, have you felt down, depressed, or hopeless? and Over the past 2 weeks, have you felt little interest or pleasure in your daily activities?) are as effective as longer inventories. If screening is positive, confirm with a more thorough assessment of neurovegetative signs (Box 32-6).

Anxious or Nervous

While there are no validated screening questions for anxiety, asking patients whether they feel anxious or nervous is useful as a general screen. Clinical experts suggest that unexplained somatic symptoms along with complaints of agitation and difficulty maintaining concentration suggest anxiety rather than depression.

A positive response to the above question can prompt further screening:
- Do you have anxiety or panic attacks?
- Have you had to limit your activities because of your anxiety?

The first question helps to differentiate anxiety from panic attacks. The second question points toward panic with agoraphobia. If the patient is not certain what you mean by the term "panic attacks," you can provide a simple description to clarify: "A panic attack is a sudden rush of fear and nervousness that makes your heart pound and makes you afraid you're going to die or go crazy" (Carlat, 1998).

Happy, Energetic, Hyper

In the presence of depressive symptoms, a positive response to the last key question is helpful in screening for bipolar disorder. If the screen is positive, the mnemonic "DIGFAST" can be used to confirm the cardinal symptoms of mania (Box 32-7).

What About Special Considerations for Adolescents?

For adolescents, a psychosocial review of systems can serve as a screen for areas that may be of concern or that have the potential to create problems. The HEEADSSS method of interviewing provides structure and a framework for focusing assessment of the **H**ome environment, **E**ducation and employment, **E**ating, peer-related **A**ctivities, **D**rugs, **S**exuality, **S**uicide/depression, and **S**afety from injury and violence (Goldenring & Rosen, 2004).

Key Questions

The HEEADSSS interview progresses from less intimidating questions about home, family members, and the past to more personal and private issues (Box 32-8). While the HEEADSSS interview is designed to be used in a reasonably short period of time, in many instances you will not be able to ask all the questions and have time for the adolescent to respond. Some questions are considered essential, while other questions can be asked as time permits or as the situation demands.

Is This Patient at Risk For Suicide?

Key Questions

■ Have you been feeling that life is not worth living or that you are better off dead?

> ### Box 32-7 | **DIG FAST**
>
> **Cardinal symptoms of bipolar disorder**
> **D :** Distractibility
> **I :** Indiscretion (excessive involvement in pleasurable activities)
> **G:** Grandiosity
> **F :** Flight of ideas
> **A:** Activity increase
> **S :** Sleep deficit (decreased need for sleep)
> **T :** Talkativeness (pressured speech)

From Carlat DJ: The psychiatric review of symptoms: a screening tool for family physicians, *Am Fam Physician* 58:1617, 1998.

■ Sometimes when a person feels down or depressed he or she might think about dying. Have you been having thoughts like that?

If yes, to the above questions:
■ Do you have a plan?
■ What is the plan?
■ Do you have the means to carry it out?
■ What would cause you to carry out your plan or keep you from carrying it out?
■ Have you ever attempted suicide in the past?

Initial Questions

The first set of questions helps determine if the patient is at risk. Patients rarely volunteer thoughts of suicide, so it is important to ask directly. There is no evidence to suggest that asking about suicide precipitates suicidal thinking or acts.

Follow-Up Questions

The second set of questions helps you evaluate how imminent the risk is. Patients at high risk for suicide should be referred for psychiatric evaluation; those at imminent risk should be admitted for evaluation and treatment. Major risk factors for suicide include hopelessness, substance abuse, and prior suicide attempts.

How Do I Evaluate for a Diagnosable Psychological Disorder?

All positive screening tests for mental health disorders require follow-up with a full diag-

Box 32-8	The HEEADSSS Psychosocial Interview for Adolescents

ESSENTIAL QUESTIONS	AS TIME PERMITS	FOR MORE IN-DEPTH
Home		
Who lives with you? Where do you live? Do you have your own room?	Have you ever run away? (Why?) Is there any physical violence at home?	
What are relationships like at home?		
To whom are you closest at home?		
To whom can you talk at home?		
Is there anyone new at home? Has someone left recently?		
Have you moved recently?		
Have you ever had to live away from home? (Why?)		
Education and Employment		
What are your favorite subjects at school? Your least favorite subjects?	Tell me about your friends at school. Is your school a safe place? (Why?)	Do you feel connected to your school? Do you feel as if you belong?
How are your grades? Any recent changes? Any dramatic changes in the past?	Have you ever had to repeat a class? Have you ever had to repeat a grade? Have you ever been suspended?	Are there adults at school you feel you could talk to about something important? (Who?)
Have you changed schools in the past few years?	Expelled? Have you ever considered dropping out?	
What are your future education/ employment plans/goals?	How well do you get along with the people at school? Work?	
Are you working? Where? How much?	Have your responsibilities at work increased?	
Eating		
What do you like and not like about your body?	Do you worry about your weight? How often?	What would it be like if you gained (lost) 10 pounds?
Have there been any recent changes in your weight?	Do you eat in front of the TV? Computer?	
Have you dieted in the last year? How? How often?	Does it ever seem as though your eating is out of control?	
Have you done anything else to try to manage your weight?	Have you ever made yourself throw up on purpose to control your weight?	
How much exercise do you get in an average day? Week?	Have you ever taken diet pills?	
What do you think would be a healthy diet? How does that compare to your current eating patterns?		
Activities		
What do you and your friends do for fun? (With whom, where, and when?)	Do you have any hobbies? Do you read for fun? (What?)	
What do you and your family do for fun? (With whom, where, and when?)	How much TV do you watch in a week? How about video games?	
Do you participate in any sports or other activities?	What music do you like to listen to?	
Do you regularly attend a church group, club, or other organized activity?		

Continued

Box 32-8	The HEEADSSS Psychosocial Interview for Adolescents—cont'd

ESSENTIAL QUESTIONS

AS TIME PERMITS

FOR MORE IN-DEPTH

Drugs

Do any of your friends use tobacco? Alcohol? Other drugs?

Does anyone in your family use tobacco? Alcohol? Other drugs?

Do you use tobacco? Alcohol? Other drugs?

Is there any history of alcohol or drug problems in your family? Does anyone at home use tobacco?

Do you ever drink or use drugs when you are alone?

(Assess frequency, intensity, patterns of use or abuse, and how youth obtains or pays for drugs, alcohol, or tobacco.)

(Ask the RAFFT questions, Box 32-5.)

Sexuality

Have you ever been in a romantic relationship?

Tell me about the people that you've dated. OR Tell me about your sex life.

Have any of your relationships ever been sexual relationships?

Are your sexual activities enjoyable?

What does the term "safer sex" mean to you?

Are you interested in boys? Girls? Both?

Have you ever been forced or pressured into doing something sexual that you didn't want to do?

Have you ever been touched sexually in a way that you didn't want?

Have you ever been raped, on a date or any other time?

How many sexual partners have you had?

Have you ever been pregnant or worried that you may be pregnant? (females)

Have you ever gotten someone pregnant or worried that this might have happened? (males)

What are you using for birth control? Are you satisfied with your method?

Do you use condoms every time you have intercourse?

Does anything ever get in the way of always using a condom?

Have you ever had a sexually transmitted infection (STI) or worried that you had an STI?

Suicide and Depression

Do you feel sad or down more than usual? Do you find yourself crying more than usual?

Are you "bored" all the time?

Are you having trouble getting to sleep?

Have you thought a lot about hurting yourself or someone else?

Does it seem that you've lost interest in things that you used to really enjoy?

Do you find yourself spending less and less time with friends?

Would you rather just be by yourself most of the time?

Have you ever tried to kill yourself?

Have you ever had to hurt yourself (by cutting yourself, for example) to calm down or feel better?

Have you started using alcohol or drugs to help you relax, calm down, or feel better?

Box 32-8	**The HEEADSSS Psychosocial Interview for Adolescents—cont'd**

ESSENTIAL QUESTIONS	AS TIME PERMITS	FOR MORE IN-DEPTH
Safety (Savagery)		
Have you ever been seriously injured? (How?) How about anyone else you know?	Have you ever been in a car or motorcycle accident? (What happened?)	
Do you always wear a seatbelt in the car?	Have you ever been picked on or bullied? Is that still a problem?	
Have you ever ridden with a driver who was drunk or high? When? How often?	Have you gotten into physical fights in school or your neighborhood? Are you still getting into fights?	
Do you use safety equipment for sports and/or other physical activities (for example, helmets for biking or skateboarding)?	Have you ever felt that you had to carry a knife, gun, or other weapon to protect yourself? Do you still feel that way?	
Is there any violence in your home? Does the violence ever get physical?		
Is there a lot of violence at your school? In your neighborhood? Among your friends?		
Have you ever been physically or sexually abused? Have you ever been raped, on a date or at any other time? (If not asked previously)		

From Goldenring J, Rosen D: Getting into adolescent heads: an essential update, *Contemp Pediatr* 21:64, 2004.

nostic interview using standard diagnostic criteria such as those from the text revision of the fourth edition of the *Diagnostic and Statistical Manual of Mental Disorders* (*DSM-IV-TR*) to determine the presence or absence of specific disorders. The manual describes specific symptom criteria for mental disorders and psychosocial problems. While primary care providers often diagnose and treat patients with symptoms of depression and anxiety, serious impairment of mental or emotional functioning, psychoses, bipolar disorder, and substance abuse disorders require evaluation, diagnosis, and treatment by qualified mental health specialists. Primary care is not a substitute for psychiatric care. Once a patient has been screened and is suspected to be at high risk for a condition, the primary care practitioner has a responsibility to refer the patient to an appropriate resource. See the differential diagnosis table at the end of this chapter for the diagnostic criteria for some common psychological disorders.

DIAGNOSTIC REASONING: FOCUSED PHYSICAL EXAMINATION

Physical examination may yield little additional data that are of diagnostic value. No physical finding is specific for any psychological disorder. The physical examination should be directed at identifying organic-based conditions that mimic psychological disorders. Perform a comprehensive and thorough physical examination if the patient has not had one since the onset of symptoms. This chapter presumes that you have performed the physical evaluation for specific presenting symptoms as part of your process to rule out a physiological cause.

Assess Vital Signs

When substance abuse is suspected, vital signs can quickly confirm the presence of an organic condition related to substance intoxication or withdrawal. Abnormal values for body temperature, blood pressure, heart rate, or respiratory rate indicate a need for a thorough evaluation.

Observe General Appearance

Look for signs of depression or substance abuse, such as an unkempt personal appearance, unusual dress, and general state of poor nutrition—skin condition and appearance of hair and nails. Observe the patient's demeanor and appearance for signs of neglect or a facial expression that might indicate depression. Observe for behaviors such as finger tapping and pacing that indicate anxiety. Methamphetamine users will often have self-induced facial lesions secondary to scratching.

Adolescents who are using substances may wear clothing or jewelry that displays drug-oriented graffiti.

Observe Mental Status

Perform a mental status examination if you suspect cognitive losses or confusion (see Chapter 30).

Note Speech and Thought Process

Speech tone, quality, and rate reflect mental status. In depression, the speech may be soft and monotonous with little spontaneity. In mania, the speech may be rapid, pressured, and loud, and the speech content consists of a flight of ideas.

Examine the Eyes

Substance users may have eyes that are injected, jaundiced, puffy, or glassy. Pupils may be dilated or constricted. The patient may have droopy eyelids and a sleepy appearance or a fixed stare. He/she may have difficulty controlling eye movements.

Examine the Nose and Mouth

Substance users may have chronic rhinorrhea, frequent nosebleeds, or lesions in the nose or around the nostrils. The patient may have dry lips, halitosis, or an odor of alcohol, marijuana, or tobacco.

Examine the Skin

Look for skin lesions that may reflect depression or anxiety, such as neurogenic scratching, nail biting, and hair pulling. Look for evidence of attempted self-injury or suicide.

Adolescents may show evidence of "cutting" scars or superficial cuts on areas of the body. While typically not suicide attempts, the cutting serves as a coping mechanism for unrelieved feelings.

In substance users, the skin may be cold and clammy, itching and burning, tight, swollen, or puffy. The person may perspire excessively and have discolored fingers or injection marks along the veins. Tattoos or burn marks, possibly done while under the influence, may disguise injection marks. The patient may have injuries or bruises from falling or fighting.

Assess Balance and Gait

The patient who has a substance use problem may have a slow gait or poor balance.

LABORATORY AND DIAGNOSTIC STUDIES

There are no laboratory tests to assist in the diagnosis of most psychological conditions. Focus the laboratory and diagnostic studies based on the presenting complaints (see specific chapters).

Commonly performed tests to help identify underlying conditions include the following:

Complete Blood Count (CBC) With Indices and Differential

The CBC will provide information about the presence of infection or anemia.

Serum Electrolytes

Hyponatremia or hypernatremia can exacerbate symptoms of depression. Hypercalcemia and hyperphosphatemia can exacerbate depression.

Thyroid Function Tests

An elevated level of thyroid-stimulating hormone (TSH) is related to chronic symptoms of depression. A hyperthyroid state may be associated with anxiety.

Toxicology Screen and Blood Alcohol Level

Urine and blood screening tests can be used to determine alcohol or drug intoxication as a cause of psychological symptoms.

DIFFERENTIAL DIAGNOSIS

Normal Stress

Stress is the nonspecific response of the body to any demand. The perception of a demand as stressful depends upon the individual's experience of how much demand for adaptation an event or situation requires. Stressors can be acute or chronic. External stressors include adverse physical conditions (such as pain) or stressful psychological environments (such as poor working conditions, abusive relationships, or major life events). Internal stressors can be physical (such as infections or inflammation) or psychological (such as worry). Daily hassles or situational factors influence the stress load because minor annoyances that happen daily can accumulate. Situational factors can exacerbate a depressive disorder in significant ways. Symptoms of stress include mental, physical, and behavioral symptoms. Common physical symptoms include responses of the autonomic nervous system and musculoskeletal system.

Normal Grief

Grief is a subjective feeling precipitated by the loss of someone or something important to the individual. Normal grief is a process of emotional upheaval, distress, and eventual resolution. Individuals who are grieving often experience both physical and psychological symptoms and may have difficulty functioning. Grief and depression share many of the same characteristics, and normal grief can become clinical depression. An individual with a history of depression is at risk of becoming depressed in times of significant loss. The mood disturbance in depression is typically pervasive and unrelenting. In normal grief, fluctuations in mood are common. Although the pain of grief is intense, the individual is able to experience moments of less intensity or even happiness.

Domestic Violence

Domestic violence is a pattern of assaultive and coercive behaviors that include physical, sexual, psychological, and economic attacks by adults or adolescents against their intimate partners. Individuals who have experienced abuse may present with an injury that is not consistent with the description of how the injury occurred. The individual may be seen frequently for undiagnosed psychosomatic concerns. This patient may appear depressed or show evidence of suicide attempts.

Substance Use Disorders

Substance use disorders are divided into two groups: substance abuse and substance dependence. The categories of substances included are alcohol, amphetamines, cannabis, cocaine, hallucinogens, inhalants, opioids, phencyclidines, sedatives, and hypnotics. Substance abuse occurs when repeated use of alcohol or other drugs leads to significant impairment in functioning and relationships, but does not include compulsive use or addiction, or withdrawal symptoms when stopping the substance. Substance dependence includes a history of substance abuse plus continued use despite related problems, an increase in substance tolerance, and withdrawal symptoms if the substance use is stopped.

Adjustment Disorders

There are several adjustment disorder diagnoses. All of the disorders in this category relate to a significantly more difficult adjustment to a life situation than would normally be expected considering the circumstances. The condition is acute if the disturbance lasts less than 6 months and chronic if it lasts for 6 months or longer in response to a chronic stressor or one that has enduring consequences.

The disorders in this category can present themselves quite differently. The key to diagnosis is to examine the issue that is causing the adjustment disorder and to determine the primary symptoms associated with the disorder (e.g., anxiety or depression).

Anxiety Disorders

There are several types of anxiety disorders and multiple diagnoses. An anxiety disorder should not be confused with everyday stress and worry. Anxiety disorders are persistent conditions that require careful diagnosis. Anxiety is a group of disorders characterized by a number of both mental and physical symptoms, with no apparent explanation.

The primary feature is abnormal or inappropriate anxiety. Apprehension, fear of losing control, fear of going "crazy," fear of impending danger or death, and uneasiness are among the most common psychological symptoms. Common physical symptoms include dizziness, lightheadedness, chest/abdominal pain, nausea, increased heart rate, and diarrhea.

Generalized Anxiety Disorder (GAD)

Chronic anxiety, also referred to as generalized anxiety disorder, manifests as persistent worries, fears, and negative thoughts lasting a minimum of 6 months. Excessive worry over daily activities and a tendency toward headache and nausea are seen. Typically, GAD develops over a period of time and may not be noticed until it is significant enough to cause problems with functioning.

Panic Disorder

Panic disorder is manifested by sudden attacks of fear accompanied by symptoms that may resemble a heart attack (e.g., palpitations, chest pain, dizziness). Often the symptoms develop rapidly and without an identifiable stressor. The individual may have had periods of high anxiety in the past, or may have been involved in a recent stressful situation; however, the underlying cause is typically subtle. Panic attacks subside as abruptly as they begin, typically lasting a few minutes, although they can last several hours. The frequency of these attacks may vary from several times a day to only once or twice a year.

Social Phobia (Social Anxiety Disorder)

Symptoms include extreme anxiety and fear associated with social or performance situations in which the patient is exposed to unfamiliar people or to scrutiny. The patient recognizes that the fear is excessive or unreasonable but avoids the social or performance situations or endures them with intense distress or anxiety.

Mood Disorders

Mood disorders contain several categories including dysthymia, depression, and bipolar disorder.

The disorders in this category include those in which the primary symptom is a disturbance in mood with inappropriate, exaggerated, or a limited range of affect. The feelings are extreme, pervasive, and unrelenting.

Dysthymia

The patient experiences feelings that are less intense than major depression but still disrupt everyday life. The patient experiences a depressed mood for most of the day and for more days than not, for at least 2 years. During this time, there must be two or more of the following symptoms: undereating or overeating, sleep difficulties, fatigue, low self-esteem, difficulty with concentration or decision making, and feelings of hopelessness.

Major Depressive Disorder

The hallmark symptom of depression is either a depressed mood or a loss of interest or pleasure in usual activities. Major depression can significantly impair a person's ability to function in family, work, and social situations. Patients with depression experience deep, unshakeable sadness and diminished interest in nearly all activities. Crying and feeling depressed or suicidal occur frequently.

Bipolar Disorder

Bipolar disorder has two types. Bipolar I requires the occurrence of at least one manic episode even though other episodes such as major depressive, hypomanic, or mixed may have occurred. Bipolar II requires at least one hypomanic episode. Mania is sometimes referred to as the other extreme of depression. The patient experiences an elevated, expansive, or irritable mood with behaviors and symptoms that reflect a "high." The symptoms are sufficient to interfere with usual social activities and relationships with others In bipolar II disorder, there are periods of highs, as described previously, often followed by periods of depression. The "high" episodes are hypomanic rather than manic. The symptoms are similar but are not severe enough to cause marked impairment in social or occupational functioning and typically do not require hospitalization to ensure the safety of the person.

Box 32-9 | **DSM-IV-TR Criteria for Diagnosis of Major Depressive Disorder**

A. Five or more of the following symptoms have been present during the same 2-week period and represent a change from previous functioning; at least one of the symptoms is either (1) depressed mood or (2) loss of interest or pleasure:
1. Depressed mood most of the day, nearly every day (or irritable mood if a child or adolescent)
2. Markedly diminished interest or pleasure in all, or almost all, activities of the day, nearly every day
3. Significant weight loss when not dieting, or weight gain, or a decrease or increase in appetite nearly every day
4. Insomnia or hypersomnia nearly every day
5. Psychomotor agitation or retardation nearly every day
6. Fatigue or loss of energy nearly every day
7. Feelings of worthlessness or excessive or inappropriate guilt nearly every day
8. Diminished ability to think or concentrate, or indecisiveness, nearly every day
9. Recurrent thoughts of death (not just fear of dying), or suicide
B. The symptoms are not due to a psychotic condition.
C. There has never been a manic episode, a mixed episode, or a hypomanic episode.
D. The symptoms are not a result of the direct physiological effects of a substance (e.g., a drug of abuse, a medication) or a general medical condition (e.g., hypothyroidism).
E. The symptoms are not related to bereavement.

From the American Psychiatric Association: *Diagnostic and statistical manual of mental disorders, fourth edition, text revision: DSM-IV-TR,* Washington, DC. 2000, American Psychiatric Association.

DIFFERENTIAL DIAGNOSIS OF *Common Causes of Psychological Disorders*

CONDITION	HISTORY	PHYSICAL FINDINGS	DIAGNOSTIC STUDIES
Normal stress	Perceived stress related to external or internal stressors such as daily life events or situations, psychological environments, relationships May be acute or chronic May feel unable to cope or adapt May have mental, physical, and behavioral symptoms	May appear unkempt, with unusual dress May have depressed demeanor Facial expression (e.g., dejected, sad, downcast) Tearing, crying Adolescents may show evidence of cutting	None
Normal grief	Loss of someone or something of importance May have physical and psychological symptoms Mood fluctuations; may feel depressed May have difficulty functioning	May appear unkempt, with unusual dress, general state of poor nutrition Depressed demeanor Facial expression (e.g., dejected, sad, downcast) Tearing, crying Speech may be soft and monotonous with little spontaneity Adolescents may show evidence of cutting	None

Continued

DIFFERENTIAL DIAGNOSIS OF *Common Causes of Psychological Disorders—cont'd*

CONDITION	HISTORY	PHYSICAL FINDINGS	DIAGNOSTIC STUDIES
Domestic violence	Reports physical, sexual, psychological, emotional, or economic attacks from family or partners May seek care frequently for undiagnosed psychosomatic concerns May report suicide attempts	May have injuries inconsistent with history Adolescents may show evidence of cutting	None
Substance use disorders*	Reports recurrent substance use that may result in failure to fulfill major obligations at work, school, or home and substance-related legal problems Use in situations that are physically hazardous (e.g., driving while intoxicated) Continued use despite significant social or interpersonal problems caused or exacerbated by effects of the substance May report increased tolerance of and need for increased amounts of substance May report withdrawal symptoms May report unsuccessful efforts to cut down or control substance use	Skin may be cold and clammy, itching and burning, tight, swollen, or puffy Excess perspiration Discolored fingers or injection marks along the veins Tattoos or burn marks, injuries or bruises Methamphetamine users may have self-induced facial lesions secondary to scratching Eyes may be injected, jaundiced, puffy, or glassy Pupils may be dilated or constricted Eyelids may be droopy with sleepy appearance or fixed stare May have difficulty controlling eye movements May have chronic rhinorrhea, lesions in the nose or around the nostrils May have dry lips, halitosis, or an odor of alcohol, marijuana, or tobacco	Toxicology screen Blood alcohol level
Anxiety Disorders			
Adjustment disorder*	The development of emotional or behavioral symptoms in response to an identifiable stressor(s) occurring within 3 months of the onset of the stressor(s) Distress that is in excess of what would be expected from exposure to the stressor Significant impairment in social or occupational (academic) functioning	None	Refer for psychological evaluation

DIFFERENTIAL DIAGNOSIS OF *Common Causes of Psychological Disorders—cont'd*

CONDITION	HISTORY	PHYSICAL FINDINGS	DIAGNOSTIC STUDIES
Generalized anxiety disorder*	Excessive anxiety and worry for most days of past 6 months, about a number of events or activities (such as work or school performance) Difficult to control the worry Associated physical symptoms such as restlessness, edginess, fatigue, difficulty concentrating, irritability, sleep disturbance Significant impairment in social, occupational, or other areas of functioning	Behaviors such as finger tapping and pacing that indicate anxiety Adolescents may show evidence of cutting	Refer for psychological evaluation
Panic disorder*	Recurrent unexpected panic attacks: discrete period of intense fear or discomfort with physical symptoms such as palpitations, pounding heart, or accelerated heart rate, sweating, trembling or shaking, sensations of shortness of breath or smothering, feeling of choking, chest pain or discomfort, nausea or abdominal distress, feeling dizzy, unsteady, lightheaded, or faint, paresthesias, chills or hot flushes May report fear of losing control or going crazy, fear of dying Persistent concern about having additional attacks	None except during attack	Refer for psychological evaluation
Social phobia (Social anxiety disorder)*	Marked and persistent fear of one or more social or performance situations Anxious that will act in a way that will be humiliating or embarrassing	None	Refer for psychological evaluation

DIFFERENTIAL DIAGNOSIS OF *Common Causes of Psychological Disorders—cont'd*			
CONDITION	**HISTORY**	**PHYSICAL FINDINGS**	**DIAGNOSTIC STUDIES**
	May report panic attack related to exposure to the situation Avoids the situation Avoidance, anxiety, and distress interferes significantly with the person's normal routine, occupational (academic) functioning, or social activities or relationships		
Mood Disorders Dysthymic disorder*	Depressed mood for most of the day, for more days than not, for at least 2 years Reports symptoms of depression such as appetite and sleep disturbance, low energy or fatigue, low self-esteem, poor concentration or difficulty making decisions, feelings of hopelessness	May appear unkempt, with unusual dress; general state of poor nutrition Depressed demeanor Facial expression (e.g., dejected, sad, downcast) Tearing, crying Speech may be soft and monotonous with little spontaneity Adolescents may show evidence of cutting	Refer for psychological evaluation
Major depressive disorder (see Box 32-9)	Reports acute symptoms of depressed mood most of the day, nearly every day, or loss of interest or pleasure in all or almost all activities of the day, nearly every day Experiences other symptoms most every day such as appetite disturbance, sleep disturbance, psychomotor agitation or retardation, fatigue or loss of energy, feelings of worthlessness or excessive or inappropriate guilt, diminished ability to think or concentrate, recurrent thoughts of death or suicide	May appear unkempt, with unusual dress; general state of poor nutrition Depressed demeanor Facial expression (e.g., dejected, sad, downcast) Tearing, crying Speech may be soft and monotonous with little spontaneity Adolescents may show evidence of cutting	Serum electrolytes CBC Thyroid function tests Refer for psychological evaluation

DIFFERENTIAL DIAGNOSIS OF *Common Causes of Psychological Disorders—cont'd*

CONDITION	HISTORY	PHYSICAL FINDINGS	DIAGNOSTIC STUDIES
Bipolar disorder*	History of at least one manic episode or hypomanic episode A distinct period of abnormally and persistently elevated, expansive, or irritable mood, lasting at least 1 week Accompanying symptoms of inflated self-esteem or grandiosity, decreased need for sleep, more talkative than usual or pressure to keep talking, insomnia or hypersomnia nearly every day, psychomotor agitation or retardation, flight of ideas or racing thoughts, easy distractibility, increase in goal-directed activity, excessive involvement in pleasurable activities that have a high potential for painful consequences May report history of one or more major depressive episodes (see above)	In mania, the speech may be rapid, pressured, and loud, and the speech content consists of a flight of ideas.	Refer for psychological evaluation

*For specific diagnostic criteria see American Psychiatric Association: *Diagnostic and statistical manual of mental disorders*, ed 4, text revision, 2000, Washington, DC, The Association.

CHAPTER RESOURCES

American Psychiatric Association: *Diagnostic and statistical manual of mental disorders, fourth edition, text revision: DSM-IV-TR.* Washington, DC, 2000, American Psychiatric Association.

Bastiaens L, Francis G, Lewis K: The RAFFT as a screening tool for adolescent substance use disorders, *Am J Addict* 9:10, 2000.

Carlat DJ: The psychiatric review of symptoms: a screening tool for family physicians, *Am Fam Physician* 58:1617, 1998.

Citrome L, Goldberg JF: The many faces of bipolar disorder: how to tell them apart, *Postgrad Med* 117:15, 2005.

Depression Guideline Panel: *Depression in primary care: volume 1. Detection and diagnosis. Clinical practice guideline,* No. 5, Rockville, Md, 1993, U.S. Department of Health and Human Services; AHCPR Publication No. 93-0550.

Dunphy LM, Winland-Brown JE: *Primary care: the art and science of advanced practice nursing,* Philadelphia, 2001, FA Davis.

Ewing JA: Screening for alcoholism using CAGE. Cut down, annoyed, guilty, eye opener, *JAMA* 280:1904, 1998.

Feldhaus KM, Koziol-McLain J, Amsbury HL et al: Accuracy of 3 brief screening questions for detecting partner violence in the emergency department, *JAMA* 277(17):1357, 1997.

Goldenring J, Rosen D: Getting into adolescent heads: an essential update, *Contemp Pediatr* 21:64, 2004.

Goolsby MJ, Grubbs L: *Advanced assessment: interpreting findings and formulating differential diagnoses,* Philadelphia, 2006, FA Davis.

Lieberman JA III: BATHE: an approach to the interview process in the primary care setting, *J Clin Psychiatry* 58(suppl 3):3, 1997.

Mersy DJ: Recognition of alcohol and substance abuse, *Am Fam Physician* 67:1529, 2003.

Sokol RJ, Martier SS, Ager JW: The T-ACE questions: practical prenatal detection of risk-drinking, *Am J Obstet Gynecol* 160:863, 1989.

Stein M: Attending to anxiety disorders in primary care, *J Clin Psychiatry* 64(suppl 15):35, 2003.

Whooley MA, Avins AL, Miranda J et al: Case-finding instruments for depression: two questions are as good as many, *J Gen Intern Med* 12:439, 1997.

Williams JW, Hitchcock NP, Cordes JA et al: Rational clinical examination. Is this patient clinically depressed? *JAMA* 287:1160, 2002.

XIII

Common Systemic Problems

Fever

Fever is an elevation of temperature above the normal daily variation and is a symptom of an underlying process. The major common cause of fever is infection; however, noninfectious processes may present with fever. Fever of unknown origin (FUO) occurs in a small percentage of cases. These fevers are usually caused by an infection that has not yet been identified. A meticulous history and physical examination supported by laboratory investigation are necessary to find the origin of the fever.

There are three types of fevers, each caused by a specific pathophysiological process. The first involves the raising of the hypothalamic set point. The receptors in the area of the hypothalamus regulating body temperature are triggered to reset at a higher core body temperature. This results in an elevation of the helper T-cell production and an elevation in the effectiveness of interferon. Infection, collagen disease, vascular disease, and malignancy are commonly responsible for these fevers.

A second type of fever is a result of heat production exceeding heat loss. Here the set point is normal, and heat loss mechanisms are active. Fever occurs either because the body raises its metabolic heat production or because the environmental heat load exceeds normal heat loss mechanisms. Aspirin overdose, malignant hyperthermia, hyperthyroidism, or hypernatremia may cause this type of fever.

A third type of fever is caused by a defective heat loss mechanism that cannot cope with normal heat load. Heat stroke, poisoning with anticholinergic drugs, ectodermal dysplasia, and burns are causes of this kind of fever.

For the first type of fever, antipyretics are given to lower the hypothalamic set point. Antipyretics are ineffective for the second and third types of fever.

DIAGNOSTIC REASONING: FOCUSED HISTORY

Is This Really a Fever?

Key Questions
- How do you know you have a fever?
- Has the temperature been measured? How was it measured?

Occurrence of Fever
Fever is a common presenting problem and a cardinal manifestation of disease. Patients often report a subjective fever (i.e., clinical symptoms such as flushing, chills, shaking chills, headache, malaise, or muscle aches) that is assumed by the patient to be a fever although not validated with a thermometer. Nevertheless, the absence of fever in a single patient visit does not eliminate a febrile illness.

Measurement of Temperature
Many people use touch to determine if a fever is present. Although not a precise indication, touch can signal a high fever. During the early stages of fever, perfusion to the skin is decreased and skin temperature falls. In later stages, when temperature within the muscles has risen significantly, increased body temperature is reflected by increased skin temperature. In children, hands and feet should not be used to gauge a fever because they may be vasoconstricted and feel cold.

Accurate temperature should be measured using a thermometer. Because of the diurnal variation in normal body temperature and the effect of physiological factors and body rhythms, frequent recordings throughout the day are needed to monitor fever.

Should Sepsis or Meningitis Be of Concern?

Key Questions
- Has there been any recent head trauma?
- Have you had recurrent ear infections?
- Have you had contact with anyone who has had meningococcal disease?
- Have you had any headache, lethargy, confusion, or stiff neck?
- If an infant: How old is the baby?

Head Trauma, Otitis Media, and Contact
Recent head trauma, especially at the base of the skull, may provide an entrance for infectious organisms. Children with recurrent or chronic otitis media may have mastoiditis spreading to the meninges. Contact with anyone with meningococcal disease and/or *Haemophilus influenzae* places the individual at risk for contracting the disease.

Headache, Vomiting, Lethargy, or Stiff Neck
Meningitis is characterized by headache, fever, lethargy, confusion, vomiting, and stiff neck. However, the presentation is highly variable. Any patient with even minimal neurological signs and symptoms should be evaluated for meningitis.

Infant
Fever in children less than 2 months of age is uncommon but must be viewed as serious. Generally neonates and young infants are less able to mount a febrile response; when they do, it is a significant finding. Fever can be viral or bacterial in nature. Fevers in the neonate may also be an indication of an underlying anatomical defect. Urinary tract infection and bacteremia are often the first indications of a structural abnormality of the urinary tract. Also, infants with galactosemia may present in the first weeks to 1 month of life with gram-negative sepsis. Occasionally, infants present with sepsis associated with delivery (prolonged rupture of membranes) or acquired from instrumentation used during delivery, such as scalp electrodes, or from a procedure performed in a neonatal intensive care unit.

All infants younger than 2 months with fever are considered to have sepsis or meningitis until proved otherwise.

What Does the Pattern of Fever Tell Me?

Key Questions
- How long have you had the fever?
- What has been the highest temperature reading? When did this occur?

Length of Fever
In adults, fevers from an acute process usually resolve in 1 to 2 weeks. Fevers that last 3 weeks or longer, that exceed temperatures of 38.4° C (101.1° F), and that remain undiagnosed after 1 week of intensive diagnostic study are classified as FUOs.

Fevers in children can be grouped into three categories: short-term fever, fever without localizing signs, and fever of unknown origin. Short-term fever is defined as a fever of short duration, readily diagnosed, that resolves within 1 week. Fever without localizing signs is a fever with no localizing sign and of brief duration (usually <10 days) that is not explained by findings on history or physical examination. FUO is a fever usually greater than 38.5° C (101.2° F) that lasts longer than 2 weeks on more than four occasions.

Height of Fever
Dehydration and febrile seizures are related to the height of the fever. Generally, body temperatures greater than 41.1° C (106° F) are seen in heat illness, central nervous system disease, or a combination of these with infection. The higher the fever, the greater is the likelihood of bacteremia.

Is the Fever Caused by a Localized Infection?

Key Questions

- Do you have any frequency, burning, or urgency with urination?
- Are you having any unusual vaginal/penile discharge?
- Do you have any face or sinus pain?
- Do you have nasal discharge? If so, what color is the discharge?
- Do you have a cough? Is it productive? What color is the sputum?
- Do you have ear pain?
- Is your throat sore?
- Do you have any aphthous ulcers?
- Are you having any nausea/vomiting or diarrhea?
- Do you have any joint pain?

Localizing symptoms will point to the site of the infection. These diagnostic clues include headache or sinus pain, purulent nasal discharge, ear pain, toothache, sore throat, breast tenderness, chest pain, cough, dyspnea, abdominal pain, flank pain, dysuria, vaginal discharge, pelvic pain, rectal pain, testicle pain, calf pain, neck stiffness, joint stiffness, pain or heat, or focal neurological deficits (see appropriate chapters).

Genitourinary Tract

Upper urinary tract infection (UTI) in adults commonly produces systemic symptoms with flank pain and fever (see Chapters 17 through 21). Fever with cystitis is uncommon in adults, but children with UTIs present with systemic rather than localized signs and symptoms. UTI is the most common infection in girls younger than 2 years who present with a high fever and in all infants younger than 90 days with fever. Pelvic inflammatory disease in women may cause fever as well as an increased amount of vaginal discharge and bleeding after intercourse. Men who have an acute UTI often present with chills, high fever, urinary frequency and urgency, perineal pain, and low back pain. They may also have penile discharge.

Ear, Nose, and Throat Symptoms

Viral infections of the upper respiratory tract are common and usually produce fever (see Chapters 2 through 6). Otitis media is common in children. Fever may accompany both viral and bacterial pharyngitis. Pharyngitis is frequently manifested only by fever, with the infection localizing 1 or 2 days later. Acute sinusitis can produce a fever. Aphthous ulcers with pharyngitis and cervical lymphadenopathy are seen in children with periodic fevers.

Respiratory or GI Symptoms

Most febrile illnesses are caused by viral upper respiratory tract infection, lower respiratory tract infection, or gastrointestinal (GI) tract infection (see Chapters 11 through 13 and Chapter 16). Localized symptoms can help pinpoint the cause of the fever. Vomiting occasionally signals pneumonia.

Joint Pain

Joint pain may indicate connective tissue disorders in adults and in children more than 6 years of age (see Chapter 26). Osteomyelitis or septic arthritis may also produce fever.

Can the Diagnostic Possibilities Be Narrowed or a Cause Be Eliminated?

Key Questions

- Have you noticed a rash?
- Do you ache all over?

Skin Rash

The prodromal period of a rash is an important historical clue to diagnosis (see Chapter 8). The common fever and eruption periods of rashes are as follows.

- Varicella, rubella, erythema infectiosum—1 day
- Scarlet fever—2 days
- Rocky Mountain spotted fever—3 days
- Measles—4 days
- Roseola infantum—5 days

Ache

Fevers localized to a site without general body manifestations are often bacterial in nature. Fevers accompanied by muscle aches (myalgias), malaise, and/or respiratory symptoms are often viral in nature.

Does the Patient Have an Increased Risk for Complications?

Key Questions

- Do you have any chronic health problems?
- Have you had any recent surgery?
- Have you been diagnosed with an infectious disease recently?
- Are you sexually active? How many partners do you have?
- Are your immunizations up to date?
- Does anyone in the family have tuberculosis (TB) or hepatitis?

Chronic Disease

Chronic conditions and systemic disorders, such as diabetes mellitus, human immunodeficiency virus (HIV), malignancies, neutropenia, and sickle cell anemia, compromise host resistance and increase susceptibility to infection. Prosthetic devices, such as heart valves or joint prostheses, also increase susceptibility to infection.

Health Problems, Surgery, and Recent Infection

Current health problems, recurrent infection, or incomplete treatment of infection may be the cause of fever. Risk factors such as diabetes mellitus, neutropenia, and sickle cell anemia heighten the likelihood of bacterial infection. Patients with a past history of infection such as upper respiratory tract infection (URI) or streptococcal pharyngitis may be prone to relapse or recurrence. Recent surgical procedures can provide a locus for occult infection; however, a surgical procedure can also induce an inflammatory response, which causes a fever without infection.

Sexual Activity

High-risk sexual activity may raise the index of suspicion for HIV infection and additionally for pelvic inflammatory disease (PID) in women.

Immunizations

Children and adults who have not been properly immunized are more at risk for infectious diseases.

Tuberculosis or Hepatitis Exposure

Exposure to populations with a high incidence of TB or viral hepatitis increases the risk of infection. Inquire further about constitutional symptoms such as cough or night sweats (TB) or malaise and abdominal discomfort (hepatitis).

Does the Parent Report a Behavior Change in the Child?

Key Questions

- Is the child sleepier than normal?
- Is the child more irritable?
- How is the child acting?

In infants and children, behavior changes may be the only indication that the child is ill. Mildly ill infants may act alert, be active, smile, and feed well. Moderately ill infants may be fussy or irritable but continue to feed, be consolable, and may smile. Severely ill infants appear listless, cannot be consoled, and feed poorly or not at all.

Could the Fever Be Caused by Something Acquired While Traveling?

Key Question (to self)

- Has this patient been exposed to an emerging infectious disease based on his or her travel activities or exposure?

Key Questions

- Have you been out of the country recently?
- Have you spent time in the woods or been camping recently?

A history of travel out of the country presents the possibility of infection with amebiasis, malaria, schistosomiasis, typhoid fever, or hepatitis A and B. Epidemiological surveillance data continually provide updates on patterns of occurrence of infections such as severe acute respiratory distress syndrome (SARS), avian influenza or "bird flu," and West Nile virus (see Box 33-1). Camping or exposure to wooded areas may indicate exposure to ticks, Q fever, tularemia, Rocky Mountain spotted fever, *Giardia,* or Lyme disease.

Box 33-1	**Emerging Infectious Diseases Associated With Fever**

Avian Influenza ("Bird Flu")

A highly pathogenic strain of avian influenza A virus, H5N1, infects birds and mutates rapidly to acquire genes from viruses infecting other animal species. "Bird flu" is transmitted to humans usually through the slaughtering and processing of infected birds. Symptoms of infection can range from flulike symptoms (e.g., fever, cough, sore throat, muscle aches) to pneumonia and severe respiratory distress. Outbreaks that began in Asia in 2003 have spread to parts of Europe. Suspect infection in persons showing flulike symptoms such as high fever and cough who have confirmed contact with birds in an area where confirmed outbreaks have occurred. Clinical deterioration is rapid over 4 to 13 days. Laboratory findings include leukopenia, thrombocytopenia, and elevated levels of aminotransferases. Although avian influenza is a rare disease, more than half of reported cases have been fatal and there is great potential for this virus to evolve into a world pandemic.

SARS (Severe Acute Respiratory Distress Syndrome)

Severe acute respiratory distress syndrome (SARS) is a febrile severe lower respiratory tract illness that is caused by infection with SARS-associated coronavirus (SARS-CoV). From 2002 through 2003, The World Health Organization received reports of more than 8000 cases and nearly 800 deaths. No specific laboratory test distinguishes SARS-CoV from other febrile respiratory illness. Lymphopenia and elevated levels of hepatic transaminases, creatinine, and C-reactive protein have been seen in some patients. Diagnosis is based on clinical features (e.g., fever, difficulty breathing, pneumonia) and epidemiologic history of exposure either to a SARS patient or to a setting in which the SARS-CoV transmission is occurring.

West Nile Virus (WNV)

West Nile virus is a potentially serious illness most often caused by the bite of an infected mosquito. It occurs most often in summer and fall in North America. Symptoms develop 3 to 14 days after being bitten. Approximately 80% of people who are infected with WNV will not show symptoms; however, up to 20% have symptoms called West Nile fever, characterized by fever, headache, fatigue, truncal rash, lymphadenopathy, and eye pain lasting from days to several weeks. People more than 50 years old are more likely to develop serious symptoms. A positive IgM antibody test of serum or cerebral spinal fluid is needed to confirm the disease. The test is positive in most patients within 8 days of onset of symptoms.

NOTE: The most current information on these diseases can be found online at the Centers for Disease Control and Prevention, http://cdc.gov, and The World Health Organization, http://who.int.

Could the Fever Be Medication Related or Caused by Poisoning?

Key Questions

- What medications have you taken recently?
- Describe the foods you have eaten in the past 3 days.
- Could the child have eaten a poisonous plant?

Medications may hide an occult infection. Many drugs (e.g., penicillin, atropine, sulfonamides, streptomycin, and diphenylhydantoin) can induce fever in predisposed individuals. The fever starts about 7 days after the drug is taken for the first time or soon after the first dose in a patient previously sensitized. Any patient who is taking immunosuppressive agents is at a higher risk for infection. Some medications interfere with thirst recognition (e.g., sedatives, haloperidol) or sweating (e.g., anticholinergics, phenothiazines).

Aspirin overdose can also cause fever. Earliest signs are vertigo and tinnitus, but fever can occur shortly thereafter and may be the only symptom that patients recognize.

Food Poisoning

Food poisoning fevers may occur up to 72 hours after ingestion of contaminated food.

Plants

Plants containing alkaloid atropine (deadly nightshade, jessamine, and thornapple) cause dilated pupils, flushed skin, and fever because they interfere with the normal heat loss mechanism.

Could Exposure to Animals Explain the Fever?

Key Questions

- Has a cat scratched you recently?
- Have you been around any animals?

Cat-Scratch Disease

Cat-scratch disease is a bacterial infection transmitted by cats. The etiological agent is a gram-negative bacillus. Single-node or regional adenopathy is the dominant clinical feature. A low-grade fever is also present.

Animal Exposure

Also possible are brucellosis and leptospirosis from dogs, tularemia from rabbits, ornithosis, histoplasmosis, or psittacosis from birds, and lymphocytic choriomeningitis from hamsters or cats. Exposure to infected animals can produce infection and fever in humans. Occupational exposure to pathogens such as brucellosis should be investigated in patients who work with animals or animal products.

Could This Be the Result of a Recent Immunization?

Key Question

■ What immunizations have you had recently? Adverse effects of immunization are rare but do occur. History of recent immunization followed by 4 hours of high temperature (39.5° C, 103° F) may indicate such an adverse reaction. Measles/mumps/rubella (MMR) immunization may cause elevation of temperature 10 to 14 days after the inoculation.

Could the Fever Be Caused by Heat Exposure?

Key Questions

■ Were you overdressed? If an infant: Is the infant overbundled?
■ Do you have air conditioning or windows that open?
■ How warm is the room you live/sleep in?

Overdressing

Classic heatstroke occurs when the person is unable to dissipate the environmental heat burden. Mothers may inadvertently overdress children or cover them in blankets; the elderly may not be able to get out of bed when hot. Obese persons have extra adipose tissue that insulates the body, preventing loss of heat. Some cultures treat illnesses with bundling, which can cause high fevers.

Air Conditioning and Room Temperature

During heat waves, persons may become overheated in apartments without air conditioning or with windows that will not open or are not opened because of safety concerns. The high ambient temperatures in those apartments produce elevations in core body temperature that cannot be compensated for, leading to hyperthermia.

DIAGNOSTIC REASONING: FOCUSED PHYSICAL EXAMINATION

Most fevers have an obvious cause, so look initially for localizing symptoms or clusters of symptoms that point to the cause. Remember that in both children and adults, bacterial and viral upper respiratory tract infections (URIs), lower respiratory tract infections (LRIs), and gastrointestinal (GI) tract infections are the most common causes of fevers. Look for and rule out the common causes before investigating more unlikely causes. Boxes 33-2 and 33-3 list the common causes of fever in children and adults.

Fever in a Child Less Than 2 Months Old

The younger the child, the greater is the cause for concern in the presence of fever. Neonates and young infants are less able to mount a febrile response and therefore are more vulnerable to meningitis and other hematogenous complications. The infrequency of high fever in this age-group relates to innate differences in the ability to mount a febrile response. The data suggest that fever in the first 2 to 3 months of life is relatively uncommon but that when it does occur, it is usually significant and often ominous.

Observe the Patient

General appearance is a most important aspect of physical examination. Note how the patient looks—does he or she appear acutely ill, look dehydrated, seem lethargic, respond appropriately?

Responsiveness in children older than 2 months of age has been used by pediatricians to identify febrile children with serious

---

Box 33-2 Common Causes of Fever in Children

Acute Fever
Upper respiratory tract disorders
  Viral respiratory tract diseases
  Otitis media
  Sinusitis
Lower respiratory tract disorders
  Bronchiolitis
  Pneumonia
Gastrointestinal disorders
  Bacterial gastroenteritis
  Viral gastroenteritis
Musculoskeletal infections
  Septic arthritis
Osteomyelitis
Cellulitis

Urinary tract infections
Bacteremia
Meningitis

Fever of Unknown Origin
Infectious diseases (localized and systemic)
Collagen/inflammatory diseases
Neoplastic diseases
Miscellaneous disorders
  Drug fever
  Factitious fever
  Kawasaki disease
  Inflammatory bowel disease
  Immunodeficiency
  Central nervous system dysfunction

Box 33-3 Common Causes of Fever in Adults

Acute Fever
Upper respiratory tract infections
  Tonsillitis
  Sinusitis
  Pneumonia
Gastrointestinal disorders
  Bacterial gastroenteritis
  Viral gastroenteritis
  Acute abdomen
Urinary tract infection
Pelvic inflammatory disease

Prostatitis
Drug reactions
Alcohol withdrawal

Fever of Unknown Origin
Infectious disease
Neoplasm
Collagen/vascular; other multisystem disease
Drug fever
Factitious fever

---

illness. The Yale Observation Scale for severity of illness in children is commonly used to quantify observations (Table 33-1). The scale has six general areas related to the child's appearance and behavior. Two thirds of children with acute illness have scores of less than 10 and, of these, only 3% were found to have serious illness. Scores greater than 10 predicted serious illness, and a score of 16 was associated with serious illness 92% of the time.

Take Vital Signs and Note Temperature

The incidence of bacteremia, as well as specific infections, increases with the magnitude of fever. A temperature greater than 40° C (104° F) seems to be the marker for occult bacteria. However, many patients with high fever do not have major diseases. In adults, take an oral temperature; in infants and children, a rectal temperature is more reliable.

Most infectious diseases produce temperatures between 37.2° C and 41° C (99° F and 106° F). However, some patients with infectious diseases remain afebrile; these include neonates, immunocompromised hosts, patients with chronic renal insufficiency, and the elderly. Extreme pyrexia (i.e., temperatures exceeding 41.5° C [106.7° F]) rarely occurs with an infectious disease. Conditions in which extreme pyrexia is seen include drug fevers, central nervous system injury, malignant hyperthermia, stroke, and HIV.

Hypothermia is always an unfavorable prognostic sign in the presence of infectious

Table 33-1	Yale Observation Scale Predictive Model: Six Observation Items and Their Scales		
OBSERVATION ITEM	1 NORMAL	3 MODERATE IMPAIRMENT	5 SEVERE IMPAIRMENT
Quality of cry	Strong with normal tone *or* content and not crying	Whimpering *or* sobbing	Weak *or* moaning *or* high-pitched
Reaction to parent stimulation	Cries briefly and then stops *or* content and not crying	Cries on and off	Continual cry *or* hardly responds
State variation	If awake, stays awake *or* if asleep and stimulated, wakes up quickly	Eyes close briefly, not awake *or* awakes with prolonged stimulation	Falls to sleep *or* will not rouse
Color	Pink	Pale extremities *or* acrocyanosis	Pale *or* cyanotic *or* mottled *or* ashen
Hydration	Skin normal, eyes normal, *and* mucous membranes moist	Skin and eyes normal *and* mouth slightly dry	Skin doughy *or* tented *and* dry mucous membranes *and/or* sunken eyes
Response (talk, smile) to social overtures	Smiles *or* alerts (<2 mo)	Brief smile *or* alerts (<2 mo)	No smile, face anxious, dull, expressionless *or* no altering (<2 mo)

From McCarthy PL, Sharpe MR, Spiesel SZ et al: Observation scales to identify serious illness in febrile children, *Pediatrics* 70(5):806, 1982.

disease. This condition is seen with overwhelming sepsis (most commonly in the elderly and neonates), uremia, cold exposure, and hypothyroidism.

Observe Skin and Mucous Membranes

A macular/papular rash may indicate a viral exanthema, infectious disease, or a drug sensitivity reaction (see Chapter 8). Vesicular rashes occur with viral infection. A petechial skin rash indicates meningococcemia or Rocky Mountain spotted fever. Petechial eruptions on the hard and soft palate may indicate mononucleosis. Splinter hemorrhages found in the nail beds and petechiae of the conjunctivae indicate endocarditis.

The presence of a petechial skin rash indicates a serious infection that requires immediate referral and hospitalization.

Examine the Head and Neck

Percuss the sinuses and transilluminate for evidence of sinusitis (see Chapters 2 through 6). Examine and palpate the teeth for abscesses. Palpate the salivary glands for tenderness. Examine the throat and tonsils for signs of infection, specifically enlarged or red tonsils, lymphadenopathy, or tonsillar or pharyngeal exudate. Examine the mouth for aphthous ulcers.

Inspect the ears and tympanic membrane (TM) for effusion, erythema, fluid, or purulent secretion. Inspect the optic fundi for changes associated with infectious endocarditis (i.e., Roth's spots—small, pale retinal lesions with areas of hemorrhage with white centers, usually located near the optic disc).

In the infant, feel for a tense or bulging anterior fontanel. This is best noted if the patient is in the sitting position. The normal fontanel may feel questionably tense if the infant is supine. Tenseness may be noted in the crying child but only during expiration; this physiological bulging disappears when the patient relaxes or inspires.

Palpate the Lymph Nodes

Palpate all lymph nodes for enlargement and tenderness.

■ Anterior cervical—Suspect viral or bacterial pharyngitis.

- Preauricular or postauricular—Suspect ear infection
- Posterior cervical—Suspect mononucleosis
- Supraclavicular—Suspect neoplasms
- Axillary—Suspect breast inflammation, local infection, or neoplasm
- Localized lymphadenopathy—Suspect local infectious process
- Generalized lymphadenopathy—Suspect immunosuppression, such as being HIV positive, or neoplasm.

Examine the Lungs and Chest

Percuss and auscultate the lungs (see Chapters 11 and 12). Adventitious sounds, decreased breath sounds, or areas of consolidation may indicate LRI or pneumonia.

Examine the sputum for color, consistency, and presence of blood or odor.

- Yellow/green sputum—bacterial infection
- Brown sputum—check smoking history
- Blood-streaked sputum—indicates URI and bronchitis
- Hemoptysis—suspect tumor, trauma, or pulmonary embolism

Palpate Breasts if Indicated

Inspect the breasts for signs of inflammation (see Chapter 24). Palpate for masses, tenderness, and discharge. Palpate axillary lymph nodes for presence of tenderness.

Examine Genitourinary System if Indicated

Palpate for suprapubic tenderness, which may indicate PID or UTI, and for costovertebral angle (CVA) tenderness, which suggests pyelonephritis (see Chapters 17 through 22). Perform a pelvic examination in women without another obvious source of fever. Cervical motion tenderness, discharge, or adnexal tenderness and lower abdominal tenderness may indicate PID. In men, examine for penile discharge, suggesting a sexually transmitted disease, UTI, or prostatitis.

Perform a rectal examination to evaluate for tenderness and discharge, which may indicate rectal abscess or infection as well as retrocecal appendicitis.

Perform a prostate examination in men without another obvious source of fever

because prostatitis may be the cause. If you suspect prostatitis, do not perform a vigorous examination or massage the prostate as this can release bacteria and produce septicemia.

Examine Musculoskeletal System if Indicated

Examination may suggest inflammation or infection of bone or joints if there is swelling, increased warmth, or tenderness (see Chapters 26 and 27). Infants may present with poor feeding, irritability, fever, or vomiting. Examination should reveal decreased mobility of the affected bone or joint area, increased heat, tenderness, and swelling.

Examine the lower extremities for asymmetrical swelling, calf tenderness, or palpable vessels as an indicator of deep vein phlebitis.

Osteomyelitis may occur in young children, most commonly between 3 and 10 years of age. Septic arthritis can occur in children under the age of 3 and in young women who are sexually active.

Perform Neurological/Mental Status Examination

Evaluate for signs of meningeal irritation (see Chapters 28 and 30). Inflammation of the meninges from infection or blood evokes reflex spasm in the paravertebral muscles. In the cervical area, this manifests as neck stiffness. Normally the chin can be flexed passively to touch the chest. If neck stiffness is present, this maneuver is not possible. With the patient supine, attempts to flex the neck cause the knees and hips to rise from the bed (Brudzinski's sign) to reduce the pull on the meninges. In the lumbar region, meningeal irritation also causes spasm and can be demonstrated by passive movement of the lower limbs. Attempts to extend the knee joint when the hip joint is flexed are resisted, and the other limb may flex at the hip (Kernig's sign). Neck stiffness (nuchal rigidity) or resistance to neck flexion or rotation is a late sign and not a true sign of meningitis in infants less than 3 months old, the very old, or the severely obtunded patient. Vomiting, headache, and photophobia may also be present.

Note the presence of focal deficits, which suggests vascular occlusion or abscess formation. Assess for disturbances in mentation, irritability, lethargy, somnolence, or coma, which indicates increased intracranial pressure. Seizures occur in 20% to 30% of children with meningitis.

A seizure in a febrile infant less than 6 months old suggests meningitis rather than a simple febrile seizure. Benign febrile seizure is uncommon in very young infants.

LABORATORY AND DIAGNOSTIC STUDIES

Laboratory studies can be used selectively to confirm or negate the clinical diagnosis, especially if the history and physical examination findings provide strong indication of a particular infectious process. In patients with obvious viral URI, no studies are necessary. Patients with a sore throat may require a throat culture, Monospot, or rapid strep test, depending on the clinical findings. In patients with urinary symptoms, a urinalysis and culture may be sufficient unless clinical findings indicate an upper urinary tract infection, which would warrant further diagnostic testing such as radiography, ultrasonography, or intravenous pyelography.

Also see appropriate chapters for specific presenting problems and discussion of diagnostic tests.

Complete Blood Cell Count

Leukocytosis with a left shift suggests a bacterial infection. Atypical lymphocytes are characteristic of systemic viral infection. Immature neutrophils suggest leukemia.

Anemia may be seen in inflammatory conditions such as juvenile arthritis, malaria, and parvovirus B19 infections. Low platelet counts may be associated with Epstein-Barr virus infection, histoplasmosis, tuberculosis (TB), and spirochetal infections or may be drug induced. Thrombocytosis is common in Kawasaki disease (an acute febrile illness in children that resembles scarlet fever) and some viral infections.

Erythrocyte Sedimentation Rate

An elevated erythrocyte sedimentation rate (ESR) indicates an inflammatory condition. However, the test is nonspecific and does not indicate the source or cause of inflammation.

Antistreptolysin Titer

An increase in the antistreptolysin (ASO) titer is detectable by comparing two blood samples more than 2 weeks apart (see Chapter 3). An elevated titer indicates immunological response of the host after exposure to streptococcal antigen.

HIV Testing

There are two tests used to diagnose HIV infection. The enzyme-linked immunosorbent assay (ELISA) detects the presence of HIV-specific antibodies that the body produces in response to the virus. A positive test may be confirmed by a second test, the Western blot. Newer, more rapid tests are being developed.

Urinalysis

Use a dipstick urinalysis (U/A) to screen for upper or lower UTI, which would reveal the presence of nitrites and leukocyte esterase (see Chapter 18). Microscopic evaluation discloses the presence of cells (white and red blood cells) and blood casts.

Urine Culture and Sensitivity

Performed on a clean catch of urine, this test will confirm a diagnosis of UTI and isolate the organism(s) (see Chapter 18).

Stool for Leukocytes

The presence of white blood cells (WBCs) may suggest invasive bacterial gastroenteritis (see Chapter 14).

Stool Culture and Sensitivity

Use stool culture and sensitivity to detect the presence of *Salmonella* or *Shigella* (see Chapter 14).

Stool Sample for Ova and Parasites

Have the patient collect three stool samples over a 5-day period (see Chapter 14). The first morning stool is preferred and must be delivered to the laboratory in 30 minutes or less after defecation.

Sputum for Acid-Fast Bacilli

A sputum sample to test for acid-fast bacilli (AFB) is used to diagnose respiratory TB (see Chapter 12). A smear is prepared from a series of three first-morning specimens collected on 3 separate days to catch the sporadic discharge of the bacilli from the tubercle.

Sputum for Gram Staining

A smear is prepared from a sputum sample and stained with Gram stain. Gram-positive organisms stain purple; gram-negative organisms stain red.
- Gram-positive cocci or diplococci—indicate pneumococcal, staphylococcal, or streptococcal infections
- Gram-negative cocci—indicate meningococcal or gonococcal infections
- Enteric gram-negative bacilli—indicate *Escherichia coli, Proteus, Bacteroides, Klebsiella,* typhoid, *Salmonella,* or *Shigella*
- Other gram-negative bacilli—indicate *Haemophilus,* pertussis, chancroid, brucellosis, tularemia, or plague

Sputum for Culture and Sensitivity

Use a sputum culture to isolate a specific organism (see Chapter 12). Have the patient rinse the mouth well with water without swallowing before coughing to produce a specimen; this decreases the amount of saliva present. Do not use mouthwash because this can kill the bacteria. An early morning sample is best. The sample must contain mucoid or mucopurulent material.

Cultures of Discharge

Cultures can be prepared from any source with a discharge (e.g., vaginal, urethral, wound). Place the culture in the transport medium indicated. Culture is used to isolate causative organisms.

Collect a specimen of vaginal or penile discharge on a sterile swab and place in the medium provided. For penile discharge, use a sterile urethral swab to collect a specimen from the anterior urethra by gentle insertion and scraping of the mucosa. For wound culture, use a sterile swab or aspirate with a sterile needle and syringe from the moist area. Bacteria from the center of a wound may be nonviable; culture near the periphery.

Molecular Testing for Infectious Organisms

Molecular testing using a sample taken from the vagina provides rapid, sensitive, and specific results. A number of products are available. Follow manufacturer directions to collect and transport the sample.

DNA probes and nucleic acid amplification tests (NAATs) are available to test for *Chlamydia trachomatis* and *Neisseria gonorrhoeae*. Single or dual organism tests are available.

Blood Cultures

Two culture specimens are obtained at two different venipuncture sites. If one culture produces bacteria and the other does not, the positive culture is likely from a contaminant and not the infecting agent. Culture specimens drawn through an intravenous catheter are frequently contaminated. All cultures should be drawn before initiation of antibiotics if possible. Most organisms require approximately 24 hours to grow in the laboratory, and a preliminary report can be given at that time. Often 48 to 72 hours are required for growth and identification of organisms. Blood cultures may be positive in bacteremia.

Lumbar Puncture

A lumbar puncture is indicated if you suspect meningitis (see Chapter 28). Laboratory data on cerebrospinal fluid (CSF) always include leukocytes, protein, glucose, Gram stain, cell count, and culture and sensitivity. In meningitis, expect cloudy CSF fluid with many polymorphonuclear cells containing bacteria. Glucose level in CSF is decreased compared with blood glucose level, protein is increased, and the culture will be positive.

Radiographic Imaging

Chest radiographs may detect infiltrates, effusions, masses, or nodes. Kidney, ureter, and bladder (KUB) and upright abdominal films can reveal air-fluid levels in the bowel. Computed tomography (CT) scan may be used to detect abscess or tumor. Radiographs are useful for detecting bone and joint involvement in osteomyelitis. Radionuclide scanning is also beneficial in detecting osteomyelitis.

DIFFERENTIAL DIAGNOSIS
Upper Respiratory Tract Infection
Viral infections can occur in any age-group and are more prevalent during winter months (see Chapter 12). The temperature is usually less than 38.7° C (101.5° F). Systemic symptoms are common. Known contact with others who have had similar symptoms or illness is typical but not necessary. The patient usually has a cough; any sputum is nonpurulent. Pharyngitis may be present with erythema of the oral pharynx.

Gastroenteritis
Nausea, vomiting, and diarrhea are the hallmarks of a GI infection (see Chapter 14). Fever is usually mild. Abdominal cramping may be present.

Urinary Tract Infection
UTIs are more common in females (see Chapter 18). Localized urinary tract symptoms are common in adults; systemic symptoms are more common in children. CVA tenderness indicates upper UTI. The temperature associated with an upper UTI is likely to be a high fever, and the patient feels systemically ill. Urinalysis can support a clinical diagnosis of UTI. Urine for culture and sensitivity usually confirms the diagnosis.

Pelvic Inflammatory Disease
Suspect PID in women with a fever for which there is no other explanation (see Chapter 21). There may be vague complaints of lower abdominal pain; suprapubic tenderness may be present on abdominal examination. Pelvic examination reveals cervical motion tenderness, discharge, and/or adnexal tenderness.

Prostatitis
In men without another obvious source of fever, suspect prostatitis (see Chapter 19). The prostate will be exquisitely tender to gentle palpation. Other system examinations will be normal.

Pharyngitis
The patient complains of a sore throat (see Chapter 3). In children, fever may precede throat complaints by 1 or 2 days. The pharynx is red, and the tonsils may be enlarged or have exudate. For differential diagnosis of bacterial and viral pharyngitis, see Chapter 3. Mononucleosis occurs most often in young adults and may present with palatine petechiae, tonsillar exudate, and posterior cervical lymphadenopathy.

Sinusitis
Sinuses that are tender to percussion or do not transilluminate may indicate sinusitis, especially in the presence of purulent nasal discharge. Patients often complain of a frontal headache, which worsens as the patient leans forward (see Chapter 4). Patients sometimes experience a sore throat and cough from postnasal discharge, which may be apparent in the posterior pharynx.

Ear Infections
Otitis media is more common in children (see Chapter 2). The tympanic membrane will appear red and may bulge. The light reflex will be absent or diminished. Tympanic membrane mobility will be limited. The child may tug at the ear and act restless or irritable. The young child or infant may feed poorly. The temperature may be a high- or low-grade fever. Respiratory symptoms occur if the patient has a concomitant respiratory tract infection. Ear infections are commonly associated with other upper respiratory tract symptoms.

Meningitis
The signs and symptoms of meningitis are related to nonspecific findings associated with bacteremia or a systemic infection or to specific manifestation of meningeal irritation with central nervous system inflammation (see Chapter 28). Inspect the skin for petechiae, cyanosis, and state of hydration and peripheral perfusion. Nuchal rigidity, back pain, Kernig's sign, Brudzinski's sign, nausea, vomiting, and bulging fontanel (in infants) may be seen. Papilledema is rarely seen. If it is present, look for other processes

such as brain abscess or subdural empyema. Ataxia may be a presenting sign. Lumbar puncture confirms the diagnosis.

Osteomyelitis

Bone infection is usually caused by bacteria and may arise from a clinically evident infection or from general bacteremia (see Chapter 26). Patients complain of pain in the affected bone or joint and may exhibit soft tissue tenderness and swelling. Children demonstrate localized tenderness near the epiphysis. Diagnosis requires isolation of the responsible organism via blood cultures, pus from tissue abscesses, synovial fluid aspirate, or material from needle aspiration or bone biopsy. Radionuclide scanning, CT, or magnetic resonance imaging (MRI) may be helpful in determining the extent of infection and destruction.

Kawasaki Disease

Kawasaki disease is an acute mucocutaneous lymph node syndrome that is classified as a vasculitic syndrome (of which fever is only one sign) affecting infants and young children under age 9 (see Chapter 8). It is more common in males and often occurs in fall and spring. The etiology is unknown. Fevers are of a high-spiking remittent pattern in the range of 38° C to 40° C (100.4° F to 104° F, with some to 107° F) and persist despite the use of empiric antibiotics and antipyretics. Seizures may be present, and other neurological causes must be ruled out. The febrile phase lasts from 5 to 25 days with a mean of 10 days. Because of the associated rash with fever, Kawasaki disease resembles scarlet fever.

To make the initial diagnosis of Kawasaki disease, fever lasting at least 5 days with at least four of the following signs, in the absence of a known diagnosis or infection, must be present:
- Bilateral conjunctival hyperemia
- Mouth lesions—dry fissured lips and injected pharynx or strawberry tongue
- Change in peripheral extremities, edema, erythema, desquamation of skin at 10 to 14 days
- Nonvesicular erythematous rash
- Cervical lymphadenopathy

Factitious Fever

Suspect factitious fever when there is a discrepancy between oral or rectal temperature and urine temperature. The pulse rate will be inconsistent with elevated temperature. The patient has no weight loss. Repeated monitored temperature-taking does not support previous readings.

Roseola Infantum

Roseola infantum is the most common exanthema of children younger than 3 years of age. Symptoms include an irritable child who has high fever, with rapid defervescence when the rash appears on day 3 or 4. The rash is maculopapular and lasts 1 to 2 days.

Fevers Without Localizing Signs

Often examination fails to disclose any specific signs or symptoms other than the fever itself. Most children who have a fever without localizing signs have neither an unusual nor a serious disease. In many cases, the fever will clear within a few days without a specific diagnosis. However, the longer the child has a fever without localizing signs, the less likely the fever is the result of infectious disease. Viral illness or malignancy must be considered.

Always investigate in the history and physical examination any abnormal growth suggesting any possibility of preexisting chronic disease. Morning stiffness suggests rheumatoid arthritis, weight loss or abdominal pain suggests inflammatory bowel disease, and frequent respiratory tract infection suggests cystic fibrosis or immunodeficiency.

Enterovirus

All enteroviruses may cause a mild, nonspecific, febrile illness that lasts 2 to 5 days. Most are seasonal, occurring in late summer and early fall. Herpangina, nonexudative pharyngitis with or without lymphadenopathy, generally occurs.

Occult Bacteremia

Occult bacteremia is diagnosed in children older than 3 months who have positive blood cultures but do not have the usual clinical manifestation of sepsis or septic shock. Occult means "hidden from view"; the child looks well. The majority of children who look well and are playful are at low risk for bacteremia despite fever. Those who look ill or toxic are at significant risk. The primary concern is the small but important percentage of those children who develop secondary complications from invasive bacterial disease (i.e., meningitis, bacterial sepsis, septic arthritis, or pneumonia). Peak ages for bacteremia are between 6 and 24 months, with *Streptococcus pneumoniae* the organism most commonly responsible.

Periodic Fever in Children

This condition is characterized by an abrupt fever that occurs in children 2 to 5 years of age on a regularly recurring basis, generally every 6 weeks. The fever lasts an average of 4 days. Besides the fever, the child has malaise, sore throat, cervical adenopathy, and aphthous stomatitis. The white blood cell count may be elevated ($13,000/mm^3$) as is the sedimentation rate. There are no associated diseases or other physical examination and laboratory findings. The child has normal growth and development.

DIFFERENTIAL DIAGNOSIS OF *Common Causes of Fever*

CONDITION	HISTORY	PHYSICAL FINDINGS	DIAGNOSTIC STUDIES
URI	Any age-group; systemic symptoms; often known contact with ill others	Fever <38.7° C (101.5° F); cough; nonpurulent sputum; erythema of pharynx; viral exanthem	None
Gastroenteritis	Nausea, vomiting, diarrhea; abdominal cramping	Mild fever; abdomen may be diffusely tender	None
UTI	Females more than males; burning urgency; frequency in adults; systemic symptoms/bedwetting in children	CVA tenderness with upper UTI; fever with upper UTI	U/A; urine C & S; CBC if suspect upper UTI
PID	May have pelvic or lower abdominal pain	May have suprapubic tenderness; cervical discharge; CMT, adnexal tenderness	CBC; molecular testing
Pharyngitis	Sore throat; may or may not have other upper respiratory tract symptoms	Erythematous pharynx; may have pharyngeal or tonsillar exudates or ulcers; may have palatine petechiae in mononucleosis; lymphadenopathy	CBC; culture; rapid strep test if suspect strep; Monospot if suspect mononucleosis
Prostatitis	Perineal discomfort, frequent urination, chills and malaise	Prostate tender to palpation; fever	Segmental urine specimen; C & S of urine; C & S of prostate discharge
Sinusitis	Facial or sinus pressure or pain; headache	Purulent nasal discharge; sinuses tender to percussion; headache or pressure worsens on bending forward	Radiographs or CT scan of limited value
Ear infections	Earache, pain; may have upper respiratory tract symptoms; child tugs at ear	High- or low-grade fever; TM red, may bulge, landmarks absent; TM mobility impaired; child irritable/restless	Pneumatic otoscopy
Meningitis	Nonspecific symptoms; nausea, vomiting, irritability	Petechiae, nuchal rigidity, positive Kernig's and Brudzinski's signs, petechiae; bulging fontanel in infant	Lumbar puncture

Continued

DIFFERENTIAL DIAGNOSIS OF *Common Causes of Fever—cont'd*

CONDITION	HISTORY	PHYSICAL FINDINGS	DIAGNOSTIC STUDIES
Osteomyelitis	Pain in affected bone or joint	Swelling or tenderness over affected area of joint	Culture; CBC; radionuclide scan, CT, MRI
Kawasaki disease	Under 5 yr of age; males more than females; fall and spring	High fever, spikes; persists despite antibiotic therapy; may have seizures; fever for 5 days with at least 4 of the following: bilateral conjunctival hyperemia, mouth lesions, edema, erythema, desquamation of skin, nonvesicular erythematous rash, cervical lymphadenopathy	WBC increased, shift to left; slight anemia; thrombocytosis; positive C-reactive protein; ESR increased; serum IgM, IgE increased
Factitious fever	Vague or no symptoms	Normal physical examination; no weight loss; pulse rate normal (not consistent with temperature elevation)	Discrepancy between oral/rectal temperature and urine temperature; repeated monitored temperature-taking does not support previous readings
Roseola infantum	Irritable child with fever for 4-5 days	Normal physical examination; when fever breaks, rash appears	None
Fevers without localizing signs	No other specific symptoms	Physical examination usually normal initially; repeat examination in 24 hr and as needed	Urinalysis; urine C & S; chest x-ray; WBC; rule out systemic disease, malignancy
Enterovirus	Mild, nonspecific febrile illness lasting 2-5 days; summer and early fall peaks	Nonexudative pharyngitis with or without lymphadenopathy frequently observed	None
Occult bacteremia	Fever in children older than 3 mo	No localizing signs; child appears well	Blood culture; WBC
Periodic fever in children	Abrupt fever on periodic basis (about every 6 wk); lasts about 4 days; child aged 2-5 yr; malaise	Cervical adenopathy, aphthous stomatitis	WBC and ESR elevated

CHAPTER RESOURCES

Baraff LJ: Management of fever without source in infants and children, *Ann Emerg Med* 36:602, 2000.

Bentley DW, Bradley S, High K et al: Practice guideline for evaluation of fever and infection in long-term care facilities, *J Am Geriatr Soc* 49:210, 2001.

Long S: Distinguishing among prolonged, recurrent, and periodic fever syndromes: approach of a pediatric infectious diseases subspecialist, *Pediatr Clin North Am* 52:811, 2005.

Luszczak M: Evaluation and management of infants and young children with fever, *Am Fam Physician* 64:1219, 2001.

Norman DC: Fever in the elderly, *Clin Infect Dis* 31:148, 2000.

Fatigue

Fatigue is a constitutional symptom that can be the result of normal physiological consequences of exertion or a symptom of illness. It is defined as the sensation of profound tiredness that is not relieved by rest or sleep and is not associated with prolonged activity. Fatigue can result from any disruption of energy production. Anemia, decreased oxygenation of blood, or reduced blood flow limits the amount of oxygen available to cells. Other factors that contribute to fatigue interfere with restorative mechanisms provided by sleep and rest, nutritional state, and mechanisms to remove or regulate wastes of metabolism. When fatigue is associated with cardiovascular or respiratory symptoms, clues are present that may point to the cause. However, most patients who have the symptom of fatigue have a normal physical examination, and psychological factors are often a contributing cause.

Fatigue is classified as physiological, psychological, or acute or chronic organic. Physiological fatigue is the result of normal activities that lead to overwork or exhaustion. Psychological fatigue is often related to a stressful event. Organic causes can produce acute or chronic fatigue. Acute fatigue lasts less than 6 months and is often a prodrome to other illnesses, most often infections, such as endocarditis, hepatitis, or other acute bacterial or viral illnesses. However, fatigue can also indicate a disease state, most often related to hyperthyroidism or hypothyroidism, heart failure, anemia, chronic obstructive pulmonary disease (COPD), sleep apnea, autoimmune disorder, or cancer.

Chronic fatigue lasts longer than 6 months, and its onset is usually slow and progressive. Chronic fatigue may be an indication of depression, chronic infection, or systemic disease or it may be secondary to alcohol or medication use. Chronic fatigue syndrome is a distinct clinical entity characterized by fatigue that is persistent or relapses, is not alleviated with rest, and significantly affects the patient's ability to function.

Fatigue is uncommon in very young children; the younger the child, the more likely the cause is organic. Most cases of fatigue in school-age children are related to acute infection. Fatigue is common in adolescents because of lifestyle factors.

DIAGNOSTIC REASONING: FOCUSED HISTORY

Is This Really Fatigue?

Key Question
- Tell me what you mean by fatigue.

Fatigue Versus Weakness
It is important to discriminate between weakness and fatigue. Often, patients describe muscle weakness when speaking about fatigue such as, "I am tired all the time and I feel weak." In children with weakness, parents will say the child is floppy or "doesn't run in gym like the other children." An individual tends to tire easily with metabolic or neuromuscular diseases such as hypothyroidism or myasthenia gravis.

Young children tend not to have vocabulary that describes fatigue; often it is the parent who brings the child to the clinic. Parents may state that the child is "lying around" or "I can't get the child to do anything" or "she just doesn't have any energy." Adolescents will say they are "always" tired.

Is the Fatigue Physiological?

Key Questions

- Tell me about your lifestyle habits (e.g., exercise and diet).
- Tell me about your sleep pattern.
- Do you require naps?
- Do you feel rested when you wake up in the morning?
- When was your last menstrual period?

Lifestyle Habits

A history of the patient's daily living and working habits may reveal a physiological cause for exhaustion. Erratic eating patterns, dieting, and missed meals may result in undernutrition or overnutrition. High levels of caffeine can affect the amount of energy a person has and can affect the sleep cycle, causing fatigue. Academic stress, athletic participation, and employment further contribute to fatigue in adolescents.

Sleep Pattern

Lack of adequate amounts of sleep is often the cause of fatigue (see Chapter 31). Adults need at least 6 to 8 hours of sleep for adequate rest; adolescents, 8 to 9 hours; and children, 10 hours. Patients with sleep apnea, which is more common in men older than 45 years, may report waking up and not being refreshed. Heart failure causes postural nocturnal dyspnea, leading to difficulty breathing at night and disturbed sleep. Early morning wakening is a symptom of depression, as is excessive sleeping during the day.

Last Normal Menstrual Period

Fatigue is a common symptom in women. Fatigue is an early sign of pregnancy, a symptom post childbirth, and a symptom associated with menopause. Perimenopausal women may have fatigue as a result of disrupted sleep because of night sweats or hot flashes.

Do I Need to Consider an Organic Cause?

Key Questions

- Do you practice safe sex (if sexually active)?
- Have you ever had hepatitis?
- Do you take any medication?
- Do you drink alcohol or use street drugs?

Exposure to Body Fluids

Fatigue may be the initial and most prominent symptom of hepatitis, human immunodeficiency virus (HIV) infection, or acquired immunodeficiency syndrome (AIDS). Hepatitis B can be a sexually transmitted infection through semen or contracted from exposure to contaminated blood. Sexual practices that traumatize mucous membranes, such as anal intercourse, increase the risk of transmission of organisms. The person with HIV infection or AIDS experiences cognitive impairment that includes difficulty learning and processing complex information. These impairments are correlated with the severity of fatigue.

Medications

Almost any drug can have fatigue as a side effect. The most common drugs that cause fatigue are antihypertensive drugs, cardiovascular medications, psychotropic medications, and opiates. Side effects also occur with drugs such as sedatives and antihistamines. Many drugs that cause fatigue are over-the-counter preparations.

Alcohol and Drug Use

Alcohol abuse and use of illicit drugs may be overlooked as a cause of chronic fatigue in adolescents and school-age children. This fatigue is due directly to the substance, usually alcohol or marijuana, and to secondary factors such as associated poor lifestyle habits related to sleep, rest, and nutrition. Family and friends may express the greatest concerns about fatigue that affects the patient's ability to function. The CAGE questionnaire is a useful screening tool to assess for alcohol abuse (see Box 32-3, Mood).

What Other Clues Can Help Me Rule Out an Organic Cause?

Key Questions

- Have you noticed a change in appetite?
- Do you have any joint tenderness or pain?
- Have you noticed increased urination?
- What other symptoms have you experienced?

Appetite

An increased appetite may indicate hypoglycemia. A decreased appetite may indicate an infectious process.

Weight Loss

Weight loss may indicate malignancy or infection, or poor nutrition related to depression or lack of information about a healthy and balanced diet.

Increased Urination

Diabetes mellitus, especially type 2, often presents with fatigue along with polydypsia, polyphagia, and polyuria.

Joint Tenderness

In children with juvenile rheumatoid arthritis (JRA), severe fatigue that seems to be more than expected with the degree of joint involvement is seen.

Associated Symptoms

Psychological fatigue is often associated with nonspecific and multiple symptoms such as muscle aching, abdominal pain, and general lethargy. Organic causes of fatigue are associated with a few specific symptoms that worsen over time, such as dry skin and nails with hypothyroidism or shortness of breath with exertion or when lying flat with congestive heart failure.

Could This Have an Environmental Cause?

Key Questions

- Where do you work?
- Have you been exposed to any toxins?
- Have you been camping?

Occupational Exposure

Heavy metals and pesticides may cause fatigue and other neurological symptoms. Soldiers returning from combat zones such as the Gulf War have been found to have unrelenting fatigue from an unknown cause.

Camping

Lyme disease may present with a history of weeks of malaise and chronic fatigue before any skin manifestations appear.

What Else Do I Need to Know About the Fatigue?

Key Questions

- Describe the onset and pattern of your fatigue. When did you first notice this?
- How severe is the fatigue?
- What makes the fatigue better or worse?
- Have you had a fever?
- Have you had any bleeding?

Onset and Pattern

The onset of psychological fatigue is often related to a stressful event and may have a sudden onset. Fatigue associated with metabolic causes may have a slow and progressive onset. Significant fatigue is considered to last more than 2 weeks and is experienced by about 25% of adults. Fatigue may be an early sign of pregnancy.

Severity

Clinically significant fatigue may vary throughout the day but never completely disappears. Children with Lyme disease and JRA experience severe fatigue that is in excess of the degree of disease involvement. The patient may need to limit social functioning and recreational activities as a result of fatigue, which may then exacerbate mood disturbances, which in turn contributes to fatigue.

Aggravating/Alleviating Factors

Psychological fatigue is usually worse in the morning and physical activity may relieve the fatigue. Organic fatigue is not associated with intensity or duration of activity and is not relieved with rest or sleep.

Fever

Fever generally accompanies infectious diseases, which are common causes of fatigue (see Chapter 33). Prolonged fever may indicate chronic infection, inflammatory disease, or malignancy.

Bleeding

Heavy menstrual flow may lead to anemia (see Chapter 22). Other sources of bleeding, such as gastrointestinal ulcers, polyps, or cancer of the bowel, may result in occult blood loss and fatigue.

If I Suspect a Psychological Cause, What Else Do I Need to Know?

Key Questions

- Describe your stress level and how you cope with stress in your life.
- Have you recently had a stressful event in your life?
- Do you or anyone in your family have a problem with anxiety or depression?
- How are you doing in school?

Stress

Stressful life events increase the risk of depression in some adolescents and adults. In the presence of organic disease, stress may be secondary to pain or discomfort that may disrupt sleep and rest patterns. Deconditioning that is secondary to muscle atrophy that occurs with inactivity or bed rest can lead to fatigue (see Chapter 32).

Anxiety and Depression

Children who have family members with depression are at a greater risk for depression. Generally, the first episode of major depression occurs between the ages of 20 and 30 and more often affects women. Major depressive disorder may have a genetic component. Diagnostic criteria will point to depression or anxiety as a cause.

School Performance

Decreased academic performance and decreased productivity may be an early sign of low self-esteem and early depression. Children also may overachieve academically to compensate for their lower self-esteem and hide their depression.

DIAGNOSTIC REASONING: FOCUSED PHYSICAL EXAMINATION

A general physical examination, including psychological screening for depression and anxiety, is needed to make a differential diagnosis of fatigue. The majority of patients will have a normal physical examination, but clues can be found for the presence of systemic disease.

Note General Appearance

Observe the patient entering the examination room to note any abnormality of gait that may indicate neurological involvement or generalized weakness. Observe the patient's demeanor and appearance for signs of neglect or a facial expression that might indicate depression or generalized anxiety. In the presence of organic disease, the patient will appear ill; with psychological stress, the patient may appear depressed or anxious. Children may appear sad or irritable.

Take Vital Signs

The presence of fever suggests inflammation or infection. Blood pressure reading, pulse rate, and respiratory rate reflect the function of the cardiorespiratory system. An elevated pulse rate may be associated with anxiety, anemia, or hyperthyroidism. Evaluate the patient for orthostatic hypotension because significant fatigue may lead to bed rest and deconditioning. Weigh and measure the patient to obtain the body mass index (BMI); a BMI that is greater than or less than the normal range can indicate poor nutrition status as well as cardiovascular risk.

Inspect Skin, Hair, and Nails

Observe for signs of thyroid dysfunction. Hypothyroidism is associated with coarse, dry hair and skin and thickening of nails. Hyperthyroidism is characterized by fine, limp hair and warm skin. Look for skin lesions or rashes that may indicate infection or inflammation. A faint maculopapular rash is sometimes associated with mononucleosis. Lyme disease is associated with a macular lesion with a clear center. Atrophic skin of the lower extremities is an indication of arterial insufficiency and underlying arteriovascular disease. Patients with anxiety disorders may bite their nails or self-inflict excoriation lesions, usually over the face and extremities.

Examine the Nose, Eyes, Mouth, and Throat

Inspect for any signs of infection or inflammation secondary to an allergic response. Petechiae on the palate may be seen with mononucleosis. Palpate for cervicofacial nodes. Lymphadenopathy is seen with HIV, malignancy, and mononucleosis. Inspect mucous membranes for lesions and moisture. Dry, cracked, and ulcerated mucosa can indicate a nutritional deficiency or dehydration.

Conduct a Cardiovascular Examination

Palpate the anterior thorax for the location of the point of maximal impulse (PMI) and for lifts or heaves. Listen for carotid and thyroid bruits. Auscultate the heart, listening carefully for rate, rhythm, and murmurs, especially a late systolic murmur heard loudest over the mitral area, which may indicate mitral prolapse. An audible S_3 or S_4 in an adult may indicate heart failure.

Examine the Lungs

First, observe the patient for ease of breathing and respiratory rate. Note the antero-posterior (AP)/lateral diameter of the thorax. An increased AP diameter indicates chronic obstructive pulmonary disease (COPD). Test for egophony, and palpate and percuss the anterior and posterior thorax to listen for resonance (normal) or consolidation. Tactile fremitus will increase over areas of consolidated lung. Listen for rales and wheezes. Bilateral basilar rales indicate congestive heart failure. Barely audible breath sounds are associated with COPD.

Examine the Abdomen

Begin the examination by observing the abdomen (see Chapter 13). Observe the intactness and condition of the skin. A rigid abdomen suggests peritoneal irritation. Generalized symmetrical distention may occur with obesity, enlarged organs, fluid, or gas. Dehydration or malnutrition may present as a concave contour of the abdomen.

Listen for bowel sounds. Anxiety, gastrointestinal irritation, and hunger can increase the frequency and loudness of bowel sounds. Depression can decrease bowel sounds.

Perform general light palpation to assess the skin and abdominal musculature. Note the patient's response to the examination. Perform deep palpation over the liver, spleen, and right kidney. Fist palpation over the posterior thorax tests for kidney tenderness associated with pyelonephritis.

Perform a Musculoskeletal Examination

Observe and palpate joints for inflammation and swelling. Bilateral tenderness over the major trigger points is diagnostic of fibromyalgia. Test stamina by asking the patient to perform certain musculoskeletal movements or to walk a certain distance to evaluate changes in fatigue level. For example, ask the patient to walk a distance for 3 minutes as far and as fast as they can comfortably and then assess fatigue level.

Conduct a Neurological Examination

Assess both cognitive and physical function to evaluate attention span, judgment, memory, and affect. Abnormalities may suggest a psychiatric disorder or brain pathology. Dementia is also seen in persons with HIV/AIDS. Test cranial nerves. A change in deep tendon reflexes (DTRs) may indicate thyroid dysfunction. Cerebellar and motor testing will rule out weakness or any associated neurological pathology.

LABORATORY AND DIAGNOSTIC STUDIES

Complete Blood Cell Count With Indices and Differential

A complete blood cell count (CBC) with indices will provide information about the degree and cause of anemia. Hematocrit and hemoglobin levels reflect the degree of anemia and the indices point to a cause. Microcytic hypochromic anemia reflects chronic blood loss, whereas normocytic normochromic anemia suggests an acute blood loss.

A white blood cell (WBC) count of greater than 12,000/µl indicates inflammation or infection. Normally the circulating neutrophils are in a mature form, known as "segs" because the cell nuclei are segmented. Immature forms are known as "bands." Infection will increase the total number of neutrophils with an increase in the number of immature cells or bands.

Ferritin

Ferritin is a protein that stores iron in bone marrow, and ferritin levels most accurately reflect total body iron stores. Ferritin levels are low with iron deficiency anemia. In contrast, ferritin levels may be elevated or normal in anemia of chronic disease or in thalassemias, caused by a reduction in the life cycle of a red blood cell (RBC) and the bone marrow failing to compensate for the loss by increasing RBC production.

Total Iron-Binding Capacity

Iron is transported in plasma bound with transferrin, a serum protein synthesized in the liver. Total iron-binding capacity (TIBC) of serum is an indirect measure of transferrin. This capacity may be increased in iron deficiency anemia because although the capacity to bind with iron is high, hemoglobin is decreased and both mean corpuscular volume (MCV) and mean corpuscular hemoglobin concentration (MCHC) are decreased (e.g., microcytic, hypochromic anemia). TIBC is normal or low in chronic disease, often because of the shorter life cycle of an RBC and the body's inability to compensate.

Urinalysis

Dipstick urinalysis can rule out or point to infection or systemic disease as a cause of the incontinence. Note hematuria, pyuria, bacteriuria, or the presence of leukocyte esterase or nitrites as indicators of urinary tract infection. Glycosuria or proteinuria suggests diabetes mellitus or renal disease. The presence of bacteria, RBC casts, and WBCs on microscopic examination indicates urinary tract infection (also see Chapter 18).

Erythrocyte Sedimentation Rate

The erythrocyte sedimentation rate (ESR) measures the rate at which RBCs settle in a tube of anticoagulated blood. An increase in plasma globulins or fibrinogen causes the cells to stick together and fall faster than normal. An increased ESR is a general indication of an inflammatory process and does not identify the source. The ESR is often elevated as a result of acute or chronic infec-

tion or inflammatory conditions such as rheumatoid arthritis or temporal arteritis.

Fasting Blood Glucose

A fasting blood glucose level $\geq$126 mg/dl will identify a patient who is at risk for diabetes.

Hepatic Function

Obtain AST (aspartate aminotransferase) and ALT (alanine aminotransferase) values to assess for general inflammation of the liver, associated with hepatitis.

Thyroid-Stimulating Hormone

A serum thyroid-stimulating hormone (TSH) level identifies hypothyroidism.

HIV Infection

An enzyme-linked immunosorbent assay (ELISA) will rule out HIV infection as a cause.

Tuberculin Skin Testing

A Mantoux test is used to test for tuberculosis antibodies. See Chapter 12 for a more thorough description of skin testing for tuberculosis.

Monospot

The Monospot is a rapid slide test that detects heterophil antibody agglutination. It is not specific for Epstein-Barr virus (EBV). It is most sensitive 1 to 2 weeks after symptoms appear and remains positive for up to 1 year. If chronic fatigue syndrome is being considered as a differential diagnosis, specific EBV antibody tests should be considered.

Chest Radiograph

A chest radiograph can reveal the presence of pneumonia, a lesion in the lungs, heart size, or the presence of fluid in the lungs as a result of congestive heart failure.

DIFFERENTIAL DIAGNOSIS
Physiological Causes
Sleep and Rest

In general, total sleep time is greatest during infancy, decreases in childhood, may increase again during parts of adolescence, remains relatively stable during the adult years, and declines during the late years of adulthood (see Chapter 31).

Total sleep time for the newborn is 14 to 18 hours a day. As the child matures, the sleep cycle increases in length and the total sleep time decreases. Sleep patterns of 8 to 10 hours develop during childhood. Many adolescents need increased amounts of sleep.

Most healthy adults spend 7 to 9 hours sleeping each day. Older adults sleep less, and may experience more frequent awakenings during the night; some need to compensate for this with rest periods during the day.

Poor Nutritional Status

Assessment of nutritional risk is determined by data from the history and physical examination, food recall data, BMI (BMI <18.5 = underweight; BMI 18.5 to 24.9 = healthy weight; BMI 25 to <30 = overweight; BMI >30 = obesity), and waist circumference.

According to *Dietary Guidelines for Americans 2005,* adults are advised the following:

- Eat a variety of fruits and vegetables. Choose five or more servings a day.
- Eat a variety of grain products, including whole grain. Choose six or more servings a day.
- Include fat-free and low-fat milk products, fish, legumes, skinless poultry, and lean meats.
- Restrict total fat intake to 20% to 35% of calories, with the majority of fats consisting of polyunsaturated and monounsaturated fatty acids.
- Balance the number of calories you eat with the number you use.
- Engage in regular physical activity of moderate intensity for at least 30 minutes on most days.
- Limit your intake of high-calorie, low-nutrition foods.
- Limit your intake of foods high in saturated and trans-fatty acids.
- Eat less than 2300 mg (1 teaspoon of salt) of sodium per day.
- Drink no more than one alcohol drink a day if a woman and no more than two drinks a day if a man.

- Clean hands when handling food; cook foods to safe temperatures; chill foods promptly; and defrost foods properly.

Psychological Causes
Depression

About 30% of primary care patients will have depressive symptoms. The adult patient will most often present with a loss of interest in usual activities, feelings of worthlessness and guilt, and thoughts of suicide for more than 2 weeks' duration. The practitioner must assess the risk of suicide and intervene or refer to a mental health specialist (see differential diagnosis table in Chapter 32).

Other symptoms include sleep and appetite disturbances, malaise, and decreased libido. Patients with bipolar disease may reveal a history of a manic episode associated with increased activity, increased libido, and feelings of grandiosity. The physical examination is usually normal.

Children will appear sad, angry, or irritable. They may have somatic complaints or low self-esteem and have problems with school performance. Adolescents may exhibit euphoria, hypersomnia, and lack of interest in activities.

Anxiety

DSM-IV diagnostic criteria for anxiety will guide the diagnosis of anxiety disorder or panic attack. Patients will report a sense of doom and fear of losing control, dyspnea and chest discomfort, fatigue, restlessness, and sleep disturbance. Physical findings will include tachycardia, palpitations, and diaphoresis (see differential diagnosis table in Chapter 32).

Organic Causes of Acute Fatigue
Infection

The prodrome stage of many viral infections may produce fatigue before other symptoms, such as sore throat, nasal congestion, and myalgia. Acute hepatitis A and B can cause fatigue before symptoms of jaundice or abdominal discomfort appear. Endocarditis, an infection of the heart valves, can cause fatigue.

Drugs

Alcoholism is one of the most common causes of acute fatigue related to organic causes. Chronic alcohol abuse is associated with undernutrition, a contributing factor to fatigue.

Anemia

The fatigue associated with anemia is secondary to the body's compensation to increase oxygen in blood that is oxygen-deprived because of abnormal size or quantity of RBCs. The body compensates by increasing the heart rate and may not be able to sufficiently make up for this deficit, which leads to increased breathlessness with activity. A diet history may show inadequate dietary intake of iron or heavy menstrual bleeding. Early symptoms are fatigue, weakness, and shortness of breath. A CBC will identify the cause of anemia. Serum iron, serum ferritin, and transferrin levels may also support the diagnosis of anemia.

Hypothyroidism (Myxedema)

Patients report cold intolerance, constipation, weight gain, hoarseness, depression, and fatigue. Physical examination reveals bradycardia, dry skin, generalized edema, and delayed recovery of deep tendon reflexes. An elevated TSH level is present in primary hypothyroidism.

Hyperthyroidism (Graves' Disease)

This disorder is associated with increased sweating, heat intolerance, weight loss, irritability, disturbed sleep, and menstrual irregularity. The physical examination may disclose tachycardia, atrial fibrillation, tremor, warm moist skin, and lid lag. Graves' disease is associated with exophthalmos. Radio-iodine uptake scan will differentiate Graves' disease, toxic nodule, and thyroiditis.

Organic Causes of Chronic Fatigue
Sleep Apnea

This disorder most often affects middle-age and older men. Risk factors include obesity and hypertension. Patients describe excessive daytime fatigue, morning head-aches, and erectile dysfunction. Bed partners of patients report restless sleep, loud snoring, and periods of apnea for at least 30 seconds during the night.

Medication

Antihypertensive medications and cardiac medications such as β-blockers often are associated with fatigue. Fatigue is a side effect of some pain medications, antihistamines, and many other medications.

Heart Failure

Heart failure is associated with dyspnea, orthopnea, paroxysmal noctural dyspnea, peripheral edema, weight gain, cough with frothy sputum, palpitations, and fatigue (see Chapter 12). Persons with a history of heart disease or valvular disease are at greater risk. Physical examination may reveal an altered level of consciousness, anxiety, jugular venous distention, tachypnea, rales and rhonchi, and a displaced PMI. An S_3 and S_4 can be heard on cardiac auscultation. Chest radiographs will disclose basilar consolidation and increased heart size. An echocardiogram shows a significantly reduced ejection fraction.

Cancer

Lymphoma and leukemia may first be detected by unexplained fatigue that increases with activity and worsens over time. A CBC with differential will show any blood dyscrasias. Gastrointestinal cancer may produce occult blood loss that leads to anemia and fatigue.

Mononucleosis

Mononucleosis is often a disease of young adults that is caused by Epstein-Barr virus in 90% of cases. History discloses a gradual onset of low-grade fever, mild sore throat, posterior cervical lymphadenopathy, and fatigue and malaise. Splenomegaly occurs in 50% of cases, and palatine petechiae are a less common sign. Diagnosis can be confirmed with a positive Monospot test and a CBC that shows greater than 50% lymphocytosis. Ten percent of patients may also have concurrent β-hemolytic streptococcal pharyngitis.

Hepatitis
Generally associated with hepatitis B or C, patients will report a history of malaise, fatigue, flulike symptoms, arthralgia, and an aversion to smoking. A health history will reveal risky sexual behavior, exposure to body secretions through blood transfusion or injectable drug use, or exposure to contaminated food or water. Physical findings may include jaundice, fever, and an enlarged and tender liver. Hepatitis serology for hepatitis A, B, and C will determine the causative agent.

Fibromyalgia
This condition occurs most often in women 20 to 50 years old. It is associated with chronic pain and stiffness of the trunk and extremities, especially the neck, shoulders, low back, and hips. Patients will report fatigue, headaches, sleep disturbance, and irritable bowel symptoms. To diagnose fibromyalgia, 11 of 18 bilateral tender points must be confirmed by physical examination.

Chronic Fatigue Syndrome
There is no single pathological mechanism to explain this condition that appears as an infectious or autoimmune disorder that has neurological, affective, and cognitive symptoms. Chronic fatigue syndrome is severe fatigue lasting longer than 6 months in association with (1) impaired memory or concentration, (2) sore throat, (3) tender cervical or axillary lymph nodes, (4) muscle pain, (5) multiple joint pain, (6) new-onset headaches, (7) nonrestorative sleep, and (8) postexertional malaise.

DIFFERENTIAL DIAGNOSIS OF *Common Causes of Fatigue*

CONDITION	HISTORY	PHYSICAL FINDINGS	DIAGNOSTIC STUDIES
Physiological Causes			
	Adolescent and younger adult; history of overwork, psychological stress, disturbed sleep, poor dietary habits	Normal examination	None
Poor nutritional status	Depression, decreased appetite, lack of balanced nutrient intake, excessive alcohol intake	BMI reflecting underweight or overweight	Hematocrit increased or decreased, low serum ferritin
Psychological Causes			
Depression: children	Feeling sad, angry, irritable Decrease in academic performance Somatic complaints	None	DSM-PC, DSM-IV
Depression: adults	Loss of interest in usual activities Feelings of worthlessness Sleep problems	Depressed affect; normal examination	Depression screening instrument
Anxiety	Numerous somatic complaints, breathlessness	Tachycardia, palpitations, diaphoresis	None
Organic Causes: Acute Fatigue			
Infection	Sudden onset; history of exposure; recent viral illness	Fever; lymphadenopathy, localized signs of erythema, edema	CBC, ESR, Monospot
Drugs and alcohol	History of smoking, alcohol use; antihistamines, analgesics,	Bilaterally enhanced or depressed DTRs; pupillary changes; reduced attention span,	CAGE alcohol screening

Continued

DIFFERENTIAL DIAGNOSIS OF *Common Causes of Fatigue—cont'd*

CONDITION	HISTORY	PHYSICAL FINDINGS	DIAGNOSTIC STUDIES
	antihypertensive medications	judgment	
Anemia	Breathlessness with exertion; menstruating female; recent surgery, delivery	Increased pulse rate; pale mucosa; smooth red tongue	CBC with indices, serum iron, ferritin, transferrin
Hypothyroidism (myxedema)	Poor appetite, fatigue, weight gain, cold intolerance	Decrease pulse rate; dry skin, coarse dry hair; thyroid possibly enlarged, hoarseness	T_4 low, T_3 low, TSH elevated
Hyperthyroidism (Graves' disease)	Hyperactivity, heat intolerance, sleep problems	Lid lag, fine thinning hair, tachycardia	T_4 increased, T_3 increased, TSH depressed
Organic Causes: Chronic Fatigue			
Sleep apnea	Male, middle-age or older; partner reports periods of no breathing during sleep, fatigue	Hypertension, obesity, narrowed upper airway	Sleep studies
Medications	History of allergies treated with antihistamines; medications for hypertension, heart disease, chronic pain	Nasal congestion, cough, injected conjunctiva	Evaluate medication choices
Heart failure	Dyspnea, weight gain, fatigue, cough	Anxiety, jugular venous distention, displaced PMI, rales	ECG, chest radiograph, ABGs
Cancer	Fatigue, unexplained weight loss	Observe, palpate, and percuss all systems for lumps, lesions, or consolidation; physical examination may be normal	CBC to rule out anemia; leukocyte count
Mononucleosis (Epstein-Barr virus)	Young adult; slow onset of malaise, low-grade fever, mild sore throat	Palatine petechiae, posterior cervical lymphadenopathy, splenomegaly	Positive Monospot; CBC with differential; >50% leukocytes
Hepatitis	Jaundice, anorexia, fatigue; fever may be reported	Jaundice, weight loss, arthralgia, skin rash	Bilirubin increased; hepatitis panel
Fibromyalgia	Female 20 to 50 yr; history of depression, sleep disturbance, chronic fatigue, general muscle and joint aches	Palpation of trigger points will produce pain; normal physical examination	None
Chronic fatigue syndrome	Fatigue lasting longer than 6 mo; sudden onset of flulike symptoms that persist or recur	Physical examination may be normal; cervical and axillary lymphadenopathy	CBC, ESR

T_3, Triiodothyronine; T_4, thyroxine; *ECG*, echocardiogram; *ABGs*, arterial blood gases.

CHAPTER RESOURCES

Cavanaugh R: Evaluating adolescents with fatigue: ever get tired of it? *Pediatr Rev* 23:337, 2002.

Craig T, Kakumanu S: Chronic fatigue syndrome: evaluation and treatment, *Am Fam Physician* 65:1083, 2002.

Morrison RE: Fatigue in primary care, *Obstet Gynecol Clin North Am* 28:225, 2001.

Rodriguez T: The challenge of evaluating fatigue, *J Am Acad Nurs Pract* 12:329, 2000.

Solomon L, Reeves WC: Factors influencing the diagnosis of chronic fatigue syndrome, *Arch Intern Med* 164:2241, 2004.

U.S. Department of Agriculture: *The dietary guidelines for Americans 2005*, Washington, DC, 2005. The full document is available at www.healthierus.gov/dietaryguidelines.

The Chest Film

X-rays are high-speed light energy produced by an x-ray tube. The short wavelength produced by this light energy is unique in that it penetrates opaque objects. Releasing the beam onto a photosensitive surface causes a photochemical reaction, which results in an image on the x-ray film in conventional systems or on an image receptor in digital systems. For ease of reference, the term "film" will be used throughout the chapter. The density of the material determines the penetration of the light energy. The image on the film is therefore a result of the amount of x-rays being absorbed by the density of the tissue/organ as it passes to the film. Two terms are used to describe this absorption. The first is radiolucent, which means there is no interference with the flow of the x-ray particles. The result is a black or very dark film. The second term is radiopaque; in this instance, something lies between the beam and the cassette that causes the beam to absorb or disperse, thereby not allowing the beam to reach the cassette and making the film appear white.

Decreasing density | Increasing density
(black) | (white)

→

Radiolucent | Radiopaque

Gradations of gray result from variations in density of the tissue or organ. There are four basic roentgen densities, and all films include one or more of these densities (Table 35-1). A chest film demonstrates all four densities: from the black of the air in the lung tissue to the full white density of the rib bones. The densities of the objects result in the shadows on the film.

The radiograph film is a two-dimensional shadow picture of a three-dimensional object. Because the film is two-dimensional, it is important that the clinician think three-dimensionally when viewing a film. This thinking requires knowledge of the normal anatomy of the area being x-rayed and transference of this knowledge to the shadows on the film.

DIAGNOSTIC REASONING: VIEWING THE CHEST FILM

What Are the First Steps in Reviewing a Film?

Key Questions

- Are the films of the correct patient being examined?
- Do I have two views of the area being examined?
- Is the film correctly displayed on the view box?
- Are the films of good quality?
- Do I know the anatomy of the chest?

Identification of Film and Patient

Before viewing a film it is important to acknowledge that the film being viewed is from the patient being evaluated. Pertinent information about the patient should be found on the film in the upper corner and should be verified.

Views

Generally, two films are taken when examination of the chest is requested. One is a frontal view; it is usually a posteroanterior (PA) view, where the patient is standing 6 feet from the cassette and the film is taken from

Table 35-1	Chest Film Densities	
DENSITY	DESCRIPTION	EXAMPLES
Gas (air)	Black, radiolucent	Lung tissue, trachea, bronchi, gas in stomach or intestine
Fat	Gray, less radiolucent	Soft tissue around muscle
Water	Whitish, slightly radiopaque	Heart, blood vessels, muscle, diaphragm
Metal	All white, radiopaque	Calcium of ribs, vertebrae, scapulae, clavicles, other bones, prostheses, contrast media

From Kersten L: *Comprehensive respiratory nursing*, Philadelphia, 1989, Saunders, p. 402.

back (posterior) to front (anterior) (Figure 35-1, *A*). A second film is the lateral view (Figure 35-1, *B*). In a lateral view, the patient is standing with the hands held above the head and the lateral thorax is against the cassette. A left lateral view (where the left thorax is against the film cassette) is usually ordered instead of a right lateral view because it provides a better view of the area behind the heart and bases of the lower lungs.

Additional views are occasionally ordered for specific reasons:

- **Anteroposterior (AP) chest film:** This view is created when the beam passes from the anterior to the posterior surface of the chest and then onto the film. Patients who are in bed or who cannot stand usually have these films ordered. When viewing the AP films, the heart and mediastinum appear larger because they are located in the anterior chest, and in this position the chest is farther from the film cassette.
- **Expiration film:** This type of film is ordered when a pneumothorax is suspected. A maximum expiration by the patient will cause the lung tissue to compress. The lung tissue is then compared to the pleural air. With a pneumothorax, the pleural air will occupy more space.
- **Lateral decubitus film:** This view is used to assess fluid and air levels in the pleural spaces. The patient is lying on his/her side with the film cassette upright against the patient's chest. The beam is sent perpendicular to the film cassette. Air rises and fluid falls to the dependent area.

- **Oblique film:** The oblique film is used to distinguish anterior from posterior lesions by avoiding bony structures. It is also used for examining the trachea. Oblique films can be right or left obliques. In a right oblique, the patient's anterior right side is against the film cassette.
- **Lordotic film:** The lordotic film identifies right and left middle lung fields. The x-ray machine is tilted to a 45-degree angle. This position offers a better view of lung apices that can otherwise be obscured by clavicles and upper ribs on the PA view.

Film Box Placement

Place the PA film on the lightened view box with the patient's left side facing the reader's right side. The film is labeled with an R or L. If there is no labeling, look for the aortic arch. The arch is the first bump seen on the film and is on the patient's left or the viewing clinician's right. In the rare patient with dextrocardia, the reverse is true.

The left lateral film should be placed on the view box such that the left side of the patient is facing the reader.

Film Quality

The amount of x-ray beamed through the patient onto the film affects the details seen on the film. If not enough beams were delivered, the film will be underexposed and appear lighter than normal. If too many beams were delivered, the film will become overexposed and will be darker than normal. On the PA view, thoracic vertebral bodies should be

A

B

FIGURE 35-1   Patient positioning for AP and left lateral chest films. **A,** A patient positioned for a posteroanterior projection of the chest. **B,** Proper patient position for a left lateral chest view. Note the left side of the patient is placed against the image receptor. (From Ballinger PW, Frank ED: *Merrill's atlas of radiographic positions and radiographic procedures,* ed 10, Vol 1, St Louis, 2003, Mosby.)

barely visible through the heart shadow; on the lateral view, the spinal bodies should be visible.

To obtain a good chest film, the x-ray is taken with the patient in full inspiration. If the film is taken on expiration or poor inspiration, the heart appears larger and the lungs look cloudy. Identification of the 10 posterior ribs above the diaphragm should be evident in a good quality film.

The angle of the beam should be direct and the patient should be positioned properly. If the patient is at an angle, the beam will be more scattered and details will be lost. To determine if the patient is positioned correctly, note the clavicles. The medial heads of the clavicles should be positioned over the spine. If the heads are not centered, alignment may not be correct, causing the film to be slightly oblique. The costophrenic angle as well as the lateral lung fields should be visible.

Reviewing Anatomy

Reviewing the normal anatomy of the structures of the chest is helpful when learning how to interpret a chest film.

Superimposing the anatomy onto a chest film will help to correlate the normal structures to the shadows (Figure 35-2).

What Approach Should Be Used When Viewing a Film?

Key Questions

- What is your initial impression?
- Are you using a systematic examination technique?

Initial Impression

Most clinicians view films initially by standing 6 to 8 feet from the film and giving the film a once-over glance. The purpose of this activity is to observe for any obvious abnormality as well as to obtain an overall impression of the thorax for size, shape, and symmetry.

Systematic examination of the film after an initial overview is mandatory. All parts of the chest anatomy are evaluated at 2 to 4 feet from the film, concentrating on one part of the film at a time, to observe any abnormalities. A suggested systematic examination follows.

FIGURE 35-2 Normal PA film. (From Fraser R, editor: *Fraser and Paré's diagnosis of diseases of the chest*, ed 4, Vol 1, Philadelphia, 1999, Saunders.)

DIAGNOSTIC REASONING: SYSTEMATIC EXAMINATION

How Do I Assess the PA View?

Soft Tissue

Examine the periphery of the film to evaluate the amount of soft tissue present (obesity or cachexia), calcifications, or gas collections indicating subcutaneous emphysema. Note the presence of breasts in female patients. Be aware that breast tissue may cover the lower lung fields.

Trachea

Located in the anterior mediastinum, the trachea should be checked for size and position. The trachea will appear deviated in a rotated patient. Abnormal pathological deviations may be a result of the effect of pressure on the mediastinum, including tumors, pneumothorax, or emphysema. A mass will push the trachea away from midline. The trachea will deviate toward a large pneumothorax and away from a tension pneumothorax. Thickening of the trachea may indicate lymph node enlargement or an upper mediastinal tumor.

Clavicles

The clavicles should be present and symmetrical and located at the second and third intercostal spaces. Scrutinize for fracture lines, which appear black on the film because of air space surrounded by white bone and tissue.

Bony Thorax

Note the size and shape of the thorax. Scoliosis is visible on the frontal film whereas kyphosis and funnel chest are best seen on the lateral view. Examine individual shoulder girdles for shape, size, and contour. Bony structures are evaluated for deformity, mineralization, density, and cortical thickness, as well as for fractures.

Scapulae

The distance between the scapulae is increased when the shoulders are rotated forward in the PA film. This position also ensures that the scapulae will be out of the lung fields. Observe for fractures and symmetry.

Thoracic Spine

Look through the mediastinum and lungs to view the spine and observe for symmetry of the rib cage. Vertebral evaluation is best done on the lateral film. Look for compression fractures, height of vertebral bodies, disk spaces, and density of bones.

Ribs and Intracostal Spaces

Count the posterior ribs; 10 should be visible. If 8 or fewer ribs are visible, this is either a poor film or an expiratory film. Be careful to begin the rib count at the first thoracic vertebra. Locate the anterior end of the first rib just below the medial end of the clavicles, follow it back to its posterior end, and start counting ribs. The posterior ribs are more superior than the anterior ribs. Check ribs side to side and completely to the lateral end. Most fractures occur on the lateral parts of the ribs. Normal ribs appear sloped at the edges; ribs that are horizontal or flattened indicate emphysema or chronic obstructive pulmonary disease (COPD) (Figure 35-3).

Describe abnormalities using ribs or interspaces as location markers horizontally and chest lines as vertical markers. Interspaces are numbered using the posterior rib and according to the rib above. Observe the widths of the intracostal spaces, which should be equal bilaterally.

Decreased lung volume narrows the intracostal spaces. Conditions that cause this include interstitial fibrosis (bilateral) or a foreign body (unilateral). Increased lung volume increases the intracostal spaces in such conditions as asthma and COPD.

Diaphragm

The diaphragm separates the abdominal contents from the pleural cavity. Any changes in these areas can be seen radiographically to affect the diaphragm. Count down the posterior ribs near the spine; the diaphragm should be at the tenth or eleventh rib. The diaphragm should have a curve that is shaped upward. The right side is usually higher (1 to 2 cm) than the left because the liver is located under the right hemidiaphragm; this will be more visible on a lateral film of the diaphragm. Note if the diaphragm is elevated or flattened.

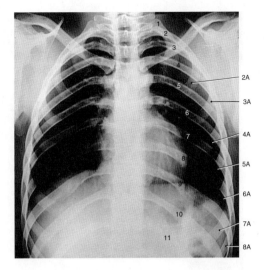

FIGURE 35-3 Respiratory lung movement. Full expiration with the ribs numbered. The anterior ribs are labeled with a suffix. (From Ballinger PW, Frank ED: *Merrill's atlas of radiographic positions & radiologic procedures,* ed 10, St Louis, 2003, Mosby.)

Suspect hepatomegaly in patients who have marked asymmetry of the right diaphragm. A unilateral elevation of the diaphragm is seen with a pneumothorax.

Patients who do not take a deep breath, who have ascites or intestinal obstruction, or who are in the third trimester of pregnancy will have elevated diaphragms. A diaphragm that is low and flat indicates structures within the thorax are enlarged, as seen in COPD.

Note any free air in the peritoneum visible below the right lower diaphragm edge. The air appears as lucency (decreased opacity) under the crescent of the hemidiaphragm typically as result of a perforated viscus.

Costophrenic Angle

The edge of the diaphragm curves downward at the costophrenic junction, meeting the ribs and forming an angle that is sometimes referred to as the letter "V" on its side. This angle should be sharp. Blunting of the angle is caused by pleural effusion, pneumonia, neoplasm, or fibrosis (Figure 35-4).

Gastric Air Bubble

The gastric air bubble should always be on the examiner's right side as the film is viewed (the patient's left side). The stomach lies close beneath the left diaphragm. The liver, spleen, and kidneys are occasionally visible and should be noted for size.

Mediastinum

The mediastinum is located between the sternum anteriorly, the vertebral bodies posteriorly, and the lungs laterally. It encompasses a number of structures including the heart and its large vessels as well as the trachea, thymus, and lymph nodes.

A prominent structure is the aortic arch. The arch is the first prominent bulge along the left mediastinal border. Assess for size and length. As patients age, the aorta increases in thickness and length. An increase in size is also seen in an aortic aneurysm.

The ascending aorta is the small bulge on the right.

Hilar Area

The hilar area contains the roots of the lungs and is where the major bronchi and pulmonary vessels project outward.

Note the size of the hilar area. Increased fullness or size generally indicates lymphoma, metastatic carcinoma, tuberculosis, or fungal (*Histoplasma*) adenopathy.

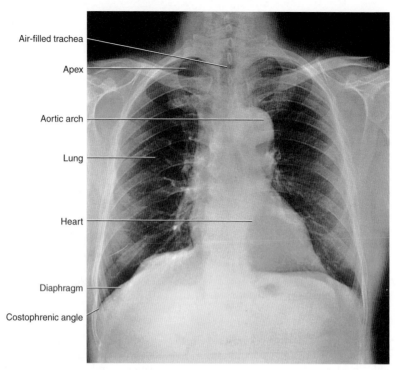

Air-filled trachea

Apex

Aortic arch

Lung

Heart

Diaphragm

Costophrenic angle

FIGURE 35-4   Normal costophrenic angle. (From Ballinger PW, Frank ED: *Merrill's atlas of radiographic positions and radiologic procedures*, ed 10, Vol 1, St Louis, 2003, Mosby.)

Pulmonary Vasculature

Pulmonary arteries become smaller as they progress out to the chest periphery, ending approximately 1.5 cm from the pleural surface. Normal markings extend approximately one third of the way into the lung fields.

Increased pulmonary pressure causes engorgement of the pulmonary vessels, and increased markings are seen that resemble a branching tree. When engorgement occurs, a butterfly appearance is seen. Pulmonary edema causes blurred borders and hilar clouding.

Heart

Measure the size of the heart using a ruler. The heart should be less than 50% of the transverse diameter of the thorax. The measurement should be compared to the widest thoracic diameter (found below the diaphragm and between the ribs), resulting in the cardiac/thoracic (C-T) ratio. The normal ratio is 1:2 (Figure 35-5).

Left ventricular hypertrophy extends the heart border to the left, increasing the size of the heart and decreasing the C-T ratio.

Look for the silhouette sign, which occurs when two structures have the same density and are in contact with each other, resulting in a loss of borders on the x-ray. Because the right and left borders of the heart are air-filled,

FIGURE 35-5   The normal cardiac-thoracic ratio is 1:2.

lesions in the lung cause the differentiation of the heart border to be lost.

Pleura

Follow the pleura around the lungs and note any thickening, calcification, effusion, or pneumothorax.

Pleural thickening is seen as increased soft tissue around the periphery of the lung. An effusion will blunt the costophrenic angle. A pneumothorax will pull the visceral pleura into the lung field, away from the chest wall.

Lungs

Examine the lungs from central to peripheral. The lungs will appear whiter when looking from top to bottom because of the increasing thickness of the chest areas. The lung markings will decrease by thirds as the viewer goes from central to peripheral. The markings are also more prominent in the bases of the lungs than in the upper lung fields.

Compare right and left lung fields, starting at the top and continuing across and down. Do this in small segments, evaluating each area carefully. Look for lesions, lung markings, and density changes such as areas of opacity (seen in white), which represent consolidation, nodules, and calcifications. Note the lung volume. Decreased volume is seen with atelectasis. Large-volume lungs with a narrow mediastinum and a flat diaphragm are typically viewed in the patient with emphysema.

Final Look

Research has shown that there are three high-risk locations where pathology is often missed. They are the following: the upper lobes of the lungs, costophrenic areas, and peripheral lung margins. Take one more look at each of these areas.

How Do I Assess the Lateral View?

Key Questions

- What position is the patient in?
- How do I know the film quality is good?
- What are the indications for a lateral film?
- Am I using a systematic approach to reviewing the film?

The common position for the lateral view is with the patient's left chest against the film cassette. The beam passes from right to left through the patient. Remember that the right side of the patient is closer to the beam and therefore images are magnified on the right side as compared to the left. The left lateral position is preferred because the heart is less magnified and the bases of the lungs are more easily seen.

A right lateral film is ordered when the right side of the lung needs to be less magnified and sharper, such as when a tumor is suspected. In the lateral position, the ribs will seem to be superimposed on each other and the sternum will appear thin.

A good quality lateral film shows lung markings, fissures (the septa that divide the lobes of the lung), and good visualization of the spine.

A lateral film can help localize a lesion seen on the PA view or it may verify lobar consolidation. In addition, the lateral film allows the viewer to see behind the sternum and cardiac shadow.

Use a systemic approach to viewing the lateral film, similar to the PA review.

DIAGNOSTIC REASONING: SYSTEMATIC EXAMINATION

Anatomy

Review the anatomy of the lateral chest (Figure 35-6).

Vertebral Bodies

The amount of soft tissue is greater at the lung apices than at the lung bases; therefore the vertebral bodies appear darker as they approach the diaphragm. Kyphosis is noticeable on the lateral film. Examine each vertebra for fractures, and scrutinize the intervertebral disk spaces.

Diaphragm

The right diaphragm is visualized and is higher than the left because of the heart. On the left, the latter two thirds of the diaphragm should be visible. The gastric bubble is below the left diaphragm.

FIGURE 35-6 Lateral chest film. **A,** Unlabeled. **B,** Labeled. (From Fraser R, editor: *Fraser and Paré's diagnosis of diseases of the chest*, ed 4, Vol 1, Philadelphia, 1999, Saunders.)

Costophrenic Angle
The angle is seen in the most dependent part of the lung. Both angles should be visualized and sharp.

Fissures
Fissures are septa that divide the lobes of lungs. The major oblique fissure separates the left upper lobe from the left lower lobe. The right major fissure separates the right upper and middle lobes from the right lower lobe. The right minor fissure separates the right upper lobe from the right lower lobe. Fissures are generally not seen on plain films because their small surface provides no shadow or interface. However, these fissures may be seen when pathology occurs in the lung.

Pleura
Follow the pleura around the lungs from the posterior costophrenic area to the posterior sternal margin and posterior ribs.

Retrosternal Area
The retrosternal space is usually dark because of the presence of air. It is the lower one third of the sternum and appears in contact with the right ventricle. When this area is seen as opaque, air has been replaced with solid material, and anterior mediastinal disease should be considered. The area is enlarged when pulmonary overinflation occurs, as in emphysema. The retrosternal space will not be visible with an enlarged heart.

Heart/Retrocardiac Area
Identify the right ventricle, left ventricle, and left atrium. The retrocardiac area of the lateral chest film is normally dark due to air. If the space is opaque, then the air has been replaced with an effusion, consolidation, or mass.

Lungs
The scapulae make visualizing the upper lobe difficult in the lateral film. Lung lesions are

often hidden by the heart on the PA view. Localizing a lesion in the left lung is best accomplished with the lateral film.

Final Look

Take a last look at each of the areas where lesions are often missed: the upper lobes, peripheral lung margins, retrocardiac area, and costophrenic area.

What Other Imaging Studies Should I Consider?

Key Questions

- What other common imaging studies are available for the chest?
- What imaging studies would give me the best information for a particular complaint?

Computed Tomography

Computed tomography (CT), sometimes called computed axial tomography (CAT), provides a cross-sectional slice of the area examined. Unlike plain films, which superimpose structures onto a film, a CT scan gives only one slice. The beams of x-rays pass through the body in an axial plane as the x-ray tube moves in a continuous arc around the patient. Detectors are placed opposite the beam to catch the electrical pulses. The image is the result of the x-rays that are not absorbed by the tissues between the beam and the detectors. Detectors pick up the electrical impulses that are fed into a computer that provides the "picture." CT is used to distinguish overlapping shadows from the chest film. It is also very useful in showing fine details of the pulmonary parenchyma and hilum.

MRI

Magnetic resonance imaging (MRI) produces a computer-based sectional image that does not use ionizing radiation. MRI uses the hydrogen molecules in the body to produce the image. A radio frequency pulse transmitted through coils causes some of the hydrogen molecules to absorb energy and spin in a different direction from the other hydrogen ions (resonance). When the radio frequency pulse stops, the hydrogen molecules stop spinning and release their excess stored energy. A gradient magnet located inside the main magnet, which provides the slicing capability of the image, picks up the change. The results are sent to the computer system, providing a two-dimensional image. MRI of the chest is used to view lesions of the chest wall and is less useful for examining the lungs.

PET Scan

Positron emission tomography (PET) provides information on the biochemical metabolism of an organ or tissue. Positrons come from the nucleus of a proton as it decays to a neutron. Once released, the positron eventually collides with an electron, resulting in the release of two high-energy gamma photons. These gamma photons are released at 180 degrees from each other. The PET scan patient is given a radiotracer that follows the destruction of the positron and the resulting gamma photons. PET scans are built with hundreds of detectors on circular rings that are located directly across from each other. The detectors allow the localization, in three-dimensional space, of the decay of the gamma photons. PET scans show the chemical function of an organ or tissue rather than its structure; very highly active metabolism is seen with cancer cells. PET scans are ordered for evaluating the effects of lung cancer therapy.

Echocardiogram

High-frequency sound waves are directed into the body, which are then recorded as they deflect off organs and structures. These deflections are transmitted back to a transducer that records the difference in acoustic impedance. This recording is changed into an electrical signal, which is then analyzed by a computer to produce an image. Echocardiograms are useful to evaluate heart size and valvular function.

DIFFERENTIAL DIAGNOSIS OF *Common Causes of the Chest Film*

WHAT TO LOOK AT	NORMAL FINDING	ABNORMAL FINDING	SUGGESTED CAUSE
Clavicles	Midline, symmetrical, intact	Dark lines; clavicles not centered	Fracture; patient rotated; film taken off center
Chest wall	Chest wall has rounded contour	Sternum pushed outward (lateral film)	Pectus carinatum
		Sternum pushed inward (lateral film)	Pectus excavatum
Inspiration	Adequate inspiration	Less than 10 ribs identified	Inadequate inspiration
Vertebral column	Straight, equal disk spaces	Curved	Kyphoscoliosis (lateral view); scoliosis (PA view)
		Collapsed disk spaces	Degenerative disk disease
Ribs	All ribs intact and able to count 10	Rib fractures present; unable to count all 10 ribs	Trauma; less than 10 ribs, poor inspiration
	Ribs sloped at edges	Ribs horizontal or flattened	Hyperinflated lungs, acute asthma, COPD
Trachea	Midline	Deviation from midline	Atelectasis: trachea deviated toward area of atelectasis; pneumothorax: air, fluid, tumor, lymph node enlargement push trachea away from center; rotated film
Hilar region	Size, centrally located	Area enlarged	Pulmonary artery congestion; lymph node enlargement
	Vascular markings extend <$^1/_3$ out into lung field	Vascular markings >$^1/_3$ into lung field	Bronchopneumonia or pulmonary congestion
	Bronchi invisible because air-filled bronchi have same density as air in lungs	Bronchograms present (bronchi become visible when lung tissue filled with fluid is contrasted with air-filled bronchi)	Infiltration; pulmonary edema
		Infiltrates or consolidation of lung tissue	Pneumonia
Gastric air bubble	Present on right	Not visible	Film placement error; film label error
Diaphragm	Right higher than left; right at level of sixth rib	Elevated	Collapsed lobe or multisegmental collapse; pleural effusion
		Radiolucent line present that follows curvature of diaphragm	Free air present
		Flattened diaphragm	Emphysema, asthma, tension pneumothorax
		Elevation on left	Perforated ulcer or gas distention of stomach
		Bilateral elevation	Pregnancy, obesity, peritoneal fluid
Costrophrenic angle	Present, sharp edges	Blunted edges or absent	Pneumonia, pleural effusion
Visceral pleura	Traced around chest wall	Hairline shadow, dark black with no lung markings	Pneumothorax

Continued

DIFFERENTIAL DIAGNOSIS OF *Common Causes of the Chest Film—cont'd*			
WHAT TO LOOK AT	NORMAL FINDING	ABNORMAL FINDING	SUGGESTED CAUSE
Heart size	Cardiac ratio <50%	Ratio >50%	Enlarged heart, patient rotated
Heart borders	Presence of heart borders	Loss of border	Infiltrates
Lungs	Translucent	Fluffy appearance	Engorged vasculature
		Honeycomb appearance	Acute respiratory distress syndrome
		Butterfly appearance	Pulmonary edema
		Density changes to consolidation	Bacterial pneumonia
		Web-shaped density	Pulmonary embolism

CHAPTER RESOURCES

Dettenmeier P: *Pulmonary nursing care,* St Louis, 1992, Mosby.

Fraser R, editor: *Fraser and Paré's diagnosis of diseases of the chest,* ed 4, Vol 1, Philadelphia, 1999, Saunders.

Gaber KA, McGavin CR, Wells IP: Lateral chest X-ray for physicians, *J Royal Soc Med* 98(7):310, 2005.

Kersten L: *Comprehensive respiratory nursing: a decision making approach,* Philadelphia, 1989, Saunders.

Landay M: *Interpretation of the chest roentgenogram,* Boston, 1987, Little Brown and Co.

Novelline R: *Squire's fundamentals of radiology,* ed 5, Cambridge, Mass, 1997, Harvard University Press.

Wilson S, Thompson J: *Respiratory disorders,* St Louis, 1990, Mosby.

Appendix A

Conversion Tables

LENGTH				WEIGHT			
IN	CM	CM	IN	LB	KG	KG	LB
1	2.54	1	0.4	1	0.5	1	2.2
2	5.08	2	0.8	2	0.9	2	4.4
4	10.16	3	1.2	4	1.8	3	6.6
6	15.24	4	1.6	6	2.7	4	8.8
8	20.32	5	2.0	8	3.6	5	11.0
10	25.40	6	2.4	10	4.5	6	13.2
20	50.50	8	3.1	20	9.1	8	17.6
30	76.20	10	3.9	30	13.6	10	22
40	101.60	20	7.9	40	18.2	20	44
50	127.00	30	11.8	50	22.7	30	66
60	152.40	40	15.7	60	27.3	40	88
70	177.80	50	19.7	70	31.8	50	110
80	203.20	60	23.6	80	36.4	60	132
90	228.60	70	27.6	90	40.9	70	154
100	254.00	80	31.5	100	45.4	80	176
150	381.00	90	35.4	150	66.2	90	198
200	508.00	100	39.4	200	90.8	100	220

1 in = 2.54 cm
1 cm = 0.3937 in

1 lb = 0.454 kg
1 kg = 2.204 lb

From Seidel HM et al: *Mosby's guide to physical examination,* ed 5, St Louis, 2003, Mosby.

Appendix B

Temperature Equivalents			
CELSIUS*	**FAHRENHEIT†**	**CELSIUS***	**FAHRENHEIT†**
34.0	93.2	38.6	101.4
34.2	93.6	38.8	101.8
34.4	93.9	39.0	102.2
34.6	94.3	39.2	102.5
34.8	94.6	39.4	102.9
35.0	95.0	39.6	103.2
35.2	95.4	39.8	103.6
35.4	95.7	40.0	104.0
35.6	96.1	40.2	104.3
35.8	96.4	40.4	104.7
36.0	96.8	40.6	105.1
36.2	97.1	40.8	105.4
36.4	97.5	41.0	105.8
36.6	97.8	41.2	106.1
36.8	98.2	41.4	106.5
37.0	98.6	41.6	106.8
37.2	98.9	41.8	107.2
37.4	99.3	42.0	107.6
37.6	99.6	42.2	108.0
37.8	100.0	42.4	108.3
38.0	100.4	42.6	108.7
38.2	100.7	42.8	109.0
38.4	101.1	43.0	109.4

From Hoekelman RA et al: *Primary pediatric care,* ed 4, St Louis, 2001, Mosby.

*To convert Celsius to Fahrenheit: $(^9/_5 \times$ Temperature$) + 32$.

†To convert Fahrenheit to Celsius: $(^5/_9 \times$ Temperature$) - 32$.

Appendix C

Body Mass Index Chart

ARE YOU AT A HEALTHY WEIGHT?

BMI measures weight in relation to height. The BMI ranges shown above are for adults. They are not exact ranges of healthy and unhealthy weights. However, they show that health risk increases at higher levels of overweight and obesity. Even within the healthy BMI range, weight gains can carry health risks for adults.

Directions: Find your weight on the bottom of the graph. Go straight up from that point until you come to the line that matches your height. Then look to find your weight group.

Healthy Weight BMI from 18.5 up to 25 refers to healthy weight.

Overweight BMI from 25 up to 30 refers to overweight.

Obese BMI 30 or higher refers to obesity. Obese persons are also overweight.

Source: Report of the Dietary Guidelines Advisory Committee on the Dietary Guidelines for Americans, 2000, page 3.

Bibliography

Aldmen W: The adolescent male genital examination: what's normal and what's not, *Pediatr Rev* 20:125, 1999.

American Cancer Society: *Cancer facts & figures;* available online at http://www.cancer.org/docroot/STT/stt_0.asp.

Armon K et al: An evidence and consensus based guideline for acute diarrhea management, *Arch Dis Child* 85:132, 2001.

Barkauskas VH, Baumann LC, Darling-Fisher CS: *Health and physical assessment,* ed 3, St Louis, 2002, Mosby.

Beers MH, Porter RS, Jones TV: *The Merck manual of diagnosis and therapy,* ed 18, Rahway, NJ, 2006, Merck & Co.

Berg D, Worzala K, editors: *Atlas of adult physical diagnosis,* Philadelphia, 2005, Lippincott Williams & Wilkins.

Bowden CL, Hirschfeld RM, Shahady EJ: Biploar disorder: keys to diagnosis—strategies for effective management, *Consultant* 45(suppl 14):51, 2005.

Brouillette R: Noctural pulse oximetry as an abbreviated testing modality for pediatric obstructive sleep apnea, *Pediatrics* 105:405, 2001.

Daly KA: Chronic otitis media with effusion, *Pediatr Rev* 20:85, 2001.

DeCherney AH, Nathan L, editors: *Current obstetric and gynecologic diagnosis and treatment,* ed 9, Norwalk, Conn, 2004, Appleton & Lange.

Ebell MH: *Evidence-based diagnosis,* New York, 2001, Springer.

Edwardson BM: *Musculoskeletal disorders: common problems,* San Diego, 1995, Singular Publishing Group.

Forsyth R, Farrell K: Headache in childhood, *Pediatr Rev* 20:39, 1999.

Fox J: *Primary health care of infants, children, and adolescents,* ed 2, St Louis, 2002, Mosby.

Goroll AH, Mulley AG, editors: *Primary care medicine: office evaluation and management of the adult patient,* ed 5, Philadelphia, 2005, Lippincott Williams & Wilkins.

Gross CW: Tonsils and adenoids, *Pediatr Rev* 21:75, 2000.

Guerrero RA, Cavender CP: Constipation: physical and psychological sequelae, *Pediatr Ann* 28:312, 1999.

Habif TP: *Clinical dermatology: a color guide to diagnosis and therapy,* ed 4, St Louis, 2004, Mosby.

Ham RJ, Sloane PD, Warshaw G: *Primary care in geriatrics: a case based approach,* ed 5, St Louis, 2001, Mosby.

Hay W et al: *Current pediatric diagnosis and treatment,* ed 18, Norwalk, Conn, 2002, Appleton & Lange.

Hoekelman R et al: *Primary pediatric care,* ed 4, St Louis, 2001, Mosby.

Huges E: Otitis externa, *Pediatr Rev* 22:191, 2001.

Ian G: Scrotal swelling in children, *Pediatr Rev* 21:311, 2000.

LeBlond RF, DeGowin RL, Brown DD: *DeGowin diagnostic examination,* ed 8, New York, 2004, McGraw-Hill.

Leitman M: *Manual for eye examination and diagnosis,* ed 5, Boston, 2001, Blackwell Scientific.

Lewis D: Syncope in the pediatric patient, *Pediatr Clin North Am* 46:205, 1999.

Loretz L: *Primary care tools for clinicians,* St Louis, 2005, Mosby.

Luszczak M: Evaluation and management of infants and young children with fever, *Am Fam Physician* 64:1219, 2001.

Malhotra A: Viral croup, *Pediatr Rev* 22:5, 2001.

Mengel MB, Schwiebert LP: *Ambulatory medicine: the primary care of families,* ed 3, Stamford, Conn, 2001, Appleton & Lange.

Morton RL: Evaluation of the wheezy infant, *Ann Allergy Asthma Immunol* 86:251, 2001.

Noble J: *Textbook of primary care medicine,* ed 3, St Louis, 2001, Mosby.

Oakley LD: Psychosocial problems. In Dunphey LM, Winland-Brown JE, editors: *Primary care: the art and science of advanced practice nursing,* Philadelphia, 2001, FA Davis.

Pagana K, Pagana T: *Diagnostic and laboratory test reference,* ed 7, St Louis, 2005, Mosby.

Patel D, Wasserman A: Chest pain: is it life threatening—or benign? *Consultant* 45(1):21, 2005.

Peral H et al: The approach to common abdominal diagnoses in infants and children, *Pediatr Clin North Am* 45:1287, 1998.

Rakel RE: *Saunders manual of medical practice,* ed 2, Philadelphia, 2000, Saunders.

Rakel RE: *Textbook of family practice,* ed 6, Philadelphia, 2002, Saunders.

Riggio S, Jagoda A: What you forgot about the neurologic exam, part 2, *Consultant* 45(1):53, 2005.

Ruckenstein MJ: The dizzy patient: how you can help, *Consultant* 46(2):145, 2006.

Sabatini S: The female athlete triad, *Am J Med Sci* 322:193, 2001.

Santiago-Rosado L: Syncope: step-by-step through the workup, *Consultant* 45(6):759, 2005.

Seidel HM et al: *Mosby's guide to physical examination,* ed 6, St Louis, 2006, Mosby.

Seller RH: *Differential diagnosis of common complaints,* ed 4, Philadelphia, 2000, Saunders.

Sloane PD et al: *Essentials of family medicine*, ed 4, Philadelphia, 2002, Lippincott Williams & Wilkins.

Weisleder P, Fife TD: Dizziness and headache: a common association in children and adolescents, *J Child Neurol* 16:727, 2001.

Werner HA: Status asthmaticus in children: a review, *Chest* 119:1913, 2001.

Wiatrak BJ: Congenital anomalies of the larynx and trachea, *Otolaryngol Clin North Am* 33:91, 2000.

Williams JW, Simel DL: Does this patient have sinusitis? Diagnosing acute sinusitis by history and physical examination, *JAMA* 270:1242, 1993.

Zeiter DK, Hymas JS: Recurrent abdominal pain in children, *Pediatr Clin North·Am* 49:53, 2002.

Index

Accurately assess and treat patients... *at any age!*

Practice Guidelines for
Family Nurse Practitioners, 3ʳᵈ Edition

*By Karen Fenstermacher, MS, RN, CS;
and Barbara Toni Hudson, MSN, RN, CS*

Quickly find thorough and detailed assessment
information for all common primary care conditions,
including signs and symptoms, diagnostic methods, drug
therapies, and treatment in any clinical setting. Written by
expert nurse practitioners, it features complete, practical,
up-to-date information on diagnosing and treating primary
care disorders in the family practice setting.

2004 • 528 pp., illustd. • ISBN: 0-7216-0345-9
• ISBN-13: 978-0-7216-0345-2

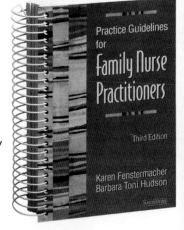

Practice Guidelines for
Pediatric Nurse Practitioners

By Beth Richardson, DNS, RN, CPNP

This portable quick-reference book is filled with valuable
assessment and management information for both
pediatric and family nurse practitioners. Information is
presented in a clear, concise outline format beginning
with growth and development and moving on to key
issues such as nutrition, immunizations, and anticipatory
guidance. Coverage also includes common childhood
conditions affecting each body system.

2006 • 560 pp., illustd. • ISBN: 0-323-02977-9
• ISBN-13: 978-0-323-02977-3

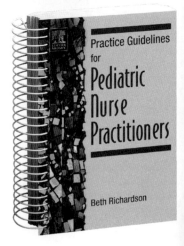

Ordering is easy!
ONLINE: **www.elsevierhealth.com**
PHONE: **toll-free 1-800-545-2522**

NM-06294